AN INTRODUCTION TO

Drugs AND THE Neuroscience OF Behavior

Adam J. Prus
Northern Michigan University

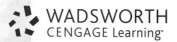

WADSWORTH
CENGAGE Learning·

Australia • Brazil • Japan • Korea • Mexico • Singapore • Spain • United Kingdom • United States

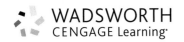

WADSWORTH
CENGAGE Learning·

An Introduction to Drugs and the Neuroscience of Behavior, International Edition
Adam J. Prus

Publisher: Jon-David Hague

Developmental/Assistant Editor: Amelia Blevins

Media Editor: Jasmin Tokatlian

Senior Brand Manager: Elisabeth Rhoden

Market Development Manager: Christine Sosa

Content Project Manager: Charlene Carpentier

Art Director: Vernon Boes

Manufacturing Planner: Karen Hunt

Rights Acquisitions Specialist: Dean Dauphinais

Production Service: MPS Limited

Photo/Text Researcher: Q2A/Bill Smith

Copy Editor: S.M. Summerlight

Art Editor: Precision Graphics

Illustrator: Argosy Publishing Inc. and Q2A/
    Bill Smith

Cover/Text Designer: Lisa Henry

Cover Image: Argosy Publishing Inc.

Compositor: MPS Limited

For product information and technology assistance, contact us at **Cengage Learning Customer & Sales Support, 1-800-354-9706**

For permission to use material from this text or product, submit all requests online at **www.cengage.com/permissions**
Further permissions questions can be e-mailed to
permissionrequest@cengage.com

International Edition:
ISBN-13: 978-1-133-93950-4
ISBN-10: 1-133-93950-3

Cengage Learning International Offices

Asia
www.cengageasia.com
tel: (65) 6410 1200

Australia/New Zealand
www.cengage.com.au
tel: (61) 3 9685 4111

Brazil
www.cengage.com.br
tel: (55) 11 3665 9900

India
www.cengage.co.in
tel: (91) 11 4364 1111

Latin America
www.cengage.com.mx
tel: (52) 55 1500 6000

UK/Europe/Middle East/Africa
www.cengage.co.uk
tel: (44) 0 1264 332 424

Represented in Canada by Nelson Education, Ltd.
www.nelson.com
tel: (416) 752 9100/(800) 668 0671

Cengage Learning is a leading provider of customized learning solutions with office locations around the globe, including Singapore, the United Kingdom, Australia, Mexico, Brazil, and Japan. Locate your local office at: **www.cengage.com/global**

For product information and free companion resources:
www.cengage.com/international

Visit your local office: **www.cengage.com/global**

Visit our corporate website: **www.cengage.com**

Printed in the United States of America
1 2 3 4 5 6 7 16 15 14 13

To Jennifer, Kendell and Daniel

AUTHOR BIOGRAPHY

Adam Prus is an Associate Professor in the Department of Psychology at Northern Michigan University, in Marquette, Michigan. He earned his Ph.D. in psychology from Virginia Commonwealth University. While in graduate school, he also worked as a research technician at a large pharmaceutical company. After earning his degree, he served as postdoctoral fellow in the Psychopharmacology Division of the Department of Psychiatry at Vanderbilt University, working under the mentorship of Herbert Meltzer, a leader in antipsychotic drug research.

Adam has published numerous original studies on psychoactive drugs and conducts research projects funded by the National Institute of Mental Health, private foundations, and pharmaceutical companies. When he is not teaching or doing research, Adam spends time with his family, fixes up their house (which he thinks has a lot of potential), and works on his golf game (which may have less potential, but is enjoyable nonetheless).

BRIEF CONTENTS

CONTENTS

PREFACE

Since my undergraduate years in psychology, I've been fascinated by how psychoactive substances produce behavioral effects. This interest led to a career in psychopharmacology research that included many graduate and postdoctoral years studying lab rats in Skinner boxes and mazes. Once I began teaching undergraduates at a university, I found that my students were also curious about how drugs altered behavior. Students wondered not only about the physiological impacts of college drug use but also about how medicines can treat psychological disorders such as depression and schizophrenia. But of particular interest were the effects of psychoactive drugs on the brain. This introductory textbook developed from my efforts to address these interests.

An Introduction to Drugs and the Neuroscience of Behavior offers an introduction to the field of psychopharmacology from the perspective of how drug actions in the brain affect psychological processes. The text approaches this rapidly advancing field by providing an introduction to major topics in psychopharmacology. I kept in mind that students have different backgrounds in neuroscience. Therefore, Chapter 2 provides an introductory overview of the nervous system, and Chapter 3 provides a basic coverage of neurotransmission.

Chapter 4 provides an overview of pharmacology principles, covering important drug properties that are necessary for understanding psychoactive drug actions and effects. By mastering these chapters on the nervous system and pharmacology, students will possess a sufficient background to comprehend subsequent chapters on psychoactive drugs.

In addition to the major drug classes in psychopharmacology, this book addresses newer drugs and recent trends in drug use. For example, the current edition includes information on bath salts, energy drinks, modern tobacco products such as tobacco orbs, medicinal marijuana, synthetic marijuana, and antidepressant drug use for treating anxiety.

How the Materials Are Organized

During the development of this textbook, I carefully attended to how this material is delivered to an undergraduate audience. My approach consists of a careful, step-by-step presentation of information supplemented by illustrations, figures, boxes, and several unique pedagogical features. These features include the following.

From Actions to Effects

Each chapter ends with a section called "From Actions to Effects." These sections cover a topic that brings together information presented in the chapter, providing a way to assemble multiple topics for addressing a single concept. In particular, these topics focus on a concept that requires understanding a drug's actions to account for its effects. These sections aid in the conceptual understanding of chapter material.

Stop & Check

Stop & Check questions conclude each section in each chapter. These questions allow students to self-assess their understanding of main points covered in the previous section.

Review!

Chapters include important reminders of facts or concepts covered in previous chapters. This helps integrate the diverse material covered in this text.

Research Techniques and Methods

Chapters include boxes that cover a research technique or method used in psychopharmacology research. These boxes model good working science and provide an easy reference when students come across research findings derived from each technique. These studies are also important in fostering critical thinking habits in students.

Key Terms

Each chapter ends with a list of key terms from the chapter. A definition is provided for each key term in a combined glossary and index at the end of the book.

Visit www.cengagebrain.com to access the free companion Web site for this text, which includes a glossary, flash cards, quizzes, and more.

Supplementary Materials

The text comes equipped with PowerPoint presentations and a test bank of exam questions organized by chapter, provided by Renee Haskew-Layton at Chimborazo Publishing, Inc. Access these supplements on the companion Web site at www.cengagebrain.com.

Acknowledgements

I warmly acknowledge the many experts who worked tirelessly to transform early drafts of well-intended ideas into a coherent collection of chapters that provide an excellent introduction to this field. I learned much from their many thoughtful critiques and perspectives, which sometimes caused sleepless nights, but always led to a better manuscript. Any errors or distortions that may be found are entirely my own.

Sharon L. Jones, Palo Verde College
William J. Jenkins, Mercer University
Sherry Tiffany Donaldson, University of Massachusetts Boston
Scott I. Cohn, Western State College of Colorado
Judith E. Grisel, Furman University
John Kelsey, Bates College
Martin Acerbo, University of Iowa

Finally, I would like to thank the many students who took the time to read these chapters. Their feedback contributed greatly to keeping this text appropriate for an undergraduate audience. In particular, I would like to acknowledge Michael Berquist, Stacy Paisley, Katelin Matazel, and Ashley Schmeling.

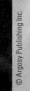

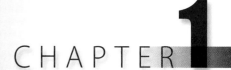

© Argosy Publishing Inc.

CHAPTER **1**

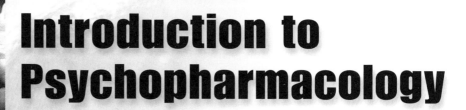

Introduction to Psychopharmacology

- ► Psychopharmacology
- ► Why Read a Book on Psychopharmacology?
- ► Drugs: Administered Substances That Alter Physiological Functions
- ► Psychoactive Drugs: Described by Manner of Use
- ► Generic Names, Trade Names, and Street Names for Drugs
- ► Drug Effects: Determined by Dose
- ► Pharmacology: Pharmacodynamics, Pharmacokinetics, and Pharmacogenetics
- ► Psychoactive Drugs: Objective and Subjective Effects
- ► Study Designs and the Assessment of Psychoactive Drugs
- ► Experimental Validity: Addressing the Quality and Impact of an Experiment
- ► Animals and Advancing Medical Research
- ► The Regulation of Animal Research
- ► Researchers Consider Many Ethical Issues When Conducting Human Research
- ► From Actions to Effects: Therapeutic Drug Development
- ► Chapter Summary

Psychoactive substances have made an enormous impact on society. Many people regularly drink alcohol or smoke tobacco. Millions of Americans take prescribed drugs for depression or anxiety. As students, scholars, practitioners, and everyday consumers, we may find that learning about psychoactive substances can be invaluable. The chapters in this book will provide a thorough overview of the major classes of psychoactive drugs, including their actions in the body and their effects on behavior.

Psychopharmacology

psychopharmacology
Study of how drugs affect mood, perception, thinking, or behavior.

psychoactive drugs
Drugs that affect mood, perception, thinking, or behavior by acting in the nervous system.

Psychopharmacology is the study of how drugs affect mood, perception, thinking, or behavior. Drugs that achieve these effects by acting in the nervous system are called **psychoactive drugs**. The term *psychopharmacology* encompasses two large fields: psychology and pharmacology. Thus, psychopharmacology attempts to relate the actions and effects of drugs to issues in psychology.

A psychopharmacologist must know how the nervous system functions and how psychoactive drugs alter nervous system functioning. This approach defines the structure of this textbook. First, this book provides an overview of brain cells and structures. Second, it covers the basic principles of pharmacology. Third, it covers the many different types of psychoactive drugs, beginning with recreational and abused drugs such as cocaine, marijuana, and LSD and ending with therapeutic drugs for treating mental disorders such as depression, anxiety, and schizophrenia.

Psychopharmacology is not the only term used to describe this field (**table 1.1**). Another term is *behavioral pharmacology*. Although behavioral pharmacology is usually considered synonymous with psychopharmacology, some professionals limit the term *behavioral pharmacology* to the psychology subfield of *behavior analysis*. In this respect, drugs serve as behaviorally controlling stimuli just like other stimuli in behavior analytic models. *Neuropsychopharmacology* is another term for psychopharmacology. The *neuro* prefix represents the nervous system. Although the terms are basically

table **1.1**

Names Used to Describe Psychopharmacology	
Field	**Description**
Psychopharmacology	The study of how drugs affect mood, perception, thinking, or behavior.
Behavioral pharmacology	The study of how drugs affect behavior. Sometimes behavioral pharmacologists emphasize principles used in field of behavior analysis.
Neuropsychopharmacology	The study of how drugs affect the nervous system and how these nervous system changes alter behavior.

similar, the neuropsychopharmacology field has a particular emphasis on the nervous system actions of drugs.

Why Read a Book on Psychopharmacology?

Beyond being a required reading as a course requirement, psychopharmacology is an incredibly important part of modern psychology. First, psychoactive drug use is highly prevalent.

Consider the following statistics in the United States:

- More than 100 million antidepressant drug prescriptions are written every year.
- More than 80 million anxiolytic, sedative, and hypnotic drugs are prescribed every year.
- More than 200 million pain-relieving drug prescriptions are written every year [Centers for Disease Control and Prevention (CDC), 2008].

When we add recreational drugs to the list, psychoactive drug prevalence in the United States increases further:

- More than 114 million adults drink on a regular basis (CDC, 2011).
- More than 25 million individuals use marijuana.
- More than 15 million individuals misuse a prescription drug.
- More than 70 million individuals use tobacco products (Substance Abuse and Mental Health Services Administration, 2010).

The World Health Organization (WHO) also reports high rates of psychoactive drug use internationally (WHO, 2012). Given this prevalence, psychology must consider what so-called normal behavior means today.

The second reason for reading this text is that the statistics just presented show how nearly all of us are consumers of psychoactive substances; as consumers, we should know about the substances we ingest. Greater knowledge of psychoactive substances improves patient understanding of prescribed medical treatments and health implications of taking recreational substances.

Third, you will come to understand how psychoactive substances provide important tools for understanding human behavior. The actions of antidepressant drugs led to understanding the roles that certain neurotransmitters and brain structures play in depression. Researchers use many experimental psychoactive drugs entirely as pharmacological tools for understanding behavior.

pharmacotherapeutics
Psychoactive treatments for disorders.

Fourth, you will see how psychopharmacologists develop psychoactive treatments for psychological disorders. As described later in this chapter, psychoactive treatments for disorders—referred to as **pharmacotherapeutics**—are not derived only from chemists. Rather, scientists trained in psychology test psychoactive drugs and determine their potential effectiveness for psychological disorders.

Drugs: Administered Substances That Alter Physiological Functions

drug Administered substance that alters physiological functioning.

In a way, you know a drug when you see one. After all, the term *drug* is part of our everyday language. We take drugs for headaches, drugs for infections, drugs for depression or anxiety, and drugs for virtually any other ailment or disorder. We even take drugs to prevent disorders. But what exactly is a drug?

To provide a simple definition, a **drug** is an administered substance that alters physiological functioning. The term *administered* indicates that a person takes or is given the substance. The phrase "alters physiological functioning" implies that the substance must exhibit sufficient efficacy to change physiological processes.

This definition has limitations. First, the term *administered* excludes substances made naturally in the body. For example, the neurotransmitter dopamine is made in the nervous system and elicits important changes in nervous system functioning. However, hospital physicians may administer dopamine to a patient in order to elevate heart rate. In this context, dopamine is an *administered* substance that *alters physiological functioning*.

Further, a naturally produced chemical important for making dopamine in the body called *levodopa* is a primary drug for Parkinson's disease. Physicians and researchers describe levedopa as a drug. Along the same lines, many of us take vitamins to ward off disease and improve health. Why not call *vitamins* drugs? We simply describe them as vitamins (**figure 1.1**). Nor do we describe herbal remedies as drugs despite their physiological effects.

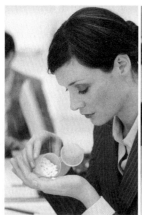 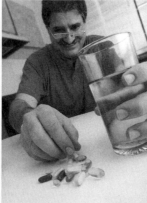 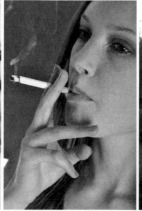 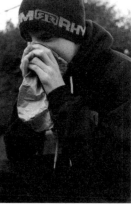

(a) Antidepressants   (b) Vitamins   (c) Smoking cigarettes   (d) Sniffing glue

The term *drug* lacks a precise definition. The antidepressant in panel A clearly seems to be a drug, but the substances in the other three panels seem less like drugs. Each substance, however, exhibits physiological changes in the body.

figure 1.1   (a) ©wavebreakmedia/Shutterstock.com. (b) ©gosphotodesign/Shutterstock.com. (c) ©Marcel Jancovic/Shutterstock.com (d) ©Janine Wiedel Photolibrary/Alamy

The emphasis on physiological functions also has limitations. Certainly drugs produce changes in the body—but is food a drug? After all, food also produces physiological changes in the body.

Do drugs have a certain appearance? Drugs come in a variety of different forms, including pills, liquids, and powders. Most people consider nicotine a drug, although nicotine molecules reside within tars in tobacco. Many adolescents sniff certain types of glue, the vapors of which contain chemicals such as toluene. In this case, drugs also come in vapor form.

Thus, although *drug* is a common term, we must not restrict our perception of a drug to a specific form or usage or we risk excluding nonconforming substances that may have powerful effects in altering behavior. As presented in Chapter 5, for example, therapists find that treating food like a drug provides a useful means of understanding food addiction.

Stop & Check

Stop & Check questions provide a quick way to self assess your comprehension of the material. These questions pertain to main points and are provided throughout the chapters of this book.

1. How prevalent are psychoactive drugs?
2. What is the definition of a drug?

1. Both therapeutic and recreational drugs are highly prevalent in society. Alcohol alone is used by more than 114 million adults in the U.S. and therapeutic drugs for depression and anxiety are used by as many as one-third of all U.S. adults.
2. A drug is a substance that alters physiological functioning. However, a more precise term is lacking.

Psychoactive Drugs: Described by Manner of Use

Psychoactive drugs broadly fall into two categories: those intended for instrumental use and those intended for recreational use. The major distinction between these categories is a person's intent or motivation for using the substance. A person uses a drug *instrumentally* toward addressing a specific purpose. For example, someone may take an antidepressant drug such as Prozac for the purpose of reducing depression. Further, most adults consume caffeinated beverages like coffee to help them wake up in the morning, another socially acceptable purpose. In psychopharmacology, instrumental use often occurs with **therapeutic drugs** for treating mental disorders such as depression and schizophrenia.

therapeutic drugs Drug used to treat a physical or mental disorder.

Recreational use refers to using a drug entirely to experience its effects. For example, recreational use of alcohol may consist of drinking alcohol purely to experience its intoxicating effects. This differs from the instrumental use of alcohol, which might consist of using alcohol for another purpose such as relieving stress after a long day of work. The term *misuse* applies to drugs that are intended for instrumental purpose but are instead used recreationally. For example, cough syrups that contain codeine or dextromethorphan are misused recreationally to achieve mind-altering effects such as euphoria or hallucinations.

Recreational use may lead to abuse or dependence. *Drug abuse* refers to drug use that causes harm to the user or others. Dependence can include the features of drug abuse, but a user also experiences a need or urge to continue using a substance. The clinical characteristics of drug abuse and dependence are expanded in Chapter 5.

Generic Names, Trade Names, and Street Names for Drugs

Individual drugs have different names. For example, people often take Tylenol to treat headaches. Although the name *Tylenol* is the most widely known name, the drug is known by a different name as well: acetaminophen. We refer to Tylenol as its trade name and acetaminophen as its generic name.

Nearly all therapeutic drugs have a generic name and at least one trade name. A pharmaceutical company that develops and markets a drug provides both trade and generic names, each for different purposes. A drug's **trade name** is developed for marketing the drug. Sometimes a trade name is designed to be memorable or emotion provoking. For example, common sleep aids include Ambien and Lunesta. The name *Lunesta* resembles the word *luna*, meaning "moon," a symbol for night. Plus, *Lunesta* has soft-sounding syllables, giving a relaxing connotation to the drug.

trade name Drug name developed for marketing the drug.

A drug's **generic name** is developed for a number of reasons, including the drug's chemical structure and similarity to other drugs. For example, note the names of the following antipsychotic drugs: chlorpromazine, clozapine, and olanzapine. All three of these drugs end in–*ine*, which corresponds to an amine chemical group in their structures. Moreover, the first two drugs, chlorpromazine and clozapine, have chloride molecules in their structures. Generic names do not follow hard rules, but as shown in this example, they do provide ways to show how drugs organizationally fit with other drugs.

generic name Names that show how drugs organizationally fit with other drugs.

Scientific reports normally refer to a drug's generic name. In these cases, the generic name is sometimes followed by the drug's trade name in parentheses. Moreover, trade names are capitalized. For example, a report might read "Physicians prescribe zolpidem (Ambien) for insomnia." The generic name is zolpidem, and its trade name is Ambien.

Recreational drugs are often referred to by street names. Street names develop by those who use, sell, or make recreational drugs. Street names can serve as benign-sounding aliases. For example, *ADAM* is a reference to the drug MDMA. Street names also reflect the drug's effects. For example, the drug MDMA is also known as *ecstasy*, which describes the drug's enjoyable effects. **Table 1.2** lists common recreational substances and their popular street names.

table **1.2**

Street Names for Selected Drugs	
Drug	**Street name**
Amphetamines	Bennies, black beauties
Benzodiazepines	Candy, downers, sleeping pills
Cocaine	Coke, rock, crack
Dextromethorphan (used in cough syrup)	Robo, triple C
Marijuana	Joint, blunt, weed
Methamphetamine	Meth, ice, crystal
MDMA	Ecstasy, Adam
LSD	Acid, blotter
Phencyclidine	PCP, angel dust

From the National Institute on Drug Abuse, http://www.drugabuse.gov.

Drug Effects: Determined by Dose

dose Ratio of the amount of drug per an organism's body weight.

Drug effects depend on the dose of a drug. **Dose** is a ratio of the amount of drug per an organism's body weight. For example, the dose of a drug given to a laboratory rat might be 1.0 gram of drug per kilogram body weight. This is written as 1.0 g/kg. To put this into context, if a rat weighed 1 kg—an incredibly large rat—then it would receive 1 gram of drug. If, instead, a rat weighed 0.3 kg, then it would receive 0.3 grams of drug.

For over-the-counter medications like Tylenol, the dosing instructions assume an average adult's body weight. If the instructions describe something like "Take one to two 325-mg tablets," then the "one to two" range refers to differences in body weight between adults. A larger individual might require two tablets, whereas a smaller individual might only require one tablet.

Many over-the-counter children's medications have medication amounts listed on a weight chart. Manufacturers do this to address a range in children's ages, such as 2 to 6 years of age, and the subsequent differences in body weights for these different ages. For example, the medication instructions might recommend one 20-mg dissolvable tablet for children weighing 20 to 40 pounds (lbs) and two dissolvable tablets for children weighing between 40 and 60 lbs. A doctor's office records your weight, in part, to calculate drug dosing. If the doctor prescribes a medication, she needs to know the dose of a drug to prescribe based on your body weight.

dose-effect curve Depicts the level of a drug effect by dose.

Generally, the higher a drug's dose, the greater its effects. Researchers determine the effects of drugs by evaluating a range of different doses. This information is plotted on dose-effect curves. A **dose-effect curve** depicts the level of a drug effect by dose. **Figure 1.2** presents two drugs plotted on dose-effect curves.

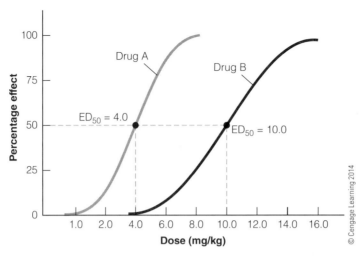

figure 1.2 Both drugs shown here achieve 100-percent effectiveness, but at different doses. Drug A is the most potent because it achieves these effects at lower doses than drug B. For drug A, the dose at which 50 percent of the effect occurs (ED_{50}) is 4.0 mg/kg. The ED_{50} for drug B is 10.0 mg/kg.

For each drug in figure 1.2, lower doses produce weaker effects and higher doses produce stronger effects. Each drug produces a full effect at a high enough dose. Yet notice that both drugs achieve full effectiveness at different doses. For drug A, 100-percent effectiveness occurs at a dose of 8.0 mg/kg dose, whereas 100-percent effectiveness for drug B occurs at a 16.0 mg/kg dose. In fact, the entire dose-response curve for drug A is located to the left of drug B (i.e., the curves do not overlap).

To describe the position of a dose-effect curve, researchers calculate an ED_{50} value. An **ED_{50} value** represents the dose at which 50 percent of an effect was observed. As shown in figure 1.2, drug A's ED_{50} value is 4.0 mg/kg. This corresponds to a dose that matches with the 50-percent effect point on the dose-effect curve.

ED_{50} values also provide a means to compare the potency of drugs. **Potency** refers to the amount of drug used to produce a certain level of effect. A "highly potent drug" means that low doses produce significant drug effects. Researchers use potency to compare different drugs that produce similar effects.

Consider again the drugs in figure 1.2. Drug A produces effects at lower doses than drug B does. Thus, drug A has a higher potency than drug B. By representing a dose-response curve, an ED_{50} value allows a way to calculate the relative level of potency between different drugs. Drug A has an ED_{50} value of 4.0 mg/kg, and drug B has an ED_{50} value of 10.0 mg/kg. The potency difference is calculated from dividing drug B, the compound with the highest ED_{50} value, by drug A, the compound with the lowest ED_{50} value. In this example, drug A is 2.5 times more potent than drug B.

During **drug development**, researchers must determine a drug's lethal dose. Lethality studies also produce dose-effect curves. The ED_{50} for lethality

ED_{50} value Represents the dose at which 50% of an effect was observed.

potency Amount of drug used to produce a certain level of effect.

drug development Multistep process of developing an effective, safe, and profitable therapeutic drug.

dose-response curves is referred to as an LD_{50} value (LD stands for *lethal dose*) or a TD_{50} value (TD stands for *toxic dose*). LD_{50} values allow for the determination of a therapeutic index.

therapeutic index
Ratio of a drug's a lethal dose-effect value relative to therapeutic dose-effect value.

A **therapeutic index** is a ratio of a drug's a lethal dose-effect value relative to a therapeutic dose-effect value. One way to calculate a therapeutic index is to divide an LD_{50} value by an ED_{50} value. A therapeutic index answers this question: How different is a dose that kills half of the subjects from a dose of the same drug that produces a full therapeutic effect in half of the subjects?

Although ED_{50} and LD_{50} values provide a means to calculate therapeutic indexes, they are not ideal for identifying safe drugs. **Figure 1.3** shows a drug's therapeutic dose-effect curve and lethal dose-effect curve. The LD_{50} dose is three times greater than the ED_{50} dose. Is that good? Notice that approximately 15 percent of all subjects died at the ED_{50} dose. If you look further, a fully effective therapeutic dose killed half of the subjects. This is clearly not a safe drug.

To avoid any overlapping therapeutic and lethal dose-effect curves, drug developers adopt a far more conservative calculation for a therapeutic index. They often identify a lethal dose that caused only 1 percent of subjects to die—which is referred to as LD_1—and divide this by a dose that achieved a 99-percent therapeutic effect—an ED_{99}. Large therapeutic indexes derived from this safer calculation describe very separate therapeutic and lethal dose-effect curves.

The U.S. Food and Drug Administration (FDA) and similar regulatory bodies in other countries require conservative therapeutic indexes for drugs

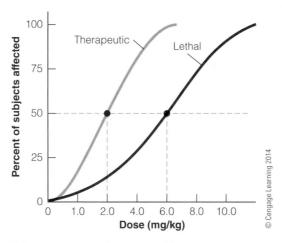

This drug produces therapeutic effects at doses lower than those that produce lethal effects. The LD_{50} value ($LD_{50} = 6.0$ mg/kg) is three times greater than the ED_{50} value ($ED_{50} = 2.0$ mg/kg). Is this drug safe to use? Notice that at an ED_{50} dose (2.0 mg/kg), approximately 15 percent of the subjects died. At a dose where full therapeutic effects were shown (6.0 mg/kg), approximately 50 percent of the subjects died. Thus, although the therapeutically effective doses are lower than the lethal doses, a number of subjects will die at those doses—clearly this is not a safe drug to use.

figure 1.3

they approve. However, this is not to say that every drug on the market has a large therapeutic index. For example, the mood stabilizer lithium has a lethal dose near the therapeutic dose, and for some individuals, taking only twice the recommended dosage might lead to life-threatening adverse effects.

Stop & Check	1. What determines if a drug is a therapeutic drug or a recreational drug?
	2. What are the two different names provided for therapeutic drugs?
	3. What is a dose?
	4. What is the best approach for calculating a therapeutic index?

1. The manner of usage. Individuals use therapeutic drugs instrumentally toward treating a disorder or ailment, whereas individuals take recreational drugs entirely to experience the drug's effects. **2.** Therapeutic drugs are provided a generic name, which refers to the organizational fit of a drug with similar acting drugs, and a trade name, which a company provides for marketing a drug. **3.** A dose is a ratio of the amount of drug per amount of body weight. Most of the instructions provided with over-the-counter drug packages advise taking pills based on an average adult weight. **4.** Conservative therapeutic indexes are derived from dividing a lethal dose for 1 percent of subjects, referred to as an LD_1, by a 99-percent effective dose, referred to as an ED_{99} value. When this calculation produces large therapeutic indexes, the lethal doses are much higher than therapeutically effective doses.

Pharmacology: Pharmacodynamics, Pharmacokinetics, and Pharmacogenetics

pharmacodynamics
mechanisms of action for a drug.

pharmacokinetics A drug's passage through the body.

pharmacogenetics
The study of how genetic differences influence a drug's pharmacokinetic and pharmacodynamic effects.

Pharmacodynamics and pharmacokinetics represent two major areas in pharmacology. **Pharmacodynamics** is the study of how drugs affect biological actions. For psychoactive drugs, the biological actions include the drug actions on the nervous system. Most addictive recreational drugs, for example, act on the brain's reward pathways to produce pleasurable effects. Chapter 4 provides an overview of many pharmacodynamic processes.

Pharmacokinetics is the study of how drugs pass through the body. This field considers different ways to administer a drug, how long a drug stays in the body, how well the drug enters the brain, and how it leaves the body. For example, pharmacokinetic properties explain why smoked cocaine reaches the brain more rapidly than snorted cocaine.

Although pharmacodynamics and pharmacokinetics define the classical broad categories in pharmacology, a subfield of pharmacology—**pharmacogenetics**—affects both categories. Pharmacogenetics is the study of how genetic differences influence a drug's pharmacokinetic and pharmacodynamic effects. This field provides the basis for differences in drug response between individuals. As we well know, a single therapeutic drug does not work for everyone. In fact, for psychoactive therapeutic drugs such as antidepressants, a physician often switches through several different medications until finding an effective one.

Genetically related differences in drug responsiveness may affect a drug's actions in the nervous system or passage through the body. In particular, many individuals are "fast metabolizers" for many drugs, meaning that certain drugs are quickly broken down in their livers. When this occurs, less of a drug stays intact in the body, resulting in weaker drug effects. Knowing that a patient is a fast metabolizer for certain drugs enables physicians to alter treatment plans. For example, a physician may prescribe a separate treatment that reduces metabolism of the drug or may prescribe an alternative drug that the person will metabolize slower.

Psychoactive Drugs: Objective and Subjective Effects

objective effects
Pharmacological effects that can be directly observed by others.

subjective effects
Pharmacological effects that cannot be directly observed by others.

To characterize the spectrum of a drug's pharmacological effects, researchers must measure the drug's objective and subjective effects. **Objective effects** are pharmacological effects that can be directly observed by others. In other words, a researcher can independently measure the drug's effects. For example, psychostimulant drugs increase heart rate. A researcher can objectively measure an individual's heart rate by taking the person's pulse (**figure 1.4**).

Subjective effects are pharmacological effects that cannot be directly observed by others. In other words, we cannot observe or measure another's drug experience. Researchers measure subjective effects by asking study participants to describe a drug's effects. The inability to independently observe subjective effects provides important scientific limitations. In particular, the drug's subjective effects may vary from person to person. To address this, researchers must develop a consensus about a drug's effects among many individuals and assume this consensus accurately reflects the drug's effects.

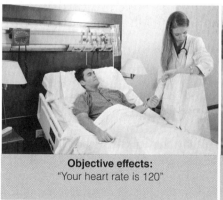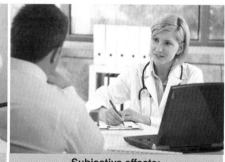

Objective effects:
"Your heart rate is 120"

Subjective effects:
"Describe the drug's effects?
Do you like the effects?"

Objective effects (left) are pharmacological effects that can be directly observed by others, whereas subjective effects (right) are pharmacological effects that cannot be directly observed by others.

figure 1.4   (a) ©Tyler Olson/Shutterstock.com. (b) ©StockLite/Shutterstock.com

Despite scientific limitations, a psychoactive drug's subjective effects are more important to understand than its objective effects. Subjective effects explain the purpose of recreational and addictive drug use. Subjective effects also explain the therapeutic value of antidepressant, anti-anxiety, and antipsychotic drugs. Only the patient can say if medications truly help depressed feelings, anxiety, and paranoid thoughts.

Stop & Check

1. How do pharmacodynamic effects differ from pharmacokinetic effects?
2. How might pharmacogenetic factors alter a person's response to a psychoactive drug?
3. What is the challenge in studying subjective drug effects?

1. Pharmacodynamic effects refer to the biological effects of a drug, whereas pharmacokinetic effects refer to the movement of a drug through the body, including a drug's entry into the nervous system. **2.** One's genetic makeup may alter a drug's passage through the body or alter a drug's actions in the nervous system. **3.** Subjective effects represent an individual's personal and nonpublicly observable effects from a drug. Yet for recreational drugs, subjective effects are the most important.

Study Designs and the Assessment of Psychoactive Drugs

dependent variable A study variable measured by a researcher.

independent variable Study conditions or treatments that may affect a dependent variable.

correlational study Study in which an investigator does not alter the independent variable.

The logic behind study designs provides the means to assess a drug's behavioral effects. Studies attempt to answer scientific questions about drug effects and the nervous system by using dependent and independent variables. A **dependent variable** is a study variable measured by a researcher. In psychology, dependent variables usually consist of behavioral measures, such as how many words an individual recalls from a list or an evaluation of one's level of depression.

Independent variables are study conditions or treatments that may affect a dependent variable. Independent variables for the previous examples might include teaching individuals a memorization technique or providing depressed individuals an antidepressant drug. In each case, study researchers sought to determine if an independent variable produced changes to a dependent variable.

Research studies fall into two categories: correlational studies and experimental studies (see **table 1.3**). In a **correlational study**, an investigator does not alter the independent variable.* For example, to study the effects of long-term MDMA use on memory, a researcher might recruit participants with experiences with MDMA and then measure each participant's ability to recall words from list. Duration of MDMA use serves as the *independent variable*, and each participant's level of memory serves as the *dependent variable*. The investigators did not alter the independent variable, but instead studied duration of MDMA use and memory ability as they already existed. Researchers

---

*Alternatively, correlational studies can use the term *predictor* instead of *independent variable*.

table **1.3**

Correlational and Experimental Studies	
Study type	**Description**
Correlational study	No alteration of study conditions. Changes in study variables are observed, and relationships are inferred.
Experiment	The study's independent variable is altered by researchers, and changes in a dependent variable are observed. Experiments can identify causal relationships between an independent variable and a dependent variable.

© Cengage Learning 2014

experimental study Study in which investigators alter an independent variable to determine if changes occur to the dependent variable.

placebo Substance identical in appearance to a drug but physiologically inert.

treatment arms Number of treatments and doses provided to patients described in a clinical study.

clinical study reports Detailed summaries of a clinical study's design and results.

might infer a relationship between MDMA use and memory if long-term MDMA users exhibited poor word recall, but infrequent MDMA users exhibited good word recall. However, correlational studies do not indicate that a variable *causes* changes to another variable.

In an **experimental study**, investigators alter an independent variable to determine if changes occur to the dependent variable. For example, many clinical studies use experiments to evaluate drug effects. In a standard experimental study design, individuals sharing a type of disorder are separated into two groups: a control group and a treatment group. The treatment group receives the treatment, but the control group does not. Instead, the control group may be given a **placebo**, or a substance identical in appearance to a drug but physiologically inert. Researchers may also refer to a placebo as a *vehicle*. If individuals in the treatment group improve over the course of this study and those in the control group do not, then researchers attribute improvements to the treatment. Experiments such as these indicate that the independent variable *caused* changes to the dependent variable.

Clinical drug studies use other terminology to describe an experiment. Drug experiments in clinical trials describe the number of treatments and doses provided to patients as **treatment arms**. A two-arm design refers to two patient experimental groups. Often, one group, or arm, receives an experimental drug and the other group receives a placebo.

Many times, researchers require more than a dose-versus-placebo comparison. In these cases, researchers may use a three- or four-arm design. For example, a three-arm design may consist of a high-dose drug group, a low-dose drug group, and a placebo group. Or a treatment arm may include an entirely different drug. Testing an experimental drug in comparison with a standard treatment and placebo provides a valuable assessment of drug efficacy compared to existing medications or no medications, respectively.

Why call study group arms? Look at the two-arm and three-arm designs in **figure 1.5**. This is the standard style of presenting multigroup study designs in **clinical study reports**, the detailed summaries of a clinical study's design and results (International Conference on Harmonization, 1996). As shown in figure 1.5, the different groups appear on separate lines like arms or branches.

Two-arm Study

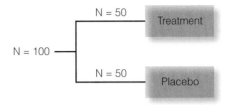

Three-arm Study

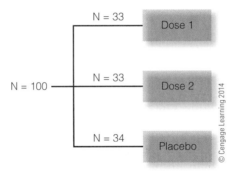

Clinical drug study designs describe treatment conditions as *arms*. The left portion of each design shows the total number of participants recruited for the study, and each arm shows the number of participants assigned to each study condition.

figure 1.5

---

single-blind procedure
When researchers do not inform study participants which treatment or placebo they received.

double-blind procedure
When neither participants nor investigators know the treatment assignments during a study.

open-label studies
Assignment of study treatments without using blinded procedures.

Experiments use random sampling to assign participants to study groups. Through random assignment, researchers seek to achieve groups that have similar characteristics. Many experiments also use blinding procedures to eliminate potential biases by study participants or investigators. In a **single-blind procedure**, researchers do not inform study participants which treatment, or placebo, they received. To provide informed consent, study investigators provide participants a description of treatments that might be administered, as well as the potential for placebo administration, but they do not identify the assigned treatment to participants during the study.

In a **double-blind procedure**, neither the participants nor the investigators know the treatment assignments during the study. These procedures not only prevent potential biased responses from participants, but also prevent potential biased judgments by study investigators. Although researchers consider blinded procedures important for quality experimental studies, not all experiments allow for blinded procedures.

In clinical research, **open-label studies** refer to the assignment of study treatments without using blinded procedures. Open-label studies apply to situations where disguising study medications may have important ethical consequences or be impractical. For example, many cancer clinical trials use open-label procedures because withholding a potential effective treatment from cancer patients by using a placebo might have serious health consequences.

Experimental Validity: Addressing the Quality and Impact of an Experiment

experimental validity Addresses the logical design of effective quality experimental studies.

internal validity Control of variables with potential to influence changes in a dependent variable.

confound variables Variables other than independent variables that can cause changes to the dependent variables.

external validity Refers to how well the experimental findings generalize beyond experimental conditions.

Say you conducted an experiment and found that a newly developed drug reduced symptoms in depression. Great news, but how *valid* was the experiment? This question addresses the quality of study procedures, the appropriate choice of species tested, the ability to extend these findings to other individuals with the disorder, and many other possible experimental issues. Researchers must address questions such as these to ensure high-quality experiments (Elmes, Kantowitz, & Roediger, 2006). **Experimental validity** addresses the logical design of effective quality experimental studies. Subcategories of experimental validity include internal validity, external validity, face validity, construct validity, and predictive validity (**table 1.4**).

Internal validity refers to the control of variables with potential to influence changes in a dependent variable. Ideal experiments arrange conditions so that only changes to the independent variable will cause changes to the dependent variable. Without appropriately arranging conditions, other variables, referred to as **confound variables**, can cause changes to the dependent variable.

For example, a study designed to test new drugs for depression may involve patients checking in with a clinic physician every morning. After several weeks, the study results indicate a reduction in depression. Might this study have confound variables?

The daily clinic visits are a potential confound variable. The act of talking to a physician daily may also reduce depression. Without considering these variables, study investigators risk wrongly concluding that an experimental drug produces therapeutic effects. To avoid this potential confound variable, researchers blind participants to the study medications, and they may also assign placebo to one participant group. Placebo groups control for many confound variables. If placebo-treated patients also exhibited reduced depression, then researchers will conclude that variables other than the study medication caused reductions in depression.

External validity refers to how well the experimental findings generalize beyond experimental conditions. For example, many clinical antidepressant

table 1.4

Types of Experimental Validity	
Validity	**Description**
Internal validity	Adequacy of controlling variables that may influence a dependent variable.
External validity	Ability to extend findings beyond experimental conditions.
Face validity	A model appears similar to a disorder.
Construct validity	A model contains mechanisms related to those of a disorder.
Predictive validity	A model predicts characteristics of a disorder.

studies examine only adults. Such studies have poor external validity for antidepressant effects in children. In other words, the study conditions used do not provide evidence of antidepressant effectiveness in children. To improve external validity for children, clinical studies must include child participants.

animal research
Procedures that use animal subjects in scientific research.

External validity also presents limitations for **animal research** findings and their extension to effects in humans. One example of this occurred in the 1950s with the drug thalidomide. Thalidomide exhibited sedative effects and prevented nausea and vomiting. Without harmful effects to fetuses in pregnant mice, European physicians prescribed the thalidomide to pregnant women suffering from morning sickness.

However, thalidomide proved severely harmful to human fetuses. By 1962, nearly 10,000 babies were missing fingers, toes, and limbs after exposure to thalidomide during pregnancy (**figure 1.6**). In humans, but not in mice, thalidomide was metabolically broken down into **teratogens**, substances harmful to a fetus. Had drug developers tested thalidomide in rabbits, which do convert thalidomide into this teratogen, doctors would not have prescribed thalidomide to pregnant women. Thus, in this case, rabbits, not mice, provide proper external validity for this property of thalidomide (Goldman, 2001). Proper drug screening requires a thorough examination of drugs using many different models and approaches, including a variety of animal species.

teratogens Substances harmful to a fetus.

Face validity means that the model looks like the disorder the researcher intends to study. For example, researchers study drugs for Alzheimer's disease by testing mice with memory deficits. If the mice demonstrate Alzheimer-like memory loss, then this model has high face validity.

face validity Assessment of how well a model resembles the disorder a researcher intends to study.

Construct validity addresses how well a study's model approximates a disorder. Testing new drugs for Alzheimer's disease in Alzheimer's patients offers high construct validity; that is, the drug is tested in an individual who has the disease to be treated. Researchers seek to develop animal models

construct validity
Addresses how well a study's model approximates a disorder.

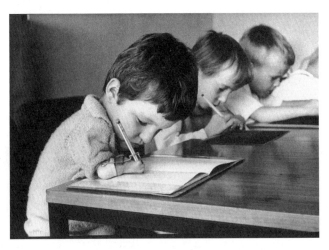

figure **1.6**

Failure to screen thalidomide in rabbits instead of mice led researchers to miss thalidomide's teratogenic effects, leading to babies born with missing digits and limbs.
Time & Life Pictures/Getty Images

with high construct validity in order to accurately screen experimental treatments during drug development. Certain genetically altered mice exhibit protein abnormalities similar to those found in Alzheimer's disease. Thus, these models offer construct validity for screening new Alzheimer's disease medications.

predictive validity
Addresses how well a model predicts characteristics of a disorder.

Predictive validity addresses how well a model predicts test results in a disorder. To continue the above example, an Alzheimer's disease treatment like the drug Aricept might improve memory in certain genetically altered mice. If this were the case, then these mice offer predictive validity for screening Alzheimer's disease medications. At times, an experimental procedure might offer high predictive validity, but fail to offer face or construct validity. Many animal models for antipsychotic drugs fail to exhibit features of schizophrenia, yet antipsychotic drugs produce unique behaviors in these models that scientists have learned to match to clinical effects in humans. Drug developers rely on models with high predictive validity when screening experimental drugs.

Stop & Check

1. How is a correlational study different from an experiment?
2. What might a three-arm clinical study consist of?
3. Why is external validity an important concern for animal experimentation?

1. Correlational studies identify potential associations between variables, whereas experiments identify causal relationships between variables. **2.** A three-arm study employs three different participant groups. Although the treatment conditions depend on the disorder and drugs being tested, a three-arm study might employ a placebo group, an experimental drug group, and a comparison drug group. **3.** Important physiological differences exist between all species, and these differences may not accurately reflect a drug's actions in humans.

Animals and Advancing Medical Research

Ethics play another important role in psychopharmacology research. Experimental treatments may have unintended effects in human participants. Ethically, researchers must fully inform participants about treatment risks and allow participants to freely end the study at their choosing. During testing, researchers take great care to monitor each participant's health. Beyond providing information to participants and monitoring their health, years of animal research went into identifying the compound as likely effective and safe.

To develop drugs for human usage, medical research relies heavily on animal testing. Not only do medical research advances depend on animal models, but also governmental regulators, such as the FDA, require proof of extensive animal research data before approving drugs for clinical testing. Medical advances rely on animal research for three major reasons: a lack of feasible alternatives, the high predictive value of animals for drug effects in humans, and drug assessment in carefully controlled laboratory environments.

A Lack of Feasible Alternatives

Treatment results from studies conducted only on cells and tissues poorly predict treatment efficacy and safety in humans. Although these biological studies provide important steps in medical development, they fail to model the complexity of living organisms. This complexity currently precludes computer simulations or mathematical models from taking the place of animal research. Animal models provide the next necessary step in drug development.

Humans also do not provide a feasible alternative to animal models. Necessary basic research procedures consist of invasive techniques that would be highly unethical to perform in humans. For example, many medical studies require euthanizing animals in order to measure drug-induced changes in cells and tissue. In addition to invasiveness, experimental drugs that have not been tested in animals carry a risk of severe and possibly irreversible adverse effects in humans.

High Predictive Value for Drug Effects in Humans

Beyond having no feasible alternatives, animal models do well in predicting drug effects in humans. During drug development, as previously presented, animal models identify effective drugs from the hundreds or thousands synthesized in a drug-development program. The FDA requires that all experimental medications be screened in animal models before testing drugs in humans. At the end of this chapter, the "From Actions to Effects" section describes the role that animals play in therapeutic drug development.

Assessing Drugs in Carefully Controlled Laboratory Environments

Like other experimental variables, drugs are best studied under well-controlled experimental conditions. For drug studies, these laboratory conditions require animal subjects. Laboratory conditions for animal studies include housing, diet, age, weight, and a consistent experimental routine.

In clinical trials, humans may be selected based on having the same disorder and possibly the same demographic characteristics such as gender, age, race, body weight, and blood pressure among others. But even controlling for such factors, humans still differ based on where they work, what they eat, hobbies, how they interact with people, when they wake up in the morning, how much they exercise, and countless other differences.

The great variety of human differences may prevent researchers from identifying an effective drug. Instead, carefully controlled animal laboratory conditions provide the ability to identify drugs with potential efficacy before evaluating them in the complex human environment. This ensures that only the most likely effective drugs reach human participants.

The Regulation of Animal Research

In Western nations, governmental and private agencies exist to oversee the responsible and humane use of animal subjects for research or teaching purposes. Journal publishers indirectly regulate nonparticipating countries by insisting that all research described in their journals abide by national regulations and policies. In short, all legitimate journals publishing scientific studies require high ethical standards for animal care and use in research.

Two government agencies regulate academic and industrial animal research in the United States: the U.S. Department of Agriculture (USDA, 2006) and the Public Health Service (PHS, 2002). The USDA enforces regulations in the Animal Welfare Act, and the Office of Laboratory Animal Welfare enforces polices of the Public Health Service. Failure to comply with federal regulations and policies results in stiff penalties, including institutional fines and withdrawal of federal grant money.

Among the many rules of institutional conduct, both the Animal Welfare Act and the Public Health Policy require that all U.S. institutions conducting federally funded animals research establish an ethics review committee called the Institutional Animal Care and Use Committee (IACUC). The Animal Welfare Act also covers many species regardless of an institution's federal funding status. Federal law not only pertains to academic institutions but also to pharmaceutical companies. The FDA will not approve any treatments resulting from animal studies that have not complied with federal regulations and policies (FDA, 2002).

The IACUC oversees an institution's entire animal care and use program, including quality of housing, veterinary practices, and research practices. All animal experiments require IACUC approval before they are started. To gain approval, researchers must submit animal research proposals to the IACUC, which reviews these protocols and determines their abidance with federal and internal policies. Moreover, the IACUC makes ethical judgments according to its "3 R's" of replacement, reduction, and refinement.

The 3 R's address the necessity of using animals (National Research Council, 2011; Russell & Burch, 1959). For replacement, the IACUC assesses the necessity of using animals for a proposed study. Drug researchers virtually never have mathematical models or computer simulations capable of replacing animals for drug testing. However, similarly useful findings may be derived by working only with cells or perhaps with invertebrates (e.g., insects) instead of animals. If this were the case, then the IACUC would reject the proposal.

The second R, reduction, refers to using the minimum number of animals necessary to achieve the study objectives. Generally, IACUCs use statistics to ensure that researchers only use the minimum number of animals necessary to detect experimental results. For the third R, refinement, the IACUC attempts to minimize any pain and distress experienced by the study animals. These attempts may include changing experimental procedures or using different testing equipment.

ethical cost Assessment that weighs the value of potential research discoveries against the potential pain and distress experienced by research subjects.

IACUCs also weigh the proposed study's ethical costs. **Ethical cost** assessments weigh the value of potential research discoveries against the potential pain and distress experienced by research animals (**figure 1.7**). For example, IACUC members easily justify painless experiments in animals that aim to develop treatments for lethal illnesses. Essentially, these studies provide tremendous gains with minimal ethical cost. On the other hand, IACUC members cannot justify studies with limited potential for discovery that uses highly painful procedures (Carbone, 2000).

Beyond federally mandated regulations and policies, many U.S. institutions seek private accreditation in order to exceed federal requirements and achieve best practices in the animal care and use. The primary private accreditor for animal care and use in research settings is the Association for Assessment and Accreditation of Laboratory Animal Care (AAALAC). AAALAC inspection teams accompany institution investigators as they tour animal facilities, talk to researchers, and oversee how animal research is approved and monitored. AAALAC is an important aid to larger institutions that use thousands of animals for research (AAALAC, 2012).

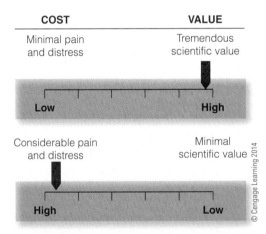

During IACUC review, researchers weigh the potential pain or distress experienced by an animal against a study's potential value. In the top panel, the scientific value outweighs the minimal pain or distress experienced by animals, whereas the bottom panel shows that the scientific value fails to outweigh considerable pain and distress expected for the animals.

figure 1.7

Animal Rights Activism Seeks to Minimize or Eliminate Animal Research

The previous section provides information about the use of animals in research and the ethical polices and legal regulations overseeing the humane use of laboratory animals. Chances are that if you have not been exposed to any of this previous information, then you have probably heard about animal rights groups such as the People for the Ethical Treatment of Animals (PETA) and the Animal Liberation Front (ALF). Groups such as these actively seek the complete cessation of animal research, either seeing no value in the work or dismissing any value as unjustified.

Historically, animal rights groups arose from concerns over animal vivisection, a procedure involving surgical procedures to living, and often conscious, animals. These concerned individuals formed antivivisection societies in the late nineteenth century. These public efforts culminated in the Cruelty to Animals Act of 1876 in Great Britain that forbade painful procedures in animals unless "absolutely necessary for the due instruction of the persons to save or prolong human life."

In the United States, animal rights groups formed by concerned citizens and animal researchers fought unsuccessfully for national animal research regulations until the 1960s. In 1966, a *Life* magazine article exposed the activities of animal research dealers (**figure 1.8**). These activities including catching stray dogs or even stealing dogs for the purpose of selling them to animal researchers. As shown in

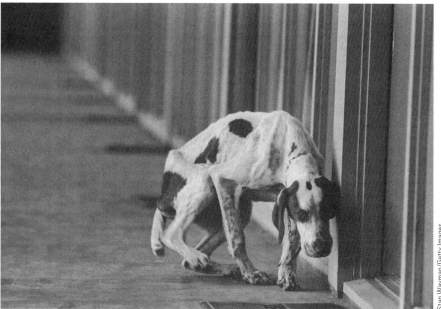

Stan Wayman/Getty Images

figure 1.8 An article in *Life* magazine in 1966 exposed the unethical activities of animal research suppliers.

figure 1.8, these dogs also lacked humane care ("Marching for science," 1966). An outraged public quickly led federal legislators to pass the Animal Welfare Act in 1966. Among other regulations, the Animal Welfare Act required researchers to obtain animals from federally approved animal dealers.

Modern animal rights activities largely began after publication of philosopher Peter Singer's book *Animal Liberation* (Singer, 1975). In short, this book is widely credited with the modern movement to cease animal research. These groups are active and well supported, and they take actions both legal and illegal against animal research.

Legal animal rights activities may include information sessions, public protests, petitions, and advertising. Illegal animal rights activities include distributing false information, illegal entering animal facilities, releasing laboratory animals, and damaging laboratory equipment. Recent years have seen terrorist activities directed at animal researchers ranging from acts of vandalism to attempted murder (**figure 1.9**). A string of incidents of vandalism and fire bombings of vehicles and homes has been linked especially to the ALF over many years (Lewis, 2005).

In response to growing threats to researchers and students, groups support-ing animal research are providing public information on the medical advances derived through animal research. The Foundation for Biomedical Research, for example, prints materials and produces television commercials that describe medical discoveries from animal research. The Pro-Test organization organizes public rallies promoting the value of animal research (Anonymous, 2009).

Researchers Consider Many Ethical Issues When Conducting Human Research

Most research investigators use animal subjects for the purpose of approximating drug effects in humans. Like animal studies, ethics committees review research practices to ensure federal regulatory and policy compliance and to weigh the ethics of human study activities. Beyond the obvious species differences, human and animal research differs according in the ability to provide informed consent. **Informed consent** consists of a participant's thorough understanding of a study's procedures, possible gains, and potential risks. In other words, human participants know what they are getting into and can freely decide to enroll in the study. Animals lack the capacity to provide informed consent (Swerdlow, 2000).

informed consent
Consent gained after a participant thoroughly understands a study's procedures, possible gains, and potential risks.

However, some human participants also lack the capacity to provide informed consent. For example, young children lack the capacity to understand what may happen during a medical study. Or an adult may be mentally incapable of providing informed consent. In these cases, informed consent is left to a legal guardian.

The informed consent principle is a relatively modern one, and there is a long history of human experimentation conducted either against the will of

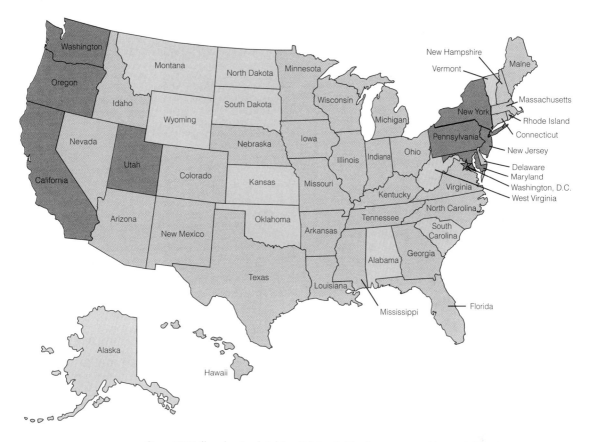

figure 1.9 Since 1997, illegal animal right activist activities have occurred in most American states. States colored blue in this map have had a high number of incidents, whereas light blue-colored states have had a low numbers of incidents. Gray indicates no reported incidents. (From www.fbresearch.org/.)

the participants or with complete dishonesty about what was being studied. The Nuremberg Principles, which arose from the Nuremberg Trials after World War II, consist of some of the first written statements about the ethical conduct of human research (**figure 1.10**). These principles provided the foundation for the Declaration of Helsinki, another set of guidelines for ethical research using humans.

In the United States, the federal Department of Health and Human Services regulates human research. This department assigns the direct responsibility of enforcing these regulations to the Office of Protection from Research Risks. These regulations require that U.S. institutions review and approve all human research in accordance with these federal regulations. U.S. institutions must file annual reports on human research activities. The penalties for violating government regulations and policies range from fines to freezing an institution's federal funding.

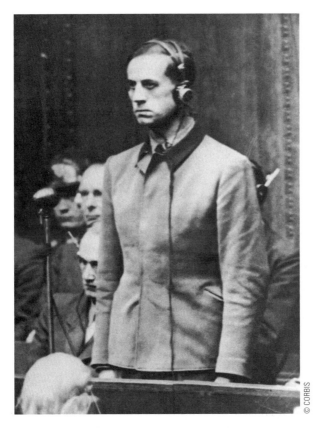

© CORBIS

figure 1.10 Karl Brandt, Adolf Hitler's personal physician and Reich commissioner for health and sanitation, was found guilty of crimes against humanity—in part because he sponsored human experimentation—during the Nuremberg Trials (1946–1947).

Stop & Check

1. Why are animal models valuable?
2. When evaluating animal research proposals, what considerations are made in an ethical cost assessment?
3. Aside from species differences, what is the major distinction between human research and animal research?

1. Although animal models present important experimental validity challenges, animal models remain the only feasible models because they are effective and provide ways to evaluate drugs under carefully controlled conditions. **2.** By considering ethical costs, an IACUC weighs the benefits of a research proposal against the potential pain and suffering experienced by animal subjects. **3.** Humans can provide informed consent whereas animals cannot.

FROM ACTIONS TO EFFECTS
Therapeutic Drug Development

Academic, government, and pharmaceutical company research contributes to the development of therapeutic drugs (e.g., Blake, Barker, & Sobel, 2006). For the most part, academic and government research consists of basic research discoveries about disorders and the development of theoretical directions for designing new treatments. This work may include characterizing a disorder's effects on the nervous system or developing a theory about chemical structures that mimic chemicals in the nervous system. Although some institutions develop new treatments, the vast majority of new treatments arrive from pharmaceutical companies.

Pharmaceutical drug research and development generally occurs in several stages (Blake et al., 2006; Dingemanse & Appel-Dingemanse, 2007; Jenkins & Hubbard, 1991) (see **table 1.5**). First, a company usually decides for which disorder to develop a treatment. This decision includes carefully considered opinions from scientists, outside consultants, and business executives. These individuals seek to develop a feasible treatment that yields a reasonable likelihood of making a significant profit.

The likelihood of a profit coincides with a disorder's prevalence. In other words, companies assess the size of the market. In this regard, rare and incurable diseases are often incurable because they are rare. To develop treatments for rare disease, there must be a high potential of developing a successful treatment. In other words, the approach must be low risk.

Feasibility and profitability often steer a research program into conservative directions, where instead of attempting treatments for currently incurable diseases, companies seek to improve treatments for currently treatable disorders. Occasionally

table **1.5**

Stage	Purpose	Description
Stages of Therapeutic Drug Development		
1	Identify disorder to treat	Decisions include feasibility and profitability concerns.
2	Drug synthesis	Chemists synthesize experimental compounds.
3	Biological experimentation	High-throughput screening methods provide basic biological information about compounds. Results are sent to chemists and guide synthesis of further compounds.
4	Refined screening methods	Refined testing occurs with most promising compounds identified during stage 3.
5	Safety pharmacology	Tests identify adverse effects and lethal doses.
6	Clinical trials	Most effective and safest compounds tested in humans. Governmental approval sought after positive clinical findings.

companies will seek a high-risk, high-reward approach. For example, developing a cure for cancer or acquired immunodeficiency syndrome (AIDS) is a currently insurmountable challenge, but the potential profit for such a treatment would be tremendous.

Drug synthesis occurs during the second drug-development stage. During this stage, a company's chemists develop experimental compounds. To do so, they may develop variations of existing therapeutic drugs for a disorder or develop drugs based on established theories.

Third, the drugs produced by the chemists during stage 2 are tested in biological experiments. For example, researchers may assess how well experimental drugs bind to certain proteins in tissue samples. Researchers prefer using **high-throughput screening** methods during these initial experiments—that is, use a rapid testing process involving a large number of experimental drugs (Garrett, Walton, McDonald, Judson, & Workman, 2003; Szymański, Markowicz, & Mikiciuk-Olasik, 2012). Generally, high-throughput tests provide quick results, but low precision. They basically determine whether the experimental drugs are close to achieving a desired biological effect.

Chemists receive these test results and use the information to develop further experimental drugs. The best drugs from the previous batch serve as the best directions for developing the next batch of experimental drugs. Then the chemists send the newest drugs back to the high-throughput screeners. The process between these drug screeners and the chemists continues as progress continues. When a drug meets their goal for a biological effect, then drug testing moves to the next stage of development.

Stage 4 represents a shift from high-throughput screening methods to refined screening methods. Compared to high-throughput screening methods, refined screening methods are slower, but offer greater precision. In particular, these refined screening methods use models that have face, construct, or predictive validity. Often these methods include animal models.

When drugs pass through refined screening tests, the next important question pertains to their safety. Thus, the fifth stage of drug development is **safety pharmacology** testing, a screening process that identifies the adverse effects of drugs (Guillon, 2010; Szymański et al., 2012). Adverse effects include mild to serious physiological effects, addiction risks, and changes in mental functioning. Safety pharmacology tests also identify a drug's lethal dose.

Many drugs determined successful in earlier stages of screening reveal a low therapeutic index—that is, the same doses that produce therapeutic effects also show serious adverse effects. For drugs to meet clinical testing approval from governmental regulatory agencies such as the FDA, safety pharmacology tests must demonstrate that a drug's harmful doses far exceed its therapeutic doses.

The sixth stage of drug development involves human drug testing. Most drugs fail to make it to this stage, having been abandoned because of a lack of efficacy or poor safety. **Clinical trials** refer to government-approved experimental drug testing in humans. In the United States and other countries, different phases describe the progression of experimental testing throughout the clinical trial process. Clinical trials begin at phase I and progress through phases II, III, and IV as long as a drug continues to prove safe and effective (National Institutes of Health, 2012).

The primary goal of a phase I clinical trial is to determine a drug's safety in humans. Phase I clinical trials employ a low dose of drug and provide it to a specific patient population for a short period of time. Unsafe drugs do not continue in clinical trial testing.

high-throughput screening Rapid testing process involving a large number of experimental drugs.

safety pharmacology Screening process that identifies the adverse effects of drugs.

clinical trials Government-approved experimental drug testing in humans.

During phase II clinical trials, researchers primarily seek to measure a drug's therapeutic efficacy. Phase II clinical trials use larger doses that are administered for longer periods of time. These trials often include an FDA-approved drug for comparison. Through using a comparison drug, drug developers determine how well their drug will compete with others on the market. Clinical trials may cease if the experimental drug fails to exhibit greater therapeutic or safer effects than drugs already on the market.

Phase III clinical trials provide greater information about the drug's therapeutic effects and potential adverse effects. These trials further increase drug doses and durations of drug treatment. Moreover, researchers recruit study participants with more diverse health backgrounds than those in previous trials. Phase IV clinical trials extend phase III clinical trial procedures to further investigate a specific patient population or evaluate longer periods of drug treatment.

‖‖‖

Stop & Check

1. What most likely happens after the first time drugs are initially screened?
2. Why might an effective and safe drug be removed from clinical trials?

1. Usually, chemists take data from the first screened batch and make further chemical compounds. The interplay between the chemists and the high-throughput screeners continues until the best drugs are made. **2.** Sometimes drugs are removed from clinical trials because they fail to be more effective than drugs that are already on the market.

▶CHAPTER SUMMARY

Psychopharmacology is the study of how drugs affect behavior. The field is largely a bridge between psychology and pharmacology. Psychoactive drug use is highly prevalent in society. Alcohol, for example, is consumed by the much of the U.S. population, and antidepressant medications are used by close to a third of the Western population. Learning about psychopharmacology provides a greater understanding of behavior and how mental disorders are treated. Defined as substances that alter physiological functioning, drugs are known by generic names, trade names, and street names. The amounts of drugs to be used are described in doses, and understanding drug effects and actions requires knowledge of pharmacokinetic and pharmacodynamic actions. Moreover, genetic differences account for varying drug effects between individuals. Drugs fall into two categories: therapeutic drugs and recreational drugs. However, many drugs cross both categories, depending on their usage. Drugs come from three different sources: plants, industry, and clandestine laboratories. Researchers study the objective and subjective effects of drugs in studies that address important experimental validity concerns, pertaining to quality of study conditions and reliable value of the study findings. These studies employ either animal or human subjects, in abidance with regulatory and ethical guidelines. The drug-development process employing these studies begins with the decision to pursue a disorder through a process of drug synthesis, efficacy and safety experiments, and human clinical trials.

KEY TERMS

Psychopharmacology

Psychoactive drugs

Pharmacotherapeutics

Drug

Therapeutic drugs

Trade name

Generic name

Dose

Dose-effect curve

ED_{50} value

Potency

Drug development

Therapeutic index

Pharmacodynamics

Pharmacokinetics

Pharmacogenetics

Objective effects

Subjective effects

Dependent variable

Independent variable

Correlational study

Experimental study

Placebo

Treatment arms

Clinical study reports

Single-blind procedure

Double-blind procedure

Open-label studies

Experimental validity

Internal validity

Confound variables

External validity

Animal research

Teratogens

Face validity

Construct validity

Predictive validity

Ethical cost

Informed consent

High-throughput
  screening

Safety pharmacology

Clinical trials

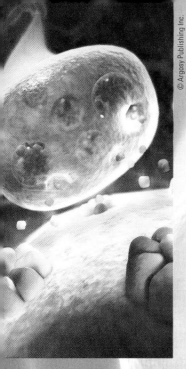

CHAPTER **2**

The Nervous System

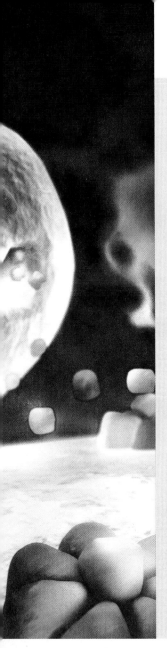

Is There More to the Story of Phineas Gage?

Psychology students are familiar with the story of Phineas Gage, a railway construction foreman who, in 1848, survived an accident when a 3-foot tamping iron shot through his skull. As the familiar story goes, his behavior radically transformed from a "mild-mannered...[and] friendly" man to "a restless, moody,...depraved, slovenly, [and] violently quarrelsome" man. The incident shows that one's personality can dramatically change from injury to the brain.

Yet we may not know the complete story of Phineas Gage (MacMillan, 2008). After recovery from the incident, for example, Gage's mother remarked that he "entertained his little nephews and nieces with the most fabulous recitals" and that he "conceived a great fondness . . . for children, horses and dogs." Moreover, a seemingly industrious Gage had traveled to New York, Boston, and other New England towns to show his injury at medical lectures and at the Barnum's American Museum in New York. He also spent 18 months as a stage coach driver, a job that required physical stamina and high cognitive functioning social skills in order to prepare horses, keep to a schedule, collect fares, be polite to hotel guests, and successfully navigate miles of winding poor roads.

These characteristics differ dramatically from popular perceptions of Gage. That Phineas Gage's personality perhaps did not switch so abruptly and that his cognitive and social abilities appeared intact is a tacit reminder about the brain's complexity and adaptability to injury.

The study of psychoactive drugs requires knowledge about how drugs act on the nervous system. This chapter provides a basic overview of the nervous system, with an emphasis on cells and structures important for psychoactive drug effects.

Cells in the Nervous System

neurons Cells in the nervous system that receive and transmit information to other neurons.

glia cells (or glial cells) Cells that support the function of neurons.

Each structure of the brain contains a dense ensemble of neurons and glia cells. **Neurons** are cells in the nervous system that receive and transmit information to other cells. Neurons serve as the principal players for behavior and have many unique characteristics that set them apart from other cells in the body. **Glia cells,** or glial cells, are cells that support the function of neurons. General estimates give the brain approximately 100 billion neurons, but 10 times as many glial cells (Herculano-Houzel, 2009).

Neuron Communication in the Nervous System

Neurons comprise dense communication networks in the brain. These networks support the function of individual brain structures and facilitate communication between brain structures. Like other cells in the body, neurons have basic characteristics such as a membrane, nucleus, ribosomes, and an endoplasmic reticulum (**figure 2.1**), yet they have many unique characteristics for cellular communication.

Neurons have four major components: a soma, dendrites, axon, and axon terminal (**figure 2.2**). The soma is the body of the neuron. It also contains the nucleus, which holds DNA. Overall, components within the soma support a neuron's basic physiological processes.

dendrites Parts of a neuron that receive information from other neurons.

Generally, a neuron has many dendrites that branch off from the soma. The **dendrites** of a neuron receive information from other neurons. Small stems called *dendritic spines* grow along the length of dendritic branches. The membranes of dendrites and dendritic spines contain proteins called *receptors*

Nucleus

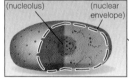

(nucleolus)   (nuclear envelope)

Membrane-enclosed region containing DNA

Plasma membrane

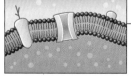

Control of material exchanges, mediation of cell-environment interactions

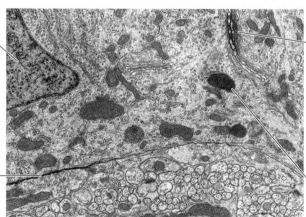

Endoplasmic reticulum

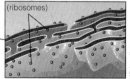

(ribosomes)

Isolation, modification, transport of proteins and other substances

Mitochondrion

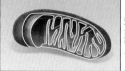

Aerobic energy metabolism

© Cengage Learning 2014; Micrograph courtesy of Dennis MD Landis

figure 2.1   The soma of a neuron contains the same basic components that other cells of the body have.

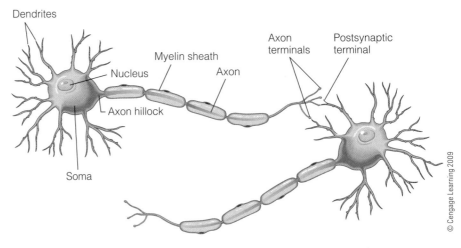

Dendrites

Myelin sheath

Axon terminals

Postsynaptic terminal

Nucleus

Axon

Axon hillock

Soma

© Cengage Learning 2009

figure 2.2 The four major components of a neuron are the soma, dendrites, an axon, and an axon terminal. Dendrites receive information, and axons send information.

---

axons Part of a neuron that sends neurotransmitters to other neurons.

synapse Components that comprise a connection between two neurons that includes the axon terminal, postsynaptic terminal, and synaptic cleft.

interneuron Neuron with the soma and axon found within the same structure.

sensory neurons Neuron that conveys sensory information via axons to the central nervous system.

motor neurons Neuron that conveys motor information via axons from the central nervous.

that neurotransmitters can activate. When activated, receptors cause changes in the functioning of the neuron. The overall coverage of dendrites for a neuron is called the *receptive area*; the more dendrites a neuron has, the more input it can receive from other neurons.

Axons send neurotransmitters to other neurons. Most neurons have only one axon, which branches from the soma, usually opposite from the dendrites. An axon begins at a part of the soma called the *axon hillock* and ends with multiple branches containing axon terminals. These branches are called *axon collaterals*. An axon terminal contains and releases neurotransmitters at a part of a dendrite called a *postsynaptic terminal*. The postsynaptic terminal contains receptors for neurotransmitters. The small space between the axon terminal and postsynaptic terminal is called the *synaptic cleft*. The term **synapse** refers to the components that comprise this connection, and these include the axon terminal, postsynaptic terminal, and the synaptic cleft.

Neuroscientists use different terms to describe the location of a neuron and the direction of its axon. The term **interneuron** describes a neuron with the soma and axon found within the same structure. An afferent neuron has an axon *going to* another structure. **Sensory neurons**, which convey sensory information via axons to the central nervous system, are considered *afferent* neurons. An *efferent* neuron has an axon *coming from* a structure. **Motor neurons**, which convey motor information via axons from the central nervous system, are considered efferent neurons (**figure 2.3**). Thus, the terms *afferent* and *efferent* neurons can refer to any structure being studied. For example, the thalamus, a structure that routes sensory information to different parts of the cerebral cortex, has both types of neurons: afferents send axons *to* the thalamus, and efferents send axons *from* the thalamus.

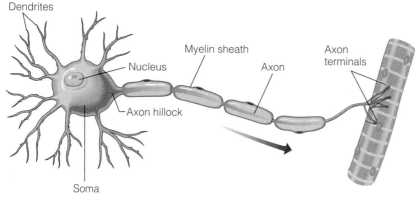

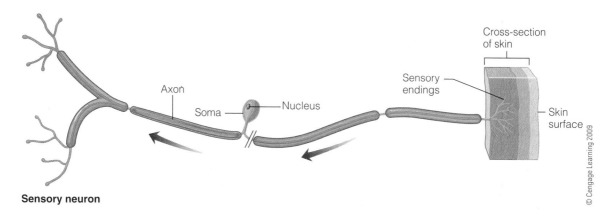

Motor and sensory neurons   Motor neurons convey movement information to muscles in the body, and sensory neurons convey sensory information to the central nervous system (CNS). Relative to the central nervous system, motor neurons are efferent neurons (going away from the CNS), and sensory neurons are afferent neurons (going to the CNS).

figure 2.3

Glial Cells: Facilitating Nervous System Functions

Glial cells consist of three different types: (1) oligodendrocytes, (2) astrocytes, and (3) microglial cells (**figure 2.4**). Oligodendrocytes produce a material called *myelin* around the axons of neurons that functions like an insulating material to facilitate the movement of electrical impulses down an axon (more on this in Chapter 3). Schwann cells are like oligodendrocytes, but are found in the peripheral nervous system. The motor dysregulation, paralysis, and other symptoms of multiple sclerosis result from degeneration of myelin sheaths that surround axons in the nervous system.

Astrocytes play a role in forming the blood–brain barrier, facilitating neuronal function, and responding to injury. Astrocytes form the blood–brain barrier by forcing endothelial cells to fit tightly together. Astrocytes support neuronal function through acting at synapses during neurotransmission, which we consider in Chapter 3.

oligodendrocytes Glia cell that produces a material around the axons of neurons called myelin.

astrocytes Glia cell that plays a role in the forming the blood-brain barrier, facilitating neuronal function and responding to injury.

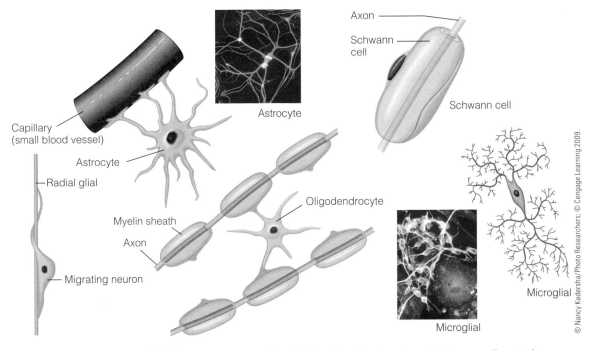

Glial cells support neuronal functioning. Oligodendrocytes and Schwann cells provide myelin sheathing for axons. Astrocytes form the blood–brain barrier, break down certain neurotransmitters, and respond to injury in the nervous system. Microglial cells remove cellular waste.

figure 2.4

gliosis Process involving the swelling of glia cells in response to injury.

Astrocytes respond to injury in the brain through a process called **gliosis**. Gliosis is also referred to as a *glial scar*. During gliosis, glial cells swell in response to injury. By surrounding damaged tissue, glial cells segregate damaged tissue from undamaged tissue. When this occurs, however, gliosis severely limits the ability of regenerated axons to reach healthy tissue and then how well an individual recovers from brain injury. The final type of glial cell, the microglial cell, removes normal cellular waste from neurons and glial cells. In addition to this role, microglial cells also contribute to gliosis (Matsumoto, Ohmori, & Fujiwara, 1992).

Stop & Check

1. What are the two types of cells found in the brain?
2. _____ receive information from other neurons, and _____ send information to other axons.
3. Sensory neurons are also called _____ neurons because axons go to the central nervous system.
4. Which types of glial cells provide myelin sheathing for axons?

1. Neurons and glial cells **2.** Dendrites, axons **3.** afferent **4.** Oligodendrocytes produce myelin sheathing around axons in the central nervous system, and Schwann cells produce myelin sheathing around axons outside of the central nervous system.

The Nervous System: Control of Behavior and Physiological Functions

Learning the basic terms used to describe where nervous system structures are located is an important first step for learning about structures of the brain. Standard terms describe the location of structures in the nervous system. For example, we refer to the front portion of the brain as *anterior* and the back portion of the brain as *posterior*. The bottom of the brain, the side that faces toward the stomach, is referred to as the *ventral* side, and the top of the brain is referred to as the *dorsal* side. We refer to structures near the sides of the brain as *lateral*; structures near the middle of the brain are described as *medial*. **Table 2.1** lists these and other terms that describe structures in the nervous system.

Looking at structures inside the brain may be accomplished through any of three basic types of dissection planes. Slicing the brain from anterior to posterior produces a *coronal*, or *frontal*, section. We produce horizontal sections by slicing the brain from dorsal to ventral and sagittal sections by slicing the brain side to side. Dissection planes provide different perspectives of a structure. For example, the thalamus appears as a circular structure on a sagittal plane at the midline, but it appears larger on coronal and horizontal sections as shown in **figure 2.5**.

table 2.1

Common Neuroscience Terms			
Term	**Definition**	**Term**	**Definition**
Dorsal	Toward the back, away from the ventral (stomach) side. The top of the brain is considered dorsal because it has that position in four-legged animals.	Medial	Toward the midline, away from the side
Ventral	Toward the stomach, away from the dorsal (back) side	Proximal	Located close (approximate) to the point of origin or attachment
		Distal	Located more distant from the point of origin or attachment
Anterior	Toward the front end	Ipsilateral	On the same side of the body (e.g., two parts on the left or two on the right)
Posterior	Toward the rear end	Contralateral	On the opposite side of the body (one on the left and one on the right)
Superior	Above another part	Coronal plane	A plane that shows brain structures as seen from the front (or frontal plane)
Inferior	Below another part	Sagittal plane	A plane that shows brain structures as seen from the side
Lateral	Toward the side, away from the midline	Horizontal plane	A plane that shows brain structures as seen from above (or transverse plane)

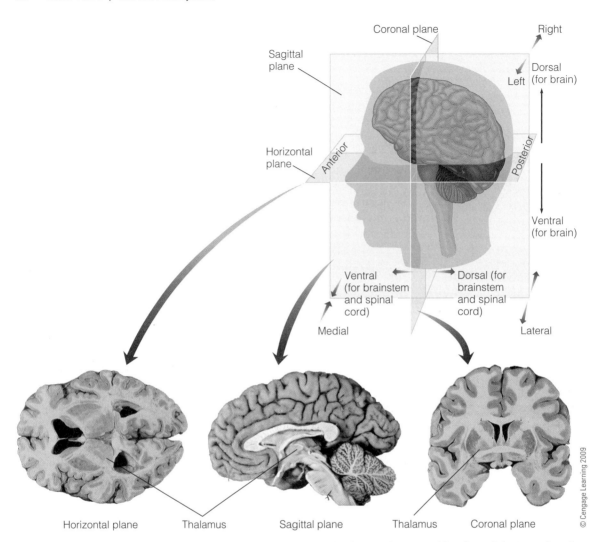

figure 2.5 **The Human Brain** The human brain can be dissected in coronal (i.e., frontal), horizontal, and sagittal sections.

The Peripheral Nervous System: Controlling and Responding to Physiological Processes in the Body

The nervous system consists of two systems: (1) the peripheral nervous system and (2) the central nervous system (CNS). Much of what we will discuss in this book pertains to the central nervous system, which consists of the brain and spinal cord. Drugs also have many effects on the peripheral nervous system, which contains two subsystems called the *somatic nervous system* and *autonomic nervous system*.

The Somatic Nervous System: Delivering Motor Signals to Muscles and Sensory Signals to the Spinal Cord

somatic nervous system
System responsible for delivering voluntary motor signals from the central nervous system to muscles throughout the body and for conveying sensory information from the body to the central nervous system.

The **somatic nervous system** is responsible for delivering voluntary motor signals from the CNS to muscles throughout the body and for conveying sensory information from the body to the CNS. Thus, the somatic nervous system is comprised of motor neurons and sensory neurons. Sensory neurons send information to the dorsal part of the spinal cord (referred to as the *dorsal horn* or *dorsal root*), whereas motor signals are sent to muscles from the ventral part of the spinal cord (referred to as the *ventral horn* or *ventral root*) (**figure 2.6**). The point where a motor neuron meets a muscle fiber is called the *neuromuscular junction*. Muscles contract when motor neurons release the neurotransmitter acetylcholine at neuromuscular junctions.

The Autonomic Nervous System: Controlling Vital Functions

autonomic nervous system System that controls involuntary movements for vital functions, such as heartbeat, breathing, and swallowing.

sympathetic nervous system System that prepares the body for rigorous activity by increasing heartbeat, inhibiting digestion, and opening airways, among many other involuntary functions.

parasympathetic nervous system
Subsystem of the autonomic system that is dominant during relaxed states, including decreases in heartbeat, stimulation of digestion, and the closing of airways.

Whereas the somatic nervous system produces voluntary movement, the **autonomic nervous system** controls involuntary movements for vital functions such as heartbeat, breathing, and swallowing. The autonomic nervous system consists of two systems: (1) the sympathetic nervous system and (2) the parasympathetic nervous system (**figure 2.7**). The **sympathetic nervous system** prepares the body for rigorous activity by increasing heartbeat, inhibiting digestion, and opening airways, among many other involuntary functions. The **parasympathetic nervous system** is dominant during relaxed states and decreases heartbeat, stimulates digestion, and closes airways.

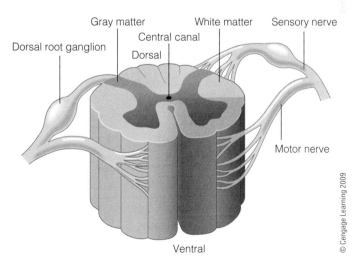

© Cengage Learning 2009

figure 2.6 Sensory neurons send information to the dorsal part of the spinal cord, whereas motor signals are sent to muscles from the ventral part of the spinal cord. Gray matter appears in the middle portion of the spinal cord forming an H shape. White matter appears in the outermost portions of the spinal cord.

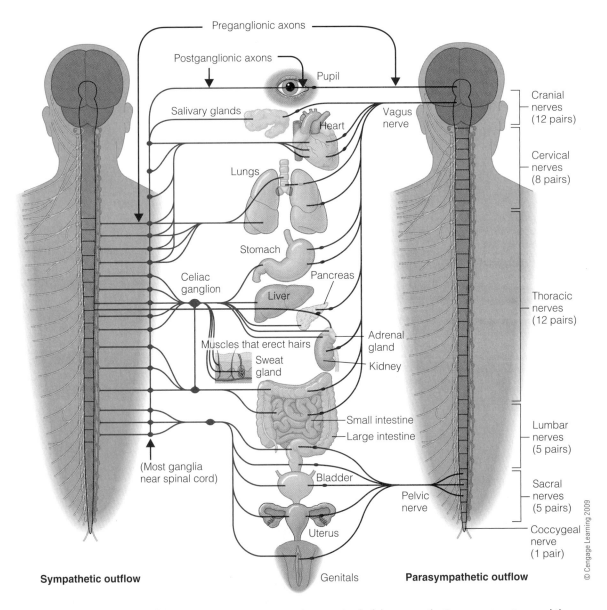

Preganglionic axons
Postganglionic axons
Pupil
Salivary glands
Heart
Vagus nerve
Lungs
Stomach
Pancreas
Celiac ganglion
Liver
Muscles that erect hairs
Adrenal gland
Sweat gland
Kidney
Small intestine
Large intestine
(Most ganglia near spinal cord)
Bladder
Pelvic nerve
Uterus
Genitals

Cranial nerves (12 pairs)
Cervical nerves (8 pairs)
Thoracic nerves (12 pairs)
Lumbar nerves (5 pairs)
Sacral nerves (5 pairs)
Coccygeal nerve (1 pair)

Sympathetic outflow   **Parasympathetic outflow**

© Cengage Learning 2009

figure **2.7**

The autonomic nervous system is comprised of the sympathetic nervous system and the parasympathetic nervous system. The sympathetic nervous system has activating effects on organs in the body because of the release of norepinephrine. The parasympathetic nervous system has deactivating effects on these same organs from the release of acetylcholine.

Stop & Check

1. Brain sections produced by slicing the brain from anterior to posterior are referred to as _____ sections.

2. The somatic nervous system delivers movement signals to muscles by releasing acetylcholine at _____ .

3. The _____ system controls vital functions such as breathing and heartbeat.

1. coronal 2. neuromuscular junctions 3. autonomic

The Central Nervous System: Controlling Behavior

cerebral cortex The surface of the brain; comprised of gyri and sulci.

The brain and spinal cord comprise the central nervous system. Look at the brain's surface in figure 2.8. The surface of the brain—the **cerebral cortex**—has hills called *gyri* (singular *gyrus*) and crevices called *sulci* (singular *sulcus*). The base of the brain, where the spinal cord meets, is called the *brain stem*. Above the brain stem sits a structure called the *cerebellum* that is itself brainlike in appearance.

The brain is divided into two hemispheres, left and right. Structures found in one hemisphere have a matching structure in the other hemisphere. Cross communication occurs between the hemispheres primary through the corpus callosum. To a lesser extent, cross communication occurs through other structures called *commissures*—for example, the anterior commissure.

The brain also contains three different divisions called the *hindbrain*, *midbrain*, and *forebrain* (**figure 2.8**). The hindbrain is the lower part of the

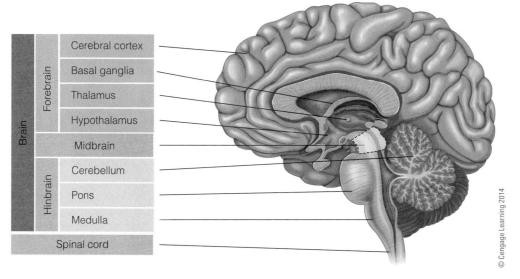

© Cengage Learning 2014

figure 2.8   The CNS is divided into three different divisions or regions of the brain called the *hindbrain*, *midbrain*, and *forebrain*.

brain stem, and it begins where the spinal cord meets the brain stem at a structure called the *medulla*. The midbrain comprises a region between the hindbrain and forebrain; it includes the *inferior colliculus*, which plays a role in auditory processing, and the *superior colliculus*, which directs eye movement. The forebrain includes the rest of the brain and contains the cerebral cortex and structures beneath the cerebral cortex such as the *corpus callosum*, *basal ganglia*, *thalamus*, and *hypothalamus*.

The Medulla and Hypothalamus: Controlling Unlearned Behaviors

medulla Structure that controls the autonomic nervous system and is situated where the spinal cord meets the hindbrain.

We previously discussed the autonomic system, which maintains vital functions in the body. The autonomic nervous system is controlled by the medulla (**figure 2.9**). As already described, the **medulla** rests where the spinal cord meets the hindbrain. In fact, from the surface, the medulla looks like a thicker section

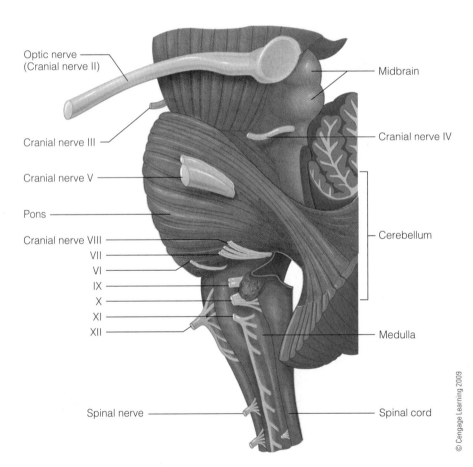

© Cengage Learning 2009

figure 2.9   Many structures in the brain stem, particularly the medulla, play a critical role in autonomic functions.

table **2.2**

Cranial Nerves

Cranial Nerve	Function
I. Olfactory	Smell
II. Optic	Vision
III. Oculomotor	Control of eye movements; pupil constriction
IV. Trochlear	Control of eye movements
V. Trigeminal	Skin sensations from most of the face; control of jaw muscles for chewing and swallowing
VI. Abducens	Control of eye movements
VII. Facial	Taste from the anterior two-thirds of the tongue; control of facial expressions, crying, salivation, and dilation of the head's blood vessels
VIII. Statoacoustic	Hearing; equilibrium
IX. Glossopharyngeal	Taste and other sensations from throat and posterior third of the tongue; control of swallowing, salivation, throat movements during speech
X. Vagus	Sensations from neck and thorax; control of throat, esophagus, and larynx; parasympathetic nerves to stomach, intestines, and other organs
XI. Accessory	Control of neck and shoulder movements
XII. Hypoglossal	Control of muscles of the tongue

of spinal cord. Through controlling the autonomic nervous system, the medulla controls basic autonomic functions such as breathing, heart rate, and vomiting.

Many of the cranial nerves also come from the medulla. These nerves are devoted to movement and sensations of the head (**table 2.2**). There are 12 cranial nerves, each noted by its name and a number. The vagus nerve (roman numeral X) differs from the functions of the other cranial nerves because it controls and receives sensory information from various internal organs in the body, including the heart, liver, and intestines.

Clearly, damaging the medulla can be life threatening, and suppressing its functioning can be just as dangerous. Narcotics and central nervous system depressants suppress medullary functions, which can be fatal at high enough doses. Moreover, mixing two or more CNS depressants at otherwise safe amounts can produce combined suppressant effects on medullary functions.

hypothalamus Structure found in the forebrain that maintains important physiological conditions.

The **hypothalamus**, a structure found in the forebrain, maintains important physiological conditions (**figure 2.10**). The hypothalamus maintains many physiological processes through motivating an organism's behavior. When the body requires food, for example, the hypothalamus elicits feelings of hunger. Similarly, the hypothalamus elicits thirst when we become dehydrated. The hypothalamus also facilitates a motivation for sexual activity, which maintains the survival of a species. Other processes the hypothalamus regulates include body temperature and sleep.

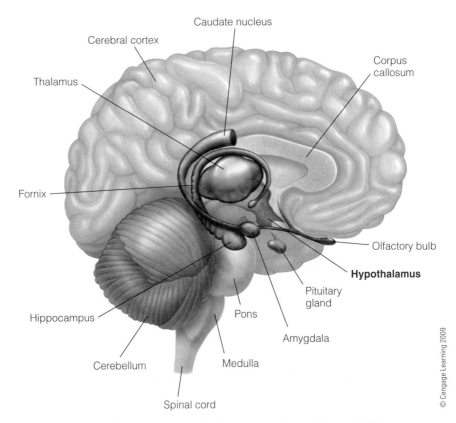

Caudate nucleus

Cerebral cortex

Corpus callosum

Thalamus

Fornix

Olfactory bulb

Hypothalamus

Pituitary gland

Hippocampus

Pons

Amygdala

Cerebellum

Medulla

Spinal cord

© Cengage Learning 2009

figure **2.10**   The hypothalamus plays an important role for homeostasis, partly through eliciting motivation for various physiological activities such as eating and drinking.

The hypothalamus also controls the *pituitary gland*, which sits on the ventral surface of the brain. The pituitary gland releases several hormones into the bloodstream, affecting organ functions in the body. These effects include water absorption into the kidneys, growth, thyroid function, and reproductive functions. The hypothalamus also controls the *pineal gland*, another forebrain structure that is responsible for the release of *melatonin*, a sleep-regulating hormone.

Stop & Check

1. The central nervous system contains the brain and _____ .
2. What are the lobes of the cerebral cortex?
3. What is the primary structure in the brain for controlling autonomic functions?
4. How does the hypothalamus alter hormone levels in the body?

1. spinal cord **2.** The lobes consist of the frontal, temporal, parietal, and occipital lobes. **3.** The medulla **4.** The hypothalamus controls the pituitary gland, which releases many hormones throughout the body.

The Limbic System: Controlling Emotional Behaviors

limbic system Series of structures that together appear to form a ring around the thalamus and hypothalamus.

The **limbic system** is a series of structures that together appear to form a ring around the thalamus and hypothalamus. These other structures include the *cingulate gyrus*, *hippocampus*, *amygdala*, *nucleus accumbens*, and *olfactory bulb* (**figure 2.11**). Many structures within the limbic system control emotional

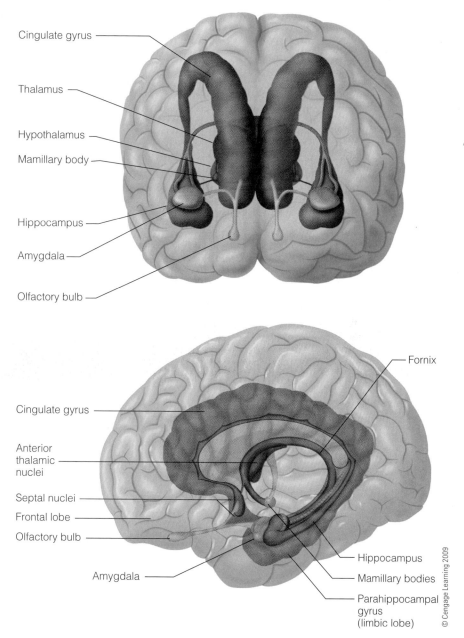

figure 2.11   The limbic system generally is important for emotion, although the hippocampus also plays an important role in long-term memory.

behaviors. The amygdala, for example, facilitates fear and aggression. Many drugs that reduce anxiety reduce the activity of neurons in the amygdala.

The **nucleus accumbens** facilitates reinforcing effects. For this reason, we refer to the nucleus accumbens as the brain's *reward center*. The nucleus accumbens belongs to a network of other structures referred to as the *reward circuit*. Chapter 5 presents more information on the brain's reward circuitry and the role this circuitry plays in the reinforcing effects of abused substances.

The Cerebral Cortex: Processing Sensory Information, Controlling Cognitive Functions, and Eliciting Movement

Four lobes divide the cerebral cortex (**figure 2.12**). The **occipital lobe** is the most posterior portion of the cerebral cortex and processes visual information. The **temporal lobe** is anterior to the occipital lobe and below the parietal lobe. The temporal lobe processes auditory information and supports language comprehension and production. This area of the cerebral cortex also processes certain aspects of vision, including shape and color analysis. The **parietal lobe** includes the *primary somatosensory cortex*, the structure responsible for processing touch information from the body. The parietal lobe also analyzes visual information that contains movement.

nucleus accumbens Limbic system structure that facilitates reinforcing effects.

occipital lobe Region of the cerebral cortex important for processing visual information.

temporal lobe Region of the cerebral cortex important for processing auditory information and supporting language comprehension and production.

parietal lobe Region of the cerebral cortex important for processing touch information.

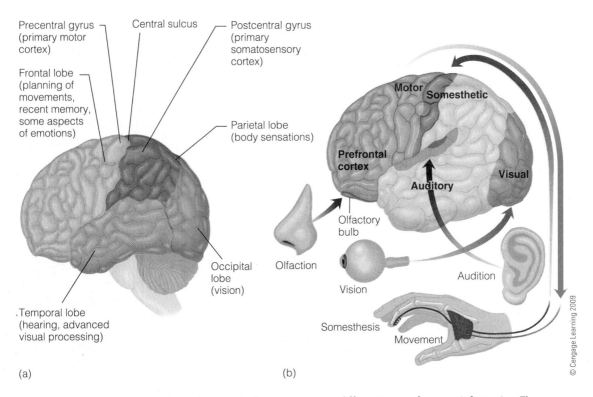

(a)

(b)

© Cengage Learning 2009

figure 2.12 Each lobe of the cerebral cortex processes different types of sensory information. The prefrontal cortex, within the frontal lobe, is an integration center for all types of sensory information.

frontal lobe Region of the cerebral cortex important for decision making and movement.

prefrontal cortex Most anterior part of the frontal cortex; an integration area for all types of sensory input; is involved in initiated movements.

thalamus Forebrain structure that routes sensory information from the body to the appropriate lobes.

The **frontal lobe**, which is at the anterior of the brain, supports decision making and movement. The frontal lobe contains the primary motor cortex. The most anterior part of the frontal lobe is called the **prefrontal cortex** and is an integration area for all types of sensory input and where the signal to produce movement occurs. Prefrontal cortical function also supports short-term memory and attention.

The **thalamus** routes sensory information from the body to the appropriate lobes. For example, visual information is sent from the eyes through the thalamus and to the occipital lobe, whereas auditory information is sent from the ears through the thalamus and to the temporal lobe. After processing, all sensory information integrates in the prefrontal cortex.

Stop & Check

1. What are the primary functions of the amygdala and nucleus accumbens?
2. Which lobe analyzes sound, including language?
3. What role does the thalamus play in processing sensory information?

1. The amygdala elicits feelings of fear, anxiety, and aggression, whereas the nucleus accumbens elicits reinforcing effects. **2.** Temporal lobe **3.** The thalamus routes sensory information to the appropriate lobes of the cerebral cortex.

The Frontal Lobe and Basal Ganglia: Controlling Voluntary Movement

primary motor cortex Part of the frontal lobe that sends movement signals to the body through the pyramidal system.

After the prefrontal cortex signals a movement to occur, the **primary motor cortex** sends movement signals to the body through the *pyramidal system*, which comprises the lateral corticospinal tract and the medial corticospinal tract. The lateral corticospinal tract crosses from one hemisphere of the brain to the opposite side of the body. This tract sends motor information to the limbs, hands, and feet. The medial corticospinal tract sends information from each hemisphere mostly to the same side of the body. This tract functions mainly for middle parts of the body, providing for posture and balance (**figure 2.13**).

basal ganglia Aids in the stabilization of movement.

substantia nigra Aids in regulating activity in the basal ganglia.

Other structures—including the basal ganglia, thalamus, and substantia nigra—act to stabilize voluntary movements (**figure 2.14**). The **basal ganglia**, also called the *striatum*, has three major structures: the *caudate nucleus*, the *putamen*, and the *globus pallidus*. The **substantia nigra** aids in regulating activity in the basal ganglia. The primary symptoms of Parkinson's disease, a disorder characterized by muscle rigidity, tremor, and resistance to voluntary movement, occurs from the destruction of substantia nigra neurons that go to the basal ganglia. Many of the first drugs to treat schizophrenia, called *antipsychotic drugs*, disrupt these neurons, leading to Parkinson-like symptoms called *extrapyramidal side effects*.

Some other components of the overall motor system must be noted. The *pons*, a structure located just above the medulla in the hindbrain, elicits startle reflexes. The *cerebellum* facilitates balance and the timing of movements.

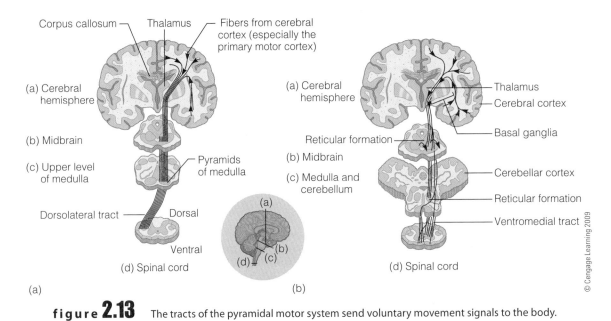

f i g u r e 2.13   The tracts of the pyramidal motor system send voluntary movement signals to the body.

Learning and Memory Processes in the Brain

Psychologists characterize short- and long-term memories in different ways. Most consider short-term memory as working memory. **Working memory** consists of short-term verbal or nonverbal memories employed when carrying out a task. In essence, we are "working" with memory. **Long-term memory**, which is also referred to as *reference memory*, consists of stored verbal and nonverbal information. Long-term memories include information that we can declare such as the capital of the United States or information we can demonstrate such as how to swing a golf club.

The prefrontal cortex facilitates working memory function. Recall that information from all sensory modalities integrates in the prefrontal cortex. The prefrontal cortex uses this information to control behavior when engaging in a task.

Long-term memory formation and retrieval requires the *hippocampus*. The hippocampus then sends information to the prefrontal cortex, possibly for use during working memory function. Damage to the hippocampus in Alzheimer's disease may account for impairments in long-term memory. Long-term motor memories, also referred to as *procedural memories*, may depend on the basal ganglia. Motor memories include skills such as riding a bike.

Other parts of the brain indirectly aid memory formation by keeping the brain active. Many of these parts are found in the **reticular activating system**, which includes the *reticular formation*, *tegmentum*, thalamus, and hypothalamus. The activity within these structures ultimately support arousal in the cerebral cortex. Another structure important for cortical arousal is the basal forebrain area. Drugs that increase cortical arousal include psychostimulant

working memory Consists of short-term verbal or nonverbal memories employed to carry out a task.

long-term memory (or reference memory) Consists of stored verbal and nonverbal information.

reticular activating system System of structures that support arousal in the cerebral cortex.

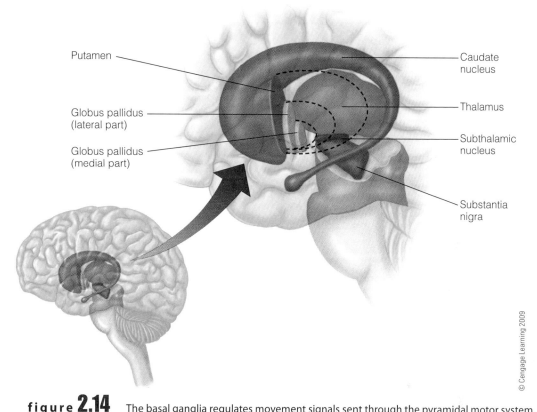

figure 2.14   The basal ganglia regulates movement signals sent through the pyramidal motor system.

drugs, whereas drugs that depress cortical arousal include benzodiazepines, barbiturates, and alcohol.

Nutrient levels also alter our ability to learn and remember. Neurons, like other cells, require a constant supply of glucose and oxygen, particularly when engaging in highly demanding tasks. Poor diet or low oxygen supply impairs our ability to concentrate, learn, and remember.

Stop & Check

1. Which part of the cerebral cortex sends movements signals to the body?

2. What parts of the brain are damaged in Parkinson's disease?

3. Which structures are linked to working memory and long-term memory, respectively?

1. The primary motor cortex. **2.** Parkinson's disease arises from damage to neurons that begin in the substantia nigra and end in the basal ganglia **3.** The prefrontal cortex is particularly important for working memory, whereas the hippocampus is important for long-term memory.

Blood Flow in the Brain

cerebral blood flow
Blood flow throughout
the brain.

Proper blood flow throughout the brain, called **cerebral blood flow**, is critical for neuron and glial cell function. Highly active brain areas require increased blood flow. When you are working hard on a task such as an exam, your prefrontal cortex is very active. Blood flow increases to the prefrontal cortex to sustain this activity.

Blood flow changes throughout the brain when blood capillaries dilate and contract. Highly active cells release a chemical called *nitric oxide* that dilates blood capillaries, which in turn delivers more oxygen. Oxygen uptake in the brain can be imaged using *functional magnetic resonance imaging* (fMRI). Brain areas with high amounts of oxygen uptake imply high levels of brain activity (**figure 2.15**).

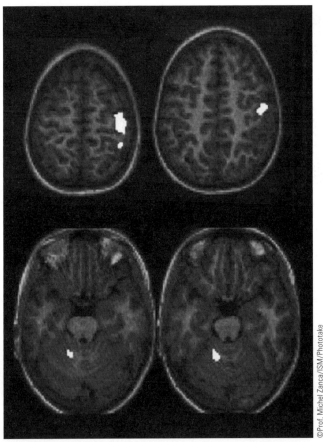

©Prof. Michel Zanca/ISM/Phototake

figure **2.15**   Magnetic resonance imaging (MRI) provides detailed images of the brain, and functional MRI (fMRI) superimposes neuronal activity information over these images.

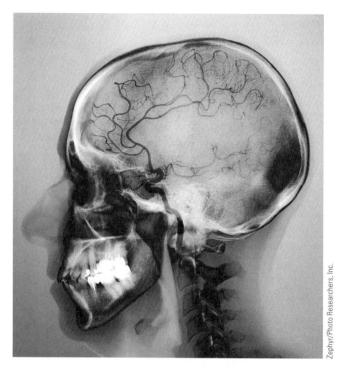

Zephyr/Photo Researchers, Inc.

figure 2.16   An angiogram provides an image of blood vessels.

Abnormal blood flow in the brain may lead to medical problems. *Ischemia* is a term used to describe too little cerebral blood flow, potentially causing cell death if severe or persistent enough. Stroke, which occurs from the blockage of brain vessels, is a serious type of ischemia. *Hyperemia* means there is too much cerebral blood flow, which may increase intracranial pressure and damage brain tissue. Physicians diagnose many abnormal blood flow concerns by conducting *angiograms*, which provide pictures of parts of the circulatory system by taking X-ray images of blood vessels that contain an X-ray absorbing agent (**figure 2.16**).

The brain is supplied with blood through two major arteries: the carotid artery and the vertebral artery (**figure 2.17**). The carotid artery runs up the front of the neck and is the one we commonly press down on to measure our heart rate. The vertebral artery runs through the back of the neck. The vertebral artery flows into a collection of arteries in the brain stem called the Circle of Willis.

Cerebrospinal Fluid

cerebrospinal fluid
Clear fluid that surrounds cells in the brain.

Cerebrospinal fluid is a clear fluid that surrounds cells in the brain. Cerebrospinal fluid provides a medium through which nutrients, a sugar called *glucose*, hormones, and other chemicals access brain cells (**figure 2.18**).

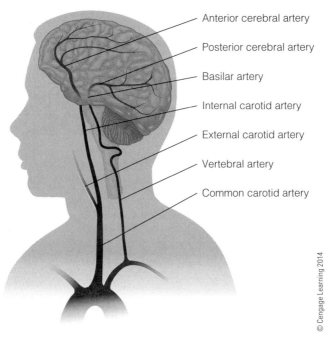

© Cengage Learning 2014

figure 2.17 Blood is supplied to the brain through the internal carotid artery and the vertebral artery.

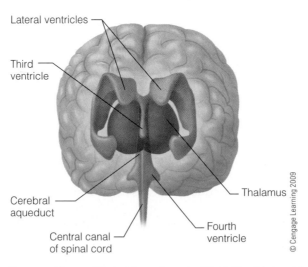

© Cengage Learning 2009

The ventricles are filled with cerebrospinal fluid. The third and fourth ventricles are connected by the cerebral aqueduct. Within the spinal cord, the central canal is filled with cerebral spinal **figure 2.18** fluid.

In addition to surrounding cells in the brain, cerebrospinal fluid fills many spaces and canals in the brain. The central canal of the spinal cord is filled with cerebrospinal fluid, and there is a smaller canal-like structure in the brain called the *cerebral aqueduct*. The cerebral aqueduct is surrounded by a small layer of tissue called **periaqueductal gray**.

periaqueductal gray Small layer of tissue that surrounds the cerebral aqueduct.

The brain also contains cerebrospinal fluid–filled cavities called **ventricles**. The fourth ventricle is found adjacent to the cerebellum in the brain stem. The third ventricle surrounds much of the thalamus. The lateral ventricles are found lateral to the third ventricle and have a large cavity at the midline.

ventricles Cerebrospinal fluid-filled cavities in the brain.

Cerebrospinal fluid is also found in the *meninges* that surround the brain. Cerebrospinal fluid forms in a layer of the meninges called the *subarachnoid space*. By filling this space, cerebrospinal fluid forms a protective cushion around the brain, protecting it from injury.

The Blood–Brain Barrier

blood–brain barrier Barrier that surrounds the blood capillaries and vessels in the brain and prevents blood from assessing brain cells.

Blood is prevented from accessing brain cells by the **blood–brain barrier** that surrounds the blood capillaries and vessels in the brain. As described previously, tight endothelial cell junctions form the blood–brain barrier. This barrier prevents pathogens, hormones, and other substances from entering the brain. Nutrients and other important molecules pass through this barrier through either passive diffusion or active transport.

Molecules must possess three properties to passively diffuse through the blood–brain barrier (**figure 2.19**). First, the chemical should be lipid soluble, meaning that it can pass through cell membranes. Second, the chemical should be uncharged, which is an important reason why many neurochemicals cannot pass from the bloodstream into the brain. Instead, neurochemicals must be made within cells in the brain. Third, the chemical should be relatively small.

However, many nutrients lack the necessary properties for passive diffusion and must instead use active-transport mechanisms. Active-transport mechanisms consist of channels that penetrate endothelial cell membranes. For example, the sugar glucose passes through a channel in the blood–brain barrier in order to access cells within the brain.

Stop & Check

1. Reduced blood flow to a part of the body is referred to as _____.
2. The meninges protect the brain from injury because they contain a clear fluid called _____ .
3. Given the protective properties of the blood–brain barrier, many important sugars and nutrients must enter the brain using _____ mechanisms such as channels.

1. ischemia **2.** cerebrospinal fluid **3.** active-transport

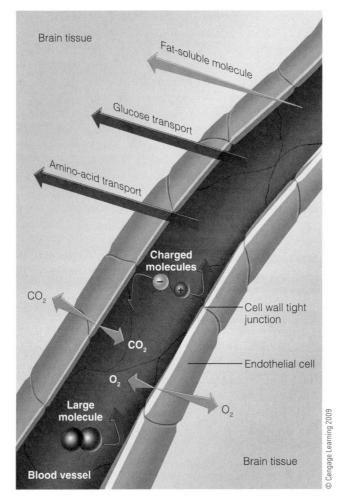

The blood–brain barrier prevents blood from accessing brain cells directly. The barrier surrounds the blood capillaries and vessels that wind throughout the brain. The various nutrients and other molecules needed for cells must pass through this barrier through either passive diffusion or active transport.

figure **2.19**

The Nervous System: Rapid Development After Fertilization

teratogenic effects
Harmful and potentially lethal effects for a fetus.

Rapid and complex neural growth occurs over the course of a 9-month pregnancy. Many drugs have harmful and potentially lethal effects for a fetus. These drug effects are known as **teratogenic effects**. For example, heavy alcohol consumption during pregnancy may lead to fetal alcohol syndrome. Chapter 1 presented another known teratogen called *thalidomide*. Thalidomide's teratogenic effects led to thousands of birth defects during the 1950s.

Another teratogen is isotretinoin, better known by the trade name Accutane. Isotretinoin is effective for treating acne but is also a well-known teratogen associated with high abortion risk and birth defects (Stern, Rosa, & Baum, 1984). Given this, women taking Accutane must agree to use birth control, have pregnancy tests, and, in the United States, be registered with iPLEDGE, which has entrance criteria and monthly monitoring programs.

A full-term human pregnancy is 9 months, or 40 weeks, and the stages of pregnancy are characterized in trimesters. The first trimester begins at conception and ends after 12 weeks. The second trimester begins at week 13 and continues through week 27, and the third trimester begins at week 28 and continues until birth. The nervous system rapidly develops throughout the entire 40 weeks of pregnancy, but the primary features of the central nervous system are produced during the first trimester (**figure 2.20**).

The fertilized egg, or *zygote*, becomes an *embryo* once it implants within the wall of the uterus. The embryo quickly develops multiple layers of cells and within about 4 weeks exhibits the basic divisions of the central nervous system, including a forebrain, midbrain, and hindbrain region as well as a spinal cord and central canal. However, a discernible brain, with prominent forebrain, develops between 8 and 10 weeks. After 10 weeks, the term *fetus*

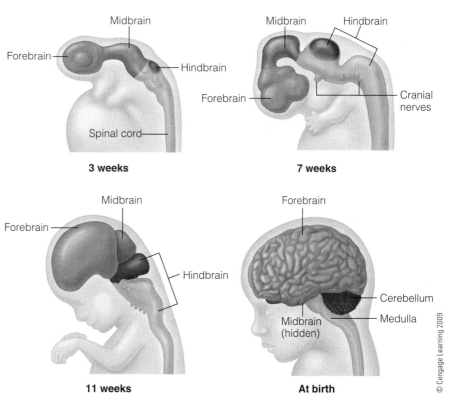

© Cengage Learning 2009

figure 2.20   The central nervous system grows rapidly during pregnancy.

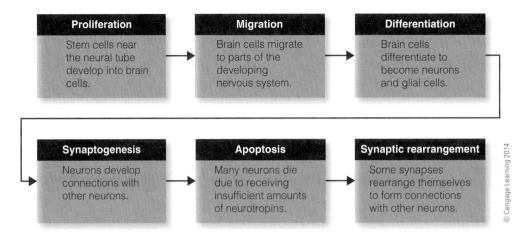

The nervous system begins with stem cells and continues through the migration of cells, their differentiation into neurons and glial cells, and then finally functioning as communication networks between neurons.

figure **2.21**

proliferation
Neurodevelopment phase involving generation of brain cells.

migration
Neurodevelopment phase involving the moving of newly generated cells to parts of the nervous system.

synaptogenesis
Development of connections with other neurons through forming axons and dendrites.

neurotrophins Chemicals that promote the survival of neurons.

apoptosis Cell death during neurodevelopment that occurs because of insufficient levels of neurotrophins.

synaptic rearrangement
The rearrangement of synaptic connections during neurodevelopment.

is used, rather than *embryo*. The gyri and sulci of the cerebral cortex become most apparent between 24 and 30 weeks into a pregnancy.

Brain-cell development underlies the central nervous system changes taking place during pregnancy. Very early in development, stem cells near the neural tube, which eventually becomes the ventricles and central canal of the CNS, develop into brain cells. We call this phase **proliferation**. During the next phase, **migration**, these brain cells migrate to parts of the developing central nervous system (**figure 2.21**). The differentiation phase begins once these brain cells reach the appropriate part of the central nervous system. During this phase, the brain cells differentiate to become either neurons or glial cells. Afterward, neurons develop connections with other neurons through forming axons and dendrites, a phase referred to as **synaptogenesis**. Neurons release **neurotrophins**, which are chemicals that promote the survival of neurons. Neurotrophins include neural growth factor, *brain-derived neurotrophic factor* (abbreviated as BDNF), neurotrophin-3, and neurotrophin-4. Many neurons also die during this stage of development because they do not receive sufficient amounts of neurotrophins. The process is referred to as **apoptosis**. Further, synapses may rearrange themselves to form other connections with neurons, a process referred to as **synaptic rearrangement**.

Stop & Check

1. The drugs alcohol, thalidomide, and isotretinoin all share a risk for _____ effects.

2. How many weeks into prenatal development does the forebrain become prominent?

1. teratogenic 2. After 8 to 10 weeks

Genes and the Development and Physiological Processes of Cells

The blueprints for a cell and its functions reside within the nucleus. The nucleus of every cell for humans contains 46 chromosomes. A child inherits 23 chromosomes from each parent. Two of the 46 chromosomes consist of X and Y chromosomes, which determine an individual's sex. If both of these sex chromosomes are X's, then an individual is genetically female. However, if one of these sex chromosomes is a Y, then the individual is genetically male. All of the other chromosomes are called *autosomal chromosomes*.

Each chromosome contains a strand of *deoxyribonucleic acid* (DNA), which contains the specific coding instructions for the basic functions of cells called genes. Genes are encoded with the traits we have (**figure 2.22**). Within this role, genes contain information to build and maintain cells. Researchers can alter genetic information in animals to study the nervous system (**Box 2.1**).

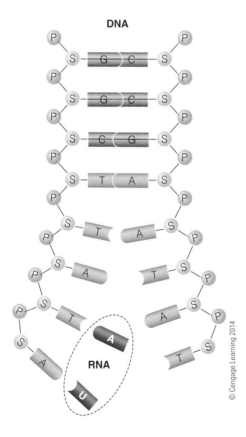

In gene activation, a specific DNA segment is unraveled and transcribed onto ribonucleic acid (RNA), which may then leave the nucleus and carry the transcribed information to ribosomes that synthesize proteins as instructed.

figure **2.22**

box **2.1 Genetically Modified Organisms**

Genetic technologies allow researchers to characterize the role between genes and behavior. These advances led to the creation of genetically modified invertebrate and vertebrate organisms. For vertebrates, most genetic modification research uses mice.

The genetic-modification process starts by injecting genetic material into a pregnant mouse. After the mouse has a litter, researchers test the *genotype*, or genetic makeup, of each mouse pup to identify those with the targeted genetic change. Genetically modified mice fall largely into two categories: transgenic animals and *knock-out* animals. A **transgenic mouse** has either altered genes or additional genetic information. For example, researchers alter amyloid precursor protein genes in transgenic mice to cause production of amyloid plaques, a key neurobiological characteristic found in Alzheimer's disease. A **knock-out mouse** fails to express traits from a particular gene; in essence, the gene is "knocked out."

Scientists use a notation system to describe different genotypes for knock-out animals. A heterozygous genotype is noted by a "−/+," with the "−" sign indicating the removed or deactivated gene on one chromosome and the + indicating the unaffected gene on the other chromosome. A "+/+" notation, indicating unaffected genes on both chromosomes, describes a nongenetically modified animal, also referred to as a *wildtype*. Animals with a homozygous genotype for a certain trait are noted with a "−/−," indicating a deactivated gene on each chromosome. For example, serotonin transporter −/− knock-out mice exhibit greater levels of serotonin in the synaptic cleft and show anxious behavior (Holmes, Li, Murphy, Gold, & Crawley, 2003). The −/− describes

the deactivation of the serotonin transporter gene on both chromosomes. Thus, these mice completely lack serotonin transporters. A **phenotype** describes the physiological or behavioral changes caused by a genetic alteration. In this example, enhanced serotonin levels and increased anxiety describe the phenotype for a serotonin transporter knock-out mouse.

Although transgenic and knock-out data provide important links between genetics and physiological and behavioral activity, scientists keep in mind that genetic alterations may cause unexpected changes during neurodevelopment. In fact, a study by Zhou, Lesch, and Murphy (2002) demonstrated a unique and unexpected consequence of knocking out the serotonin transporter.

In this study, researchers compared serotonin levels in serotonin transporter knock-out mice and confirmed that greater serotonin levels occurred at serotonin synapses, as described previously. However, these researchers also discovered serotonin neurotransmitters inside of dopamine neurons. Exploring further, the team found that dopamine transporters had adapted to allow entry of serotonin into dopamine neurons (Zhou et al., 2002). Thus, instead of having mice with an altered serotonin system, they unintentionally produced mice that also had an altered dopamine system (figure 1).

For these caveats and other reasons, researchers seek to refine and develop new approaches for developing genetically modified organisms. In a variation of the knock-out mouse, researchers have developed **conditional knock-out mice** that have normally functioning genes until a researcher administers a type of enzyme that deactivates a gene. Thus, these mice

polymorphism
Differences in the gene that encodes for a trait within a species.

Although genes contain codes to express certain traits such as eye color or production of a particular enzyme, the coding sequence for genes may not be precisely the same from individual to individual. We term these differences *polymorphisms*. A **polymorphism** is a difference in the gene that encodes for a trait such as a protein. Polymorphisms are common, and determining what type of polymorphism an individual has can aid greatly in understanding a person's response to drug effects.

For example, some individuals have polymorphisms that cause them to produce more of a certain type of liver enzyme. For these individuals, the

develop normally but still allow researchers to assess the effects of gene deactivation on some physiological or behavior characteristic. During a study, researchers might wait until mice reach an adult age before administering the enzyme. This technology also allows researchers to specify a particular part of the body to alter the gene, such as a structure within the central nervous system. These and other genetic modification procedures have important implications for understanding the nervous system and for characterizing drug actions and their effects.

transgenic mouse Mouse with either altered genes or additional genetic information.

knock-out mouse Mouse that fails to express a particular gene.

phenotype Physiological or behavioral changes caused by a genetic alteration.

conditional knock-out mice Mice that have normally functioning genes until a researcher administers a type of enzyme that deactivates a gene.

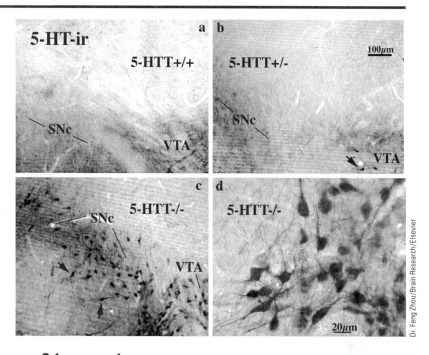

Dr. Feng Zhou/Brain Research/Elsevier

box 2.1, figure 1

Few neurons reveal the neurotransmitter serotonin in the dopamine-rich ventral tegmental area and substantia nigra in wild-type mice (top panel, a). However, in serotonin transporter knock-out mice (bottom panel, c & d), many dopamine neurons contain serotonin. These findings suggest that removal of serotonin transporters led to the nervous system adapting to the loss of serotonin by using dopamine neurons for synthesizing serotonin. VTA = ventral tegmental area; 5-HT = serotonin; 5-HTT, = serotonin transporter; ir = immunoreactive; the labeling technique used to identify serotonin; SNc = substantia nigra. From Zhou et al., 2002.

extra enzymes may reduce a particular drug's effects. If this is the case, then a physician may opt to prescribe a drug unaffected by these enzymes.

Activating genes leads to the release of genetic information, a process referred to as *gene transcription*. A **transcription factor** consists of a substance that increases or decreases gene transcription. During gene transcription, the coding sequence of a gene copies onto ribonucleic acid (RNA). The type of RNA used to trigger protein synthesis is called *messenger RNA* because it leaves the nucleus and binds to ribosomes in the cell. Ribosomes produce the type of protein specified in the message.

transcription factor Substance that increases or decreases gene transcription.

Stop & Check	**1.** How many chromosomes does a human cell contain?
	2. A _____ is a protein that activates a gene.
	3. Genetic code is copied onto _____, which delivers the code to ribosomes outside the nucleus.

1. 46 **2.** transcription factor. **3.** messenger RNA

FROM ACTIONS TO EFFECTS
Glial Scars and Recovery from Brain Injury

Traumatic brain injury occurs from a severe blow to the head. Mild traumatic brain injury includes a range of potential symptoms including cognitive and mood changes. Moderate and severe traumatic brain injuries also include seizures, vomiting, and sustained headache. Approximately 1.7 million Americans experience a traumatic brain injury each year (CDC, 2010).

Treatments for traumatic brain injury seldom provide full recovery. The first approach consists of limiting further injury. These efforts may include surgeries to reduce brain swelling or medications to sustain blood flow throughout the brain. Although these approaches may limit further brain injury, they do not restore lost brain function.

An important challenge in brain injury recovery consists of a natural response to injury called a *glial scar* or *gliosis* (Silver & Miller, 2004). A glial scar consists of reactive astrocytes—that is, astrocytes that swell in response to injury. The resulting glial scar from traumatic brain injury segregates damaged tissue from healthy tissue. The action serves to repair the blood–brain barrier. In doing so, however, glial scars prevent neurons in damaged tissue from regaining connections to other structures in the nervous system.

Regaining connectivity after injury involves the sprouting of severed axons. **Figure 2.23** provides an image of regenerating axons near an area of damaged tissue surrounded by a glial scar. Because of the barrier created, the glial scars caused regenerating axon terminals to divert from the damaged tissue. These conditions result in misaligned patterns of growth, including retractions into balls called *dystrophic end bulbs*.

Astrocytes in glial scars prevent axon growth through an inhibitory extracellular matrix. The **inhibitory extracellular matrix** consists of chemicals that inhibit axon growth, including proteoglycans, secreted protein semaphorin 3, and ephrin-B2. Each molecule prevents the growth or penetration of axons into damaged tissue (Silver & Miller, 2004).

inhibitory extracellular matrix Part of gliosis consisting of chemicals that inhibit axon growth.

Experimental treatments for traumatic brain injury recovery focus on ways to improve axon regeneration into damaged brain areas. One approach uses the enzyme chondroitinase to break down proteoglycans. Related approaches seek to reduce other inhibitory components in the inhibitory extracellular matrix.

Other treatments focus on improving the availability of growth material for axons. These strategies often involve neural growth factors, such as neurotropin-3 and brain-derived neural growth factor. The delivery of neural growth factors promotes the growth of axons into damaged tissue.

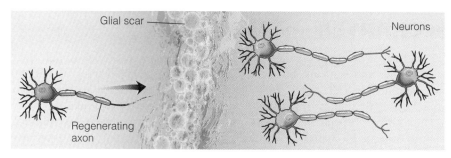

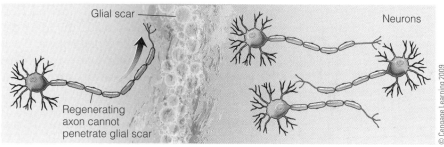

figure **2.23**

Regenerating axons from dorsal root ganglion (arrow) can grow next to a damaged area (shown in the left side of the image), but cannot penetrate damaged tissue surrounded by gliosis (right side of the image).

Finally, researchers have combined both of the preceding strategies to reduce inhibitory extracellular matrix components while promoting the growth of axons. For example, Tropea and colleagues (2003) assessed the effects of each approach on damaged retinal neurons that terminate in the superior colliculus. The application of either chondroitinase or BDNF promoted the regrowth of these neurons into the superior colliculus. Yet far greater neuronal growth was demonstrated by using both chrondroitinase and BDNF.

|||||||||||||||||||||||||||||||||||||||||||||||||||||||||||||||||||||||||||||||||||||||||||||||||||||||||||||||||||||||||||||||||||||||||||||||||||||||||

Stop & Check

1. What functions does a glial scar serve?
2. How does an inhibitory extracellular matrix impair recovery from brain trauma?
3. How might a neural growth factor such as BDNF aid in neural recovery?

1. Glial scars form from swelled astrocytes in response to injury. Glial scars repair blood–brain barrier damage and separate damaged tissue from healthy tissue. **2.** The inhibitory extracellular matrix contains molecules that inhibit the growth of regenerating axons through the glial scar. **3.** Neural growth factors promote the growth of axons into damaged brain areas.

▶ CHAPTER SUMMARY

The cells in the central nervous system consist of glial cells and neurons. Most neurons consist of dendrites, a soma, an axon, and an axon terminal. Signals from other neurons are received through dendrites, and the message is sent to other neurons from the axon terminal. Glial cells play an important role in supporting the function of neurons. Oligodendrocyte and Schwann glial cells form myelin sheathing around the axons of neurons, and astrocytes play an important role in supporting neuronal communication and responding to injury. Microglial cells remove cellular waste from all central nervous system cells.

We divide the brain into subdivisions called the *hindbrain*, *midbrain*, and *forebrain*. The forebrain division is the largest and encompasses the four cortical lobes in the brain called the *occipital lobe* (for vision), the *parietal lobe* (mainly for processing touch information), the *temporal lobe* (for audition and language), and the *frontal lobe* (for cognition and movement). The limbic system includes the nucleus accumbens, amygdala, hippocampus, cingulate gyrus, thalamus, and hypothalamus. Together these limbic system structures play an important role in emotion. Sensory information is received from the head and body and routed through the thalamus to the appropriate lobe for processing. The prefrontal cortex is the most anterior portion of the frontal lobe and the integration center for all sensory information. Motor signals are sent down to the body beginning in the primary motor cortex and through the lateral corticospinal tract and the medial corticospinal tract. This system of voluntary movement is called the *pyramidal motor system*. The extrapyramidal motor system regulates voluntary movements and includes the basal ganglia, thalamus, substantia nigra, and other structures.

The cells in the brain receive important sugars and nutrients from the cerebrospinal fluid surrounding these cells and oxygen from blood vessels. Cerebrospinal fluid exists throughout the central nervous system through the central canal in the spinal cord and through a network of ventricles and the cerebral aqueduct in the brain. Cerebral blood flow increases in active parts of the brain. The brain's blood supply comes from the carotid and the vertebral arteries.

During the first 10 weeks of embryonic development, the brain and spinal cord form from the outer layers of the embryo. Within this developing tissue, there is the rapid production and migration of brain cells. Neurons develop axons and dendrites and form complex neural networks, whereas glial cells develop to support the function of these neurons.

The basic functions and development of cells are directed by genes, which are small portions of DNA strands. Molecules that activate genes are called *transcription factors*. Gene activation causes a copy of the gene to be imprinted on RNA. RNA directs the production of protein synthesis through ribosomes found outside of the cell's nucleus.

KEY TERMS

Neurons	Sensory neurons	Autonomic nervous system	Cerebral cortex
Glia cells (or glial cells)	Motor neurons	Sympathetic nervous system	Medulla
Dendrites	Oligodendrocytes		Hypothalamus
Axons	Astrocytes	Parasympathetic nervous system	Limbic system
Synapse	Gliosis		Nucleus accumbens
Interneuron	Somatic nervous system		Occipital lobe

Temporal lobe

Parietal lobe

Frontal lobe

Prefrontal cortex

Thalamus

Primary motor cortex

Basal ganglia

Substantia nigra

Working memory

Long-term memory (or reference memory)

Reticular activating system

Cerebral blood flow

Cerebrospinal fluid

Periaqueductal gray

Ventricles

Blood–brain barrier

Teratogenic effects

Proliferation

Migration

Synaptogenesis

Neurotrophins

Apoptosis

Synaptic rearrangement

Polymorphism

Transcription factor

Inhibitory extracellular matrix

Transgenic mouse

Knock-out mouse

Phenotype

Conditional knock-out mice

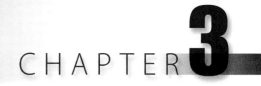

CHAPTER **3**

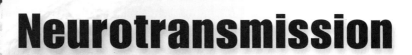

Neurotransmission

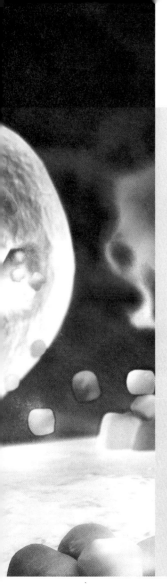

Drugs for Alzheimer's Disease Alter Acetylcholine Neurotransmission

Jessica's memory loss at age 46 was completely unexpected. In fact, she had an impeccable memory until this point. Yet even the simplest memories caused Jessica to struggle. When filling up her car, she forgot if she was going to work or coming from work. Also, she forgot her phone number and the names of co-workers. Finally, after getting lost in a grocery store, she contacted her doctor.

Jessica's physician diagnosed her with early stage Alzheimer's disease (AD), a neurobiological illness characterized by a progressive decline in cognitive functioning. To slow her cognitive decline, her physician prescribed an acetylcholinesterase inhibitor, a drug that enhances levels of a neurotransmitter called *acetylcholine* in the brain. Although not a cure, the medication restored cognitive functioning for almost a year before her symptoms became untreatable.

Many treatments for neurological disorders address neurotransmission abnormalities in the nervous system. Unfortunately, many of these disorders provide daunting challenges for scientists, and there remains a great need for new treatments in neurology.

Story adapted from anonymous personal accounts at **www.alz.org**.

neurotransmission
Transmission of information between neurons.

Neurotransmission is the transmission of information between neurons. Neurotransmission typically involves a neuron releasing chemicals called *neurotransmitters* into a synapse, which allows these neurotransmitters to act on sites on another neuron. The study of neurotransmission includes looking at events inside the neuron that cause the production and release of neurotransmitters as well as the actions neurotransmitters have on sites situated on other neurons.

Electrical Events Within a Neuron and the Release of Neurotransmitters

electrical transmission Series of electrical events that begin at an axon hillock and proceed down the length of an axon.

electrical potential Difference between the electrical charge within a neuron versus the electrical charge of the environment immediately outside the neuron.

depolarization Reduced difference between the positive and negative charges on each side of a membrane.

hyperpolarization Increased difference between the positive and negative charges on each side of a membrane.

local potential Electrical potential on a specific part of a neuron.

ion channels Pores in a neuronal membrane that allow the passage of ions.

excitatory postsynaptic potential (EPSP) Stimulus that depolarizes a local potential.

inhibitory postsynaptic potential (IPSP) Stimulus that hyperpolarizes a local potential.

Certain electrical events within a neuron must take place before neurotransmitters can be released. These events are referred to as **electrical transmission**, which is a series of events that begin at an axon hillock and proceed down the length of an axon. These events depend on electrical potentials.

For a neuron, an **electrical potential** is a difference between the electrical charge within a neuron and the electrical charge of the environment immediately outside the neuron. Normally, the electrical charge within a neuron is negative compared to the outside environment. This characteristic leaves the neuron's membrane polarized, meaning that on one side the charge is negative, but on the other side the charge is positive, similar to the negative and positive poles of a magnet (**figure 3.1**). The term **depolarization** describes a reduced difference between the positive and negative charges on each side of a membrane. The term **hyperpolarization** describes an increased difference between the positive and negative charges on each side of a membrane.

REVIEW! A neuron has many dendrites and a single axon. A synapse consists of an axon terminal, the synaptic cleft, and the postsynaptic terminal. Chapter 2 (pg. 31).

The term **local potential** refers to an electrical potential on a specific part of a neuron. The local potential changes in response to events within a neuron and with communication from other neurons. Local potentials change as charged particles called *ions* move in and out of the neuron through pores called **ion channels**. The influence on local potentials from other neurons occurs as either an excitatory postsynaptic potential or an inhibitory postsynaptic potential. An **excitatory postsynaptic potential** (**EPSP**) depolarizes a local potential, whereas an **inhibitory postsynaptic potential** (**IPSP**) hyperpolarizes

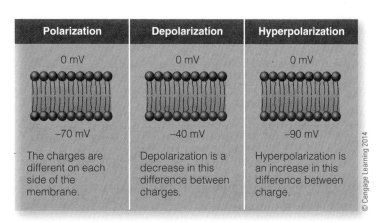

Polarization	Depolarization	Hyperpolarization
0 mV	0 mV	0 mV
−70 mV	−40 mV	−90 mV
The charges are different on each side of the membrane.	Depolarization is a decrease in this difference between charges.	Hyperpolarization is an increase in this difference between charge.

© Cengage Learning 2014

figure **3.1** An electrical polarization is a difference between two electrical charges. Depolarization is a decrease in this difference, whereas hyperpolarization is an increase in this difference.

box **3.1** Electrophysiology and Microdialysis

A research technique called *electrophysiology* uses electrodes to measure potentials on neuronal membranes. Electrophysiology procedures use either macroelectrodes or microelectrodes. **Macroelectrodes** record the activity of thousands of neurons within a structure. They also can be used as a stimulator to activate thousands of neurons within a structure. **Microelectrodes** provide a precise assessment of either just a few or even single neurons. The use of a microelectrode to measure potentials within a single neuron is called **intracellular recording**. In particular, researchers use intracellular recording to measure action potentials. This technique allows a neuron's firing rate to be calculated. Although electrophysiological techniques can assess the activity of neurons, they cannot determine the amount of neurotransmitter released from a neuron.

Microdialysis procedures, however, can be used to sample neurotransmitter levels. Microdialysis probes have a semipermeable membrane. When implanted into a structure of the brain, a probe's membrane allows some of the surrounding cerebrospinal fluid to pass through. Researchers then analyze the collected cerebrospinal

box **3.1**, figure **1**

Each line on this graph represents the number of action potentials detected over a 10-second period (i.e., spikes/10 sec). The arrows indicate the precise moment when β-PEA (β-phenylethylamine) (followed on the graph by the amount given) was administered. After every administration of β-PEA, a decrease in the firing rate (i.e., the rate of spikes) was shown. Subsequent administrations of β-PEA were given after the firing rate recovered. As greater amounts of β-PEA were administered, greater decreases in the firing rate were observed. (Figure 1 from Kota Ishida, Mikio Murata, Nobuyuki Katagiri, Masago Ishikawa, Kenji Abe, Masatoshi Kato, Iku Utsunomiya, and Kyoji Taguchi, Effects of β-Phenylethylamine on Dopaminergic Neurons of the Ventral Tegmental Area in the Rat: A Combined Electrophysiological and Microdialysis Study, J Pharmacol Exp Ther August 2005 314:916-922.)

a local potential (**figure 3.2**). Researchers study local potential changes using electrophysiological procedures as described in **Box 3.1**.

Nerve Impulses: Electrical Potential Changes in Neurons

An important way in which neurons release neurotransmitters from the axon terminal is through electrochemical signals called *nerve impulses*. Nerve impulses are comprised of changes from resting potentials to action potentials.

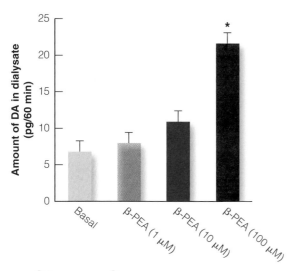

box **3.1**, figure **2**

Each bar on this graph represents the amount of dopamine sampled from microdialysis probes in the ventral tegmental area during a 60-minute period. The amount of dopamine collected was much higher after administration of a 100-micromole amount of β-phenylethylamine compared to the baseline condition and before β-phenylethylamine was administered. (Figure from Kota Ishida, Mikio Murata, Nobuyuki Katagiri, Masago Ishikawa, Kenji Abe, Masatoshi Kato, Iku Utsunomiya, and Kyoji Taguchi, Effects of β-Phenylethylamine on Dopaminergic Neurons of the Ventral Tegmental Area in the Rat: A Combined Electrophysiological and Microdialysis Study, J Pharmacol Exp Ther August 2005 314:916-922.)

macroelectrodes Electrode used in electrophysiology that records the activity of thousands of neurons within a structure.

intracellular recording Use of a microelectrode to measure potentials within a single neuron.

fluid for levels of certain chemicals such as neurotransmitters. Microdialysis probe size limits neurotransmitter detection to an entire structure rather than a specific neuron. Thus, increases in neurotransmission must be large enough to cause neurotransmitters to cause significant overflow from synapses.

Microdialysis procedures lack the precision that electrophysiology can achieve, yet microdialysis can answer important questions about neurotransmitter release that electrophysiology cannot. Both procedures complement each other. The effective use of both procedures together is shown in a study by Ishida and colleagues (2005).

In this study, the effects of β-phenylethylamine (β-PEA) (which is synthesized from phenylalamine) on dopamine neuron firing rates and dopamine release was assessed in rats. The application of β-PEA onto dopamine neurons in the ventral tegmental area caused a decrease in firing rates as determined through electrophysiology (figure 1). Although a decrease in neuronal firing should be expected to decrease dopamine release from these neurons, microdialysis techniques instead revealed increased dopamine release (figure 2). Based on these findings and other information known about β-PEA, the authors concluded that increases in dopamine release were caused by β-phenylethylamine acting at dopamine D_2 autoreceptors.

microelectrodes Electrode used in electrophysiology that records the activity of only a few neurons or a single neuron.

microdialysis Procedure used to sample neurochemicals within a brain structure.

Resting Potential

A resting potential describes a negatively charged local potential that precedes an action potential. The exact negative charge of the resting potential can vary between species, nervous system structures, and the relative concentration of ions within and outside a neuron (**figure 3.3**). For example, in squid axons, which are typically used to describe action potentials, the resting potential is approximately –70 millivolts.* The resting potential exists because of negatively charged proteins within the neuron and closed ions channels that prevent the

*Millivolts are a measure of the differences in electron concentrations between two areas.

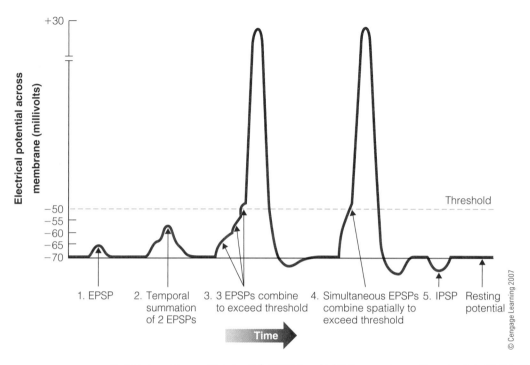

figure 3.2 Excitatory postsynaptic potentials (EPSPs) and inhibitory postsynaptic potentials (IPSPs) alter the charge within a neuron.

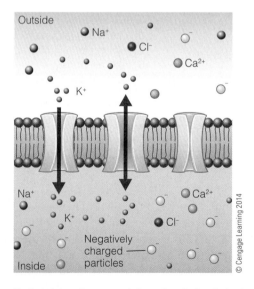

figure 3.3 During the resting potential, an electrical polarization is maintained because of a concentration of negatively charged ions and negatively charged proteins. Potassium (K⁺) ions can enter and leave the neuron through open K⁺ channels.

influx of positively charged sodium (Na^+) ions (figure 3.3). Channels *are* open for the positively charged ion potassium (K^+), however, but the influx of K^+ alone is insufficient to affect the resting potential charge.

Positively charged K^+ ions enter the neuron because they are attracted to the negative charge within the neuron, a property called **electrostatic attraction**. Yet at some point, K^+ ions cease entering the neuron because ions of the same type resist being concentrated, a property called a **concentration gradient**. Thus, as K^+ becomes more concentrated within the neuron, some K^+ ions follow a concentration gradient and exit the neuron. The balance between the electrostatic attraction and concentration–gradient repulsion facilitates a resting potential.

Although Na^+ channels are not open during the resting potential, a number of Na^+ ions still find their way in. To prevent these excess Na^+ ions from changing the resting potential, neuronal membranes contain sodium–potassium pumps. A **sodium–potassium pump** is a neuronal membrane mechanism that brings two K^+ ions into the neuron while removing three Na^+ ions out of the neuron (**figure 3.4**). By removing more Na^+ ions than the K^+ ions brought in, this pumping activity results in a net negative effect.

A resting potential changes when Na^+ channels open. Na^+ channels are **voltage-gated ion channels**, meaning that the opening or closing of these channels depends on local potential changes. Na^+ channels open in response to depolarization. When an excitatory postsynaptic potential occurs,

electrostatic attraction Attraction of ions with opposite charges.

concentration gradient Particles of the same type resist being concentrated.

sodium–potassium pump Neuronal membrane mechanism that brings two K+ ions into the neuron while removing three Na+ ions out of the neuron.

voltage-gated ion channels Channels that open or close, depending on local potential changes.

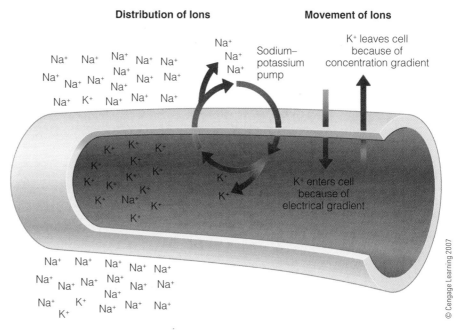

figure **3.4** Sodium–potassium pumps help maintain a resting potential by removing three Na^+ ions for every two K^+ ions brought in.

© Cengage Learning 2007

temporal summation
Short succession of excitatory postsynaptic potentials from the same source.

spatial summation
Excitatory postsynaptic potentials occurring from multiple sources.

depolarization causes local Na⁺ channels to open, allowing Na⁺ ions to enter the neuron. If no other EPSPs occur, then depolarization quickly ends and a resting potential resumes.

Combined excitatory postsynaptic potentials produce greater depolarization in one of two ways. First, several EPSPs may be produced in short succession from the same source, a process called **temporal summation**. Second, several EPSPs may occur simultaneously from multiple sources, a process called **spatial summation**. If a series of EPSPs causes depolarization to reach a certain threshold value, then an action potential will occur (figure 3.2).

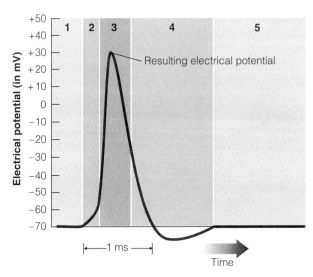

❶ During the resting potential stage, the membrane is only pemeable to K+ through having open K+ channels.

❷ As depolarization occurs, the membrane becomes permeable to Na+ ions through opening Na channels.

❸ An action potential occurs if polarization meets a specific threshold. During the action potential stage all Na+ channels open, causing rapid Na+ influx. Then Na+ channels reclose.

❹ During the refractory period the K+ ions rapidly exit the neuron, returning a negative charge within the neuron. During the refractory period, the neuron resists producing another action potential.

❺ After the refractory period, the neuron returns to a resting potential.

© Cengage Learning 2014

figure 3.5 Electrical impulses within neurons occur in several stages, and each stage depends on the opening or closing of voltage-gated ion channels.

Action Potential

action potential Rapid depolarization, causing the potential in the neuron to become temporarily more positive than the outside environment.

An **action potential** is a rapid depolarization that causes the potential in the neuron to become temporarily more positive than the outside environment (**figure 3.5**). The action potential occurs when all Na^+ ion channels open. These Na^+ channels remain open for only 1 to 3 milliseconds, and this limits the change in potential to a certain value. As the example shows in figure 3.5 the action reaches +30 mV. These properties support the **all-or-none law**, which states that the magnitude of an action potential is independent from the magnitude of potential change that elicited the action potential. The action potential ends immediately after the Na^+ channels close.

all-or-none law Magnitude of an action potential is independent from the magnitude of potential change that elicited the action potential.

Refractory Periods

refractory period Period following an action potential when the neuron resists producing another action potential.

The refractory period begins after the action potential ends (figure 3.5). During the **refractory period**, the neuron resists producing another action potential. The refractory period is divided into two phases.

The first phase is the **absolute refractory period**, which lasts approximately 1–2 milliseconds after the action potential ends. During this period, K^+ channels are opened, and the concentration of positively charged ions causes K^+ ions to rapidly exit the neuron. The rapid exit of K^+ ions causes the potential to become negative again. In fact, the negative charge is initially more negative than the resting potential charge. Because the Na^+ channels remain closed during the absolute refractory period, no amount of depolarization can produce another action potential.

absolute refractory period First phase of the refractory period, during which no amount of depolarization can produce another action potential.

Stop & Check

1. Depolarization is a decrease in potential, whereas hyperpolarization is a(n) _____ in potential.
2. To prevent leaked Na^+ from altering a resting potential, a(n) _____ expels Na^+ from the neuron.
3. When membrane depolarization meets a specific threshold value, all Na^+ channels open, resulting in a massive depolarization called a(n) _____.
4. After the action potential, K^+ channels open, causing K^+ to rapidly _____ the neuron.

1. increase **2.** sodium–potassium pump **3.** action potential **4.** exit

relative refractory period Second phase of the refractory period, during which greater depolarization is necessary to reach threshold and produce another action potential.

The second phase is called the **relative refractory period** and lasts 2–4 milliseconds. During this period, Na^+ channels can be opened, and the local potential remains hyperpolarized. Because of hyperpolarization, greater depolarization is necessary to reach the threshold and produce another action potential. Unless excitatory postsynaptic potentials occur during the relative refractory period, the membrane returns to a resting potential.

Propagation of Action Potentials Down Axons

propagation of action potentials Series of action potentials occurring in succession down an axon.

The **propagation of action potentials** refers to a series of action potentials occurring in succession down an axon. The propagation of action potentials begins at the axon hillock. Once this begins, each depolarization produced by an action potential causes another action potential to occur further down the axon (**figure 3.6**). This series of action potentials continues until an action potential occurs at the axon terminal. Action potentials propagate in only one direction because the preceding portion of an axon is in a refractory period.

nodes of Ranvier Uncovered sections of axons between myelin sheaths.

Myelin sheathing increases the speed of conductance down the axon. Sections of myelin sheaths surround most vertebrate axons. The uncovered sections of axons between myelin sheaths are called **nodes of Ranvier** (pronounced RAHN-vee-ay). Each node contains Na⁺ and K⁺ channels. When

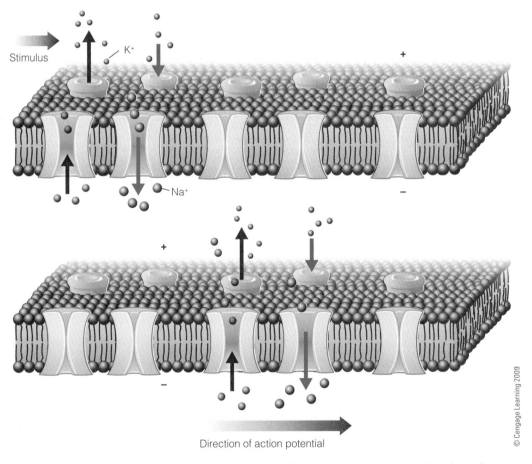

Stimulus

K^+

Na^+

Direction of action potential

© Cengage Learning 2009

figure 3.6 Action potentials only propagate down the axon because the previous Na⁺ channels remain in a refractory period.

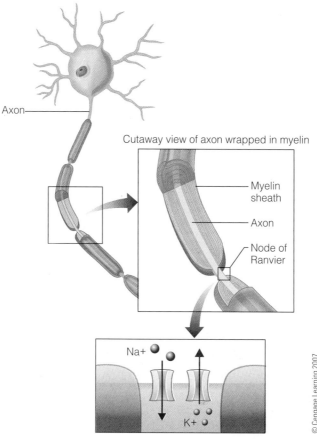

Cutaway view of axon wrapped in myelin

Axon

Myelin sheath

Axon

Node of Ranvier

Na+

K+

© Cengage Learning 2007

figure 3.7   On myelinated axons, action potentials occur at each node of Ranvier.

firing rate Number
of action potentials
occurring per unit of time,
usually in milliseconds.

an action potential occurs at one node, depolarization is carried through the myelin sheathing to the next node, where another action potential occurs (**figure 3.7**). The jumping of action potentials from one node to another is referred to as *saltatory conduction*. The number of action potentials occurring per unit of time, usually milliseconds, is called a **firing rate**.

Stop & Check

1. Sodium and potassium channels are located down the length of an axon, facilitating the propagation of _____ potentials.
2. Axons with _____ sheathing have a greater speed of conductance compared to axons without myelin sheathing.
3. The number of action potentials occurring during a certain period of time is called a(n) _____.

1. action **2.** myelin **3.** firing rate

Neurotransmitters: Signaling Molecules for Neuronal Communication

neurotransmitters
Signaling chemicals that are synthesized within neurons, are released from neurons, and have effects on neurons or other cells.

Action potentials at an axon terminal trigger a series of events that ultimately cause the release of neurotransmitters. **Neurotransmitters** are signaling chemicals that are synthesized within neurons, are released from neurons, and have effects on neurons or other cells. Neurotransmission between neurons involves a series of stages, beginning with the synthesis of neurotransmitters and ending with the release of neurotransmitters (**figure 3.8**).

Neurotransmitter Synthesis

Neurotransmitters are synthesized from other molecules with the aid of enzymes. Neurotransmitters may be synthesized anywhere within the neuron.

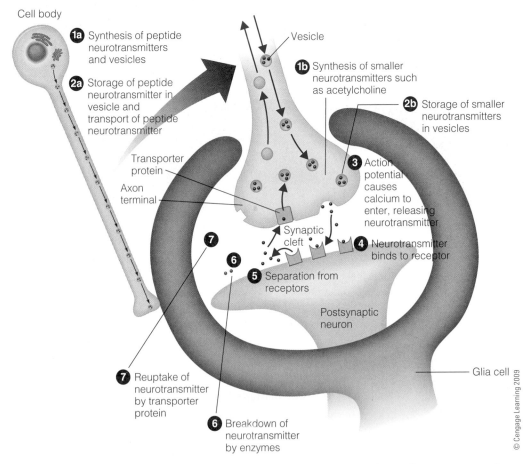

Cell body

1a Synthesis of peptide neurotransmitters and vesicles

2a Storage of peptide neurotransmitter in vesicle and transport of peptide neurotransmitter

Vesicle

1b Synthesis of smaller neurotransmitters such as acetylcholine

2b Storage of smaller neurotransmitters in vesicles

3 Action potential causes calcium to enter, releasing neurotransmitter

Transporter protein

Axon terminal

Synaptic cleft

4 Neurotransmitter binds to receptor

5 Separation from receptors

Postsynaptic neuron

Glia cell

7 Reuptake of neurotransmitter by transporter protein

6 Breakdown of neurotransmitter by enzymes

© Cengage Learning 2009

Chemical neurotransmission occurs in many steps, including neurotransmitter synthesis, release, receptor binding, and termination. Please see the text for a description of each stage of this process.

figure 3.8

Generally, smaller neurotransmitter molecules such as acetylcholine and dopamine are synthesized in the axon terminal. Larger neurotransmitter molecules such as neuropeptide neurotransmitters are synthesized in the soma.

Neurotransmitter Storage

vesicular transporter
Channel located on a vesicle that allows passage of neurotransmitters.

After synthesis, neurotransmitters are stored in protective vesicles. Neurotransmitters enter vesicles through a **vesicular transporter** (figure 3.8). Synaptic vesicles protect neurotransmitters from being destroyed by enzymes, and synaptic vesicles prevent neurotransmitters from being released prematurely. Synaptic vesicles also allow neurotransmitters to be pooled in the axon terminal, allowing for immediate neurotransmitter release during neurotransmission.

However, not every neurotransmitter is stored after synthesis. For example, the endocannabinoid neurotransmitter anandamide is not stored in vesicles (Placzek, Okamoto, Ueda, & Barker, 2008). Without a storage mechanism, anandamide escapes from the neuron immediately after synthesis.

Calcium Influx and Neurotransmitter Release

exocytosis Fusing of synaptic vesicles to the axon membrane and release of stored neurotransmitters into the synaptic cleft.

Once an action potential occurs in the axon terminal, voltage-gated calcium $(Ca)^{2+}$ channels open and allow Ca^{2+} to enter the axon terminal. Calcium causes **exocytosis**, the fusing of synaptic vesicles to the axon membrane and release of stored neurotransmitters into the synaptic cleft (figure 3.8). After fusing with the membrane, the vesicles are brought back into the terminal and then refilled with neurotransmitters. However, vesicle recycling does not occur for neuropeptide neurotransmitters, which must be stored in vesicles produced in the soma.

Neurotransmitters Bind to Receptors

volume neurotransmission
Type of neurotransmission involving the binding of neurotransmitters to receptors outside of the synapse.

Neurotransmitters released into the synaptic cleft bind to receptor proteins (described shortly) which may be located on the postsynaptic terminal, axon terminal, or both (figure 3.8). Neurotransmitters may also bind to receptors outside of the synapse, a process called **volume neurotransmission**. Volume neurotransmission occurs from the overflow of neurotransmitters from a synaptic cleft, which generally results from high neuronal activity.

Termination of Neurotransmission

catabolism Process involving the enzymatic breakdown of neurotransmitters and other molecules.

After a neurotransmitter releases from a receptor, one of a number of processes occur to prevent the neurotransmitter from binding to other receptors in the synapse (figure 3.8). These processes serve to end neurotransmission. For one of these processes, enzymes break down a neurotransmitter into different molecules, a function referred to as **catabolism**. Because these new molecules do not match to a neurotransmitter's receptor, neurotransmission effectively stops.

During another process called *reuptake*, transporter channels on axon terminals return neurotransmitters to the axon terminal. Vesicles then store the neurotransmitters for later release. In essence, reuptake serves as a recycling program for neurons. Finally, neurotransmitters may be transported from the synaptic cleft into an astrocyte glial cell. Afterward, enzymes within the glial cell catabolize the neurotransmitters.

Stop & Check

1. After synthesis, a neurotransmitter may be stored in a(n) _____ until released from the neuron.

2. Neurotransmitters are released from a neuron on the influx of _____.

3. Neurotransmitters bind to and activate _____.

4. Neurotransmission can be terminated through enzymatic breakdown, transportation into a glial cell, or through _____ of neurotransmitters.

1. vesicle 2. calcium 3. receptors 4. reuptake

Neurotransmission: Neurotransmitter Binding to Receptors

receptors Proteins located in neuron membranes that can be bound to and activated by neurotransmitters.

Receptors are proteins located in neuron membranes that can be bound to and activated by neurotransmitters. Receptors match to a specific neurotransmitter. Thus, the neurotransmitter dopamine cannot bind to receptors for the neurotransmitter acetylcholine, and vice versa. Researchers not only characterize receptors by the neurotransmitter they match to but also by their location within a synapse and basic molecular structure. The terms *presynaptic* and *postsynaptic* describe the locations for receptors in a synapse. Receptors that are located on the postsynaptic terminal are called *postsynaptic receptors*, and receptors located on the axon terminal are called *presynaptic receptors*.

autoreceptor Presynaptic receptor that is activated by neurotransmitters released from the same axon terminal.

Presynaptic receptors have two types. The first type is an **autoreceptor**, a presynaptic receptor that is activated by neurotransmitters released from the same axon terminal (**figure 3.9**). Activating an autoreceptor usually inhibits neurotransmitter release. This action serves to limit the amount of neurotransmitter released. A receptor for the neurotransmitter dopamine functions as an autoreceptor. When released from an axon terminal, dopamine binds to this autoreceptor, reducing the amount of dopamine released.

heteroceptor Presynaptic receptor that is activated by neurotransmitters different from those released from the axon terminal.

The second type of presynaptic receptor is a **heteroceptor**, a presynaptic receptor that is activated by neurotransmitters different from those released from the axon terminal (figure 3.9). Heteroceptors may increase or decrease neurotransmitter release. For example, a heteroceptor for the neurotransmitter norepinephrine is located on axon terminals for the neurotransmitter serotonin. Binding to this receptor reduces serotonin release.

Receptors: Ionotropic or Metabotropic

In addition to synaptic location, receptors also are identified by their structure. We distinguish between two primary types of neurotransmitter receptors: ionotropic receptors and metabotropic receptors. **Table 3.1** summarizes the differences between these two types of receptors.

ionotropic receptors Ion channels that open when a matching neurotransmitter binds to a site on the channel.

Ionotropic receptors are ion channels that open when a matching neurotransmitter binds to a site on the channel (**figure 3.10**). An ionotropic receptor is comprised of subunits that span the neuronal membrane. The subunits

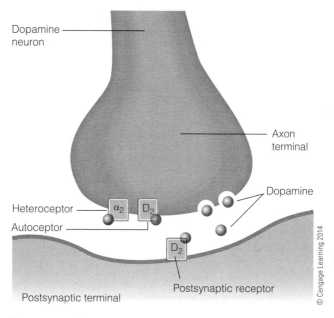

Receptors on the presynaptic terminal influence the amount of neurotransmitter released. Autoreceptors are activated by the neurotransmitter released from the terminal, whereas a heteroceptor is activated by a different neurotransmitter. On the dopamine neuron shown here, the D$_2$ autoreceptor is activated by dopamine, whereas the α_2 heteroceptor is activated by norepinephrine.

figure 3.9

table **3.1**

Differences Between Ionotropic and Metabotropic Receptors		
	Ionotropic receptor	**Metabotropic receptor**
Physical proximity to parts of neuron where effects exerted	Attached to ion channel	Separated from ion channels and other proteins
Type of effect	Open ion channel	Uses G protein to activate ion channels and effector enzymes
Duration of effect	Ends when neurotransmitter leaves binding site	Effector enzymes engage a cascade of events that persist after neurotransmitter leaves receptor
Impact on a neuron	Influx of ions changes local potential	Can affect local potentials; also has other effects, including enzyme regulation, gene expression, and protein synthesis

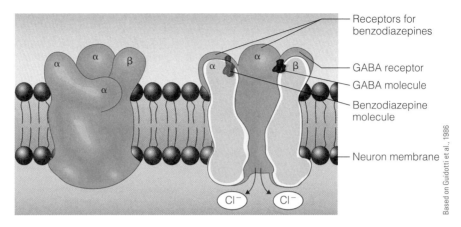

An ionotropic receptor consists of an ion channel with a neurotransmitter binding site. The receptor shown here is activated by the neurotransmitter γ-aminobutyric acid (GABA) and is called the GABA$_A$ receptor. GABA$_A$ receptor activation causes an IPSP by allowing negatively charged chloride (Cl$^-$) ions into the neuron. The GABA$_A$ receptor shown here also has binding sites for different chemical substances, such as benzodiazepines. These other binding sites serve to modify the receptor's function, including how well GABA activates the receptor.

figure 3.10

metabotropic receptor Receptors physically separated from parts of the neurons where the receptors exerts its effects.

form a ring that comprises the channel. The shifting of these subunits causes the channel to open or close. A **metabotropic receptor** is physically separated from parts of the neurons where the receptor exerts its effects (**figure 3.11**). Unlike an ionotropic receptor, which contains an ion channel, a metabotropic receptor relies on a G protein to convey effects to channels or other parts of the neuron.

A G protein resides within a neuron in close proximity to the receptor. G proteins have three subunits: alpha (α), beta (β), and gamma (γ). These subunits remain attached to each other until a neurotransmitter activates the receptor. Activating the receptor causes a separation of the G protein into two sections, one consisting of the α subunit and the other consisting of the $\beta\gamma$ subunit. After a period of time, the subunits return to a three-subunit state. Box 4.1 in Chapter 4 describes a research technique used to characterize the activation and inactivation process for G proteins.

After an activated receptor causes G protein subunits to separate, the separated subunits may cause a variety of effects within a neuron (figure 3.11). First, the free subunits can activate ion channels such as K$^+$ or Ca^{2+} ion channels. Second, the free subunits can activate **effector enzymes**. Common effector enzymes include adenylyl cyclase, phospholipase C, phospholipase A2, and phosphodiesterase. Usually, an effector enzyme activates a *second messenger*. Common second messengers include cyclic adenosine monophosphate (cAMP), cyclic guanosine monophosphate (cGMP), phosphoinositide, and calcium. A second messenger, in turn, activates a protein kinase.

A **protein kinase** is an enzyme that causes phosphorylation of a substrate protein. Phosphorylation is a common process for activating proteins, which

effector enzymes Enzyme that usually activates a second messenger.

protein kinase Enzyme that causes phosphorylation of a substrate protein.

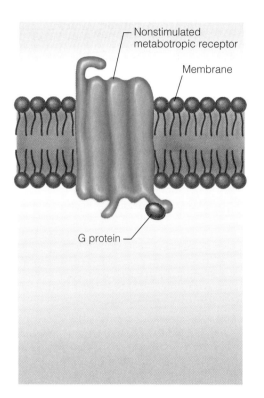
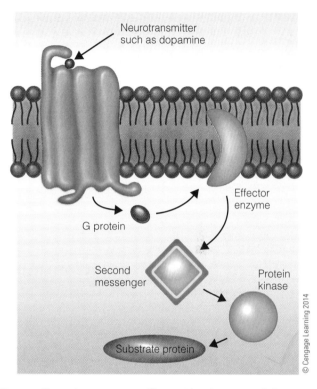

A metabotropic receptor relies on a G protein to carry out effects within the neuron (left). Through the activation of a G protein, a cascade of biological events may occur within the neuron, including the activation or inhibition of ion channels, second messengers, protein kinases, and substrate proteins (right).

figure 3.11

© Cengage Learning 2014

involves adding at least one phosphate group ($-PO_4^{2-}$) to a protein. Common protein kinases include protein kinase A, protein kinase G, protein kinase C, and calcium/calmodulin kinase.

A protein kinase activates a substrate protein. A **substrate protein** can be an ion channel, an enzyme involved in the making of neurotransmitters, a neurotransmitter receptor, or other proteins within the neuron. A substrate protein also can be a transcription factor. Two common transcription factors for neurons are c-Fos and cAMP response element-binding (CREB) protein. The activation of genes may lead to the synthesis of proteins within the neuron, including receptors for neurotransmitters and enzymes used in neurotransmitter synthesis. Given that a series of events may occur after activating a metabotropic receptor, effects within a neuron continue after the neurotransmitter leaves the receptor.

substrate protein
Protein that may consist of an ion channel, enzyme, neurotransmitter receptor, or other proteins involved in neuronal processes.

REVIEW! A transcription factor activates or deactivates a gene. Chapter 2 (pg. 57).

Stop & Check

1. Receptors located on a post synaptic terminal are called _____ receptors.
2. Where is an autoreceptor located?
3. Although G proteins may directly activate ion channels, other intracellular effects are carried out by activating _____ such as cAMP or cGMP.
4. After being activated by a second messenger, a protein kinase can affect the functioning of a neuron in a variety of ways, including acting as a _____ to alter gene expression.

1. postsynaptic receptors **2.** An autoreceptor is located on an axon terminal and is activated by the neurotransmitters released from the same axon terminal. **3.** second messengers **4.** transcription factor

Different Types of Neurotransmitters and Communication

Table 3.2 lists the neurotransmitters most important for psychoactive drugs, but this list is only a subset of the dozens of neurotransmitters currently known. Table 3.2 groups neurotransmitters by chemical structure. For example, glutamate and γ-aminobutryic acid (GABA) are both amino acids and thus belong to the amino acids category of neurotransmitters. Dopamine, norepinephrine, and serotonin belong in the monoamine category because they have a single amine chemical group, $-NH_2$, in their structures.

table **3.2**

Neurotransmitter Categories and Selected Neurotransmitters	
Category	**Neurotransmitter**
Amino acids	Glutamate GABA
Modified amino acids	Acetylcholine
Monoamines	Indoleamines Serotonin Catecholamines Dopamine Norepinephrine Epinephrine
Neuropeptides	Endorphins
Gases	Nitric oxide

© Cengage Learning 2009

Glutamate and GABA Are the Most Abundant Neurotransmitters

glutamate Excitatory amino acid neurotransmitter.

excitatory amino acid neurotransmitters An amino acid neurotransmitter family that tends to elicit excitatory effects on neurons.

GABA Inhibitory amino acid neurotransmitter.

inhibitory amino acid neurotransmitters An amino acid neurotransmitter family that tends to elicit inhibitory effects on neurons.

NMDA An ionotropic receptor for the neurotransmitter glutamate.

AMPA The α-amino-3-hydroxy-5-methyl-4-isoxazolepropionic acid (AMPA) receptor is an ionotropic receptor for the neurotransmitter glutamate.

kainite An ionotropic receptor for the neurotransmitter glutamate.

The amino acids glutamate and GABA are found throughout the nervous system. The amino acid neurotransmitter **glutamate** is the most prominent member of a small amino acid family called **excitatory amino acid neurotransmitters**. The amino acid **GABA** is the most prominent member of a small amino acid family called **inhibitory amino acid neurotransmitters**.

Glutamate

Glutamate is synthesized within axon terminals from the amino acid glutamine. The enzyme glutaminase converts glutamine to glutamate (**figure 3.12**). After synthesis, vesicular transporters carry glutamate into protective vesicles, where it resides for later release into the synapse. Glutamate is released from *pyramidal neurons*, so named for the pyramid shape of the soma. The cerebral cortex is rich in pyramidal neurons, and the groupings of pyramidal neurons partly define different layers of the cerebral cortex.

Within the synaptic cleft, glutamate binds to any of four types of receptors. Three of these receptors—NMDA, AMPA, and kainite receptors—are ionotropic. The fourth receptor type, the mGlu receptor, is metabotropic.

When activated, the ionotropic **NMDA, AMPA,** and **kainite** receptors allow positively charged ions to enter a neuron (**figure 3.13**). The influx of positively charged ions function as excitatory postsynaptic potentials. The names for these receptors come from the chemical substances used to discover them. NMDA stands for N-methyl-D-aspartate, which is a drug that serves as an agonist, a

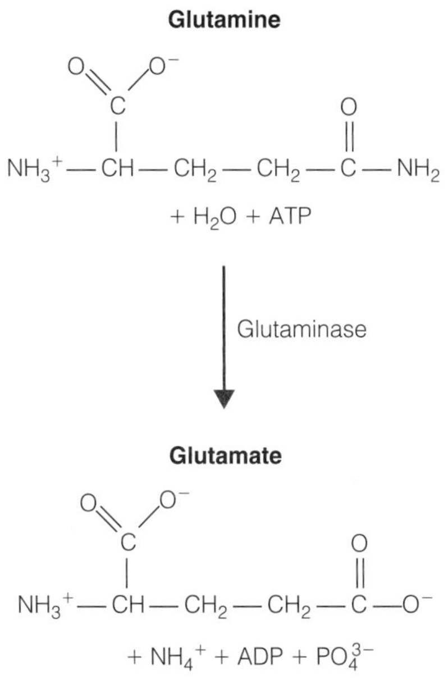

Glutamine

$$NH_3^+ - CH - CH_2 - CH_2 - C - NH_2$$
$$+ H_2O + ATP$$

↓ Glutaminase

Glutamate

$$NH_3^+ - CH - CH_2 - CH_2 - C - O^-$$
$$+ NH_4^+ + ADP + PO_4^{3-}$$

figure 3.12   Glutamate is synthesized from glutamine using the enzyme glutaminase.

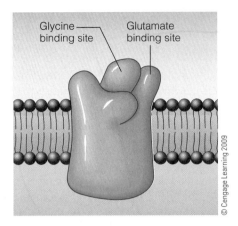

Glycine binding site

Glutamate binding site

© Cengage Learning 2009

figure 3.13   The glutamate NMDA receptor produces excitatory effects by allowing positively charged ions to enter a neuron.

drug that mimics a neurotransmitter, at these receptors. AMPA stands for α-amino-3-hydroxy-5-methyl-4-isoxazole proprionic acid, a receptor agonist used to discover this receptor. Finally, the kainate receptor is named from the receptor agonist kainic acid. Agonist drug effects are described in Chapter 4.

Glutamate is not the only endogenous chemical that binds to the NMDA receptor. One site on the NMDA receptor is called the *glycine* or *D-serene* site. Either glycine or D-serine must be bound to this site for glutamate to activate the receptor. Another site is located inside the channel and can be bound to by magnesium, Mg^{2+}. Because of the location of this site, Mg^{2+} prevents the influx of ions even when glutamate activates the receptor.

Several subtypes of mGlu receptors include group I, II, and III receptors. Group I mGlu receptors enhance neuronal activity by activating signaling molecules such as second messengers and protein kinases. However, groups II and III mGlu receptors differ from other glutamate receptors by causing inhibitory effects on neurons. Groups II and III mGlu receptors produce inhibitory effects by inhibiting signaling molecules.

After glutamate has been released from a receptor, it is removed from the synaptic cleft through any of several excitatory amino acid transporters. These transporters for glutamate are found on the axon terminal that released glutamate, effectively recycling glutamate for release at a later time. Excitatory amino acid transporters are also located on astrocytes near the synaptic cleft. Within an astrocyte, glutamate is broken down by the enzyme glutamine synthetase into the amino acid glutamine. The astrocyte then releases glutamine near the axon terminal, where it can be brought into the terminal through glutamine transporters and then used for glutamate synthesis.

GABA

The inhibitory amino acid neurotransmitter γ-aminobutyric acid is found in most structures in the nervous system. GABA, like other neurotransmitters,

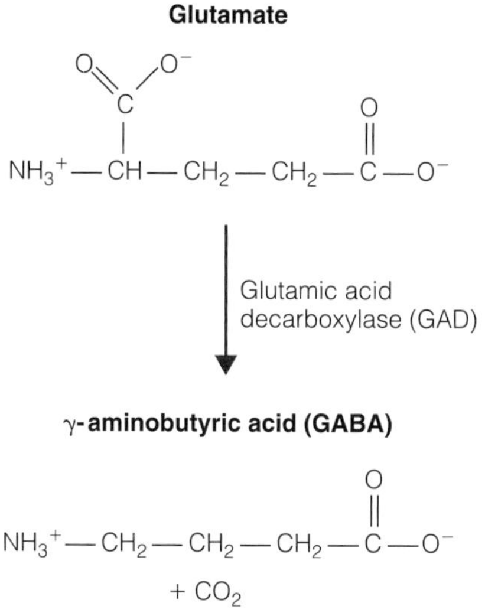

Glutamate

$$\begin{array}{c}
\overset{O}{\underset{}{\diagdown}}\overset{}{C}\overset{O^-}{\diagup} \\
| \\
NH_3{}^+ - CH - CH_2 - CH_2 - \overset{O}{\overset{||}{C}} - O^-
\end{array}$$

Glutamic acid
decarboxylase (GAD)

γ-aminobutyric acid (GABA)

$$NH_3{}^+ - CH_2 - CH_2 - CH_2 - \overset{O}{\overset{||}{C}} - O^-$$

$$+ CO_2$$

figure 3.14　The enzyme glutamic acid decarboxylase converts glutamate to GABA.

is synthesized from other molecules using enzymes. GABA is converted from glutamate with the enzyme glutamic acid decarboxylase (GAD). After synthesis, vesicular transporters bring GABA neurotransmitters into synaptic vesicles (**figure 3.14**).

There are two GABA receptors, named $GABA_A$ and $GABA_B$. The $GABA_A$ receptor is ionotropic, whereas the $GABA_B$ receptor is metabotropic. Both receptors produce inhibitory effects when they are bound by GABA. Of these two receptors, the $GABA_A$ receptor has been the most studied and is important for the effects of central nervous system depressants, such as alcohol (ethanol), barbiturates, and benzodiazepines.

Figure 3.10 illustrated binding sites for GABA and other substances on the $GABA_A$ receptor. The $GABA_A$ channel contains a site for GABA, and the receptor will open when GABA binds to the GABA site. Once the channel is open, negatively charged chloride (Cl^-) ions enter the neuron, resulting in inhibitory postsynaptic potentials. As previously described, inhibitory postsynaptic potentials cause hyperpolarization to local potentials and reduce the likelihood of action potentials.

As also shown in figure 3.10, the $GABA_A$ channels contain binding sites for other molecules. When molecules bind to these other *allosteric sites*, they negatively or positively alter the effects of GABA on the $GABA_A$ receptor. Positive modulation increases the length of time GABA activates the receptor, whereas negative modulation decreases the length of time GABA activates the receptor.

One of these binding sites is called the *barbiturate site*, so named because barbiturates, such as phenobarbital, bind to this site. By binding to this site, barbiturates positively modulate GABA's effects on the receptor. Another site is called the *benzodiazepine site*, again so named because benzodiazepines such as Valium and Xanax bind to this site. Benzodiazepines also enhance GABA's effects on the GABA$_A$ receptor.

The GABA$_A$ receptor also contains a *picrotoxin site*. This site can be a bound to by picrotoxin, the drug used to discover this site, and certain seizure-producing drugs such as pentylenetetrazol. The picrotoxin site resides inside the GABA$_A$ receptor's ion channel, and substances that bind to this site block the channel.

After GABA neurotransmitters release from receptors, astrocytes terminate neurotransmission by transporting GABA into astrocytes. Within an astrocyte, the enzyme GABA aminotransferase breaks GABA down to glutamate. In some situations, enzymes further break glutamate down into glutamine, which may be released near GABA neurons, which bring in glutamine for glutamate and then GABA synthesis.

Stop & Check

1. Glutamate is the most common excitatory neurotransmitter in the nervous system, whereas _____ is the most common inhibitory neurotransmitter in the nervous system.

2. Glutamate is synthesized and released from _____ neurons.

3. Of the two types of GABA receptors, the GABA$_A$ receptor is ionotropic whereas the GABA$_B$ receptor is _____.

4. The inhibitory effects of GABA that occur at GABA$_A$ receptors result from the influx of _____ charged ions such as chloride.

1. GABA **2.** pyramidal **3.** metabotropic **4.** negatively

---

Monoamine Neurotransmitters: Dopamine, Norepinephrine, Epinephrine, and Serotonin

Chances are that you have already learned something about the neurotransmitters serotonin, dopamine, or norepinephrine in other college courses. Selective serotonin reuptake inhibitors (SSRIs), such as Prozac, for example, treat depression by increasing serotonin levels in synapses. The dopamine system plays an important role in reinforcing the effects of recreational drugs and in the symptoms of schizophrenia. These neurotransmitters belong to the *monoamine* class of neurotransmitters, which includes two subgroups, the catecholamines and the indoleamines.

The catecholamines include the neurotransmitters dopamine, norepinephrine, and epinephrine. Each of these neurotransmitters share a catechol chemical structure and have a single amine chemical group (**figure 3.15**). The same synthesis process produced these neurotransmitters, as shown in **figure 3.16**. This synthesis pathway begins with the amino acid phenylalanine. Phenylalanine is an **essential amino acid**, an amino acid that is not produced in the human body and must come from our diet.

essential amino acid
Amino acid that is not produced in the body and must come from diet.

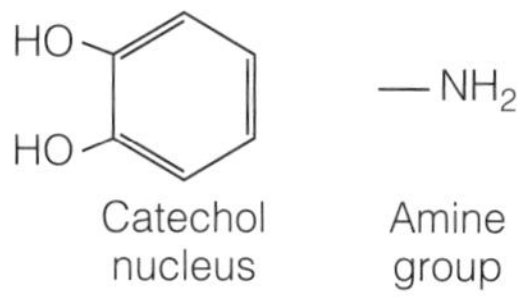

HO⟍⟋⟍   — NH₂
HO⟋⟍⟍
Catechol   Amine
nucleus   group

Every monoamine neurotransmitter has a single amine group in its structure. The catecholamines—including dopamine, norepinephrine, and epinephrine—have a catechol nucleus in their structures.

figure 3.15

Dopamine

Dopamine is the first neurotransmitter synthesized in this process. The enzyme phenylalanine hydroxylase converts phenylalamine to the amino acid tyrosine, a nonessential amino acid. Yet tyrosine, like many of the other 20 different amino acids found in the body, also comes from dietary sources. In particular, high-proteins foods such as meats, soy, and dairy products contain large amounts of tyrosine (figure 3.16).

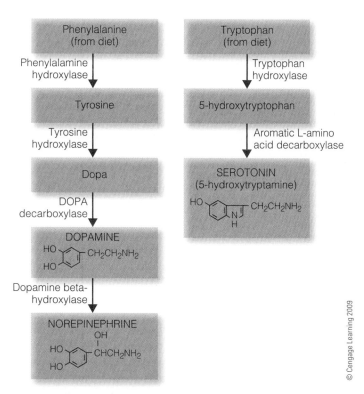

© Cengage Learning 2009

figure 3.16

Monoamine neurotransmitters are synthesized through a series of steps beginning with an amino acid.

The enzyme tyrosine hydroxylase converts tyrosine to L-DOPA (L-3,4-di-hydroxyphenylalanine). The enzyme DOPA decarboxylase then produces dopamine from L-DOPA. In the many synthesis steps for dopamine, tyrosine hydroxylase serves as the **rate-limiting step** because it has the slowest conversion rate. Increasing tyrosine levels is not an effective means of increasing dopamine levels because the relatively slower conversion rate of tyrosine hydroxylase acts as a bottleneck for this synthesis pathway. On the other hand, increasing L-DOPA levels will increase dopamine levels because the conversion of L-DOPA to dopamine does not depend on tyrosine hydroxylase. After synthesis, vesicular monoamine transporters (VMATs) deliver dopamine into vesicles for storage.

Once released from an axon terminal, dopamine may bind to any of several types of **dopamine receptors**, which are classified by two families: the D_1 receptor family and the D_2 receptor family. The D_1 receptor family includes the D_1 and D_5 receptors, and the D_2 receptor family includes the D_2, D_3, and D_4 receptors. All dopamine receptors are metabotropic, G-protein–coupled receptors. The D_1 family of receptors tend to have excitatory effects on neurons, whereas the D_2 family of receptors have inhibitory effects on neurons.

Once dopamine releases from a dopamine receptor in the synaptic cleft, termination of dopamine transmission occurs in either of two ways. First, dopamine may be catabolized by an enzyme. One type of catabolic enzyme is **monoamine oxidase** (**MAO**), which has two types—MAO_A and MAO_B. Both types of MAO are capable of breaking down dopamine, as well as norepinephrine and serotonin. Another type of catabolic enzyme is **catechol-O-methyltransferase** (**COMT**). COMT catabolizes catecholamine neurotransmitters, including dopamine, norepinephrine, and epinephrine.

Second, reuptake transporters also terminate dopamine neurotransmission. Reuptake occurs through the **dopamine transporter**. After dopamine molecules pass through this transporter, vesicles store dopamine for later release.

Two brain-stem structures—the *ventral tegmental area* and the *substantia nigra*—and the hypothalamus contain most of the brain's dopamine neuron cell bodies (**figure 3.17**). Bundles of dopamine axons from these structures terminate in other parts of the brain. The dopamine pathways most important for psychoactive drugs are the mesolimbic, mesocortical, nigrostriatal, and tubero-infundibular dopamine pathways.

The **mesolimbic and mesocortical dopamine pathways** originate in the ventral tegmental area. The axons in the mesolimbic pathways terminate in the nucleus accumbens as well as other limbic system structures, including the amygdala and hippocampus. The axons in the mesocortical pathways terminate in the frontal cortex, particularly the prefrontal cortex. The **nigrostriatal dopamine pathway** originates in the substantia nigra and terminates in the basal ganglia. The tubero-infundibular dopamine pathway originates in the hypothalamus and terminates in the pituitary gland, where it plays an important role in the secretion of prolactin, an important hormone for maternal behavior. In the peripheral nervous system, dopamine activates dopamine receptors found in the heart and certain arteries that enhance blood flow from increased cardiac output and dilated arteries. However, enhanced dopamine levels may not necessarily achieve these effects because of the conversion of dopamine to norepinephrine, which causes constriction of blood vessels.

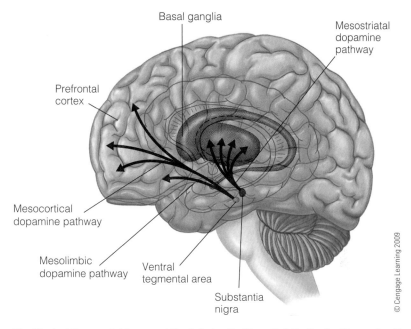

The Ventral Tegmental Area and the Substantia Nigra Cell Bodies for Dopamine Neurons
Dopamine is released in the (1) cortex from axons in the mesocortical dopamine pathway, (2) limbic system from axons in the mesolimbic dopamine pathway, and (3) the basal ganglia from axons in the nigrostriatal pathway.

figure 3.17

Norepinephrine and Epinephrine

Norepinephrine represents the next step in the catecholamine synthesis process. Further synthesis leads to epinephrine. Epinephrine shares the functions of norepinephrine in the brain but has little unique impact on brain function or psychoactive drug actions of its own. Given this, epinephrine will not be further discussed in this text.

Outside of the peripheral nervous system, norepinephrine is also known as *noradrenaline*. Given this, norepinephrine describes a neurotransmitter, whereas noradrenaline describes a hormone. Yet *noradrenaline* does apply to the names of norepinephrine neurons and receptors. Norepinephrine-containing neurons are referred to as **noradrenergic neurons**, and the receptors for norepinephrine are referred to as **adrenoceptors**.

Within noradrenergic neurons, the enzyme dopamine β-hydroxylase converts dopamine to norepinephrine (figure 3.17). Like dopamine, vesicular monoamine transporters bring norepinephrine into synaptic vesicles for storage. After release from noradrenergic axon terminals, norepinephrine bind to adrenoceptors, which consist of both α and β adrenoceptors. Both types of adrenoceptors are metabotropic receptors. The α adrenoreceptors have two subtypes: α_1 and α_2. The β adrenoceptors have three subtypes: β_1, β_2, and β_3. Depending on the specific receptor, activation of adrenoceptors produce either inhibitory or excitatory effects.

noradrenergic neurons Neurons that release norepinephrine.

adrenoceptors Receptors activated by norepinephrine and consisting of the subtypes α and β adrenoceptors.

Like dopamine, norepinephrine neurotransmission is terminated by the catabolic enzymes MAO or COMT or through reuptake into the axon terminal. Reuptake occurs through the norepinephrine transporter. Noradrenergic neurons are concentrated in the locus coeruleus, a structure located in the brain stem near dopamine-containing structures. Noradrenergic pathways innervate many structures throughout the brain, including the cerebral cortex, hippocampus, and amygdala (**figure 3.18**). In the peripheral nervous system, norepinephrine activates cells in the sympathetic nervous system.

Serotonin

Serotonin is part of the indoleamine class of monoamines. Serotonin is also known as 5-hydroxytryptamine, or 5-HT for short. Given that serotonin belongs to a different category of monoamines, serotonin's synthesis pathway differs from the catecholamines. The synthesis of serotonin begins with the essential amino acid tryptophan. The enzyme tryptophan hydroxylase converts tryptophan to 5-hydroxytryptophan. From here, the enzyme aromatic L-amino acid decarboxylase converts 5-hydroxytrypt*ophan* to 5-hydroxytrypt*amine* (figure 3.16).

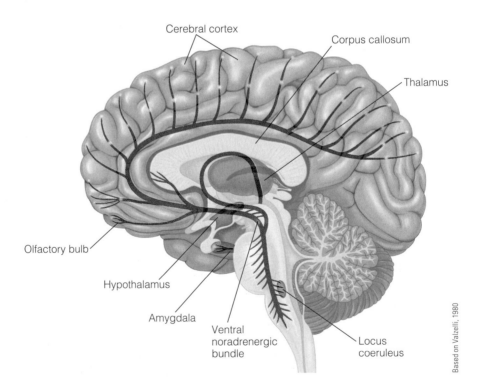

Based on Valzelli, 1980

figure 3.18 The cell bodies for norepinephrine are mostly found in the locus coeruleus, and axons from these neurons are sent to many areas throughout the brain, including the cortex, amygdala, and structures in the hindbrain.

Once synthesized, vesicular monoamine transporters, the same vesicular transporters for dopamine and norepinephrine, bring serotonin into synaptic vesicles via the VMAT2 transporter, the same vesicular transporter used for dopamine and norepinephrine storage. The major types of serotonin receptors include 5-HT$_1$ through 5-HT$_7$. Each receptor type includes multiple subtypes.

The termination mechanisms for serotonin includes enzymatic breakdown and reuptake. Like dopamine and norepinephrine, the enzyme MAO catabolizes serotonin. Otherwise, serotonin neurotransmitters are brought back into the axon terminal through reuptake via the serotonin transporter. Like dopamine and norepinephrine, serotonin is then stored in vesicles for later release.

The cell bodies for serotonergic neurons are located in the raphe nuclei, which are found in the brain stem near structures for dopaminergic and noradrenergic neurons. Serotonin pathways terminate in structures all throughout the brain.

Stop & Check

1. The monoamine include the neurotransmitters dopamine, norepinephrine, and _____.
2. How might one's diet influence dopamine neurotransmission?
3. Unlike dopamine and norepinephrine, serotonin can only be broken down by the enzyme _____.

1. serotonin **2.** A poor diet reduces the availability of amino acids important for dopamine synthesis. For example, a protein-impoverished diet reduces tyrosine levels in the body, in turn reducing the amount of dopamine synthesized. **3.** MAO

Acetylcholine

vesicular acetylcholine transporter A protein that transports acetylcholine into a synaptic vesicle.

nicotinic receptors Receptors activated by acetylcholine with subtypes derived from α and β subunits.

muscarinic receptors Receptors activated by acetylcholine with subtypes named M$_1$, M$_2$, M$_3$, M$_4$ and M$_5$.

Acetylcholine is listed alone in table 3.2 for neurotransmitters. Acetylcholine is derived from a single synthesis step by assembling *choline* and *acetyl* coenzyme A using the enzyme choline acetyltransferase (**figure 3.19**). Acetylcholine neurons are referred to as *cholinergic* neurons, owing to choline's role in acetylcholine synthesis. After synthesis, the **vesicular acetylcholine transporter** brings acetylcholine into synaptic vesicles.

The receptors for acetylcholine, called *cholinergic receptors*, have two major classes: **nicotinic receptors** and **muscarinic receptors**. The receptor names come from compounds used to discover them. Nicotine selectively acts on nicotinic receptors. Similarly, muscarine, a toxin found in the mushroom *Amanita muscaria*, was found to act on a separate class of class of cholinergic receptors.

Nicotinic receptors are ionotropic; when activated, they cause the influx of positively charged sodium (Na$^+$), potassium (K$^+$), and calcium (Ca^{2+}) ions. Five subunit structures make up nicotinic receptors. The names of the primary subunits are the Greek letters α and β. Other subunits include δ and ε. Each subunit has multiple subtypes, which are described by placing a numbered

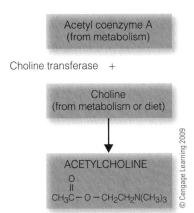

Acetylcholine is synthesized from acetyl coenzyme A and choline with the enzyme choline acetyltransferase.

figure 3.19

subscript after the subunit name. For example, one type of subunit is α_4. So far researchers have discovered nine α subunits (α_2 through α_{10}) and three β subunits (β_2 through β_4).

The configuration of nicotinic receptor subunits serves as the receptor's subtype. For example, the receptor comprised of α_4 and β_2 subunits is called the $\alpha_4\beta_2$ *nicotinic receptor*, whereas the receptor comprised only of α_7 subunits is called the α_7 *nicotinic receptor*. Numerous nicotinic receptor subtypes are based on these subunit configurations.

Muscarinic receptors are metabotropic and coupled to G proteins. There are two families of muscarinic receptors: the M_1 and M_2 families. The subtypes of the M_1 receptor family are M_1, M_3, and M_5, and the subtypes of the M_2 receptor family are M_2 and M_4. In general, activation of M_1 family receptors produces excitatory effects within a neuron by activating second messengers. Activation of M_2 family receptors produce inhibitory effects within a neuron by inhibiting second messengers.

After acetylcholine is released from the receptor, it is broken down into choline and acetic acid by the enzyme **acetylcholinesterase**. There is no reuptake transporter for acetylcholine. However, there is a reuptake transporter for choline. Once choline is transported via the choline transporter into the axon terminal, choline acetyltransferase enzymes facilitate acetylcholine synthesis.

Many structures in the brain contain cholinergic neurons, including the nucleus basalis magnocellularis, pons, hippocampus, and tegmentum. Cholinergic axons from the nucleus basalis magnocellularis innervate the cerebral cortex. Cholinergic axons from the pons also innervate the cerebral cortex as well as the thalamus. Most cholinergic axons from hippocampal neurons remain in the hippocampus, and tegmental cholinergic axons innervate other brain-stem structures, including the dopamine-rich substantia nigra and ventral tegmental area structures (**figure 3.20**). Acetylcholine is also the key neurotransmitter for the parasympathetic nervous system. Increased parasympathetic nervous

acetylcholinesterase
Enzyme that breaks down acetylcholine.

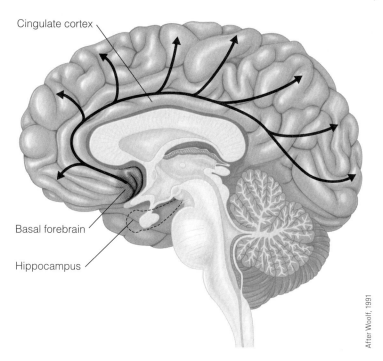

Cingulate cortex

Basal forebrain

Hippocampus

After Woolf, 1991

figure **3.20**   Acetylcholine cell bodies are located in the basal forebrain, and acetylcholine is released in the cerebral cortex and hippocampus.

system activation accounts for many of the effects of muscarine poisoning such as increased salivation, diarrhea, blurred vision (through pupil constriction), and labored breathing.

The cholinergic nervous system is the target of both chemical warfare and therapeutic drugs. The chemical weapon sarin gas potently inhibits acetylcholinesterase, causing a massive build up of acetycholine. Sarin gas overactivates the parasympathetic nervous system. Inhaling sarin gas causes constriction of the lungs, leading to suffocation and death. This weapon was developed in Nazi Germany in the 1930s and was most recently used by Saddam Hussein during the Iran–Iraq War and on ethnic Kurds in northern Iraq (Ganesan, Raza, & Vijayaraghavan, 2010). Sarin was also the agent used in the Japanese subway terrorist attacks in the 1990s (Yanagisawa, Morita, & Nakajima, 2006).

Significantly less potent inhibitors of acetylcholinesterase provide a means to treat some forms of dementia such as Alzheimer's disease. One of the most prescribed acetylcholinesterase inhibitors is donepezil (Aricept). These medications compensate for cholinergic loss found in Alzheimer's disease. The "From Actions to Effects" section in this chapter describes the use of these inhibitors and other medications for the treatment of Alzheimer's disease.

Neuropeptides: A Large Class of Neurotransmitters

Neuropeptides make up a large class of neurotransmitters. Opioids are the most studied neuropeptides in psychopharmacology. The opioid system is acted on by opioid drugs such as heroin and morphine, and neurons for opioids terminate in parts of the brain stem and the limbic system. Chapter 10 covers the opioid system as well as the use and actions of opioid drugs. Other neuropeptides are often found in neurons that contain another neurotransmitter. For example, dopamine neurons also synthesize and release the neuropeptide neurotensin (Ervin & Nemeroff, 1988).

Nitric Oxide: A Unique Neurotransmitter

nitric oxide (NO) Gas that functions as a neurotransmitter.

Many of the criteria that define a neurotransmitter have changed over the years. Until recently, a neurotransmitter had to be released in a Ca^{2+}-dependent manner and then had to have receptors specific to the neurotransmitter. Fewer criteria exist today, due in no small part to **nitric oxide (NO)**.

NO is a gas that functions as a neurotransmitter. Unlike conventional neurotransmitters, however, NO is not stored in a vesicle; instead, it is immediately released after synthesis. NO synthesis occurs from L-arginine in the presence of the enzyme nitric oxide synthase. In this synthesis reaction, the oxidation of L-arginine by nitric oxide synthase causes a nitrogen atom and an oxygen atom to break away and form a NO bond. Although Ca^{2+} does not trigger the release of NO, Ca^{2+} does facilitate nitric oxide synthase activity.

Once synthesized, NO diffuses through the neuronal membrane and permeates the membranes of nearby neurons and glial cells. Furthermore, unlike conventional neurotransmitters, NO does not bind to membrane receptors. Instead it forms bonds with various intracellular proteins, including second messengers and substrate proteins. In addition to effects within neurons, NO

Stop & Check

1. The receptor types for acetylcholine are muscarinic receptors, which are metabotropic, and _____, which are ionotropic.

2. Acetylcholine activity in the cortex and _____ has important effects on cognitive function.

3. _____ neurotransmitters are often in neurons that synthesize another type of neurotransmitter.

4. Although nitric oxide is considered a neurotransmitter, it is neither stored in vesicles released in a calcium-dependent manner nor bound to _____ on the surface of neurons.

1. nicotinic receptors **2.** hippocampus **3.** Neuropeptide **4.** receptors

also causes blood vessels to dilate. NO, therefore, may facilitate increased blood flow to highly active neurons in the brain.

Other Types of Chemical Transmission in the Nervous System

Neurotrophins

Neurotrophins are a family of neurotrophic factors that promote the survival and plasticity of neurons during development and in adulthood. The class of neurotrophins includes neural growth factor (NGF), brain-derived neurotrophic factor (BDNF), neurotrophin-3, and neurotrophin-4. Neurotrophins are synthesized after expression of a particular gene such as the BDNF gene for BDNF.

There are several receptors for neurotrophins, including TrkA (pronounced "track A"), TrkB, and TrkC receptors. Among these receptors, NGF binds selectively to TrkA receptors, NT-3 binds selectively to TrkC receptors, and both BDNF and NT-4 bind selectively to TrkB receptors. Trk receptors are neither associated with ion channels nor G proteins. However, activation Trk receptors may produce an entire cascade of intracellular effects. These can influence the strength of synaptic connections and may account for the long-term effects of some psychoactive drugs. For example, Trk receptor activation may facilitate hippocampal synaptic changes associated with antidepressant drug treatment (Li et al., 2008).

Hormones

hormones Signaling molecules derived from cholesterol and released from glands.

Hormones are signaling molecules derived from cholesterol and released from glands. They differ from neurotransmitters in several ways. First, hormones have widespread effects on target areas, whereas neurotransmitters are often released into tight synaptic junctions to carry out specific effects at postsynaptic terminals. Second, hormones bind not only to membrane receptors but also to intracellular receptors and act as transcription factors (**figure 3.21**). Neurotransmitters, on the other hand, primarily bind to receptors located on the surface of a neuron. Third, hormones can be delivered throughout the body via the bloodstream, whereas neurotransmitters generally act on receptors in the close vicinity where the neurotransmitter was released. Neurotransmitters, however, are synthesized and released in the nervous system.

The central nervous system uses hormones to regulate the endocrine system. The hypothalamus directly controls the pituitary gland. The pituitary gland is sometimes referred to as the *master gland* because it releases several hormones into the bloodstream that control the release of hormones from other endocrine system glands (**figures 3.22 and 3.23**).

REVIEW! The hypothalamus regulates body temperature, thirst, hunger, and other internal regulatory functions. Chapter 2 (pg. 41).

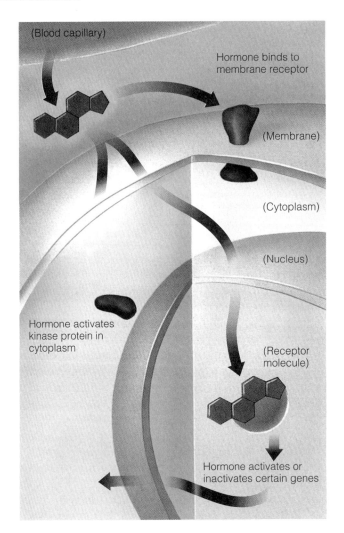

(Blood capillary)

Hormone binds to
membrane receptor

(Membrane)

(Cytoplasm)

(Nucleus)

Hormone activates
kinase protein in
cytoplasm

(Receptor
molecule)

Hormone activates or
inactivates certain genes

figure 3.21 Hormones influence neuronal function by either binding to areceptor on the neuronal membrane or acting as transcription factors. (Source: Revised from Starr & Taggart, 1989.)

oxytocin Pituitary hormone important for uterine contraction during childbirth; also contributes to milk letdown during breast-feeding.

vasopressin Antidiuretic hormone that causes the kidneys to absorb water from the bloodstream.

Neurons from the hypothalamus release two hormones into the pituitary gland: vasopression and oxytocin. Through the pituitary gland, these two hormones enter the bloodstream and are delivered throughout the body. **Oxytocin** is particularly important for uterine contraction during childbirth, and it also contributes to milk letdown during breast-feeding. **Vasopressin** is an antidiuretic hormone that causes the kidneys to absorb more water from the bloodstream. Alcohol suppresses vasopressin release, partly accounting for the frequent urination associated with alcohol consumption (Meier & Mendoza, 1976).

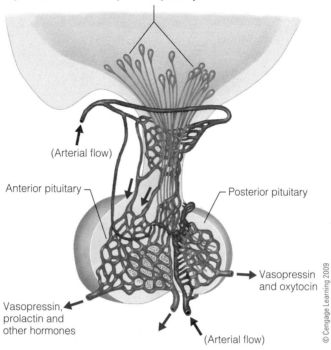

Hypothalamus secretes releasing hormones and inhibiting hormones that control anterior pituitary. Also synthesizes vasopressin and oxytocin, which travel to posterior pituitary.

(Arterial flow)

Anterior pituitary

Posterior pituitary

Vasopressin and oxytocin

Vasopressin, prolactin and other hormones

(Arterial flow)

© Cengage Learning 2009

figure 3.22   The pituitary gland is also called the *master gland* because it controls the activity of other glands in the endocrine system. The pituitary gland is controlled by the hypothalamus.

melatonin Sleep-inducing hormone that plays an important role in circadian rhythm, our natural sleep cycle.

The hypothalamus also has control over the pineal gland. The pineal gland releases melatonin, which is synthesized from serotonin. **Melatonin** is a sleep-inducing hormone that plays an important role in circadian rhythm, our natural sleep cycle (Marczynski, Yamaguchi, Ling, & Grodzinska, 1964). The sleep aid ramelteon (Rozerum) exerts its sleep-inducing effects by activating receptors for melatonin (Buysse, Bate, & Kirkpatrick, 2005; Miyamoto et al., 2004).

Stop & Check

1. Both NGF and BDNF are types of _____, which promote the survival and plasticity of neurons.

2. _____ receptors may account for the hippocampal plasticity changes caused by chronic antidepressant treatment.

3. In addition to neurotransmitters, the other major messaging chemicals in the body are _____.

1. neurotrophins 2. Trk 3. hormones

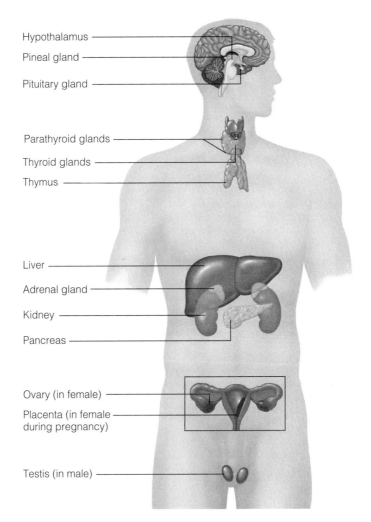

Hypothalamus

Pineal gland

Pituitary gland

Parathyroid glands

Thyroid glands

Thymus

Liver

Adrenal gland

Kidney

Pancreas

Ovary (in female)

Placenta (in female during pregnancy)

Testis (in male)

figure 3.23 The endocrine system is a network of glands that release and monitor hormone levels throughout the body. (Source: Starr & Taggart, 1989.)

FROM ACTIONS TO EFFECTS
Treating Alzheimer's Disease

Alzheimer's disease (AD) is a progressive neurological disorder characterized by severe impairments in memory, decision making, attention, motivation, language production and comprehension, and mood regulation. Alzheimer's disease affects approximately 5 million individuals in the United States. Within this estimate, AD affects approximately 5 percent of men and women between ages 65 and 74 and 50 percent of men and women 85 and older (Hebert, Scherr, Bienias, Bennett, & Evans, 2003).

Alzheimer's disease progresses through different stages, beginning with mild cognitive impairment. Mild cognitive impairment is defined as exhibiting more than age-appropriate declines in cognitive functioning. Examples of mild cognitive impairment include forgetting important appointments and difficulty following conversations. For an individual showing early signs of AD, mild cognitive impairment eventually leads to early stage AD. Early stage Alzheimer's disease represents a worsening of mild cognitive impairment symptoms. In addition, an individual with early stage AD may experience changes in mood such as irritability or depression, as well as forgetfulness about one's personal history, including the names of friends or family members or places worked. Late stage Alzheimer's disease represents severe impairments in cognitive impairment—to the extent that individuals lose touch with their environment. During late stage AD, a person cannot follow conversations or control his or her movements. These individuals need assistance for personal daily care needs.

During the course of this disease, patients commonly develop other illnesses that contribute to declining health and a shortened life span. Patients normally live for 8 to 10 years after an AD diagnosis. In most cases, an individual with Alzheimer's disease dies from pneumonia.

Alzheimer's disease causes important changes to brain. The cerebral cortex shrinks in size, as shown in **figure 3.24**. Further, the brain's lateral ventricles become enlarged by encroaching in areas of degenerated brain tissue. At the cellular level, dying and

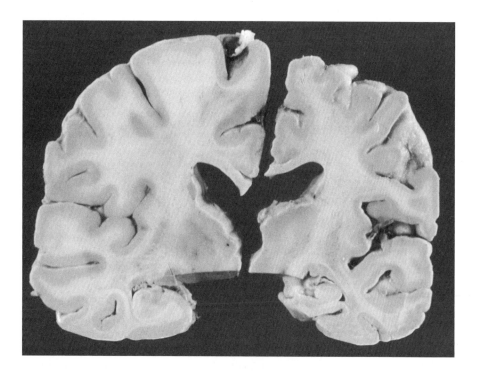

figure 3.24

The volume of cerebral cortex is reduced in Alzheimer's disease (left). Compare this to the brain of an individual without Alzheimer's disease on the right. (Jessica Wilson/Science Source/Photo Researchers)

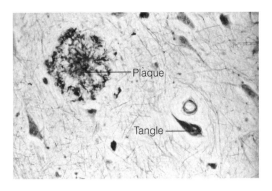

Plaque

Tangle

figure 3.25

Dying and dysfunctional neurons form neurofibrillary tangles and senile plaques in Alzheimer's disease.
© Dr. M. Goedert/Science Source/Photo Researchers, Inc.

senile plaques
Degenerated neurons formed from overproduction of amyloid beta 42 peptides, causing cell death.

fibrillary tangles Result of dysfunctional tau proteins that fail to maintain functioning and stability of axons.

degenerated neurons form aberrant cellular formations called *senile plaques* and *neurofibrillary tangles*. **Senile plaques** form from the overproduction of amyloid beta 42 peptides that impair neuronal function and cause cell death. **Fibrillary tangles** form from dysfunctional tau proteins that fail to maintain functioning and stability of axons (**figure 3.25**). Although neuronal damage occurs throughout structures in the brain, AD especially affects the basal forebrain, resulting in the degeneration of more than two-thirds of cholinergic neurons in this structure.

Although no cure exists, drug developers have targeted the destruction of cholinergic neurons for pharmacological therapies designed to reduce the progression rate of Alzheimer's disease. The brain's cholinergic system contributes to normal cognitive functioning. Drugs that impair cholinergic functions such as scopolamine selectively impair memory and other domains of attention. Currently, the first-line treatments for AD consist of acetylcholinesterase inhibitors. By inhibiting acetylcholinesterase, these drugs raise acetylcholine levels, counteracting diminished acetylcholine levels from the loss of cholinergic neurons.

The most commonly prescribed include donepezil (Aricept), galantamine (Razadyne), and rivastigmine (Exelon). As a class, acetylcholinesterase inhibitors stabilize cognitive function for as long as 3 to 6 months when given during the mild cognitive impairment or early AD stages. However, these medications fail to alter disease progression. Further, greater acetylcholine levels results enhance parasympathetic nervous system functioning, leading to risk of nausea, diarrhea, and vomiting. These risks prevent physicians from increasing drug doses as cognitive impairment worsens during the disease's progression.

REVIEW! Within the autonomic nervous system, the parasympathetic nervous system reduces heart rate, digestion, and other autonomic functions. Chapter 2 (pg. 37).

Another pharmacological strategy addresses excitotoxic destruction of neurons. Excitotoxicity derives from overstimulation of glutamate NMDA receptors. Given this, researchers have studied drugs that prevent NMDA receptor activation as treatments for Alzheimer's disease. The federal Food and Drug Administration approved the NMDA receptor channel blocker memantine (Namanda) for all stages of Alzheimer's disease. Clinical studies vary in the effectiveness of memantine for preventing cognitive decline in this disease, with some studies revealing significant treatment response and other studies reporting no perceived benefits. In a systematic review of dozens of clinical studies using memantine for AD and other dementias, McShane and colleagues (2006) found that only modest cognitive effects occurred overall.

Important scientific discoveries in neuroscience, genetics, and pharmacology will continue to improve on existing treatments. We hope that newer medications can sustain cognitive functioning not only for months but also for years. Although a cure for AD would be wonderful, simply restoring years of normal mental health would tremendously improve the quality of life for those with this disease.

| **Stop & Check** | 1. What parts of the brain are affected in Alzheimer's disease? |
| | 2. What are the first-line treatments for AD and how do they work? |

1. Key anatomical abnormalities in Alzheimer's disease consist of shrunken cerebral cortex and enlarged ventricles. Further, this disease selectively destroys cholinergic neurons in the basal forebrain. **2.** Acetylcholinesterase inhibitors. By elevating acetylcholinesterase, these drugs compensate for cholinergic neuron loss by elevating acetylcholine levels. Elevated acetylcholine levels help maintain normal cognitive functioning.

▶CHAPTER SUMMARY

Neurotransmission is a neuronal communication process that uses signaling molecules called *neurotransmitters*. Both electrical and chemical processes within a neuron facilitate neurotransmitter release. Electrical transmission conveys a signal from the soma to the axon terminal to release neurotransmitters. The nature of this transmission is a series of action potentials that first begin at the axon hillock and propagate down to the axon terminal.

Neurotransmission consists of several steps, including neurotransmitter synthesis, storage, release, receptor binding, and termination. Receptors are proteins activated by a matching neurotransmitter. There are two types of neurotransmitter receptors: ionotropic and metabotropic. Ionotropic receptors contain an ion channel, whereas metabotropic receptors utilize a G protein to convey effects. The two most common neurotransmitters in the brain are glutamate, an excitatory neurotransmitter, and GABA, an inhibitory neurotransmitter. Monoamine neurotransmitters include serotonin, dopamine,

norepinephrine, and epinephrine. Monoamine oxidase enzymes break down all monoamine neurotransmitters, whereas COMT breaks down dopamine, norepinephrine, and epinephrine. Neurotrophins are a family of neurotrophic factors that promote the survival and plasticity of neurons during development and adulthood. The class of neurotrophins includes neural growth factor (NGF), brain-derived neurotrophic factor (BDNF), neurotrophin-3, and neurotrophin-4. Hormones are chemical messengers derived from cholesterol and released from endocrine glands. The hypothalamus controls parts of the endocrine system through controlling the release of hormones from the pituitary gland. The hypothalamus also elicits melatonin secretion from the pineal gland. Alzheimer's disease results from the degeneration of neurons, as shown by senile plaques and neurofibrillary tangles. Acetylcholinesterase inhibitors can temporarily improve cognitive functioning, although these treatments fail to slow progression of the disease.

KEY TERMS

Neurotransmission	Local potential	Macroelectrodes	Concentration gradient
Electrical transmission	Ion channels	Microelectrodes	Sodium–potassium pump
Electrical potential	Excitatory postsynaptic potential (EPSP)	Intracellular recording	Voltage-gated ion channels
Depolarization		Microdialysis	
Hyperpolarization	Inhibitory postsynaptic potential (IPSP)	Electrostatic attraction	Temporal summation
			Spatial summation

Action potential

All-or-none law

Refractory period

Absolute refractory period

Relative refractory period

Propagation of action potentials

Nodes of Ranvier

Firing rate

Neurotransmitters

Vesicular transporter

Exocytosis

Volume neurotransmission

Catabolism

Receptors

Autoreceptor

Heteroceptor

Ionotropic receptors

Metabotropic receptor

Effector enzymes

Protein kinase

Substrate protein

Glutamate

Excitatory amino acid neurotransmitters

GABA

Inhibitory amino acid neurotransmitters

NMDA

AMPA

kainite

Essential amino acid

Rate-limiting step

Dopamine receptors

Monoamine oxidase (MAO)

Catechol-O-methyltransferase (COMT)

Dopamine transporter

Mesolimbic and mesocortical dopamine pathways

Nigrostriatal dopamine pathway

Noradrenergic neurons

Adrenoceptors

Vesicular acetylcholine transporter

Nicotinic receptors

Muscarinic receptors

Acetylcholinesterase

Nitric oxide (NO)

Hormones

Oxytocin

Vasopressin

Melatonin

Senile plaques

Fibrillary tangles

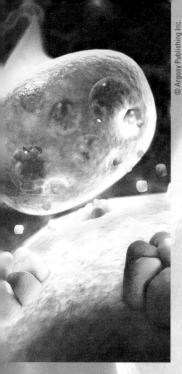
© Argosy Publishing Inc.

CHAPTER 4

Properties of Drugs

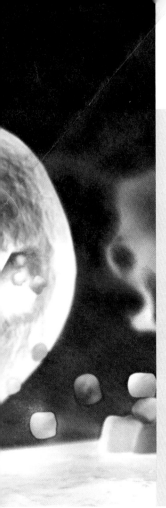

Do Environmental Stimuli Contribute to Heroin Tolerance?

In 1984, Shepard Siegel published a summary of interviews he conducted with heroin-addicted individuals who had survived an accidental heroin overdose (Siegel, 1984). Given the frequency of heroin use, one might expect heroin users to accidentally overdose from time to time. Instead, chronic heroin users have significant experience using heroin and thus exhibit an appreciable tolerance for the drug. In this respect, accidental heroin overdose may seem unlikely. Siegel's interviews sought to determine the conditions under which experienced heroin users overdosed.

Of the 10 addicts interviewed, 7 reported using a regular amount of heroin under atypical circumstances. These circumstances included unusual injection procedures or using the drug in different locations. Although seemingly benign, an earlier animal experiment reported by Siegel suggested that, in fact, these condition changes may partly account for heroin overdose in experienced users. We present the details of this prior study and the implications for human heroin addiction later in this chapter.

In previous chapters you learned about parts of the nervous system that are important for understanding drug effects. In this chapter, our attention turns to drugs themselves. We focus on how drugs move through the body and how they produce their actions.

The focus for this chapter just discussed describes the properties of drugs. As first noted in Chapter 1, pharmacology consists of two subfields called *pharmacokinetics*, which is concerned with how drugs move throughout the body, and *pharmacodyamics*, which is concerned with how drugs cause biological changes in the body. Because the focus of this textbook is on how drugs produce behavioral effects by acting in the brain, most of the material in this book concerns the pharmacodynamic effects of drugs.

Pharmacokinetic properties, however, have a lot to do with how people use drugs. For example, cocaine users prefer to smoke or snort the drug rather than consume it orally. These different methods of use do not change how cocaine acts in the brain, but they do determine how quickly cocaine reaches the brain. Thus, pharmacokinetic issues explain the common admin-istration methods for cocaine. Chapter 6 presents an overview of cocaine use, including details about cocaine's pharmacokinetic and pharmacodynamic effects.

Pharmacokinetic Properties and Drug Passage Through the Body

As first stated in Chapter 1, pharmacokinetics is the study of how drugs pass through the body. This process involves factors concerning how a drug is ad-ministered and how it is absorbed into the bloodstream, permeates different body parts, and is eliminated from the body. Designing drugs to pass through the body is a painstaking area of drug development. In fact, many therapeutic drugs fail in clinical testing because they are inadequate in reaching the areas of the body necessary for the drug's actions. A treatment is useless if the drug cannot reach its site of action. This section of this chapter provides an overview of the four primary stages of a drug's pharmacokinetic properties: absorption, distribution, metabolism, and elimination (**figure 4.1**).

Absorption

absorption Entry of a drug into the circulatory system.

The process of **absorption** refers to the entry of a drug into the circulatory system. To do so, a drug must pass through different membranes such as the mucus membranes in the mouth or the walls of the intestines. The particular membrane that a drug must pass through depends largely on the drug's route of administration. **Figure 4.2** shows examples of absorption for different administration routes, and **table 4.1** describes the characteristics of different administration routes.

PHARMACOKINETICS

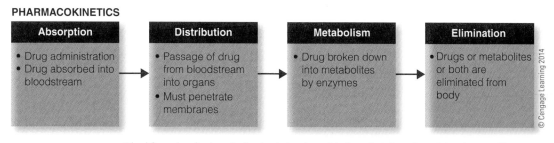

Absorption	Distribution	Metabolism	Elimination
• Drug administration • Drug absorbed into bloodstream	• Passage of drug from bloodstream into organs • Must penetrate membranes	• Drug broken down into metabolites by enzymes	• Drugs or metabolites or both are eliminated from body

© Cengage Learning 2014

figure **4.1**

The life cycle of a drug in the body begins with the administration of the drug and its absorption into the bloodstream. After entering the bloodstream, drugs diffuse through membranes and into organs. Drugs are usually metabolized by enzymes, a process that most often occurs in the liver. Finally, any remaining drug or its metabolites are eliminated from the body.

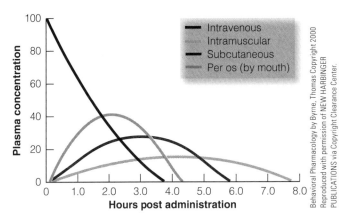

figure 4.2 The route of administration is an important determinant for how much drug reaches the bloodstream (vertical axis) and the length of time needed for drug absorption (horizontal axis). This figure shows different administration routes for a fictional drug.

Most therapeutic drugs are orally administered. As consumers, we prefer this administration route because it is easier than giving ourselves an injection. After swallowing a pill or drinking a liquid, a drug passes through the stomach and into the intestines, where the drug may absorb through stomach or intestinal walls along the way. Generally, most drug absorption occurs in the small intestine.

The oral administration route creates an important challenge for drug developers. For a drug intended for oral administration, developers must find ways to protect the drug from digestive acids in the stomach. Encasing a drug within a tablet or capsule will manage this. At the same time, however, stomach acids must dissolve enough of the tablet or capsule to free drug molecules for absorption in the intestines. This delicate balance often reduces the amount of drug that actually reaches the bloodstream.

The duration of time needed for a drug to pass through the digestive system affects the delay for drug effects. Although these delays also depend on unique chemical properties of the drug and the substance it is delivered in, most drugs take at least several minutes to reach the bloodstream; for intestinal absorption, it might take between 15 minutes and one hour. The *analgesic*—that is, pain-relieving—drug acetaminophen (Tylenol) requires about 30 minutes to provide headache relief for most people.

Users also inhale many substances, including medications such as albuterol for treating asthma or addictive substances such as tobacco. Through the inhalation route, drugs enter the circulatory system primarily through the lungs and to some degree through membranes in the nose, mouth, and throat. Therapeutically for asthma and other lung disorders, inhalation brings a drug directly to the area needing treatment. For example, albuterol treats asthma by relaxing air passages in the lungs.

Similar to oral administration, not all of an inhaled substance absorbs through tissue to reach the bloodstream. Yet inhaled substances absorb more

table **4.1**

Common Routes of Administration

Route	Form	Absorption amount	Time for absorption	Other
Oral	Pill	Variable; affected by food in stomach and digestive rates	Variable, but usually at least several minutes	Convenient for patients; most preferred and common route of administration
Intravenous	Injection into vein	100%	Immediate	Patients cannot administer drugs themselves; drug effects occur too rapidly to counteract prescribing errors or drug overdose
Intramuscular	Injection into skeletal muscle	Variable, but generally more stable than oral administration	Quicker and more even than oral administration but not as rapid as intravenous injection	Not convenient for patients and not common for drug abusers
Inhalation	Inhaled into lungs	High rate of absorption	Rapid	Convenient for patients and common for many drugs of abuse
Sublingual	Dissolved under tongue	Variable but generally more stable than oral administration	Quicker and more even than oral administration but not as rapid as intravenous injection	Can be used for individuals who may not want to take a medication (e.g., children or patients with schizophrenia)
Transdermal	Absorbed through skin, commonly through a skin patch	Variable but generally more stable than oral administration	Quicker and more even than oral administration but not as rapid as intravenous injection	Convenient and provides an even, sustained release of drug into bloodstream
Nasal and mucosal membrane	Absorbed through membranes in nasal passage or mouth	Variable but generally more stable than oral administration	Quicker and more even than oral administration but not as rapid as intravenous injection	Convenient for patients and common for drug abusers

© Cengage Learning 2014

quickly than orally administered drugs. For example, when tobacco is smoked, nicotine reaches the user's brain within 7 seconds.

Many administration methods require an injection. Intravenous injection involves drug delivery into a vein through a hypodermic needle. This route provides for rapid drug effects and avoids absorption limitations. Intravenous injections may be used in emergency medicine if physicians need a rapid drug effect or if a patient is too unresponsive to take a medication herself. For both of these reasons, a physician may give, for example, an intravenous injection of naloxone to a patient experiencing a heroin overdose (Sporer, 1999). Users of abused drugs may also prefer intravenous injections because of their speed of onset and full absorption of the drug.

Noncompliance to a medication provides another reason for delivering drugs by injection. These circumstances occur for some patients in psychiatric care. A patient with schizophrenia may refuse to swallow an antipsychotic medication out of suspicions about the motives of the medical care staff. To provide treatment to the patient, a nurse may provide an antipsychotic drug through an intramuscular injection in the arm or leg. To help psychiatric medical care staff with this particular patient noncompliance issue, many drug developers pursue antipsychotic drugs that are deliverable sublingually—that is, a pill dissolves on or under the tongue—or intranasally by using a nasal spray (Miller, Ashford, Archer, Rudy, & Wermeling, 2008; Potkin, Cohen, & Panagides, 2007).

Many other administration methods exist for drugs, each differing by speed of onset and other issues important for medical professionals and drug developers. Later in this section, discussion of another issue, first-pass metabolism, presents further differences between drug injection routes.

Stop & Check

1. What are the four primary phases of drug pharmacokinetics?
2. The administration route for a drug is important for the _____ phase of pharmacokinetics.

1. Absorption, distribution, metabolism, and elimination *2.* absorption

Distribution

distribution Passage of a drug through the circulatory system.

bioavailability Ability of a drug to reach a site of action.

Distribution, the passage of a drug through the body, is the second stage of pharmacokinetics. After absorption of the drug into the bloodstream, the drug may need to cross certain membranes in order to reach the site of drug action. The distribution phase of pharmacokinetics affects a drug's **bioavailability**, the ability of a drug to reach a site of action. For psychoactive drugs, bioavailability depends on the drug reaching the central nervous system. To enter the brain, drugs must possess sufficient properties to permeate the blood–brain barrier (covered in Chapter 2).

REVIEW! Uncharged, lipid soluble and relatively small drugs can pass through the blood–brain barrier. Chapter 2 (pg. 51).

The psychoactive drugs presented in this book pass through the blood–brain barrier, although some psychoactive drugs cross this barrier better than others. In fact, poor bioavailability often ends clinical trial testing to experimental drugs. For example, the experimental antipsychotic drug SR-142801 (Osanetant) exhibited antipsychotic-like effects during preclinical testing. After approval by the Food and Drug Administration for clinical trial testing,

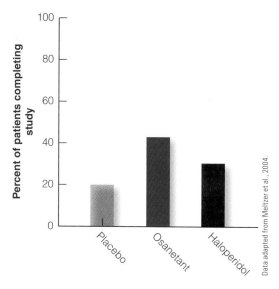

Data adapted from Meltzer et al., 2004.

figure 4.3

In a 6-week study that compared the experimental antipsychotic drug Osanetant to the antipsychotic drug Haldol and a placebo for the treatment of schizophrenia, more patients chose to remain on Osanetant during the entire study. Osanetant was later abandoned from clinical testing because higher doses failed to provide greater efficacy for schizophrenia, and this was likely the result of poor passage through the blood–brain barrier.

Osanetant proved only modestly better than haloperidol, an antipsychotic drug currently on the market (**figure 4.3**). This study revealed that Osanetant's efficacy, albeit modest, was positively correlated with blood plasma levels, indicating that Osanetant was sufficiently absorbed into the bloodstream (Meltzer, Arvanitis, Bauer, & Rein, 2004).

However, in unpublished follow-up studies, higher doses of Osanetant failed to provide any greater improvement for schizophrenia, suggesting that the drug did not permeate the blood–brain barrier sufficiently to provide stronger antipsychotic effects (Meltzer & Prus, 2006). In other words, Osanetant had poor bioavailability, which subsequently halted its further testing.

The placental barrier is also important to consider for drug effects. However, unlike the blood–brain barrier, virtually all drugs taken by the mother can permeate the placental barrier and enter the placenta. Thus, the ease of drug permeability through this barrier may allow harmful effects on a fetus.

Another factor for drug distribution is **nonspecific binding,** or the binding of the drug to sites that are not the intended target for drug effects. This may occur in the form of protein binding, which means that the drug binds to proteins in the bloodstream. By remaining bound to proteins in the bloodstream, drugs cannot cross the blood–brain barrier. Another form of nonspecific binding is depot binding, which is the binding of drugs to receptors or other parts of the body that the drug does not affect.

nonspecific binding
Binding of a drug to sites that are not the intended target for drug effects.

Metabolism

drug metabolism
Process of converting a drug into one or more metabolites.

metabolite Product resulting of enzymatic transformation of a drug.

Drug metabolism is the process of converting a drug into one or more other products called **metabolites**. This conversion most often takes place in the liver, but metabolism of a drug may also occur in other areas such as the stomach. Most drugs are broken down by members of the CYP-1, CYP-2, and CYP-3 cytochrome P450 enzymes.

These enzymes can play an important role in a person's response to a drug. For example, some individuals have a poor rate of metabolism for antidepressant drugs (Tiwari, Souza, & Muller, 2009). For these individuals, who are referred to as *poor metabolizers*, the appropriate enzymes for an antidepressant drug may either be too few or, because of gene polymorphisms, have a diminished ability to metabolize antidepressant drugs. Poor metabolizers tend to have greater treatment sensitivity for certain drugs because the drug remains for a longer duration in unmetabolized form in the body. Although some individuals may be poor metabolizers, others may be *ultrarapid metabolizers*. Ultrarapid metabolizers can exhibit opposite characteristics compared to poor metabolizers, such as greater levels of an enzyme or a greater ability of enzymes to metabolize antidepressant drugs. Unlike poor metabolizers, ultrarapid metabolizers tend to have weaker treatment sensitivity for certain drugs because the drug remains for a shorter duration in unmetabolized form in the body.

REVIEW! A polymorphism is a difference in the gene that encodes for a trait, such as a protein. Chapter 2 (pg. 56).

Learning whether someone exhibits a difference in speed of drug metabolism is important when prescribing drugs. For example, if an individual exhibits ultrarapid metabolism for antidepressant drugs metabolized by CYP2C19 enzymes, then a physician might prescribe an antidepressant drug not metabolized by CYP2C19 enzymes such as fluoxetine (Prozac). Blood testing for these enzymatic activities provides an important approach for **personalized medicine**, a method of prescribing drugs most appropriate for a patient's unique biological makeup.

personalized medicine
Method of prescribing drugs most appropriate for a patient's unique biological makeup.

first-pass metabolism Metabolism of a drug begins to occur before the drug reaches the site of action.

In some cases, metabolism of the drug begins to occur before the drug reaches the site of action. This process is called **first-pass metabolism** and most often occurs with drugs administered orally (**figure 4.4**). For example, approximately 90 percent of buspirone (BuSpar), a treatment for anxiety, converts to metabolites in the stomach before absorption occurs. Thus, for some drugs, first-pass metabolism substantially reduces the amount of drug available for biological effects.

A drug's metabolites may help to explain its effects. First, metabolites may act in the body. These actions could be harmful, or they may interact with another drug a patient is taking. Second, the metabolites of a drug may offer pharmacological effects of their own. In this case, the metabolite is referred to as an *active* metabolite. For example, enzymes convert the antipsychotic drug quetiapine (Seroquel) to the metabolite N-desalkylquetiapine, which functions as an antidepressant drug (Jensen et al., 2007). Alternatively, an active metabolite that is converted from an inert compound is called a **prodrug**.

prodrug A biologically active compound converted, through metabolism, from an inert substance.

Third, metabolites reveal the substances a person used. For example, most drug-screening tests used during job screening detect metabolites of

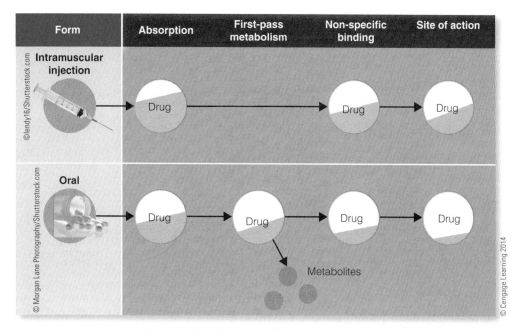

Form	Absorption	First-pass metabolism	Non-specific binding	Site of action
Intramuscular injection	Drug		Drug	Drug
Oral	Drug	Drug → Metabolites	Drug	Drug

figure 4.4 Several factors reduce the amount of drug available to produce behavioral effects as the drug is distributed through the bloodstream. After absorption, a drug may bind to nonspecific sites in the bloodstream or body, reducing how much of it is available to bind to the sites of action. Orally administered drugs are susceptible to first-pass metabolism, further reducing the amount of drug available to bind to sites of action. Finally, membrane barriers, such as the blood–brain barrier, may further reduce the amount of drug available for binding to sites of action.

controlled substances. Probation programs also employ drug tests that assess metabolites as indicators of illicit substance use.

Elimination

elimination Process for how a drug leaves the body.

Elimination is the last stage of pharmacokinetics. **Elimination** is the process by which a drug leaves the body. The body eliminates drugs through urine, feces, sweat, saliva, and breath, although the particular route of elimination depends on the drug. For example, the body eliminates alcohol partly through breath. Given this, law enforcement officials use breathalyzers to determine if an individual consumed alcohol.

elimination rate Amount of drug eliminated from the body over time.

Drugs have an **elimination rate**—that is, the amount of drug eliminated from the body over time. Physicians rely on drug elimination rates when prescribing how frequently a patient should take a medication. The elimination rate for most drugs occurs in half-lives. A **half-life** is the duration of time necessary for the body to eliminate half of a drug, usually based on measuring drug concentration in blood. A drug eliminated in half-lives is referred to as having *first-order kinetics*.

half-life Duration of time necessary for the body to eliminate half of a drug.

Figure 4.5 provides an illustration of a drug eliminated in half-lives. For the drug in the left panel, half of the drug leaves the body, as determined by

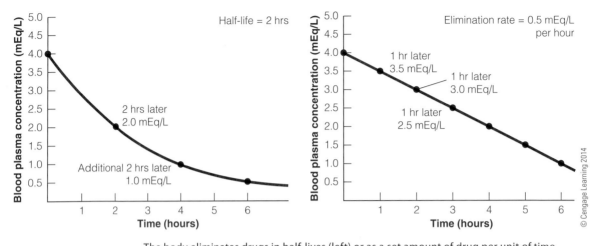

The body eliminates drugs in half-lives (left) or as a set amount of drug per unit of time (right). For elimination according to half-lives, half of a drug is eliminated from the body per unit of time. The drug in the left panel eliminates by half every 2 hours. However, the drug in the right panel eliminates 0.5 milliequivalents of blood per liter (mEq/L) every 30 minutes.

figure 4.5

concentration in blood plasma, every 2 hours. It is important to note that the amount of drug eliminated differs for every half-life. After the first half-life shown, a 2.0 milliequivalent of blood per liter (mEq/L) of drug was eliminated after 2 hours. Two hours later, 1.0 mEq/L of drug was eliminated. Two hours after this, only 0.5 mEq/L of drug was eliminated. Each time the exact amount of drug eliminated differs.

However, not all drugs follow first-order kinetics for elimination. For other drugs, the elimination rate varies by dose or drug levels in blood. For example, the body eliminates approximately 10 to 14 ml of 100 percent alcohol per hour. Thus, if someone ingested 20 milliliters of alcohol relatively quickly, the body would eliminate all of the alcohol after about 2 hours. Alcohol and other drugs that are not eliminated in set half-lives are described as having zero-order kinetics. The graph on the right in figure 4.5 shows a fictional drug eliminated according to zero-order kinetics.

The elimination rates of drugs determine how long a drug's effects will last. Physicians use elimination rate information when prescribing how frequently patients should take a medication. In doing so, they can have patients take the next dose of medication at a time when the effects from the previous treatment begin to subside. In doing so, drug effects reach a steady state.

A steady state is a sustained level of drug in the body. This is why a doctor may prescribe a drug to be taken, for example, three times a day: The drug's half-life might be about 6–8 hours. Thus, as approximately half of the drug is still in the body 6–8 hours later, the next administration of the drug would boost the drug concentrations back to therapeutically effective levels. **Figure 4.6** provides an illustration of a dosing schedule that achieves a steady state for drug concentration in blood.

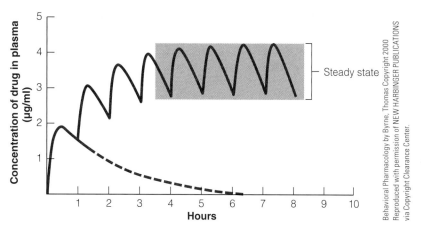

figure 4.6 The half-life of a drug can be used to determine when later administrations of the drug should be given. Eventually, a steady state can develop between the rate of drug elimination from a previous administration and the rate of drug absorption from the next administration.

Stop & Check

1. What is bioavailability?
2. What type of enzymes metabolize most drugs?
3. How might first-pass metabolism affect a drug's pharmacological effects?
4. Why is a steady state important for therapeutic drug effects?

1. Bioavailability describes a drug's ability to reach its site of action. **2.** Cytochrome P450 enzymes **3.** First-pass metabolism consists of the conversion of drug molecules to metabolites, causing less of a drug to be available for reaching its site of action. **4.** As a medical treatment, sustained drug effects are usually necessary to combat a particular illness. Thus, physicians derive a treatment schedule to achieve a steady state for drug effects.

Pharmacodynamics: Describing the Actions of Drugs

pharmacodynamics
Mechanisms of action for a drug.

Pharmacodynamics refers to the mechanisms of action for a drug. For many psychoactive drugs, particularly those covered in this text, pharmacodynamics deal largely with the actions of a drug at synapses. Psychoactive drugs alter neurotransmission at the synapses.

Depending on a drug's unique characteristics, it may alter any stage of neurotransmission. As presented in Chapter 3, neurotransmission consists of synaptic events that include action potentials reaching the axon terminal, the influx of calcium, the fusing of vesicles to membrane walls, and the emptying of stored neurotransmitters into the synaptic cleft. Within the synaptic cleft, neurotransmitters may bind to receptors. Then neurotransmission terminates. The following paragraphs provide examples of drug actions occurring at different stages of neurotransmission.

REVIEW! Termination of neurotransmission occurs when enzymes convert a neurotransmitter into metabolites, membrane transporters return neurotransmitters to the axon terminal, or transporters draw neurotransmitters into astrocytes. Chapter 3 (pg. 75).

First, certain substances can interfere with the propagation of action potentials. For example, a toxin called *tetrodotoxin*, found in the puffer fish, prevents action potentials from occurring. Tetrodotoxin does so by blocking Na^+ channels, which causes a cessation in neurotransmission. Through these actions, puffer fish paralyze any prey they successfully inject. For nervous system research, neuroscientists administer tetrodotoxin to different brain structures in animals to temporarily disable a structure's functioning. As a result, neuroscientists learn about a structure's effects on the functioning of other structures in the brain as well as the importance a structure has for behavior.

REVIEW! Action potentials consist of the rapid influx of Na^+ ions through open Na^+ channels. Chapter 3 (pg. 71).

Figure 4.7 provides examples of drug actions on dopamine neurotransmission. Many substances can alter the synthesis for dopamine. The precursor molecule for dopamine, L-3,4-dihydroxyphenylalanine, which is usually referred to as "L-DOPA," also serves as a drug for the treatment of Parkinson's disease, a movement disorder produced by the destruction of dopamine neurons in the nigrostriatal pathway. By increasing the number of L-DOPA molecules within dopamine neurons, L-DOPA administration leads to an increased production of dopamine. In doing so, L-DOPA counteracts dopamine loss in Parkinson's disease. Unfortunately, these drug effects fail to prevent further dopamine neuron loss in this progressive degenerative disease. Eventually, the neural loss reaches a point when no medication provides sufficient relief of Parkinson's symptoms.

Drugs also may interfere with neurotransmitter storage in vesicles. The psychostimulant drug amphetamine interferes with dopamine storage by entering dopamine vesicles and expelling dopamine. Subsequently, dopamine leaks out from the axon terminal and enters the synaptic cleft. Within the cleft, dopamine binds to dopamine receptors, causing an increase in dopamine transmission (Pifl, Drobny, Reither, Hornykiewicz, & Singer, 1995).

Drugs may also interfere with the binding of a neurotransmitter to a receptor. Figure 4.7 shows an antipsychotic drug called haloperidol binding to a dopamine D_2 receptor. Haloperidol acts through a basic receptor mechanism called *receptor antagonism*. As a receptor antagonist, haloperidol binds to the D_2 receptor and prevents dopamine from binding to and activating the D_2 receptor. Through this action, haloperidol prevents dopamine neurotransmission through the D_2 receptors (Seeman, Chau-Wong, Tedesco, & Wong, 1975). The next section of this chapter describes receptor antagonism, as well as other drug actions at receptors, in greater detail.

Drugs can alter the activity of enzymes that break down neurotransmitters. Figure 4.7 shows a drug bound to both the monoamine oxidase (MAO) and catechol-O-methyltransferase (COMT). For MAO, an antidepressant drug called *moclobemide* binds to and prevents MAO from breaking down dopamine (Stefanis, Alevizos, & Papadimitriou, 1982). As described in greater

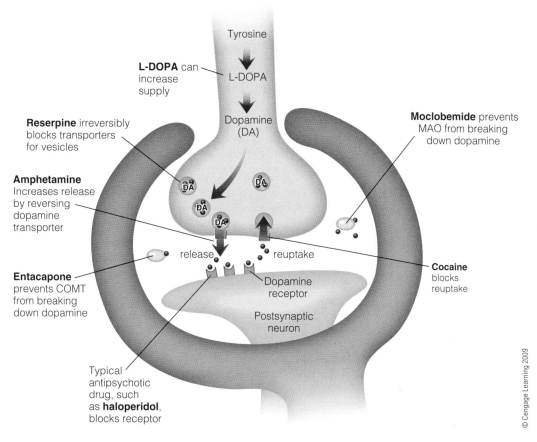

figure 4.7 Drugs can alter any step in neurotransmission, including synthesis of a neurotransmitter, storage of a neurotransmission, synaptic release of a neurotransmission, enzymatic breakdown of a neurotransmitter, and reuptake of a neurotransmitter. Drugs may also act on receptors for neurotransmitters.

detail in Chapter 14, MAO inhibitors such as moclobemide may reduce depressive symptoms by enhancing neurotransmission of dopamine, as well as the neurotransmitters serotonin and norepinephrine.

Figure 4.7 also shows a drug called *entacapone* acting on the enzyme COMT. Entacapone belongs to a class of drugs called COMT inhibitors. Like MAO inhibitors, COMT inhibitors also increase dopamine levels. COMT inhibitors serve as another treatment option for Parkinson's disease (Guttman et al., 1993).

Many drugs also interfere with the reuptake of neurotransmitters. Figure 4.7 shows the psychostimulant drug cocaine bound to the dopamine transporter. Cocaine blocks the dopamine transporter preventing dopamine from entering the axon terminal. This results in increased dopamine levels in the synaptic cleft and the continuation of dopamine neurotransmission.

REVIEW! The dopamine transporter sends dopamine from the synaptic cleft into a dopamine axon terminal. Chapter 3 (pg. 86).

Stop & Check

1. How does the drug L-DOPA increase dopamine levels?
2. How might a drug, by acting on a neurotransmitter storage vesicle, cause an elevation of the neurotransmitter in a synapse?

1. Increasing the availability of L-DOPA, a precursor of dopamine, increases the synthesis of dopamine, thus leading to greater dopamine levels in the body. 2. Like amphetamine, a drug may block the neurotransmitter transporter at the vesicle or re-place the neurotransmitter in the storage vesicle. Either way, neurotransmitters that are not stored likely permeate through the terminal membrane, leading to increased levels of the neurotransmitter in the synaptic cleft.

box 4.1 Radioligand Binding for Measuring Receptor Affinity

Radioligand binding is an important technique for studying the affinity and efficacy that drugs have for receptors. The term *ligand* refers to a chemical substance that binds to a receptor. Thus, the term refers to both drugs and neurotransmitters. A radioligand is produced by adding a radioactive element to a ligand.

Researchers conduct most radioligand experiments using dissected brain tissue that was mixed together with a chemical solution called a *buffer*, forming a homogenized solution of brain tissue and buffer. Another approach uses a large collection of cells grown in culture, referred to as *cell lines*, for radioligand experiments. After preparing the brain tissue using either method, researchers apply the radioligand to the tissue solution.

Afterward, the tissue solution, which contains both brain tissue and the radioligand, is passed through a filter. These filters allow the buffer solution to pass through but not brain tissue to pass through. After filtering, the filter contains brain tissue along with any of the radioligand bound to receptors in the brain tissue.

Researchers then use radioactivity counters on the filters. If the drug successfully binds to receptors in the brain tissue, then the researchers will find high radioactivity counts in the filters. However, if the radioligand bound to few if any receptors in the tissue, then the radioligand would have passed through the filter with the rest of the solution. In this case, researchers would detect low radioactivity counts from the filter.

Box 4.1 figure 1 shows an example of a radioligand binding experiment. This example shows, using a percentage, how many receptors the drug occupied. The y-axis of this graph shows the percentage of receptor occupied. The x-axis shows the different amounts of radioligand used, shown as the drug concentration expressed as molality. *Molality*, a term used in chemistry, refers to the number of moles (mol) per volume of

solution. A *mole* refers to the number of grams of a substance divided by the molecular weight of the substance.

The term called B_{max}, the abbreviation for *maximum binding potential*, refers the amount of drug that fully binds to population of receptors. In figure 1, the B_{max} value of the radioligand is 10^{-3} M (or 0.001 M), the concentration that occupies 100 percent of the population of receptors. The K_d value, or **dissociation constant,** refers to the amount of drug that occupies 50 percent of receptors. Drugs with low K_d values can achieve 50 percent receptor occupancy at lower drug concentrations than drugs with higher K_d values. For interpreting these data, the lower the K_d value, the greater a drug's receptor affinity.

An alternative approach for assessing receptor affinities produces an inhibition constant, or K_i value. The approach

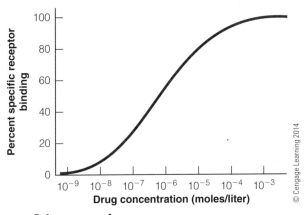

box 4.1, figure 1
This figure shows percent occupancy with the percentage of receptors for a population shown on the y-axis and the drug concentration on the x-axis, expressed in molality. See box 4.1 for further details.

© Cengage Learning 2014

Psychoactive Drugs and Receptors

As one of the many ways that a drug can alter neurotransmission described in the previous section, most psychoactive drugs act on receptors for neurotransmitters. The actions of a drug at a receptor depend on how well a drug binds to the receptor and the effects a drug has on the receptor. Researchers describe these two considerations as *binding affinity* and *receptor efficacy*. **Binding affinity** refers to a drug's strength of binding to a receptor, and **receptor efficacy** refers to a drug's ability to alter the activity of receptor.

Researchers measure a drug's binding affinity using techniques described in **Box 4.1**. These techniques result in a value for drug called a dissociation

binding affinity Drug's strength of binding to a receptor.

receptor efficacy Drug's ability to alter the activity of receptor.

---

uses similar radioligand experimental procedures, except that K_i values are derived by assessing the competition between two different drugs. Only one of the drugs serves as the radioligand; the other drug is not radioactive.

For this procedure, a researcher places both the radioligand and the nonradioactive drug into the same brain tissue solution. In this way, the researcher assesses the affinity of the nonradioactive drug by how well it binds to these receptors in the presence of the radioligand. The compound with the higher receptor affinity outcompetes the compound with the lower receptor affinity. In this case, fewer radioactivity counts indicate that the nonradioactive compound had a greater receptor affinity than the radioligand.

Box 4.1 figure 2 shows an example of a K_i experiment. Like figure 1, this graph provides the concentration of a drug—in this case, the nonradioactive drug—on the x-axis. In this figure, however, the y-axis refers to the percentage of receptors bound by the radioligand. According to the figure, greater receptor occupancy by the radioligand occurred with the lowest concentration of the nonradioactive drug, whereas lower receptor occupancy by the radioligand occurred with the highest

radioligand binding Research technique used to study the affinity and efficacy that drugs have for receptors.

concentration of the nonradioactive drug. The K_i value represents the concentration of the nonradioactive compound that caused the radioactive compound to provide 50 percent receptor occupancy.

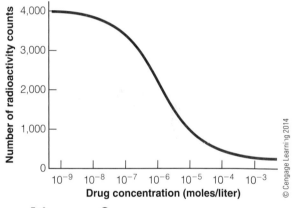

box 4.1, figure 2
This figure shows a K_i experiment as described in box 4.1. The y-axis shows radioactivity counts, and the x-axis shows the concentration for the nonradioactive drug.

dissociation constant Amount of drug that occupies 50 percent of receptors.

Stop & Check

1. By determining the drug concentration that occupies 50 percent of a specific receptor population, the _____, an index of binding affinity, can be calculated.

2. If drug A has a K_d equal to 20 nM and drug B has a K_d equal to 5 nM for a particular receptor, then which drug has a greater affinity for the receptor?

1. K_d **2.** Drug B has the greatest affinity for the receptor. The K_d value indicates that at the same concentration, drug B occupied more receptors than drug A did. As a rule, the smaller the k_D value, the greater the affinity.

table **4.2**

The Dissociation Constant (K_d) in nM* for Dopamine and Selected Antipsychotic Drugs at the Dopamine D_2 Receptor	
Substance	**K_d (in nM)**
Chlorpromazine	4.8
Haloperidol	2.6
Chlorprothixene	8.0
Dopamine	544

*n = nano, M = molality

Data from: Richelson and Nelson, 1984, Richelson and Souder 2000, Seeman 2001 and Sokoloff et al., 1992.

constant, generally noted as K_d, or an inhibition constant, noted as K_i. These values derive from the level of drug concentration necessary to bind to receptors. For both constants, *the lower the value, the greater a drug's binding affinity*.

The previous section, which presented the different ways a drug can alter neurotransmission, used the antipsychotic drug haloperidol as an example of a drug binding to a dopamine D_2 receptor. **Table 4.2** shows haloperidol's binding affinity to the D_2 receptor as well as the binding affinity of dopamine for the D_2 receptor. You may be surprised to see that haloperidol has a far greater affinity for the dopamine D_2 receptor than dopamine does. This is another important point about drugs: They can often outcompete a receptor's natural neurotransmitter.

Drugs may produce a variety of different effects on receptors. Drugs' primary receptor actions include *agonism, antagonism, partial agonism, inverse agonism, negative modulation,* and *positive modulation*. Receptor theorists have developed models in an attempt to characterize the type of receptor changes a drug can produce. Early and more basic receptor theory models described the actions of agonists and antagonists, whereas modern and more complex receptor models describe other receptor action models (Brink et al. 2004).

Many modern receptor theory models are referred to as *ternary receptor models* (*ternary* means "threefold"). These models describe receptor actions by including a drug, a receptor, and a change in G-protein activity. **Box 4.2** presents a method used to determine a drug's efficacy at a receptor. **Figure 4.8** presents the basic features of ternary models to describe the effects of drugs acting as agonists, antagonists, partial agonists, or inverse agonists. The "Before" column in figure 4.8 refers to the receptor state before a drug binds to it. The "Briefly" column illustrates a transition process that occurs when a drug first binds to the receptor, and the "After" column illustrates the subsequent changes that the drug causes to a receptor's G protein.

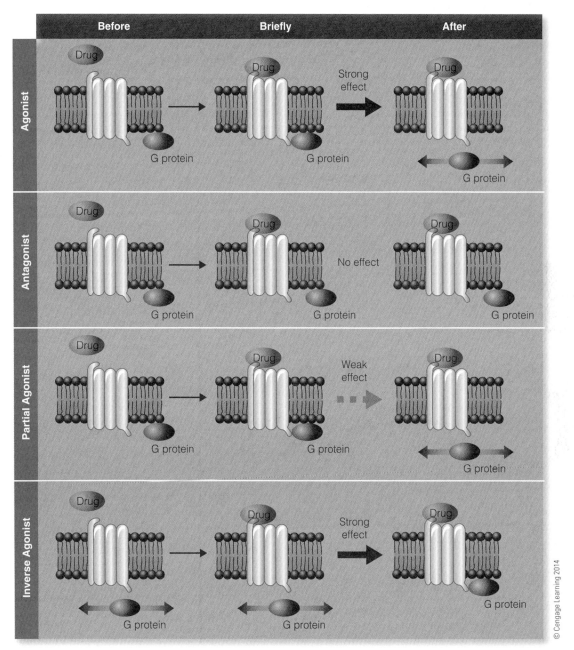

	Before	Briefly	After
Agonist	Drug / G protein	Drug / G protein	Strong effect → Drug / G protein
Antagonist	Drug / G protein	Drug / G protein	No effect — Drug / G protein
Partial Agonist	Drug / G protein	Drug / G protein	Weak effect ⇢ Drug / G protein
Inverse Agonist	Drug / G protein	Drug / G protein	Strong effect → Drug / G protein

© Cengage Learning 2014

figure 4.8 Drugs can have different types of action at receptors. An agonist (first row) will bind to a receptor (second column) and cause the receptor to shift into an active state (third column). The strong preference for the active state is indicated by the thick arrow. An antagonist (second row) will bind to a receptor but fail to shift the receptor into an active state (i.e., no effect). A partial agonist (third row) will bind to a receptor but is weaker, compared to an agonist, for shifting the receptor into an active state, as shown by the dashed line. An inverse agonist (fourth row) will bind to a receptor, but if the receptor already has constituents that are active (e.g., a G protein), then the drug will inhibit this activity.

box **4.2** The [^{35}S]GTPγS Binding Assay Assesses G-Protein Activation

The process of activating and deactivating G proteins, depends on two biochemicals: guanosine diphosphate (GTD) and guanosine triphosphate (GTP). Before receptor activation by a neurotransmitter, GDP is bound to the inactive alpha subunit of a G protein. When a neurotransmitter or agonist activates a receptor, GTP replaces GDP on the alpha subunit, and this switch from GDP and GTP characterizes an active

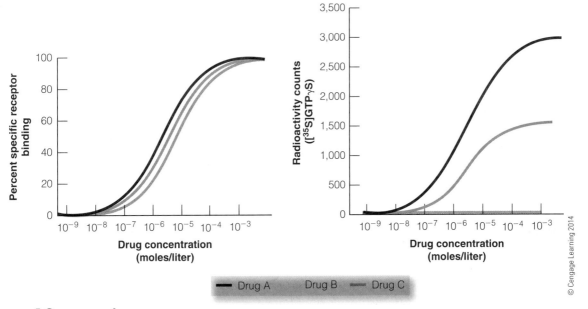

box **4.2**, figure **1**

The graph on the left shows the percentage of a receptor population occupied by three different drugs. The graph on the right shows the number of [^{35}S]GTPγS radioactivity counts. The x-axis for both figures refers to the concentration of drug expressed in molality (i.e., moles per liter). Refer to the text for further information about these figures.

REVIEW! Metabotropic receptors cause changes within neurons by activating G proteins. Chapter 3 (pg. 78).

agonist Drug that activates a neurotransmitter receptor.

An **agonist** refers to a drug that activates a neurotransmitter receptor. Researchers also refer to agonists as *full agonists* to contrast these drugs with partial agonists, described shortly. For the first line of figure 4.8, a drug acting as an agonist approaches an inactive receptor. The "Before" column represents the inactivity of the receptor by showing a stationary G protein adjacent to the receptor. When the agonist binds to the receptor, the G protein draws close to the receptor, as shown in the "Briefly" column. The "Briefly" column for an agonist shows a ternary complex consisting of both a drug and a G protein

G-protein state. This active G-protein state ends when the alpha subunit hydrolyzes GTP, causing a conversion from GTP to GDP. With GDP attached to the alpha subunit, the G protein returns to an inactive state, just as it was before the receptor was activated by a neurotransmitter.

The [^{35}S]GTPγS binding assay employs a radioactivity compound to assess the ability of drugs to activate G proteins. Because this is a binding assay, the procedure used involves tissue and radioactivity counting procedures similar to those described in box 4.1. [^{35}S]GTPγS is an analog of GTP, and as an analog it can replace GTP when the G protein is activated. However, unlike GTP, researchers can measure [^{35}S]GTPγS using radioactivity counters. Another advantage of [^{35}S]GTPγS is that the alpha subunit cannot convert it into GDP. Thus, the label of an active G protein does not vanish before researchers can measure radioactivity counts.

Box 4.2 figure 1 shows a graph providing the ability of three drugs to bind to a receptor (left) and the ability to activate the receptor as measured using [^{35}S]GTPγS (right). As shown in the left graph, each drug fully occupies the population of receptors and does so at similar doses. Yet the [^{35}S]GTPγS assay demonstrates that these drugs have different abilities to activate the receptor. At high enough concentrations, drug A exhibits full radioactivity counts, demonstrating full activation of the receptors' G proteins. Drug B achieves no more than half of drug A's radioactivity counts. Finally, drug C results in no radioactivity counts from [^{35}S]GTPγS. Try to identify the receptor actions of these drugs based on their results in the [^{35}S]GTPγS assay. Refer to figure 4.8 and box 4.1 for this. See the following Stop & Check section for these receptor actions in box 4.2, figure 1.

Stop & Check

1. How might using a [^{35}S]GTPγS assay clarify a drug's receptor actions?
2. What are the receptor actions for the drug illustrated in box 4.2, figure 1?

1. The [^{35}S]GTPγS assay assesses the level of G-protein activity engendered after receptor activation. In this way, the [^{35}S]GTPγS assay serves as a marker of receptor activation. 2. The illustration reveals that drug A functions as a full agonist because it fully activates G proteins. Drug B functions as a partial agonist because, within a population of receptors, drug B fails to activate all of the G proteins. Finally, drug C acts as an antagonist—it lacks the capacity to activate receptors.

bound to the receptor. Afterward, as shown in the after column, the G protein separates from the receptor and elicits biological actions within the neuron.

REVIEW! When activated, G proteins separate into alpha and beta-gamma subunits which activate ion channels or enzymes. Chapter 3 (pg. 78).

antagonist Drug that fails to activate a receptor.

The second row of figure 4.8 shows a drug action as an antagonist. Unlike an agonist, an **antagonist** refers to a drug that fails to activate a receptor. Referring to the model shown in figure 4.8, an antagonist fails to produce a ternary complex, meaning that an antagonist fails to cause a G protein to temporarily bind to the receptor. Without the G protein being activated, no other changes within the neuron occur.

partial agonist Drug that possesses a weaker efficacy for activating receptors than a full agonist.

inverse agonist Drug that reduces a receptor's constitutive activity.

competitive antagonists Drug that binds to the same site as a neurotransmitter, preventing a neurotransmitter from binding to the receptor.

noncompetitive antagonist Drug that does not prevent a neurotransmitter from binding to the receptor but does prevent the neurotransmitter from activating the receptor.

positive modulator Drug that binds increases the ability of a neurotransmitter to bind to and activate a receptor.

The third line of figure 4.8 presents a drug acting as a **partial agonist**—that is, it possesses a weaker efficacy for activating receptors than a full agonist. These weaker effects mean that a partial agonist may activate a receptor or it may be unable to activate a receptor. In figure 4.8, a partial agonist causes a G protein to shift toward the receptor in the "Briefly" column. After this, the G protein may remain bound to the receptor or it may separate and elicit effects within a neuron.

The drug action shown on the fourth line, inverse agonism, differs from the other actions described so far. In this case, the G protein is in an active state before a drug binds to the receptor. This baseline level of G protein activity is called *constitutive activity*, and some level of constitutive activity is not uncommon for receptors. An **inverse agonist** refers to a drug that reduces a receptor's constitutive activity. In the example in figure 4.8, the inverse agonist binds to the receptor and, as shown in the "After" column, causes the deactivation of the G protein.

Although these previous examples concerned metabotropic receptors, similar drug effects occur at ionotropic receptors. For an ionotropic receptor, an agonist causes the attached channel to open, allowing ions to pass in or out of the neuron. On the other hand, an antagonist binds to an ionotropic receptor but fails to open the channel.

For ionotropic receptors, drugs may act as competitive or noncompetitive antagonists. The antagonists defined so far served as **competitive antagonists** because they bind to the same site as a neurotransmitter, preventing a neurotransmitter from binding to the receptor. The antipsychotic drug haloperidol, as presented previously, functions as a competitive antagonist for dopamine D_2 receptors. A **noncompetitive antagonist**, however, does not prevent a neurotransmitter from binding to the receptor, but it does prevent the neurotransmitter from activating the receptor. For example, phencyclidine (PCP), a drug of abuse, functions as a noncompetitive antagonist for glutamate NMDA* receptors. Glutamate can bind to an NMDA receptor, but PCP prevents ions from passing through the receptor.

For an ionotropic receptor, the term *partial agonist* is generally used to describe drugs that occupy a receptor but do not fully activate the receptor (**figure 4.9**). In this case, the ion channel partially opens, allowing fewer ions to flow through than if the ion channel is fully open. For example, the drug kainate functions as a partial agonist for the glutamate ionotropic AMPA** $GluR_4$ receptor because the amount of ions that kainate causes to flow through the channel are far less than the full agonist AMPA or the neurotransmitter glutamate causes (Arinaminpathy, Sansom, & Biggin, 2002; Armstrong & Gouaux, 2000).

Drugs may also act as negative or positive modulators of ionotropic receptors. These drugs bind to *allosteric* sites—that is, sites different than the ones neurotransmitters bind to—on the receptor. A **positive modulator** is a chemical substance that binds to an allosteric site on the receptor and

*N-methyl-D-aspartate.
**α-amino-3-hydroxy-5-methyl-4-isoxazole proprionic acid.

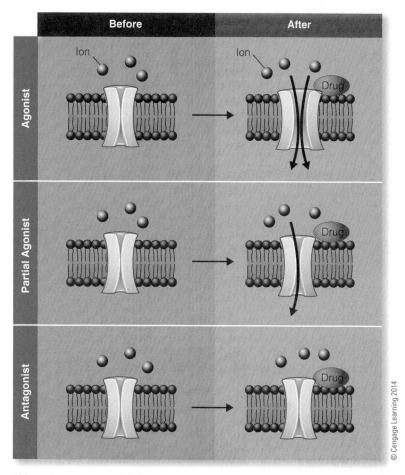

Although an agonist will fully activate an ionotropic receptor, causing the channel to fully open, a partial agonist may only partially activate an ionotropic receptor and the channel will only partially open. In these cases, more ions can flow through the fully open channel than can flow through a partially open channel. An antagonist fails to change the channel configuration at all.

figure 4.9

negative modulator
Drug that decreases the ability of a neurotransmitter to bind to and activate the receptor.

increases the ability of a neurotransmitter to bind to and activate the receptor. A **negative modulator** decreases the ability of a neurotransmitter to bind to and activate the receptor.

Many drugs act as positive or negative modulators for $GABA_A$ receptors. For example, a benzodiazepine drug such as alprazolam (Xanax) binds to a site named after these drugs called the *benzodiazepine site*. This site is physically separate from the binding site for GABA. As such, benzodiazepines fail to activate a $GABA_A$ receptor, yet by binding to the benzodiazepine site, the receptor undergoes a change that enhances its affinity for GABA. In this way, a benzodiazepine drug serves as a positive modulator for $GABA_A$ receptors.

Stop & Check

1. A drug that prevents the activation of a receptor but does not bind to the same site as a neurotransmitter is called a _____.

2. A drug that increases the ability of a ionotropic receptor to be activated by a neurotransmitter is called a _____.

1. noncompetitive antagonist *2.* positive modulator

Neurotoxins and Damage to the Nervous System

neurotoxins Substances that damage or destroy parts of the nervous system.

environmental neurotoxicology a field devoted to the study of neurotoxins in the environment.

Although this chapter pertains to the properties of psychoactive drugs, toxins also have important properties that alter nervous system functioning. **Neurotoxins** are substances that damage or destroy parts of the nervous system. Some of these toxins are found in venoms. Mentioned in this chapter, the toxin released from puffer fish called *tetrodotoxin* prevents neurotransmission by blocking Na^+ channels. Another venom called *alpha-bungorotoxin*, which is found in the Taiwanese banded krait and other types of snakes, blocks nicotinic cholinergic receptors at neuromuscular junctions. Through interfering with neurotransmission, these toxins induce paralysis to make it easier for the predator to consume its prey.

Environmental neurotoxicology is a field devoted to the study of neurotoxins in the environment. Many toxins are found in our everyday environment. Chemicals classified as *endocrine disruptors*—named for their interference with the endocrine system, including dysfunctions in the reproductive system, nervous system, and immune system—are commonly found in pesticides, plastics, flame retardants, and many types of building materials. In particular, many household plastics contain the endocrine disruptor bisphenol-A (BPA), one of the better-known endocrine disruptors.

Environmental neurotoxins also include heavy metals such as lead and mercury. Lead exposure in particular may damage neurons and can contribute to learning problems in children. We encounter lead more than we think. Aside from the lead found in computer monitors or other electronics, buildings built before the 1980s likely contain lead-based paints, and lead dust can be released in air, particularly when renovating older buildings.

Researchers study neurotoxins in the same ways that pharmacologists study psychoactive drugs. Neurotoxins may cause *neuronopathy* (the destruction of neurons), *myelinopathy* (the destruction of myelin sheathing), *axonopathy* (the destruction of axons), and *transmission toxicities*. Transmission toxicities consist of damage to processes involved in neurotransmission. Toxins for neurotransmission may destroy storage vesicles for neurotransmitters, irreversibly block receptors, or block enzymes that break down neurotransmitters. For example, sarin gas, a chemical warfare agent developed by German chemists in the 1930s, potently inhibits acetylcholinesterase, the enzyme that breaks down acetylcholine. Massive acetylcholinesterase inhibition leads to muscle constriction throughout the body and overactivation of the parasympathetic nervous system, resulting in impaired breathing and other inhibited organ functions.

Physiological Adaptations to Chronic Drug Use

Chronic drug use is the repeated, usually daily, use of a drug. The body may react differently to a drug when administered chronically compared to an acute administration. Three unique features of chronic drug use include tolerance, sensitization, and dependence (**table 4.3**).

Tolerance refers to an adaption to a drug's effects that requires a user to take greater doses of a drug to achieve the same desired drug effects. Tolerance most often occurs as a result of chronic administration, which occurred for the example of heroin noted previously. Some drugs cause tolerance after acute administration. Acute administration of nicotine, for example, causes an immediate change to nicotinic receptors that results in a temporary tolerance to nicotine's effects (Ochoa & McNamee, 1990).

Three forms of tolerance may occur from drug treatment: pharmacokinetic, pharmacodynamic, and behavioral. In the first form, **pharmacokinetic tolerance** (or *drug dispositional tolerance*), pharmacokinetic actions reduce the amount of drug reaching its site of action. Often pharmacokinetic tolerance

tolerance Adaption to a drug's effects that requires a user to take greater doses of a drug to achieve desired effects.

pharmacokinetic tolerance Pharmacokinetic actions that reduce the amount of drug reaching its site of action.

table **4.3**

Dependence, Tolerance, and Sensitization		
Function	**Type**	**Characteristics**
Tolerance		Drug adaptations require escalating drug doses to achieve desired effects
	Pharmacokinetic	Pharmacokinetic action reduces the amount of drug reaching its site of action
	Pharmacodynamic	Reduced responsiveness at a drug's site of action
	Behavioral	Decreased behavioral responsiveness
	Cross tolerance	Tolerance to other drugs in the same class
Sensitization		Increased responsiveness to a drug's effects
Dependence		Presence of withdrawal symptoms after a period of drug cessation
	Physiological	Physiological withdrawal symptoms such as nausea
	Psychological	Psychological withdrawal symptoms such as drug cravings or mood changes

© Cengage Learning 2014

causes an increased rate of drug conversion to metabolites. For example, a pharmacokinetic tolerance to alcohol occurs when increased levels of an enzyme, alcohol dehydrogenase, cause increased conversion of alcohol to its metabolite. By increasing the conversion of alcohol, alcohol dehydrogenase causes less alcohol to reach the brain.

pharmacodynamic tolerance Reduced responsiveness to a drug at the drug's site of action.

The second form of tolerance, **pharmacodynamic tolerance**, consists of a reduced responsiveness to a drug at the drug's site of action. Chronic administration of the anti-anxiety drug buspirone causes lower levels of serotonin receptors (Taylor & Hyslop, 1991). For buspirone, fewer serotonin receptors lead to weaker drug effects.

behavioral tolerance Decreased behavioral responsiveness while under a drug's effects.

The third form of tolerance, **behavioral tolerance**, produces a decreased behavioral responsiveness for a user under a drug's effects. Alcohol use provides a good example here as well. Studies show that moderate drinkers perform certain behavioral tasks under the effects of alcohol better than those who seldom drink alcohol (Goodwin, Powell, & Stern, 1971; Sdao-Jarvie & Vogel-Sprott, 1991).

cross tolerance Tolerance for other drugs with similar biological actions.

The tolerance effects for a drug may carry over to drugs with similar biological actions. For example, heroin addicts can tolerate a much higher dose of the opioid replacement drug methadone than those not addicted to heroin. This form of tolerance is called **cross tolerance**.

sensitization Increased responsiveness to a drug's effects.

Chronic drug administration may also cause **sensitization**, an increase responsiveness to a drug's effects. Researchers best study sensitization in animal models. Nicotine, which is characterized as a psychostimulant drug, first causes inhibitory effects in laboratory rats. However, after several days of administration, nicotine induces excitatory effects in rats (Rosecrans, Stimler, Hendry, & Meltzer, 1989).

dependence Needing a drug to function normally.

A drug **dependence** consists of a user needing a drug to function normally. During dependence, the absence of a drug leads to withdrawal symptoms. The term *withdrawal syndrome* refers to the collection of withdrawal symptoms for a drug. The nature of withdrawal symptoms defines the type of drug dependence. **Physical dependence** is defined by the presence of physical withdrawal symptoms. For example, physical withdrawal symptoms occurring from abrupt withdrawal of an antidepressant drug may consist of dizziness, nausea, as well as sensations of buzzing or electric shock. **Psychological dependence** is defined by the presence of psychological withdrawal symptoms, which can include drug cravings or changes in mood or behavior.

physical dependence Presence of physical withdrawal symptoms when a drug is not taken.

psychological dependence Presence of psychological withdrawal symptoms when a drug is not taken.

Withdrawal symptoms often result from the body's compensatory adaptive changes to drug actions. When a sufficient period of time without a drug administration occurs, the body's compensatory effects become evident and manifest themselves as withdrawal symptoms. For example, heroin initially produces euphoria, constipation, and pain relief, but after some period of chronic usage, the body develops a tolerance to these effects. Once a tolerance to heroin occurs, cessation of heroin use produces withdrawal symptoms that include depression, diarrhea, and exaggerated sensitivity to pain. The compensatory actions became withdrawal symptoms.

Stop & Check

1. How might a neurotoxin disrupt neurotransmission?
2. A defining feature of drug dependence is the presence of _____.
3. Adaptation to chronic drug administration, as indicated by a dose of drug no longer producing the same magnitude of effects, is called _____.

1. A neurotoxin can affect neurotransmission in a variety of ways, including irreversibly binding to enzymes or destroying synaptic vesicles. **2.** withdrawal symptoms **3.** tolerance

FROM ACTIONS TO EFFECTS
Heroin Tolerance and Environmental Factors

The beginning of this chapter described Siegel's questions about why heroin users experienced an overdose to their usual amount of heroin. Why would a chronic user's normal heroin dose cause an overdose that he apparently should have a tolerance for? From these interviews, Siegel found that most overdose victims reported a significant change in the usual drug injection routine before experiencing an overdose. Siegel suspected that a previous heroin study he conducted in rats might explain this issue.

Siegel and colleagues (1982) had given two groups of rats incrementally increasing doses of heroin during the course of a month, so that at the end of this month, rats tolerated a relatively high dose of heroin (8.0 mg/kg). However, each group of rats received these heroin injections in different environments. The first group received injections in the animal colony room in which the animals were normally housed. The other group received its injections only in a different room that contained a speaker used to generate constant white noise (like radio static).

After one month of daily repeated heroin injections ended, the researchers conducted an overdose test by giving each rat nearly double (15.0 mg/kg) the tolerated dose. In addition, the researchers switched the injection environments for half of the animals; that is, on the overdose test, half of the animals were treated in the same injection room, whereas the other half of the animals were treated in the different injection room.

Figure 4.10 shows the results of this experiment. The researchers found that a significantly greater number of rats died after receiving heroin in a different environment compared to rats receiving heroin in the same environment. Apparently, environmental stimuli facilitated a tolerance to heroin; when these environmental stimuli were removed, the rats demonstrated a weaker tolerance for heroin.

A link between environmental factors and pharmacokinetic tolerance may explain these findings. The researchers suggested

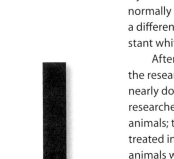

figure 4.10

More heroin-tolerant rats died when injected with high doses of heroin when they were in environments that were different from the ones in which they previously received injections.

(Adapted from Siegel et al., 1982.)

that long-term treatment with heroin resulted in pharmacokinetic tolerance because of increased enzyme activity to break down the heroin. By keeping the injection conditions constant, environmental stimuli occasioned the increased activity of these enzymes, providing for the creation of tolerance. Changing the injection environment removed the stimuli associated with heroin and possibly contributed to a reduced level of enzyme activity for heroin. With enzymes for heroin less active, less heroin was converted. Then because much of the heroin remained in nonmetabolized form in the body, the effects were similar to taking an even higher dose of heroin. Essentially, a routine dose of heroin could in fact be an overdose of heroin without sufficient activity of these enzymes. The results suggest that heroin users who have a typical place and routine for using heroin have developed a tolerance that is promoted by these environment stimuli. Removing these stimuli may result in greater drug effects, possibly accounting for the overdose cases that Siegel observed.

Stop & Check

1. What type of tolerance may have been demonstrated in the study by Siegel and colleagues (1982)?

2. How might environmental stimuli changes increase the likelihood of heroin overdose?

1. The study authors suggested that pharmacokinetic tolerance may have been weakened when the rats were injected in a different environment. **2.** If tolerance failed to sufficiently occur after heroin injection as a result of changes in environment, then the body exhibits a greater sensitivity to heroin's effects. If these differences resulted from pharmacokinetic tolerance, then greater heroin amounts were more available than usual to act within the body.

▶CHAPTER SUMMARY

The field of pharmacology is largely divided into two general areas: pharmacokinetics and pharmacodynamics. Pharmacokinetics concerns the passage of the drug through the body in four phases: absorption, distribution, metabolism, and elimination. Absorption is the ability of a drug to enter the bloodstream, and this depends on the administration route used. Distribution consists of drug passage through the bloodstream and to reaching a drug's site of action. Metabolism refers to the process of enzymatically converting a drug into metabolites. Elimination is the process of expelling drugs from the body.

Pharmacodynamics are the mechanisms of action for a drug. The pharmacodynamics of a psychoactive drug consist of altering neurotransmission, including changes in neurotransmitter synthesis, storage, release, receptor binding, and conversion to metabolites. Drugs have the ability to activate receptors or to prevent the activation of receptors. Further, drugs can alter how well a neurotransmitter binds to and activates a receptor.

Chronic drug use can lead to dependence, tolerance, or sensitization. Drug dependence is shown when abstention from a drug causes withdrawal effects. Dependence occurs as either physiological dependence or psychological dependence. Users exhibit tolerance when they require higher doses to achieve similar effects. Tolerance occurs as pharmacokinetic tolerance, pharmacodynamic tolerance, or behavioral tolerance. Sensitization consists of an increase in responsiveness to a drug over time.

KEY TERMS

Absorption

Distribution

Bioavailability

Nonspecific binding

Drug metabolism

Metabolites

Personalized medicine

First-pass metabolism

Prodrug

Elimination

Elimination rate

Half-life

Pharmacodynamics

Binding affinity

Receptor efficacy

Radioligand binding

Dissociation constant

Agonist

Antagonist

Partial agonist

Inverse agonist

Competitive antagonist

Noncompetitive
    antagonist

Positive modulator

Negative modulator

Neurotoxin

Environmental
    neurotoxicology

Tolerance

Pharmacokinetic tolerance

Pharmacodynamic
    tolerance

Behavioral tolerance

Cross tolerance

Sensitization

Dependence

Physical dependence

Psychological
    dependence

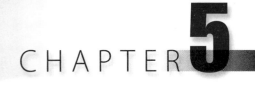

CHAPTER **5**

Drugs of Abuse

James Olds's Important Discovery

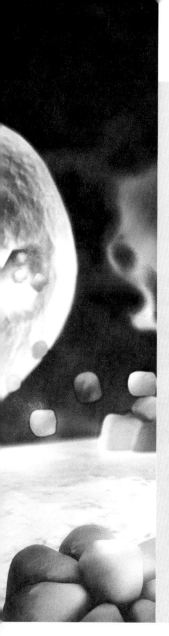

James Olds was firmly convinced when he received a PhD in psychology from Harvard University in 1952 that all valid psychological theories could be successfully linked to nervous system functioning. To further his already promising career, Olds believed he needed only to expand his experimental skill set in order to comprehensively evaluate nervous system processes. Toward this end, Olds gained a postdoctoral fellowship to study under famed psychologist Donald Hebb at McGill University in Montreal. This work would lead to a critical discovery in the field of neuroscience.

Under Hebb, Olds endeavored to study the reticular activating system by quickly contriving a rudimentary brain electrode out of wire and surgically installing it into the brain of a laboratory rat. After the rat recovered from the surgery, Olds allowed the rat to wander around a box as he toggled the connected electrode on and off. Then Olds began to notice something curious. The rat had developed a preference for areas of the box associated with the activated electrode. In fact, Old found that he could purposely attract the rat to different areas of the box with this device.

Olds's electrode had missed the reticular activating system, but instead led to the discovery of the brain's *reward center*. This accidental finding led to a fundamental understanding of a key motivational process for behavior and identified an important biological property for drugs of abuse.

From Olds (1956) and Thompson (1999).

As first presented in Chapter 1, psychoactive drugs broadly fall into two categories: those intended for instrumental use and those intended for recreational use. If you recall, the major distinction between such drugs is a person's intent or motivation for using the substance. This chapter expands on the use of recreational drugs to consider problem drug use leading to abuse and dependence.

REVIEW! A person uses a drug *instrumentally* for a socially acceptable purpose, but uses a drug *recreationally* entirely to experience the drug's effects. Chapter 1 (pg. 5).

Regulatory Agencies and Drug Classification

In addition to describing drugs based on their intended use, we also characterize drugs by their legal status. Laws at the state and national level limit the availability of drugs deemed to have a significant risk of abuse. One of the first national regulations on drugs of abuse was the Harrison Narcotics Act passed in 1915, which restricted the sale of narcotics, primarily opioid drugs, to medical uses. More important, law enforcement officials interpreted these medical uses to exclude treating withdrawal symptoms in opioid dependence.

In 1970, the Controlled Substances Act first described drugs of abuse as *controlled substances*. The act required the legal regulation of certain drugs with abuse potential, and it led to a classification system for ranking drugs by abuse potential and proven medical use. This act led to a classification system that still exists. **Table 5.1** shows a list of selected drugs of abuse controlled in the United States.

The U.S. Drug Enforcement Administration (DEA) uses five schedules to categorize drugs of abuse. Schedule V drugs have relatively low abuse potential and legitimate medical purposes. For example, the DEA assigned schedule V to codeine, an opioid drug and key ingredient in prescription strength cough syrups.

The lower the schedule number, the greater potential for abuse. Schedule II controlled substances have high abuse potential, but legitimate medical uses, according to the DEA. For example, the DEA schedules cocaine as II because of its legitimate medical use as a local anesthetic. Schedule I controlled substances have high abuse potential and no legitimate medical uses. For example, the DEA scheduled the hallucinogenic drug lysergic acid diethylamide (LSD) as schedule I, based on the agency's view of LSD's high abuse potential and lack of medical usefulness. For similar reasons, the DEA also lists cannabis as a schedule I controlled substance.

table **5.1**

Selected Controlled Substances	
Schedule	**Controlled Substance**
I	Heroin LSD Marijuana (cannabis)
II	Cocaine Morphine Phencyclidine (PCP)
III	Ketamine
IV	Alprazolam (Xanax)
V	Codeine

Adapted from the DEA Controlled Substances Schedules. (www.deadiversion.usdoj.gov/schedules/index.html)

Other countries use similar drug schedules or may take a different approach. For example, the United Kingdom assesses the harm caused by abused drugs according to three classification levels. Class A drugs cause the most harm and carry the stiffest penalties for possession and drug dealing. These drugs include MDMA (Ecstasy), cocaine, and psychedelic mushrooms. Class C drugs cause the least harm and carry the lightest penalties for possession and drug dealing. This class includes barbiturates, ketamine, and gamma-hydroxybutyric acid (GHB). Class B drugs have a moderate potential for harm. Although marijuana regulations have relaxed in most countries, including many states in the United States, the United Kingdom elevated marijuana from class C to class B in 2009.

The United Kingdom presents different considerations for certain drugs compared to the United States. For example, the United Kingdom classified GHB as a class C compound, whereas the United States classified GHB as a schedule I controlled substance. Further, the United Kingdom classified marijuana as a class B compound, but the United States classified marijuana as a schedule I controlled substance.

Although the controlled substances schedules represent a standard labeling system for drug-use risk, disagreements for drugs schedules occur among practitioners and researchers. Criticism of controlled substances schedules falls into two general categories: (1) appropriateness of drug scheduling and (2) methods used to schedule drugs.

A 1994 *New York Times* article illustrated the appropriateness of drug scheduling by gathering the opinions of two prominent drug abuse experts, Jack Henningfield and Neal Benowitz (Hilts, 1994). Both experts ranked selected abused drugs according to severity as measured by withdrawal symptoms, tolerance, reinforcing effects, addiction, and intoxication. **Figure 5.1** shows these rankings, with 1 being most severe.

In figure 5.1, both Henningfield and Benowitz agreed that nicotine presented the greatest addiction risk followed in rank order by heroin, cocaine, alcohol, caffeine, and marijuana. They generally also agreed on the other abuse areas. Both experts ranked alcohol as having the worst withdrawal symptoms and cocaine as eliciting the strongest reinforcing effects. They ranked marijuana as one of the least serious drugs among these categories. Neither alcohol nor nicotine, however, are scheduled substances, whereas marijuana and its constituents (e.g., tetrahydrocannabinol, or THC) are schedule I controlled substances.

Critics also question the methods used for scheduling drugs. One area of concern regards a slow response to new drugs of abuse. In particular, many potentially dangerous so-called club drugs are not currently scheduled substances. The DEA schedules drugs only after accumulating sufficient scientific evidence and law enforcement drug-use statistics. Thus, drug scheduling can take years. Adding to this, clandestine drug suppliers develop designer drugs, substances designed to circumvent existing drug schedules. Consider the designer drugs 1,4-butanediol, also known as *one comma four*, and gamma-butyrolactone (GBL). Neither substance is listed on DEA controlled substances listings, nor do these substances elicit rewarding effects.

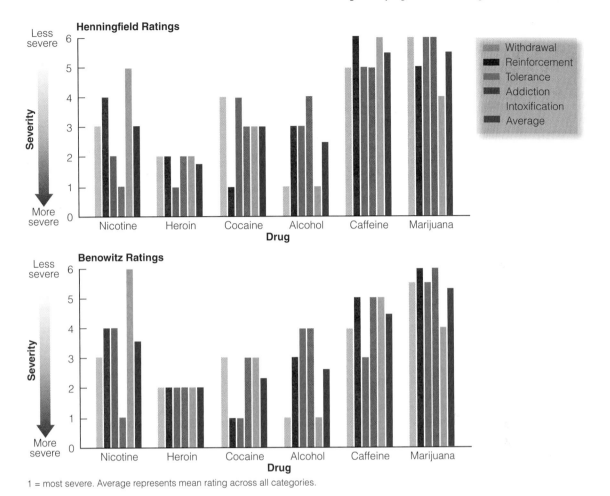

1 = most severe. Average represents mean rating across all categories.

figure **5.1** Ranked Abuse and Addiction Risk by Jack Henningfield and Neal Benowitz. (Data from Henningfield and Benowitz, 1994.)

However, these substances can metabolically convert to the schedule I drug GHB when they enter the liver.

Nutt and colleagues (2007) offered an alternative approach for drug scheduling. They defined *harm* as consisting of physical harm, addiction, or societal harm. *Physical harm* includes damage to the body such as impairment of heart or liver function. *Addiction* consists of an inability to stop taking a drug, along with other factors used in the clinical diagnosis of substance dependence. *Societal harm* ranges from harm to family and other social relationships to costs associated with health care and law enforcement. After developing these definitions, an expert panel rated 20 abused drugs according to harm subgroupings. **Table 5.2** shows ratings from this study for selected drugs.

The harm assessment by Nutt and colleagues reveals many discrepancies with regulatory scheduling. Although the drugs heroin and cocaine rated highly

table **5.2**

Harm Ratings for Selected Drugs of Abuse			
Drug	Physical harm	Addiction	Societal harm
Heroin	2.78	3.00	2.54
Cocaine	2.33	2.80	2.17
Alcohol	1.40	1.93	2.21
Tobacco	1.24	2.21	1.42
Inhaled solvents	1.28	1.01	1.52
LSD	1.13	1.23	1.32
GHB	0.86	1.19	1.30
MDMA (Ecstasy)	1.05	1.13	1.09

Higher scores = most harmful.

Nutt et al., 2007. By permission.

for harm, the drugs GHB and MDMA (Ecstasy) rated low. In contrast, the United States classifies GHB and MDMA as schedule I substances, and the United Kingdom classifies MDMA as class A, but GHB as class C. Two noncontrolled substances, alcohol and tobacco, also made the list. The harm-assessment study rated alcohol as the fourth most harmful substance and tobacco, which includes nicotine, as the ninth most harmful substance. Studies such as these have the potential to guide regulatory changes for controlling drugs of abuse.

Stop & Check

1. How might the DEA schedule a drug with high abuse potential and no perceived medical uses?
2. How does the harm scheduling for MDMA offered by Nutt and colleagues (2007) differ from the DEA's controlled substances scheduling?

1. The DEA schedules drugs with these characteristics as schedule I. **2.** Although the DEA considers MDMA a schedule I controlled substance, MDMA rated low for harm according to the study by Nutt and colleagues.

Clinical Definitions and the Diagnosis of Drug Addiction

Although regulatory agencies controlled substances based on abuse potential and potential medical uses, clinicians use precise criteria to define and diagnose drug addiction. Early clinical definitions of addiction focused on the development of tolerance, physical dependence, and craving (National Institute on Alcohol Abuse and Alcoholism, 1995). These early definitions describe an addiction to some drugs but not others. They clearly apply to heroin and alcohol, which both produce tolerance, manifest physical withdrawal symptoms, and elicit powerful cravings. Yet these definitions may fail to classify a drug such as cocaine as an addictive substances because it causes few physical withdrawal symptoms.

REVIEW! Tolerance is an adaptation to a drug that requires a user to take escalating doses to achieve desired drug effects. Chapter 4 (pg. 123).

REVIEW! A person demonstrates a dependence when he needs the drug to function normally and when removal of the drug causes withdrawal symptoms. Chapter 4 (pg. 124).

substance dependence
Maladaptive pattern of substance use.

More recent clinical definitions of drug addiction are provided in the fourth edition of the American Psychiatric Association's *Diagnostic and Statistical Manual of Mental Disorders* (DSM) (2000)* and the World Health Organization's *International Classification of Diseases* (10th edition). The definitions described in these diagnostic manuals are similar, so only the DSM criteria are described here. The DSM refers to addiction as **substance dependence**, which is defined as a "maladaptive pattern of substance use, leading to clinically significant impairment or distress as manifested by three (or more) [symptoms] occurring at any time in the same 12-month period." These symptoms include tolerance, withdrawal, taking more of the drug than intended, a persistent desire to quit, significant time spent in drug seeking and taking, replacing important activities, and continued use despite knowledge of physical or psychological problems.

It is important to note that the DSM addiction definition differs from earlier definitions because it considers drug use that persists despite a strong desire to stop. Furthermore, the DSM recognizes that drug use may continue despite the user's knowledge of physical or psychological harm to oneself and the toll that drug use takes on valuable social relationships and occupational activities.

According to the DSM's definition, both cocaine and cannabis produce substance dependence. Cocaine has the ability to produce strong cravings, produce tolerance, and compete with valuable social and occupational activities and other important natural reinforcers. Users who develop a dependence on cannabis most often report "persistent desire or unsuccessful efforts to reduce or cease use" along with other DSM symptoms such as continued use despite health problems and craving cannabis during withdrawal (Coffey et al., 2002).

substance abuse
Maladaptive pattern of substance use that does not involve tolerance or dependence.

The DSM defines *abuse* as a separate disorder from dependence. According to the DSM, **substance abuse** consists of "a maladaptive pattern of substance use, leading to clinically significant impairment or distress, as manifested by one (or more) [symptoms], occurring within a 12-month period." Although substance abuse has a definition similar to dependence, substance abuse does not include tolerance or dependence. Thus, tolerance and physical or psychological dependence are the key defining differences between the DSM's definition for substance abuse and substance dependence.

---

*The fifth edition of the DSM comes out after this textbook goes to press.

relapse Return to a chronic drug use state that meets the clinical features of addiction.

Clinicians consider addiction as a chronically relapsing disorder that may require years of treatment. **Relapse** consists of a return to a chronic drug use state that meets the clinical features of addiction. The DSM addresses remission categories after a diagnosis for substance dependence or abuse. The best outcome consists of *sustained full remission*, which is characterized by no symptoms for dependence or abuse occurring over at least a 12-month period. Patients may also improve by exhibiting fewer symptoms that no longer provide for a substance dependence or abuse diagnosis. In this case, a patient might meet the features of *sustained partial remission*, which consists of one or more symptoms occurring for dependence or abuse within 12 months.

Theoretical Models and the Features of Drug Addiction

Disease Model of Drug Addiction

On the one hand, drug-addiction models attempt to characterize and explain compulsive drug use. On the other hand, clinical definitions for addiction serve only to diagnose an addiction rather than explain the factors causing the addiction. Through developing models, researchers attempt to understand the causes and factors for facilitating addictive behavior. Addiction models largely fall into three categories: disease, dependence, and positive reinforcement.

disease model Model that characterizes drug addiction as a disease.

The **disease model** characterizes drug addiction as similar to any other disease (**table 5.3**). To put this in perspective, consider the definition for a disease offered by *Stedman's Medical Dictionary* (Stedman, 1999): "An interruption, cessation, or disorder of body function, system, or organ."

When considering drug addiction as a disease, one may thus determine how drugs of abuse may interrupt, cease, or disrupt functions in the body. Diseases also have causes, such as a pathogen, and the degree of susceptibility to disease may depend on one's unique predisposition. Those who advocate for this model affirm that the substance serves as the cause of the disease. Further, one may possess a predisposition for drug addiction. Just as a disease may disrupt physiological processes, drugs also can disrupt neurobiological

table **5.3**

Addiction Model Characteristics	
Addiction Model	**Characteristics**
Disease	Drug addiction fits the medical definition of a disease.
Drive theory	Drugs elicit powerful positive reinforcing effects that drive individuals to seek and use drugs.
Opponent-process theory	Individuals seek drugs to avoid or remove withdrawal effects.
Incentive salience	Stimuli associated with drug use receive salient incentive value. These stimuli then command a user's attention and produce a motivational state for drug seeking.

© Cengage Learning 2014

processes, which may lead to addictive behaviors. Advocates also argue that defining addiction as a disease allows the medical health-care system to address addiction toward the primary purpose of eliminating substance use. The disease model is also a central perspective for abstinence-based 12-step recovery programs such as Alcoholics Anonymous and Narcotics Anonymous, which are discussed later in this chapter.

Associative Learning Principles Used in Addiction Models

Other drug-addiction models focus on associative learning principles to characterize the behavioral features of drug use. **Associative learning** is the process in which an organism learns associations between stimuli or between behavior and stimuli. Much of associative learning theory comes from principles of operant conditioning and classical conditioning.

During operant conditioning, consequences modify the occurrence and form of behavior (Skinner, 1938). The term **reinforcement** refers to a process in which the resulting consequence from a response increases the frequency of future responses. Said another way, reinforcing outcomes strengthen behavioral tendencies. We also use the terms *negative* and *positive* when discussing reinforcers. In this usage, *negative* refers to the removal of a stimulus, and *positive* refers to the addition of a stimulus. An example of a positive reinforcement context is a hungry rat pressing a lever to earn food pellets. The food pellets serve as positive reinforcers. An example of a negative reinforcement context is a rat pressing a lever to remove some of type of aversive stimulation such as a bright light. Removal of the bright light serves as a negative reinforcer. Extinction refers to a decline in responding as the result of failing to achieve reinforcers.

A **conditioned stimulus** may develop from presenting stimuli in the presence of a stimulus involved in an associative learning process. Using one of the examples above, a tone might acquire reinforcing properties if the tone repeatedly occurs in the presence of food. If a hungry rat then emits responses in order to activate the tone, we refer to the tone as a *conditioned reinforcer*. Conditioning also takes place in classical conditioning procedures, which are described later.

Associative learning may also occur during certain conditions or environmental contexts. We describe one type of condition as a discriminative stimulus, which is a stimulus that, when present, signals the availability of reinforcement. Reinforcement processes do not occur when the discriminative stimulus is absent. For the hungry rat just described, a discriminative stimulus might consists of a light that illuminates the test chamber during experimental procedures. Lever presses result in food reinforcers when the light is on but not when the light is off.

Classical conditioning procedures describe how stimuli can elicit behavioral responses. The behaviors occur reflexively, whereas operant conditioned behaviors occur as a result of meeting past consequences. Described another way, classical conditioning consists of stimuli eliciting responses whereas operant conditioning consists of responses producing stimulus outcomes.

Russian physiologist Ivan Pavlov (Pavlov & Anrep, 1927) first described behavior in terms of classical conditioning relationships. First, we recognize that many unlearned behaviors exist, such as Pavlov's description of food in the

associative learning
Process in which an organism learns associations between stimuli or between behavior and stimuli.

reinforcement Process in which the resulting consequence from a response increases the frequency of future responses.

conditioned stimulus
A stimulus that acquires the behavioral controlling properties of another stimulus that is involved in an associated learning process.

mouth eliciting salivation. We do not learn to salivate when food is in mouth, this is simply a natural reflex. Second, Pavlov found that associations can develop, through conditioning, between other stimuli and those that produce natural reflexes. This work led to the following terms to define stimulus–response relationships.

An *unconditioned stimulus* (UCS) consists of a stimulus that elicits a reflexive response, which is referred to as an *unconditioned response* (UCR). Food in the mouth serves as a UCS, and salivation serves as a UCR. A stimulus not part of this association, such as a light or tone, will not naturally elicit salivation; given this lack of association, we refer to such stimuli as *neutral stimuli.* By repeatedly pairing a neutral stimulus with a UCS, the neutral stimulus may incur associative properties that enable the stimulus alone to elicit salivation. When this occurs, the stimulus serves as a *conditioned stimulus* (CS); to describe salivation as elicited in this conditioned associative process, salivation is identified as a *conditioned response* (CR).

The ability to condition a stimulus is subject to the principle of latent inhibition. *Latent inhibition* consists of a resistant or slower conditioning process from using a familiar stimulus as the neutral stimulus in an associative learning process. In this case, *familiar* suggests that the stimulus already belongs to at least one other associative learning process. Incorporating a familiar stimulus into a new associative learning process tends to be comparatively slower than incorporating an entirely novel stimulus into an associative learning process.

incentive salience
Attribution of salient motivational value to otherwise neutral stimuli.

Conditioning may also occur for motivational states. In particular, a motivational concept called **incentive salience** serves as important part of modern drug-addiction theory: It is the attribution of salient motivational value to otherwise neutral stimuli. These attributions can occur through associations of neutral stimuli with rewarding stimuli. When presented, incentivized stimuli command an individual's attention and elicit a motivation to pursue these and associated stimuli. The incentive-salience model for drug addiction, described later, utilizes this concept to explain compulsive drug use, where the presentation of stimuli incentivized through associations with drug use may motivate users to engage in drug seeking. The incentive-salience model also relates incentive-salience function to neural systems (Robinson & Berridge, 2003).

We also have goal-directed behaviors, which may play an important role in decision making. The topic of goal-directed behavior encompasses a large area of study approached from different areas of psychology, including cognitive and social psychology. Many frameworks for explaining and characterizing goal-directed behavior use associative learning principles, particularly in reference to drug-seeking behavior. **Goal-directed behavior** occurs when an organism engages in learned behaviors in order to achieve a desired goal.

goal-directed behavior
Behavior that occurs when an organism engages in learned behaviors in order to achieve a desired goal.

Many theorists use associative learning principles to characterize goal-directed behavior, particularly when describing this behavior during drug seeking. In this context, conditioned associations between responses and outcomes govern goal-directed behavior (de Wit & Dickinson, 2009). Neuroscientists tend to relate goal-directed behavior to the brain's reward system and the involvement of these pathways with the brain's learning and memory systems (Goto & Grace, 2005; Pennartz, Ito, Verschure, Battaglia, & Robbins, 2011).

Drive, Opponent-Process Theory, and Incentive-Salience Models of Drug Addiction

In 1952, Abraham Wikler provided one of the first drug-addiction models to consider drug effects as behavioral variables. Based on studies with individuals addicted to opioid drugs, Wikler stated that drug-addicted individuals developed a drive to achieve a drug's positive reinforcing effects (table 5.3). This drive motivates a person to engage in drug seeking. Moreover, the withdrawal effects experienced by individuals contributed to motivating a person to seek the drug's positive reinforcing effects.

opponent-process theory Holds that the effects of a drug are automatically counteracted by opposing actions in the body.

Solomon and Corbit (1974) offered the **opponent-process theory** as another explanation for drug use during addiction (table 5.3). According to this theory of drug addiction, the effects of a drug are automatically counteracted by opposing actions in the body. These opposing actions may serve to attain homeostasis or return the brain to normal functioning. During addiction, the brain may, for example, elicit anhedonic effects to counteract a drug's hedonic (i.e., pleasurable) effects.

As illustrated in **figure 5.2**, the sum of a drug's effects and its opposing processes defines an individual's subjective experience. If a drug's effects

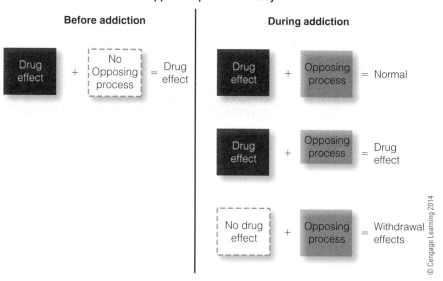

According to the opponent-process theory of drug addiction, opposing processes counter the effects of an abused drug. Before addiction occurs (left panel), few if any processes counteract a drug's effects. During addiction, opponent processes counteract a drug's effects. Equally balancing drug effects and opposing processes lead to a normal state (top, right panel), whereas overpowering drug effects can overcome opponent processes (middle, right panel). Withdrawal effects occur when opposing processes occur in the absence of drug effects (bottom, right panel). See text for further information.

figure 5.2

outweigh those from opposing processes, then an individual will experience the drug's effects. However, if effects generated from opposing processes significantly outweigh drug effects, then an individual will experience withdrawal effects. A normalized state occurs when drug effects equally balance against opponent-process effects.

The type of reinforcement governing addictive behavior also distinguishes between Wikler's drive model and Solomon and Corbit's opponent-process

box **5.1** Self-Administration

Self-administration procedures use drugs as reinforcers for operant responding in animals. In a typical self-administration procedure, an animal learns to respond on an operandum such as a lever to receive an injection of the drug. The drug is usually delivered intravenously through a surgically implanted intravenous catheter. When drugs serve as positive reinforcing stimuli, drug injections alone are entirely capable of initiating self-administration responses. For example, if a cocaine injection occurred whenever a rat pressed a lever, then cocaine's reinforcing effects would occasion further lever pressing.

The self-administration procedure provides an important analog for human drug use. As reviewed in this chapter, chronic use of an abused drug incorporates brain systems important for learning. In the self-administration procedures, animals also learn to take drugs of abuse. Beyond this, self-administration procedures provide measurements of a drug's reinforcing strength. In doing so, self-administration procedures provide an indication of a drug's potential for causing addiction.

We measure a drug's reinforcing strength by determining its **break point**, or the maximum amount of response effort an organism will devote toward receiving an administration of drug. Break-point studies normally employ progressive-ratio reinforcement schedules, which gradually increase the number of responses necessary to achieve a drug administration.

Box 5.1, figure 1 shows data from rats that self-administered any of several psychostimulant drugs on a progressive-ratio schedule (Richardson & Roberts, 1996). For d-amphetamine and methamphetamine, rats pressed the lever as many as 268 times to receive an injection. For cocaine, rats pressed the lever as many as 178 times to receive a drug injection. These maximum numbers of lever presses define each drug's break point at a given dose.

Researchers also employ other drugs to modify self-administration. For example, Maric and colleagues (2012) administered the hunger-stimulating hormone ghrelin to rats trained to self-administer heroin (box 5.1, figure 2). In this study, ghrelin administration increased the break point for heroin, suggesting that ghrelin enhanced heroin's reinforcing effects.

box **5.1**, figure **1**

Break points consist of the maximum number of lever presses an animal will emit for a drug injection. The y-axis shows the final reinforcement ratio, defined as the total number of lever presses needed to earn a reinforcer, and the x-axis shows the dose of drug administered per injection. (Richardson & Roberts, 1996. By permission.)

theory. Unlike the drive model, the opponent-process theory considers that addictive drug use occurs partly to remove or prevent withdrawal symptoms. Thus, during the development of addiction, motivations for drug use can shift achieving reinforcing effects, in a positive reinforcement context, to ridding or avoiding withdrawal symptoms, in a negative reinforcement context.

incentive-salience model Holds that drug addiction occurs after a shift from "liking" the effects of a drug to "wanting" the effects.

The **incentive-salience model** states that drug addiction occurs after a shift from *liking* the effects of a drug to *wanting* the effects of a drug. *Wanting*

Researchers also use self-administration procedures to assess *reinstatement*, the recurrence of drug self-administration responding after a period of extinction. Reinstatement may provide an analog of drug relapse in humans. The general procedure for reinstatement goes as follows. After animals learn to self-administer a drug, researchers disable the operandum, resulting in an extinction period when responding no longer achieves a drug infusion. Over time, responding reduces substantially. At this point, a researcher may cause responding to occur by giving the animal an injection of drug (drug-induced reinstatement), eliciting a stimulus previously paired with drug delivery (cue-induced reinstatement), or

delivering a brief shock or other aversive stimulus (stress-induced reinstatement).

In one of the first demonstrations of drug-induced reinstatement, Gerber and Stretch (Gerber & Stretch, 1975) extinguished self-administration responding for cocaine by replacing cocaine with saline in the chamber's infusion syringe. After responding decreased to a low level, these researchers gave the monkeys an infusion of the psychostimulant drug d-amphetamine, which resulted in a return to self-administration responding, despite having still having saline in the syringe. Box 5.1, figure 3 provides the findings from this experiment.

break point Maximum amount of response effort an organism will devote toward receiving an administration of drug.

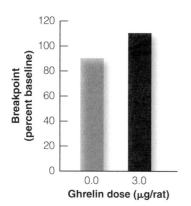

box 5.1, figure 2
The hunger-stimulating hormone ghrelin increased the break point for self-administered heroin. The *y*-axis shows the break-point value compared to baseline responding, and the *x*-axis shows the amount of ghrelin provided to the rats. (Maric, T., Sedki, F., Ronfard, B., Chafetz, D. and Shalev, U. (2012), A limited role for ghrelin in heroin self-administration and food deprivation-induced reinstatement of heroin seeking in rats. *Addiction Biology*, 17: 613–622. doi: 10.1111/j.1369-1600.2011.00396.x. Reproduced with permission of John Wiley & Sons Ltd.)

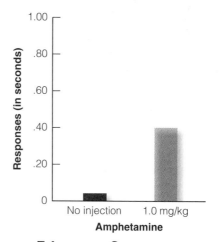

box 5.1, figure 3
A presession infusion of d-amphetamine caused monkeys trained to self-administer cocaine to resume self-administration responding. For the data shown, the infusion syringe only contained saline. The left bar shows self-administration responding and the right bar shows self-administration responding after an injection of d-amphetamine (1.0 mg/kg). (Data from Gerber & Stretch, 1975.)

occurs in an incentive-salience context, whereby stimuli associated with drug use command attention and elicit a salient motivational state toward pursuing the drug (Robinson & Berridge, 2003). In a technical sense, *wanting* in this model represents the process of developing and expressing incentive salience, whereas the term **craving**, in a basic sense, simply refers to a desire to use a drug (Sayette et al., 2000). *Liking* refers to the enjoyment of a drug's effects, which, according to this model, fails to uniquely explain drug addiction. In fact, the incentive-salience model may explain why addicted users may *want* a drug more while, as tolerance develops, *liking* the drug less (Robinson & Berridge, 2003).

craving The desire to use a drug.

Incentive salience may also offer an explanation for relapse in drug addiction. Through conditioning, such incentivized stimuli may serve as reminders of former drug use; when encountered, they may implicitly engage motivational states for drug use. As described in **Box 5.1**, researchers study conditions that reinstate drug self-administration responses in animals in an effort to better understand why relapse occurs.

Stop & Check

1. Compare the clinical definitions for addiction for cocaine.
2. How does the opponent-process theory of drug addiction account for drug withdrawal?
3. According to the incentive-salience model, what are the characteristics of drug wanting?

1. Early definitions for addiction may fail to consider cocaine as addictive because it has few physical withdrawal symptoms. However, the modern DSM definition for substance dependence incorporates other features of cocaine use, including an inability to quit despite wanting to. **2.** During drug addiction, the body automatically elicits opposing processes to regain homeostasis and normal brain functioning. When a drug is absent, effects resulting from these unchecked opposing processes occur as withdrawal effects. **3.** Drug wanting consists of a motivational state elicited by stimuli incentivized through associations with drug use.

Drugs of Abuse and Reward Circuitry

Drugs of abuse act directly or indirectly on the brain's reward circuitry (**figure 5.3**). The key structures along this circuit consist of the ventral tegmental area and the nucleus accumbens. Dopamine neurons largely compose this circuit. The ventral tegmental area contains the somas for these dopamine neurons, and the axons for these dopamine neurons terminate in the nucleus accumbens.

As described in the chapter opening, we attribute the discovery of the brain reward circuit to James Olds. In collaboration with graduate student Peter Milner, Olds first published these findings in 1954 (Olds & Milner, 1954). This experiment expanded on the serendipitous finding described previously by systemically investigating electrode-induced activation of tissue

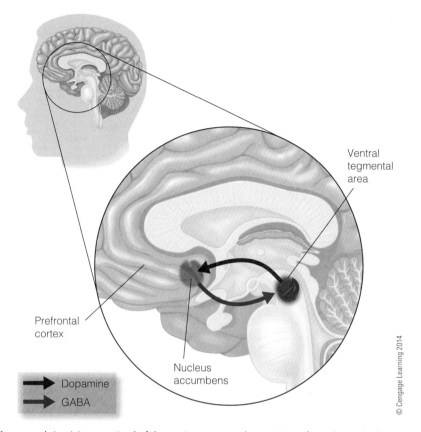

The *reward circuit* is comprised of dopamine neurons that originate from the ventral tegmental area and terminate in the nucleus accumbens. The release of dopamine in the nucleus accumbens leads to rewarding effects. GABA neurons inhibit the activity of these dopamine neurons via the activation of inhibitory GABA receptors on these dopamine neurons. Some GABA neurons form a negative feedback loop from the nucleus accumbens to the ventral tegmental area. Other GABA neurons consist of interneurons within the ventral tegmental area.

figure **5.3**

surrounding the septal forebrain area. Electrode placements found closest to the nucleus accumbens or lying between the nucleus accumbens and the ventral tegmental area led to reinforcing effects. To demonstrate these effects, Olds and Milner designed an operant chamber equipped with a lever that activated the brain electrode when pressed. In this way, the researchers provided an apparatus by which rats governed their own level of electrical stimulation (**figure 5.4**).

The study by Olds and Milner suggested a system or circuit for producing reinforcing effects, but they lacked sufficient information to understand the nature of neurotransmission for this circuit. A few years after this discovery, Kathleen Montagu reported the existence of dopamine in the brain (Montagu,

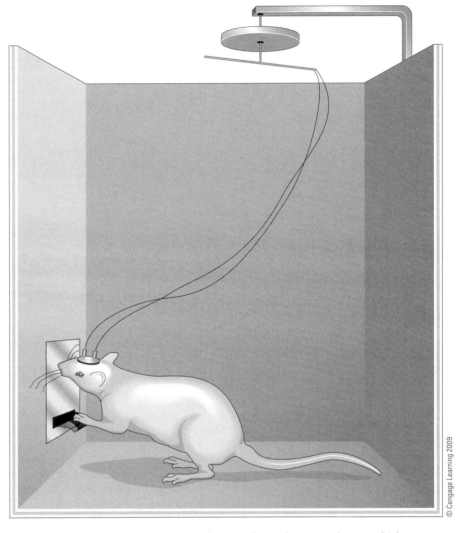

figure 5.4 In the seminal experimental by Olds and Milner, a rat learned to press a lever at a high rate to achieve the effects elicited by a septal forebrain area electrode. This electrode placement likely activated dopamine axons along the brain's reward circuit.

1957). In 1958, Arvid Carlsson first reported that dopamine had functional significance for brain function by mediating the pharmacological effects of the drug reserpine (see Chapter 13 for more on reserpine) (Carlsson, Lindqvist, Magnusson, & Waldeck, 1958). Then, during the 1960s and early 1970s, new research techniques revealed the brain's major dopamine pathways.

Today we know that reinforcing effects occur when increased dopamine release occurs in the nucleus accumbens. Later review showed that the seminal electrode experiments conducted by Olds and Milner activated these dopamine

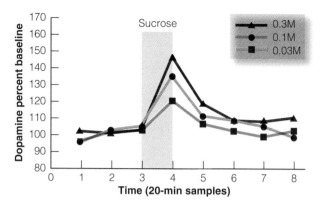

figure 5.5

Sucrose consumption elicited significant dopamine level increases in the nucleus accumbens in rats as revealed by microdialysis. M = molality, an index of concentration. (HAJNAL, András, Gerard P. SMITH, and Ralph NORGREN. "Oral sucrose stimulation increases accumbens dopamine in the rat." *American journal of physiology. Regulatory, integrative and comparative physiology* 55.1 (2004): R31- R37. By permission.)

neurons. Under natural conditions, nucleus accumbens dopamine levels elevate in the presence of stimuli that predict positive outcomes. Such stimuli include food and sex as well as complex social or cultural reinforcers such as maintaining stable personal relationships.

For example, Hajnal and colleagues (2004) used a microdialysis procedure to assess nucleus accumbens dopamine level changes elicited by food. At times during the procedure, rats consumed a sweet-tasting sucrose liquid food mix. When the sucrose mix was consumed, nucleus accumbens dopamine levels increased; dopamine levels returned to baseline levels after consumption ceased (**figure 5.5**).

We should also note that increased dopamine concentrations in the nucleus do more than elicit reinforcing effects. One perspective suggests that enhanced dopamine signaling may diminish latent inhibition effects, subsequently improving associative learning processes. De Leonibus and colleagues (2006) used a microdialysis study to examine nucleus accumbens dopamine release in rats exposed to a stimulus in the form of either a novel rat or a familiar rat introduced to the testing chamber. When the introduced rat was novel—that is, the experimental rat previously never met the introduced rat—dopamine release increased in the nucleus accumbens. However, dopamine levels did not increase when familiar rats were introduced (**figure 5.6**).

Many drugs of abuse activate reward circuits, achieving dopamine elevations far above those produced by natural reinforcers. For example, the psychostimulant drugs cocaine and amphetamine directly enhance dopamine release from axon terminals in the nucleus accumbens. In doing so, they can elevate nucleus accumbens dopamine levels many times greater than achieved by natural reinforcers and novel stimuli (Carboni, Imperato, Perezzani, & Di Chiara, 1989; De Leonibus et al., 2006; Hajnal et al., 2004; Sharp, Zetterstrom, Ljungberg, & Ungerstedt, 1987).

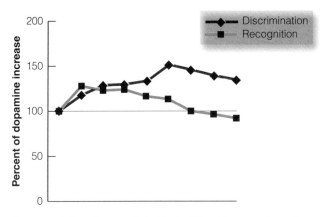

The presentation of novel rats led to significant increases in nucleus accumbens dopamine levels, whereas the presentation of familiar rats did not increase nucleus accumbens dopamine levels. (De Leonibus, E., Verheij, M. M. M., Mele, A. and Cools, A. (2006), Distinct kinds of novelty processing differentially increase extracellular dopamine in different brain regions. *European Journal of Neuroscience*, 23: 1332–1340. doi: 10.1111/j.1460-9568.2006.04658.x. Reproduced with permission of John Wiley & Sons Ltd.)

figure **5.6**

Some drugs of abuse indirectly alter dopamine neurons by acting on other neurotransmitter systems. One of these neurotransmitters is GABA, which acts to inhibit the activity of dopamine neurons in the reward circuit. First, GABA released from ventral tegmental area interneurons activate GABA receptors on dopamine neurons. Because GABA receptors have inhibitory effects, their activation decreases the activity of dopamine neurons. Decreased dopamine neuron activity reduces dopamine levels in the nucleus accumbens. Second, GABA neurons in the nucleus accumbens project to the ventral tegmental area. GABA neurotransmitters released from these axons also inhibit dopamine neuron activity (van Zessen, Phillips, Budygin, & Stuber, 2012; Xiao & Ye, 2008).

REVIEW! Interneurons are neurons that have dendrites, a soma, and an axon contained within the same structure. Chapter 2 (pg. 32).

Given these actions, GABA neurotransmission weakens reinforcing effects. Some drugs of abuse, therefore, inhibit GABA neurotransmission, subsequently causing an increase in dopamine neuron activity. For example, opioid drugs such as heroin activate inhibitory opioid receptors located on GABA neurons in the ventral tegmental area and the nucleus accumbens (Xiao & Ye, 2008). Such drugs weaken GABA's inhibitory influence on dopamine neurons, resulting in greater dopamine release in the nucleus accumbens. Chapter 9 expands on the actions that opioids have on reward circuitry.

Glutamate neurotransmission also influences the activity of the reward circuitry. Glutamate axons from the prefrontal cortex terminate in the nucleus accumbens and produce reinforcing effects. Other glutamate axons from the hippocampus terminate in the ventral tegmental area, leading to increased activation of dopamine neurons along the reward circuit. Glutamate neurons in the nucleus accumbens may increase glutamate release during the presentation of stimuli associated with previous addictive drug use (Koob & Volkow, 2009; LaLumiere & Kalivas, 2008).

Drug Abuse and Changes to Learning and Memory Systems

Acute administration of a drug of abuse produces reinforcing effects by activating reward circuitry, as described in the previous section. Chronic administration of an abused drug leads to changes in other brain systems, especially those involved in learning and memory. The interconnected structures that facilitate learning and memory include the amygdala, thalamus, prefrontal cortex, and the hippocampus. Each of these structures adapt to the chronic use of abused drugs (**figure 5.7**).

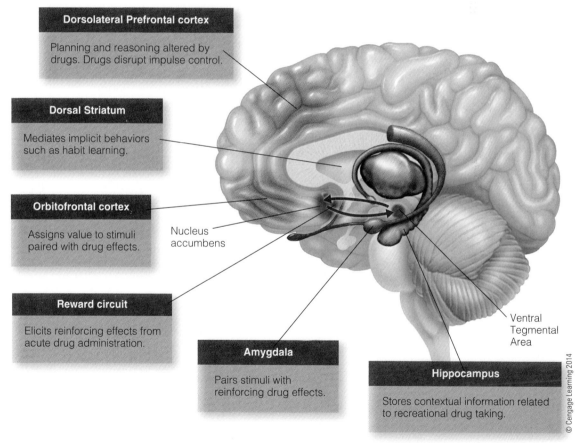

Dorsolateral Prefrontal cortex

Planning and reasoning altered by drugs. Drugs disrupt impulse control.

Dorsal Striatum

Mediates implicit behaviors such as habit learning.

Orbitofrontal cortex

Assigns value to stimuli paired with drug effects.

Nucleus accumbens

Reward circuit

Elicits reinforcing effects from acute drug administration.

Amygdala

Pairs stimuli with reinforcing drug effects.

Ventral Tegmental Area

Hippocampus

Stores contextual information related to recreational drug taking.

© Cengage Learning 2014

figure 5.7 Chronic administration of abused drugs incorporates many brain structures beyond the reward circuit. Through incorporating these structures, chronic drug administration leads to pairing stimuli with drug effects, associating an environmental context with drug effects, and inhibiting impulse control and reasoning.

The amygdala is a structure traditionally associated with fear and anxiety, yet it also supports learning and memory by associating stimuli with emotional events such as experiencing reinforcing effects from a drug. During chronic drug use, the amygdala forms associations between stimuli commonly present during drug use and the reinforcing effects of the drug. The amygdala communicates this information to two other structures important for learning and memory.

First, the amygdala is interconnected with the thalamus, a structure that routes sensory information to the cerebral cortex. Second, the amygdala interconnects with the prefrontal cortex, the brain's executive center where stimuli are processed and motor responses are initiated. These structures together form the *thalamo-cortical-amygdala pathway.*

The prefrontal cortex contains sub-structures important for normal learning processes, and these structures adapt to chronic drug use. The orbitofrontal cortex, a structure within the prefrontal cortex, receives input from the amygdala and may enhance the incentive value of stimuli associated with drug use. The orbitofrontal cortex may also elicit drug cravings when the drug is absent (Koob & Volkow, 2009).

The thalamo-cortical-amygdala pathway also has connections with the hippocampus. During chronic administration of a drug of abuse, the hippocampus provides contextual information linked with drug taking. Examples of context include the physical environment where drugs are normally taken or the types of individuals a user interacts with when obtaining and administering drugs.

The structures described above play an important role in associating stimuli with drug effects and assigning value to these associated stimuli such as conditioned reinforcing properties. Conditioned place preference procedures demonstrate these stimulus associations, as described in box 10.1 in Chapter 10. In this procedure, laboratory animals are repeatedly exposed to an environment while experiencing a drug's reinforcing effects. As a result of these exposures, animals, when given the choice, develop a preference for being in the drug-associated environment. In fact, these environmental stimuli alone can elicit enhanced dopamine levels in the nucleus accumbens (Duvauchelle, Ikegami, Asami, et al., 2000; Duvauchelle, Ikegami, & Castaneda, 2000).

In addition to a role in pairing stimuli with a drug's reinforcing effects, the amygdala-thalamo-cortical circuitry facilitates unpleasant drug withdrawal effects. Physical withdrawal effects manifest from the involvement of this circuitry with autonomic systems, particularly those involved with internal regulatory processes. The amygdala influences these functions through connections with the hypothalamus. During repeated administration, these systems adapt to a drug in the body; when the drug is absent, they elicit physical withdrawal symptoms such as decreased heart rate, gastrointestinal dysfunction, sweating, and breathing irregularities, among a variety of effects.

Chronic administration of abused drugs also alters functioning of the dorsal lateral prefrontal cortex. The dorsal lateral prefrontal cortex integrates sensory information received from other cortical areas and mediates working memory, planning, organizing, and other upper-level cognitive activities. Through these activities, the dorsal lateral prefrontal cortex is important for impulse control. Chronic use of an abused drug compromises normal functioning of the dorsal lateral prefrontal cortex. Many drug-addicted individuals exhibit a reduced ability to choose delayed larger reinforcers in place of immediate smaller reinforcers. Overall, this behavior creates a problem for drug-addiction therapy because delayed outcomes associated with being drug free may weigh poorly against immediate gratification from taking a drug of abuse. Other drugs such as depressant drugs (e.g., alcohol) or psychedelic drugs (e.g., phencyclidine) significantly impair memory function, partly through acting on the dorsal lateral prefrontal cortex (Aura & Riekkinen, 1999; Mao, Arnsten, & Li, 1999; Paulus, Tapert, Pulido, & Schuckit, 2006).

REVIEW! Working memory consists of short-term verbal or nonverbal memories employed when carrying out a task. Chapter 2 (pg. 46).

Chronic treatment with an abused drug may also recruit procedural memory systems involving dorsal parts of the basal ganglia, also referred to as the *dorsal striatum*, and interconnections between this structure and the nucleus accumbens and thalamus. As Robinson and Berridge (2003) describe, tying shoelaces involves procedural memory because once lace tying starts, the behavior continues automatically until the lace is tied. During situations in which a user commonly smokes cigarette, such as talking on the phone or having a cup of coffee, the user may engage in an automated series of behaviors involving removing a cigarette from a pack and lighting it. In other words, a user may obtain, light, and smoke a cigarette without giving it much thought. For other drugs, habits mediated by the dorsal striatum and connected circuitry might occur as rituals that drug-addicted users display during drug use.

Stop & Check

1. What effects does dopamine release in the nucleus accumbens have?
2. What role does GABA play in the reward circuit?
3. What role does the amygdala play in chronic drug actions in the brain?
4. How might altered dorsolateral prefrontal cortex functioning interfere with treating addiction?

1. Enhanced dopamine concentrations in the nucleus accumbens are linked to reinforcing effects and may facilitate certain associative learning processes involving novel stimuli. 2. GABA neurons produce inhibitory effects on dopamine neurons in the reward circuit. 3. The amygdala pairs stimuli with a drug's reinforcing effects. 4. Compromised dorsolateral prefrontal cortex functioning impairs impulse control, which may prevent drug-addicted individuals from abstaining from immediate drug use in place of delayed benefits from being drug free.

Neurobiology and the Stages of Drug Addiction

Leading authorities in drug-addiction research describe addiction as a cycle involving three primary stages (Kalivas, 2002; Koob & Volkow, 2009). The first stage of addiction is intoxication. The second stage is withdrawal, and the third stage consists of preoccupation and anticipation. These stages relate to important concepts developed from drug-addiction models and their association with drug actions in the brain (**table 5.4**).

Drug intoxication is a necessary first stage in the development of drug addiction. Drug use during this stage occurs for the purpose of achieving a drug's intoxicating and, in particular, reinforcing effects. In this way, the intoxication stage resembles the primary feature of Wikler's drive model as previously described. The actions of drugs on the brain's reward circuitry sufficiently explain drug use at this stage.

The next stage of this cycle consists of the development of dependence during chronic use. As drug use continues, the reasons for using the drug shift from purely seeking a drug's positive reinforcing effects to avoiding withdrawal effects. The opponent-process model characterizes this change in motivation for drug seeking. Neurobiologically, withdrawal effects depend largely on the amygdala. As previously described, the amygdala functions to pair stimuli with a drug's effects; when these drug effects cease, the amygdala, through connections with the hypothalamus and autonomic nervous system control centers such as the medulla, triggers an array of physical withdrawal symptoms that may include gastrointestinal effects, heart-rate changes, breathing-rate changes, body temperature dysregulation, and sleep disturbances. Further, the amygdala also facilitates negative affective symptoms such as fear, anxiety, and dread. Although the amygdala is capable of producing a wide array of withdrawal effects, the actual withdrawal effects depend on the particular drug.

As the chronic use of abused drugs continues, addiction enters a preoccupation and anticipation stage. During this stage, a person is preoccupied with seeking and using drugs. Drug use at this stage is more than simply seeking

table **5.4**

Drug-Addiction Cycle		
Addiction stage	**Characteristics**	**Neurobiology**
Intoxication	Acute drug effects	Reward circuitry
Withdrawal	Repeated drug use results in physical or psychological withdrawal effects (or both)	Amygdala, hypothalamus, and autonomic nervous system
Preoccupation and anticipation	Behavior orients from seeking natural reinforcers to seeking drug reinforcers	Prefrontal cortex, amygdala, thalamus, and hippocampus

a drug for positive reinforcing effects or to avoid aversive withdrawal effects. Rather, this stage reflects a learning pattern of drug seeking that, depending on the particular substance, can conflict with learning patterns important for normal everyday activities. Incentivization of stimuli that promote drug "wanting" may develop through the involvement of brain reward circuitry with learning systems, including the thalamo-cortical-amygdala pathway and the hippocampus. Overall, this circuitry facilitates associating drug effects with stimuli, especially in assigning incentive value to these stimuli. Through changes in the prefrontal cortex, chronic drug use affects planning and decision making, thereby facilitating a preoccupation with drug seeking and use.

Relapse represents another important feature of this third addiction stage. In a neurobiological context, relapse occurs as a result of the drug's earlier changes to the brain's learning systems. In particular, encountering stimuli once strongly paired with drug use may elicit the desire for a drug by reengaging these systems. Studies by Kalivas and colleagues show that such stimuli activate glutamate neurons that innervate the nucleus accumbens and ventral tegmental area (Kalivas, 2009; LaLumiere & Kalivas, 2008). These glutamate signals may reengage prior neural associations that facilitate the incentive value of these stimuli, essentially eliciting this wanting state. Such stimuli can include a friend the individual used drugs with in the past or physical environments similar to those in which the individual routinely used drugs. Another reminder is the drug itself. Administering only a small amount of the drug, such as a drink of alcohol, may lead to further drug use. Box 5.1 provides an example of drug-induced reinstatement in the self-administration procedure.

Psychological and Pharmacological Therapies for Treating Drug Dependence

Once established, a drug addiction is long lasting and challenging to treat. Individuals who fail to respond to treatment have a high mortality rate compared to individuals who responded to treatment and remained drug free. A longitudinal study conducted by Mützell (1998) provides an assessment of mortality rates among treated and nontreated patients with a drug addiction. In this study, Mützell conducted a 20-year longitudinal study of 284 heroin-addicted individuals. The study began with the presentation of an individual to an emergency room, usually the result of a heroin overdose. After receiving emergency care, medical staff invited these patients into a drug-addiction treatment program. Unfortunately, more than half of those attempting treatment absconded soon after.

During a follow-up study 20 years later, researchers found that more than two-thirds of the heroin-addicted individuals had died—regardless of whether or not they had attempted treatment at the hospital. The most frequent causes of death were pneumonia, suicide, physical assault, alcohol intoxication, heroin overdose, and cirrhosis of the liver. During those 20 years, two-thirds of the individuals had also committed various crimes. Only approximately

10 percent of the heroin-addicted individuals remained drug free. These results compare well to a longitudinal study conducted in the United States among individuals addicted to heroin or other opioid drugs. That study reported only 22-percent abstinence rate after a 30-year follow-up (Hser, Hoffman, Grella, & Anglin, 2001).

High mortality rates associated with drug addiction applies to legally available drugs as well. Long-term tobacco use is the greatest cause of deaths from lung cancer, chronic obstructive pulmonary disease, and heart disease annually in the United States. Alcohol causes thousands of U.S. deaths each year from liver diseases and alcohol overdose. Moreover, alcohol is a significant contributor to lethal car accidents and violence-related deaths each year.

Drug-addiction treatment options include psychotherapy, medications, or a combination of both. These forms of treatment address drug detoxification, prevention of and coping with withdrawal symptoms, and the prevention of relapse. Detoxification is the first step in any addiction treatment.

intoxication A drug's acute maladaptive or impairing effects.

Intoxication refers to a drug's acute maladaptive or impaired effects. **Detoxification** consists of process aimed at ceasing drug intoxication and reducing withdrawal symptoms. Detoxification uses two key approaches: medication and prevention of drug use. Medications provide the means to reduce or eliminate short-term withdrawal symptoms. Otherwise, a drug-addicted individual may simply refrain from using a drug or be denied access to the drug. For a treatment program, detoxification from illicit substances usually occurs in a hospital setting or an in-house treatment facility.

detoxification Process aimed at ceasing drug intoxication and reducing withdrawal symptoms.

Heroin withdrawal treatment, for example, includes medications that reduces the severity of withdrawal symptoms. These treatment options include substitute heroin-like drugs (such as methadone) or medications for specific withdrawal symptoms (such as pain-relieving drugs, anxiety-reducing drugs, and sleep aids). Severe heroin withdrawal symptoms occasionally require general anesthesia, enabling the person to sleep until the worst symptoms subside.

After completing drug detoxification, treatment options seek to reduce further withdrawal symptoms and drug cravings and to prevent relapse. Both medication and psychotherapy provide benefits for remaining drug free. Medications for treating drug addiction include those that directly address drug withdrawal and those that treat comorbid disorders such as depression and anxiety. One medicinal approach is drug-replacement therapy. **Drug-replacement therapy** exchanges the addictive drug with a similar but less harmful drug.

drug-replacement therapy Exchanging the addictive drug with a similar but less harmful drug.

Replacement therapies for tobacco include nicotine patches, nicotine gums, and nicotine-like drugs such as varenicline (Chantix). These treatments require the avoidance of tobacco use and the physically harmful tar particles released during tobacco use. Instead, nicotine or nicotine-like drugs substitute for the nicotine in tobacco. Although this strategy reduces harm from tobacco, treating a nicotine dependence using this approach requires that an individual slowly reduce the amount of nicotine used until the individual can successfully quit without the occurrence of appreciable withdrawal symptoms.

Other medications reduce cravings by acting on the same sites of action as the addictive drug. For example, the antidepressant drug bupropion (Wellbutrin) reduces cravings for tobacco and cocaine. Although bupropion is not a drug of abuse, it blocks the reuptake of dopamine and norepinephrine. In the nucleus accumbens, both nicotine and cocaine raise extracellular dopamine concentrations, which produces positive reinforcing effects. By elevating dopamine levels, bupropion substitutes for this specific pharmacological action for nicotine and cocaine, thereby reducing cravings for these drugs.

Another approach consists of psychotherapy. For drug addiction, psychotherapy includes behavioral therapies, cognitive–behavioral therapies, and social therapies. Each therapy type seeks to eliminate maladaptive behavior surrounding drug use. Toward this goal, therapy aims to reduce addictive drug use to manageable levels or to eliminate drug use altogether.

behavioral therapies
Therapies that use the principles of applied behavior analysis to analyze and develop strategies to treat drug addiction.

Behavioral therapies use applied behavior analysis principles to analyze and develop strategies to treat drug addiction. According to behavioral analyses, drugs serve as powerful reinforcing stimuli that maintain drug-seeking behavior. Behavioral therapies attempt to provide alternative reinforcers for behaviors in this drug-seeking and using process.

Behavioral therapy can include contingency-management approaches, which seek to provide healthy alternative reinforcers to those associated with addictive drug seeking. Alternative reinforcers include community reinforcers, monetary reinforcers, and voucher reinforcers. Community reinforcers include engagement in valuable and rewarding activities such as employment, volunteering, recreational activities, and improved interpersonal relationships. Monetary and voucher reinforcers are incentives for remaining drug free. In this context, a voucher is exchangeable for a tangible good in the community. Behavioral therapists may provide money or vouchers after a client provides a drug-free urine sample.

cognitive–behavioral therapies Therapies that teach drug-addicted individuals to identify and reduce urges to use a substance.

Cognitive–behavioral therapies teach drug-addicted individuals to identify and reduce their urges to use a substance. Once trained, individuals learn to avoid stimuli or situations that precipitate drug cravings and learn strategies for coping with drug cravings. For legal substances such as tobacco and alcohol, cognitive–behavioral therapy goals may consist of reduced and responsible drug use rather than completely ending drug use. In this perspective, addictive drug use is a manageable behavior, not an incurable disease.

social therapies
Therapies that consist of group therapy sessions where individuals interact with a group therapist as well as other individuals also struggling with addiction.

Social therapies consist of group therapy sessions in which individuals interact with a group therapist as well as other individuals also struggling with addiction. Group therapy facilitates a social support network whereby individuals join others in their common battle with addiction. Social therapies may also include one-on-one therapy sessions that teach coping strategies for dealing with drug cravings, including cognitive approaches such as those already described.

Twelve-step recovery programs such as Alcoholics Anonymous and Narcotics Anonymous are popular social therapies for drug addiction. These programs tend to characterize drug addiction according to the disease model and advocate complete abstention from drug use. Anonymous programs guide members, known only on a first-name basis, through 12 recovery steps, beginning with admission that drug use is out of control. The 12 steps further include acceptance of weaknesses in control of drug use as well as other parts of their life. Ultimately, these weaknesses are addressed through moral and social support by group members, a program sponsor, and family and friends. Twelve-step programs also promote members to accept a greater moral purpose or power beyond oneself, which contributes to a heightened sense of spirituality.

Although a variety of treatment options exist, none appears totally effective in treating everyone with a drug addiction. A nationwide assessment of treatment effectiveness called the Drug Abuse Treatment Outcomes Study provides one of best surveys of long-term outcomes of drug-addiction treatment. This study assessed the effectiveness of four primary treatment programs for patients who abused heroin, cocaine, marijuana, or alcohol, whether singly or in combination. The programs included outpatient methadone treatment, long-term residential treatment, outpatient drug-free treatment, and short-term inpatient treatment. Both long-term residential and short-term inpatient treatments employed some type of medication to address cravings or physiological withdrawal effects. Outpatient drug-free treatment programs provided any variety of therapeutic approaches, including 12-step programs or one-on-one therapy. Short-term inpatient programs provided some type of medical treatment to address symptoms derived from abrupt withdrawal of a drug.

Although most patients reported declines in substance use 1 year later, a follow-up with patients 5 years later revealed increased trends in substance use (Hubbard, Craddock, & Anderson, 2003). More individuals previously enrolled in methadone outpatient and long-term residential treatment programs for heroin abuse reported using heroin at a 5-year follow-up compared to a 1-year follow-up. The number of individuals previously enrolled in a long-term residential treatment program for cocaine use also increased when surveyed 5 years after treatment compared to 1 year after treatment. Fortunately, not every program saw increased relapse rates. Five-year follow-ups for both heroin and cocaine use did not increase for patients enrolled in either outpatient drug-free or short-term inpatient programs. **Figure 5.8** shows these other results with substance use before entering a program and 4 years after enrolling in a program.

Although increased substance use was reported for two programs shown in figure 5.8, many patients had relapsed and then sought treatment again during this 5-year period. Relapse is not unusual after a successful abstention from substance use. As discussed previously in this chapter, learning how to prevent relapse is an important part of drug-addiction research. To determine why some patients sought treatment again after relapse, but others did not, in the Drug Abuse Treatment Outcomes Study, Grella and colleagues (2003) conducted an analysis of the reasons patients expressed for reseeking treatment.

For this analysis, Grella and colleagues (2003) focused on cocaine-addicted users who relapsed during this study. By assessing the data gathered on these users, this research team used correlational study procedures to determine the impact of certain personal or environmental characteristics for those reseeking treatment versus those not reseeking treatment. The investigators found users reseeking treatment after relapse had an increased likelihood of being married and had experiences with drug-treatment programs before enrolling in the study. Among these prior treatment programs,

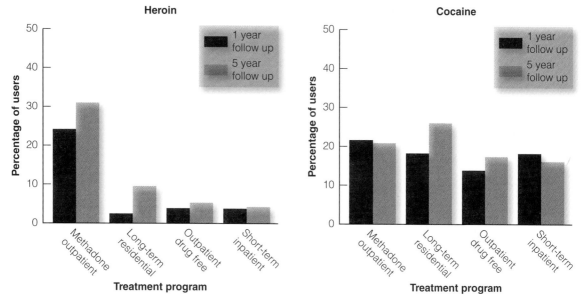

figure **5.8** One-year (dark-blue) and 5-year follow-ups (light blue) in patients seeking a treatment for heroin (left) or cocaine (right) addiction. (Data from Hubbard et al., 2003.)

most users who resought treatment had participated in a 12-step recovery program. Finally, those reseeking treatment expressed a desire for help and a readiness to accept treatment. Findings such as these provide researchers and therapists directions for improving successful treatment approaches.

REVIEW! In a correlational study, researchers do not manipulate variables. Instead, they evaluate potential relationships between variables as they already exist. Chapter 1 (pg. 12).

Stop & Check

1. Which neurobiological systems mediate rewarding effects during the intoxication of drug use?

2. How do withdrawal symptoms occur when a chronically administered drug is absent from the body?

3. What is the first step in addiction treatment?

4. What is the key difference between behavioral or cognitive–behavioral therapies versus 12-step programs such as Alcoholics Anonymous?

Anonymous programs seek the complete abstinence of the addicted drug's use.
and cognitive–behavioral therapies seek to reduce drug use to a manageable level.
system effects, leading to withdrawal symptoms. **3.** Detoxification **4.** Behavioral
negative affective state and elicits the hypothalamus to produce autonomic nervous
the nucleus accumbens **2.** When an addicted drug is absent, the amygdala elicits a
1. The reward circuit structures, which consist of the ventral tegmental area and

FROM ACTIONS TO EFFECTS
Food Addiction

||||||||||||||||||||||||||||||||||||||||||||||||||||||||||||||||||||||||||||||||||||||||||||||||||||||||||||||||||||||||||||||||||||||||||||||||||||||||||||||||||||||||||||||||||||||||||||||||||

Food addictions appear to be relatively prevalent among maladaptive disorders. Although we lack precise figures on the prevalence of food addiction, currently one-third of U.S. adults have body mass index (BMI) values over 30, the medical definition for obesity. Obesity in the United States took more than $200 billion in health-care expenses between 1998 and 2000, and obesity contributes to more than 300,000 deaths in the United States each year. Although obesity occurs from many factors, including physical inactivity, types of foods consumed, and genetic predispositions, the rewarding effects of highly palatable foods are likely contributors to obesity.

Food addiction is an emerging focus for mental health professionals. The current DSM fails to characterize food addiction as a disorder, although clinicians who work with food-addicted individuals tend to follow criteria used for diagnosing a substance dependence (Davis et al., 2011; Ifland et al., 2009). Further, we find growing scientific interest in considering obesity to be similar to substance dependence (Ifland et al., 2009; Volkow & O'Brien, 2007; Volkow & Wise, 2005). Here we consider some of the features that food addiction that shares with substance dependence.

A study by Pretlow (2011) provides an illustration for how obesity might satisfy DSM criteria for dependence. This study included a survey of anonymous qualitative statements provided by nearly 30,000 individuals ranging from ages 8 to 21. All participants had BMI levels 30 or higher and were, on average, at the 96th percentile for BMI. From reviewing statements posted on the study's Web site, Pretlow wrote that "the majority of posts exhibited at least three criteria [for substance dependence], particularly: (a) large amounts of substance consumed over a long period, (b) unsuccessful efforts to cut down, and (c) continued use despite adverse consequences." Further, participants described food use that shared many characteristics of drug tolerance, which consisted of progressively increasing food consumption over time, and drug withdrawal, as characterized by urges to overeat when attempting to diet. Among those who reported urges, nearly half described them as "intense cravings."

Overeating shares many of the neurobiological features of drug addiction (Volkow, Wang, Fowler, Tomasi, & Baler, 2011). Like drugs of abuse, foods can produce reinforcing effects by acting on brain reward circuitry. As described previously, sugary liquid food consumed by rats causes large elevations in nucleus accumbens dopamine levels (figure 5.5). Appetite hormones also regulate dopamine neurons in the reward pathway. The hunger-stimulating hormone ghrelin greatly enhances food-elicited increases in mesolimbic dopamine neuron activity, and research also shows that ghrelin enhances self-administration responding for heroin (see box 5.1). The hunger-reducing hormone leptin diminishes food-elicited increases in dopamine neuron activity. Thus, hunger enhances food's reinforcing effects, whereas satiety reduces foods' reinforcing effects. Research is ongoing to determine how addictive food use may interact with learning and memory systems in ways similar to addictive drug use.

Some food-addiction therapies resemble drug-addiction therapies, but others do not. Behavioral therapies, for example, may provide alternative reinforcers to overeating. Cognitive–behavioral approaches attempt to alter a person's view of food and then develop strategies to cope with food cravings. Just as social support drug-addiction programs include Alcoholics Anonymous and Narcotics Anonymous, social support groups exist for overeating, include Overeaters Anonymous and Food Addicts Anonymous (Johnson & Sansone, 1993; Russell-Mayhew, von Ranson, & Masson, 2010).

Medically, however, most therapies address the physical impact of food addiction rather than treating the addiction itself. For example, medical obesity treatments include appetite-reducing medications, medications that impair food absorption, and surgical procedures (Powell, Apovian, & Aronne, 2011; Stefater, Wilson-Perez, Chambers, Sandoval, & Seeley, 2012). Surgical procedures include liposuction, a fat-extracting procedure; stomach bands or staples, which reduce the size of the stomach; and temporarily wiring a patient's jaw shut to enforce a liquid diet.

Otherwise, the DSM considers overeating, or *compulsive eating*, as a symptom of another disorder such as anxiety or depression. Thus, to reduce overeating, one must treat the disorder causing overeating. For example, if overeating is a way of coping with stress or anxiety, then directly treating stress or anxiety will reduce overeating. Similarly, if overeating allows one to cope with depression, then treating depression will reduce overeating.

Thus, although psychologists and other mental health therapy providers treat overeating either as substance dependence or as a symptom of another disorder, the lack of a clear clinical definition for food addiction leaves food-addictive behaviors largely in the realm of medical symptoms for other disorders. An agreement among mental health professionals about food addiction would help clarify this diagnosis and aid in the development of appropriate treatment strategies.

Stop & Check

1. How do highly palatable foods elicit reinforcing effects?
2. How do therapists diagnose food addiction?

1. Like drugs of abuse, foods elicit increased dopamine release in the nucleus accumbens. **2.** The DSM does not include food addiction among psychological disorders. However, therapists find that the general DSM definition for substance dependence applies well to food addiction. Moreover, some therapeutic approaches for drug addiction, such as 12-step programs, also apply well to food addiction.

▶ CHAPTER SUMMARY

Regulatory agencies regulate the availability and use of drugs with abuse potential. In the United States, the Drug Enforcement Administration categorizes such drugs according to abuse potential and medical utility on a controlled substances schedule. Drug scheduling occurs in other countries, but their methods and category systems sometimes differ. Although drug scheduling provides a regulatory rating for the abuse potential of drugs, these ratings do not necessarily coincide with scientific ratings of abuse potential. A clinical diagnosis of addiction depends on medical criteria that have evolved since the first major definition offered by the World Health Organization in the 1950s. Newer clinical definitions of drug addiction include harmful effects from drug use and consider addiction as a chronically relapsing disorder.

To understand addictive behavior better, researchers use drug-addiction models. These models include considering addiction as a disease or as behavior controlled by drug-elicited variables. Drugs of abuse derive their effects through acting on the brain's reward circuit, which was first discovered by James Olds. Drugs that elicit positive reinforcing effects cause dopamine neurons in the reward circuit to release dopamine into the nucleus accumbens. Chronic usage of drugs of abuse affect brain structures for learning and memory.

We have many treatment strategies for addiction, including detoxification, medicines, and therapy—unfortunately, these strategies offer limited success. Many of the features of drug abuse and addiction relate to other addictions as well. For example, food addiction engages many of the same brain systems involved in drug addiction, satisfies clinical definitions for drug addiction, and can be treated by many approaches used for drug addiction.

KEY TERMS

Substance dependence

Substance abuse

Relapse

Disease model

Associative learning

Reinforcement

Conditioned stimulus

Incentive salience

Goal-directed behavior

Opponent-process theory

Incentive-salience model

Craving

Intoxication

Detoxification

Drug-replacement therapy

Behavioral therapies

Cognitive–behavioral therapies

Social therapies

Break point

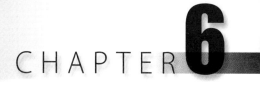

© Argosy Publishing Inc.

CHAPTER **6**

Psychostimulants

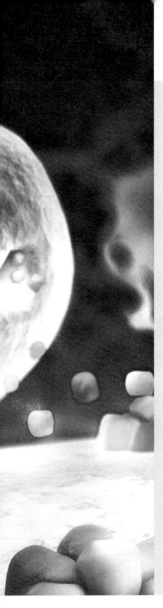

Fleischl and the Neurologist

Dr. Fleischl was a desperate man. He had painful tumors down his spine; in search of relief, he developed an addiction to morphine. Fleischl sought the help of his hospital colleagues, including a motivated young neurologist known for unique thinking and big ideas.

The neurologist visited Fleischl on many occasions and offered what advice he could. During these visits, Fleischl obsessed over suicidal thoughts, and the neurologist became convinced that unless he did something, Fleischl would kill himself. Although the neurologist was unable to treat the disease, he perhaps could rid Fleischl of his morphine addiction. In May 1884, the neurologist administered his experimental treatment: cocaine.

At the beginning of treatment, Fleischl experienced his first pain-free days without morphine in years. But only one week later his pain returned in force. Then, instead of an addiction to morphine, Fleischl developed an addiction to cocaine. The neurologist wrote that Fleischl clung to cocaine "like a drowning man," and the neurologist was horrified by the enormous doses Fleischl used and paid a fortune for.

Fleischl survived for 6 more agonizing years, dying at age 45. Fleischl's suffering and cocaine addiction made a tremendous impact on the life of this young neurologist, Sigmund Freud.

Based on Byck (1974) and Jones (1953).

Throughout the day, all of us experience moments of high alertness and arousal. You might experience this after realizing you slept through your alarm clock and have to rush out the door to avoid being late. Or you might be jolted to alertness if a car swerves in front of you and you quickly slam on the brakes. You may become more attentive if your instructor begins randomly choosing students in class to answer questions about the lecture she just gave.

Think about how you feel in these situations. Your heart rate probably becomes rapid. Your mind is racing to meet the challenge you face. You are in a state of high alertness. You might even find the experience exhilarating. All of these states activate arousal processes in the central and peripheral nervous systems. Psychostimulant drugs act on these same nervous system processes.

Psychostimulants: A Large Variety of Substances

psychostimulant Drugs that increase psychomotor and sympathetic nervous system activity as well as improve alertness and positive mood.

Psychostimulant drugs increase psychomotor and sympathetic nervous system activity as well as improve alertness and positive mood. Psychostimulants are also referred to as *sympathomimetics,* because they increase sympathetic nervous system activity. Common psychostimulants include amphetamines, methylphenidate, cathinones, and cocaine. Amphetamines represent a class of drugs, among which include amphetamine and methamphetamine. Cathinones include many drugs, such as cathinones and pyrovalerone as well as synthetic cathinones such as methcathinone and mephedrone.

Although this chapter focuses on psychostimulants as drugs, many psychostimulant drugs have legitimate therapeutic purposes. Some amphetamines have legitimate uses for the treatment of *attention deficit hyperactivity disorder* (ADHD), narcolepsy, and obesity. Cocaine was once commonly used as a local anesthetic for nasal and tear duct surgery. Given these medical uses, the U.S. Drug Enforcement Administration (DEA) assigns most psychostimulant drugs below schedule I (see **table 6.1**). However, the level of regulatory control for these drugs varies among countries. Canada, for example, assigns methamphetamine to the schedule I category, therefore preventing medicinal methamphetamine use.

Psychostimulants are well known as drugs of abuse. According to the National Institute on Drug Abuse, 1.2 million Americans used methamphetamine in 2009. In schools, 3.4 percent of 12th graders abused methylphenidate in 2008. In 2009, 4.8 million Americans used cocaine, including 1.1 million individuals who used *crack* cocaine (Substance Abuse and Mental Health Services Administration, 2010). In Europe, approximately 4 million people ages 15 and older used cocaine in 2008 (European Monitoring Centre for

table 6.1

Drug Enforcement Administration Controlled Substances Schedules for Psychostimulant Drugs	
Psychostimulant	**Schedule**
Amphetamine	III
Cathinone	I
Cathine (norpseudoephedrine)	IV
Cocaine	II
Methamphetamine	II
Methcathinone	I
Methylphenidate	II
Pyrovalerone	V

Adapted from the DEA Controlled Substances Schedules. (www.deadiversion.usdoj.gov/schedules/index.html)

Drugs and Drug Addiction, 2009). Few studies have evaluated the prevalence of cathinone or derivatives of cathinone, owing to their relatively recent emergence of popular drugs of abuse, particularly in the form of so-called bath salts, as described next. In an attempt to estimate the usage of cathinones, Winstock and colleagues (2011) conducted an anonymous online drug use survey of visitors to the Web sites for the music club scene. The results from this survey indicated that more than 40 percent of the 2,295 respondents had used methcathinone and 15 percent had used methcathinone frequently.

Designer psychostimulant drugs sold as *bath salts*—which have no legitimate use in bathing—have recently earned the attention of governmental authorities. Bath salts contain any variety of synthetic cathinones, including methcathinone, methylenedioxypyrovalerone, methylone, and mephedrone. One of the first reports in the United States to raise alarms about the growing use of bath salts occurred in Michigan's rural Marquette County, which reported 27 emergency room visits between November 2010 and March 2011 directly linked to the drugs (CDC, 2011). Two reports also describe an increased frequency of emergency room visits or calls to poison control centers in the United Kingdom because of mephedrone, suggesting that bath salt problems are not restricted to the United States (James et al., 2011; Wood, Greene, & Dargan, 2011). In September 2011, the DEA used its emergency scheduling authority to temporarily classify suspected psychoactive bath salt ingredients as schedule I controlled substances (Drug Enforcement Administration, 2011).

Psychostimulants: Herbal Remedies, Prescription Drugs, and Substances of Abuse

Ephedra

The first amphetamines were derived from ephedra, an extract of the plant *Ephedra sinica* found in dry climates in North and South America, southern Europe, central Asia, and northern Africa (**figure 6.1**). Ephedra contains two psychoactive components: *ephedrine* and *pseudoephedrine*. Many cold remedies contain these stimulants, but since 2006, U.S. pharmacies limit the number of products sold in a single purchase. By regulating the sale of ephedrine and pseudoephedrine, state law enforcement agencies hope to reduce the clandestine production of methamphetamine and other illicit psychostimulant drugs.

Amphetamines

amphetamines Class of psychostimulant drugs that share a similar structure.

Amphetamines represent a class of psychostimulant drugs that share a similar structure. The drug amphetamine has two *optical isomers*—that is, the chemical structure occurs in two different forms that are *mirror images* of

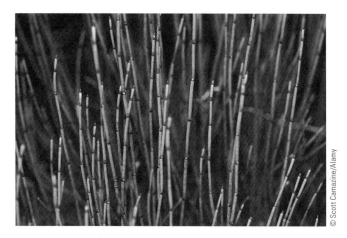

© Scott Camazine/Alamy

Ephedra sinica plants are native to dry climates in North and South America, southern Europe, central Asia, and northern Africa. (From http://home.caregroup.org/clinical/altmed/interactions /Herbs/Ephedra_sinica.htm.)

figure 6.1

each other—designated as *d* or *l*.* The drug *amphetamine* (Benzedrine) refers to *racemic* amphetamine, a mixture of both d and l optical isomers. The d-amphetamine isomer is sold as the medication Dexedrine, and the drug Adderall contains a 3:1 ratio of d-amphetamine and l-amphetamine. At one time, both racemic and d-amphetamine were approved by the Food and Drug Administration (FDA) for the treatment of attention hyperactivity disorder and narcolepsy, but currently these drugs have been pulled from the market. Adderall, however, remains on the market and has been approved by the FDA for the treatment of attention hyperactivity disorder and narcolepsy (Food and Drug Adminstration, 2007).

Methamphetamine (Desoxyn) is synthesized from ephedrine, pseudoephedrine, or the organic solvent phenylacetone (**figure 6.2**). Although methamphetamine is notoriously known as a drug of abuse, the FDA approves its use for the treatment of ADHD. The illicit production of methamphetamine occurring in a "meth lab" uses household chemicals along with either ephedrine or pseudoephedrine. In addition, meth labs may use the chemical phenylacetone in place of either ephedrine or pseudoephedrine. Meth lab synthesis methods produce a crystallized form of methamphetamine referred to as *crystal meth*, *crystal*, *speed*, *crank*, and other street names. Synthesizing methamphetamine from these methods produces toxic and flammable solvent vapors and gases, which account for a large number of third-degree burn victims in emergency care every year.

---

*The *d* and *l* designations refer to *dextrorotatory* and *levrorotary*, meaning the molecules turn to the right or left in a plane of polarized light.

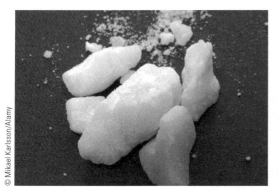
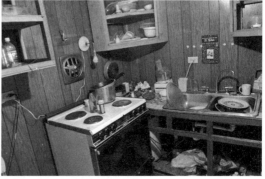

figure **6.2**   Methamphetamine crystals (left) are clandestinely made in meth labs (right) from ephedrine, pseudoephedrine, or the organic solvent phenylacetone.

Methylphenidate

Methylphenidate is a prescription psychostimulant drug used for the treatment of ADHD. Methylphenidate structurally differs from the amphetamines and cocaine and is only available in prescription form. We generally regard methylphenidate as a weak psychostimulant drug, which is probably why there is almost no illicit production of this substance. To use methylphenidate as a drug of abuse, users may often obtain methylphenidate from instrumental users. Those who are prescribed methylphenidate may choose to recreationally use the drug by grinding it up and snorting it. Because of its use for treating attention hyperactivity disorder in children, a common street name for methylphenidate is *kiddie coke*.

Cathinones

cathinone Psychostimulant derived from the leaves of Catha edulis.

The psychostimulant **cathinone** comes from the leaves of *Catha edulis*, which is also referred to as *khat*. It is found in east Africa and the Arabian Peninsula, and the traditional use of khat involves chewing the leaves or using the leaves in tea. Fresh khat leaves produce the most potent psychostimulant effects, which limits khat use to local inhabitants. Not only is cathinone used for psychostimulant effects, but also are its derivatives of cathinone, including methcathinone, methadrone, and pyrovalerones.

Clandestine laboratories produce cathinone derivatives such as methcathinone from cathinone, as well as other chemicals including the ephedra extract pseudoephedrine. As discussed previously, bath salts have recently emerged as psychostimulant drugs, which include mephedrone, methylone, and the methcathinone-like substance methylenedioxypyrovalerone (Baumann et al., 2012). Bath salts are known by many names, including *Starry Nights*, *Vanilla*, *Sky*, and *White Rush*.

Cocaine

cocaine Psychostimulant derived from the leaves of erythroxylon coca.

coca paste Liquid paste from the breaking and mixing of coca leaves.

Leaves of the *Erythroxylon coca* plant, which is found in the higher elevations of South America, provide a direct source of **cocaine** (**figure 6.3**). Cocaine is separated from these leaves and processed in either pharmaceutical or clandestine laboratories. Clandestine cocaine processing begins by breaking down and mixing coca leaves into a liquid to form a **coca paste**. The coca paste, which contains between 30 percent and 80 percent of cocaine bases, is then dried and sold for recreational use or transported to a *crystal lab* for further processing. A crystal lab represents the switch from a cottage industry to a sophisticated international industry (Casale & Klein, 1993).

Crystal labs convert cocaine from bases into a high purity salt. The labs then provide cocaine to smugglers who transport it to international clients. The salt form is produced for two reasons. First, it is a purer cocaine product than the cocaine in extracted base form. Second, the salt form allows for either *insufflating* (snorting) or intravenously injecting cocaine.

Many cocaine users, however, prefer the base form, which can be smoked. These differences are the result of the difference in vaporization points. Vaporization of the salt form of cocaine occurs at a very high temperature: 195°C (383°F). This method makes it hard not only to reach these temperatures with an ignition source but also to safely inhale the vapors without lung damage. However, the base form of cocaine has a lower vaporization point, 98°C (208°F), allowing users to easily smoke it.

Given that the smugglers often transport the cocaine's salt form, smoking cocaine requires transforming the salt form into a base form. This process requires the removal of hydrochloride (the salt) from the cocaine molecule. When cocaine salt is heated with a mixture of baking soda and water, the

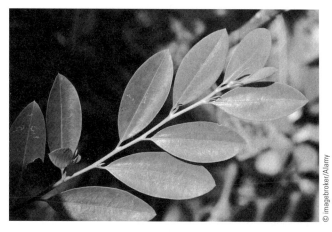

© imagebroker/Alamy

figure 6.3 Cocaine is a constituent in the leaves of the *Erythroxylon coca* plant, which is found at higher elevations in South America.

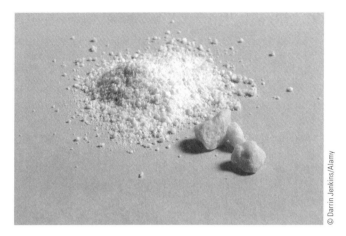

© Darrin Jenkins/Alamy

figure 6.4 Cocaine is used in both a powdered salt form (left) and a crystal or *crack* form (right). (From http://en.wikipedia.org/wiki/File:Colcoca03.jpg.)

freebasing Heating and smoking the freebase form of cocaine.

hydrochloride molecule separates from cocaine, "freeing" the base* from the salt. The *freebase* form of cocaine is called *crack* cocaine because of the crackling sound these freebase crystals make when heated (**figure 6.4**). The term **freebasing** refers to heating and smoking the freebase form of cocaine.

Stop & Check

1. What are the primary psychoactive ingredients in ephedra?
2. The sale of ephedrine and pseudoephedrine is regulated in the United States and other countries because of the clandestine production of _____.
3. Why have bath salts become a concern for law enforcement agencies?
4. Which form of cocaine can be smoked?

1. Ephedrine and pseudoephedrine **2.** methamphetamine **3.** Drugs sold as bath salts contain synthetic cathinone compounds that elicit psychostimulant effects. **4.** The freebase form, which is referred to as *crack* cocaine. The boiling point for freebase cocaine allows it to be smoked in a pipe, whereas the vaporization point for the salt form of cocaine is too high to reach without special laboratory equipment.

Instrumental and Recreational Purposes of Psychostimulants

The discovery of amphetamines, cathinones, and cocaine came from investigations into the psychoactive properties of plants. From these discoveries, entire lines of psychostimulant drugs have been developed. Newer drugs, originating

*Technically, a freebase must include an amine (NH_2) group, which cocaine does.

entirely from synthesis methods in chemical laboratories, include designer psychostimulant drugs, such as the ingredient found in bath salts, and therapeutic drugs, such as the ADHD treatment methylphenidate (Ritalin). This section describes the discovery of the first psychostimulant drugs and selected recent psychostimulant drugs.

Amphetamines

In 1887, German chemists developed amphetamine in an effort to develop a mass producible form of ephedra. In the 1920s, physicians used amphetamine as a drug for raising blood pressure; in 1937, amphetamine was first used to treat ADHD (Bradley, 1937; Brecher, 1972). Amphetamine's stimulant effects provided the first effective treatment for narcolepsy, a neurological sleep disorder characterized by extreme fatigue and excessive daytime sleep. During World War II, the U.S. military used amphetamine to improve alertness and reduce fatigue. After the war, leftover amphetamine supplies released to the general population led to a brief amphetamine-abuse epidemic in Japan (Brecher, 1972; Brill & Hirose, 1969).

In 1919, a Japanese chemist discovered methamphetamine after testing different synthesis methods that employed either ephedrine or pseudoephedrine. Another method was later developed for synthesizing methamphetamine from the organic solvent phenylacetone. In an attempt to reduce illicit methamphetamine production, the U.S. Drug Enforcement Administration first regulated the sale of phenylacetone, but this led illicit meth labs to synthesize methamphetamine from ephedrine or pseudoephedrine instead. In response to this, in 2006 the DEA began regulating the sale of ephedrine and pseudoephedrine, which as described earlier, are common ingredients in over-the-counter cold medications (Vearrier, Greenberg, Miller, Okaneku, & Haggerty, 2012).

Methylphenidate

In 1944, Leandro Panizzon, a chemist working for the Ciba Pharmaceutical Company, discovered methylphenidate, subsequently naming the drug *Ritaline* after this wife Rita. After identifying the drug's psychostimulant effects, physicians began prescribing methylphenidate for the treatment of ADHD in the 1960s. However, ADHD was not universally accepted as a disorder until the 1980s, and as ADHD diagnoses subsequently increased, so did methylphenidate prescriptions. Today, methylphenidate is prescribed to more than two-thirds of the approximately 5 million U.S. children with ADHD (Mayes, Bagwell, & Erkulwater, 2008).

Cathinones

Inhabitants of Arabia, Ethiopia, and east Africa have used khat, the source of cathinone, for centuries. The first cultivation of khat was documented in the early 1300s by King Sabr ad-Din of Ifat, who ordered its planting in the town of Marad. Europeans first discovered khat during an expedition in 1760 to Arabia ordered by King Frederick V of Denmark. During this expedition, physician and botanist Peter Forsskål discovered khat and named the plant *Catha edulis* (Al-Hebshi & Skaug, 2005; Gebissa, 2010).

Methcathinone was synthesized in the Soviet Union in 1928 and has been recreationally used since the late 1970s. Reports of methcathinone abuse began in the early 1990s (Emerson & Cisek, 1993). Currently, the origins of the recapitulated form of synthetic cathinones as bath salts is unknown.

Cocaine

Erythroxylon coca was long used by indigenous people for religious purposes, appetite suppression, and enhanced vigor and stamina. In the mid-1500s, Spanish conquistadors first discovered the plant during their conquest of the Incan empire in Peru. Cocaine was first extracted from coca leaves in 1844. In 1883, Theodor Aschenbrandt, a German Army physician, reported the anti-fatiguing properties of cocaine in soldiers. This report inspired a young physician, Sigmund Freud, to study cocaine's behavioral effects (Freud, 1974).

In 1884, Freud was fresh out of medical school and serving as a physician and lecturer at the Psychiatric Institute of the General Hospital of Vienna. Freud already had achieved a distinguished series of accomplishments in research on the nervous system. In fact, he wrote extensively in letters to his fiancé, Martha Bernays, about his desire for a career in research, but practicing medicine seemed his only option for making a living. He first chose to practice surgery because this required the least amount of interaction with his patients. A few months later, Freud obtained a psychiatric institute position, which held possibilities for research. A major discovery, he hoped, would lead to a profitable research career.

With this in mind, Freud sought a major discovery. He was intrigued by Aschenbrandt's reports on cocaine and decided to study it. In April 1884, Freud requested 1 gram of cocaine from Merck pharmaceuticals. On June 18, 1884, less than two months later, he had completed both his research and a full manuscript on his findings.

In this manuscript, *Über Coca* ("On Coca"), Freud provided the most in-depth review of cocaine at the time, which included information on coca plants, ancient human use, effects observed in animals, and his own self-reports (**figure 6.5**). Freud lauded the benefits of cocaine and pressed its usage at every opportunity. Yet Freud's interest in cocaine eventually waned. Years later Freud declared cocaine a "scourge" of humanity.

His first misgivings arose from a suffering friend, Dr. von Fleischl-Marxow, who suffered from severe pain caused by tumors along his peripheral nerves. Freud suggested that the anesthetic properties of cocaine may help, and soon Fleischl had escalated his daily dose to 1000 mg per day – approximately 20 times the amount Freud occasionally gave to himself. Eventually, Fleischl developed hallucinations and on one occasion he saw "white snakes creeping over his skin." As the adverse effects of cocaine became known, cocaine use declined in Europe and North America (Freud, 1974; Jones, 1953).

Cocaine served as a key ingredient in Coca-Cola, between 1886 and 1904 (**figure 6.6**), along with another important ingredient, caffeine. The result of this combination, as displayed in the Coca-Cola advertisement in figure 6.6, was a drink that reduced headache and relieved exhaustion. Although not a narcotic, which is defined as a sleep-inducing drug, the sale and distribution

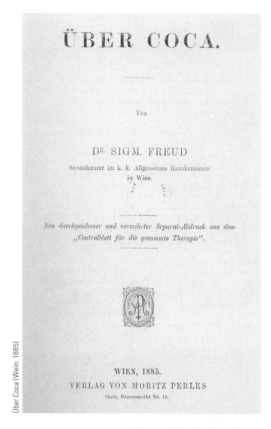

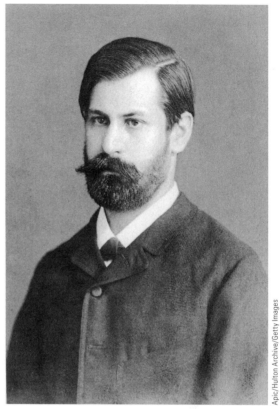

ÜBER COCA.

Von

Dᴿ SIGM. FREUD

Secundararzt im k. k. Allgemeinen Krankenhause
in Wien.

*Neu durchgesehener und vermehrter Separat-Abdruck aus dem
„Centralblatt für die gesammte Therapie".*

WIEN, 1885.
VERLAG VON MORITZ PERLES
Stadt, Bauernmarkt Nr. 11.

Über Coca (Wein: 1885)

Apic/Hulton Archive/Getty Images

figure 6.5 Sigmund Freud, shown here around the time he completed medical school, provided some of the earliest characterizations of cocaine's pharmacological effects in *Über Coca*.

of "coca leaves, their salts, derivatives, or preparations" were regulated under the Harrison Narcotics Act of 1914. The act dealt primarily with the sale and distribution of opioids, which are narcotic drugs, but the association of cocaine with opioids led to cocaine's designation as a narcotic. Cocaine remains classified as a narcotic by the U.S. Drug Enforcement Administration.

Stop & Check

1. Although amphetamine and cocaine are regarded as drugs of abuse, what were their intended purposes historically?

2. Why is Freud an important figure in the history of cocaine?

1. These psychostimulant compounds were developed as potential medicines for humans. In particular, the performance benefits of these compounds led to their use in reducing fatigue. Cocaine was used as a local anesthetic. **2.** Freud provided some of the first behavioral assessments of cocaine and was an early public advocate of cocaine use.

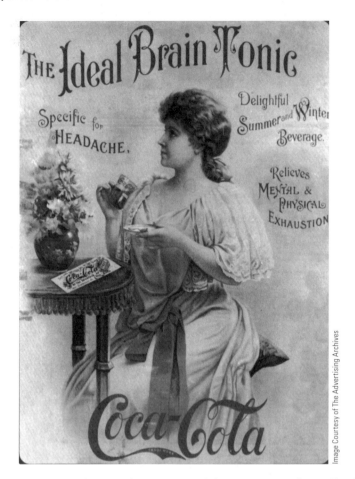

Image Courtesy of The Advertising Archives

figure 6.6 Cocaine was a key ingredient in Coca-Cola between 1886 and 1904. The drink was advertised as a tonic that reduced headache and relieved exhaustion.

Psychostimulant Administration

Routes and Forms of Psychostimulant Administration

The selected route of psychostimulant drug administration depends on the user's desired purpose for taking the drug. For achieving therapeutic effects, physicians prescribe psychostimulant drugs such as amphetamine and methylphenidate for oral administration in pill form. Methylphenidate is also available in liquid and skin-patch form. For achieving reinforcing effects, users prefer administration routes that provide rapid drug absorption, including intravenous injection, insufflation, and inhalation.

The salt forms of psychostimulant drugs tend to allow intravenous injections. To prepare amphetamine pills or methamphetamine crystals in salt form, the substance is first ground into a fine powder. Then it is mixed with a household chemical, which could be a chemical base or an organic solvent, to set the drug in a salt form. Because prescribed methylphenidate tablets contain the salt form of methylphenidate, recreational users crush the tablets in a fine powder. The cathinone drugs in bath salts already exist in salt form; for injection, users simply dissolve them in water.

The salt forms of these drugs also allow for insufflation or *snorting*. Users typically insufflate psychostimulant drugs by sharply inhaling lines of powder into a nostril through a short tube. This method places a substance into contact with membranes in the nose, throat, and lungs. The salt form is necessary for this route because drugs must be water soluble for proper absorption through these membranes.

The base forms of these drugs allow for inhalation. This is usually accomplished by heating the drug on a foil or plate or by heating the drug in a glass bulb or pipe. A *crack pipe* is a glass pipe used to smoke the freebase or crack form of cocaine. Smoking freebase cocaine can cause the release of **methylec-gonidine**, a byproduct of the freebase synthesis process that is harmful to the heart, lungs, and liver.

methylecgonidine
Byproduct of the freebase synthesis process for cocaine that is harmful to the heart, lungs, and liver.

Although intravenous injection, insufflation, and inhalation all provide quick absorption, the time courses among these routes vary. For example, Volkow and colleagues (2000) studied the peak drug effect onset times for different routes of cocaine in cocaine-addicted individuals. Through the inhalation route, cocaine's peak subjective effects occurred after only 1.4 minutes. The intravenous route took twice as long to achieve peek effects, at 3.1 minutes, and insufflation produced the longest onset time for peak subjective effects, at 14.6 minutes (**figure 6.7**). A drug's onset times can affect its

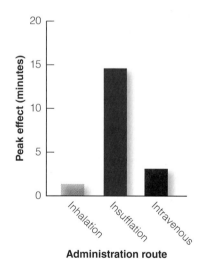

Administration route

figure 6.7   The time peak subjective effects for cocaine vary by administration route. Among the most common routes, inhalation provides a quicker onset time than either insufflation or intravenous use. (Data from Volkow et al., 2000.)

addiction liability. Hatsukami and Fischman (1996), for example, found that cocaine addiction occurred more often for users who preferred inhalation and intravenous routes compared to users who preferred insufflation routes.

Other administration routes result in poorer absorption. Inhabitants of coca plant regions have long chewed coca leaves for their rejuvenating effects and to relieve tooth pain. Because the base form poorly penetrates mucous membranes, the leaves are often chewed with lime to improve water solubility. This in turn improves mucous-membrane absorption. Even with lime, only a small portion of cocaine absorbs through the mucous membranes. On the other hand, chewing khat leaves provides an efficient means of cathinone absorption. Approximately 60 percent of cathinone absorbs through mucosa in the mouth (Toennes, Harder, Schramm, Niess, & Kauert, 2003).

Some psychostimulant drugs produce active metabolites in the liver. Many times an active metabolite exhibits the same effects as the drug. For example, liver enzymes convert methamphetamine to amphetamine. By serving as a parent drug for amphetamine, methamphetamine administration produces psychostimulant effects from both methamphetamine and amphetamine. Other parent drugs for amphetamine include the amphetamines prenylamine (Segontin) and selegiline (Anipryl).

REVIEW! A prodrug is an inert compound that produces a drug as a metabolite. This differs from a drug that produces an active metabolite. Chapter 4 (pg. 108).

Cathinone metabolism in the liver produces the active metabolite norephedrine, which is the "d" optical isomer of pseudoephedrine. As with methamphetamine, cathinone administration leads to psychostimulant effects produced by both cathinone *and* pseudoephedrine. Cocaine's active metabolite benzoylecgonine functions to constrict blood vessels (Madden, Konkol, Keller, & Alvarez, 1995). Combining cocaine with alcohol produces, through metabolism in the liver, the active metabolite cocaethylene, a compound that produces psychostimulant properties (Bradberry et al., 1993; McCance, Price, Kosten, & Jatlow, 1995; Rafla & Epstein, 1979). Through producing this psychostimulant, combined cocaine and alcohol use, otherwise referred to as *polydrug use*, may provide an enhanced pleasurable experience compared to the use of drug alone (McCance et al., 1995). A similar reaction occurs after ingesting methylphenidate and alcohol, which results in the formation metabolite and psychostimulant ethylphenidate. The formation of such active metabolites suggests that polydrug use may increase the likelihood of abuse (Grant & Harford, 1990).

Amphetamine and methamphetamine have longer elimination rates than cocaine. The half-life for amphetamine is approximately 10 hours; similarly, the half-life of methamphetamine is approximately 11 hours. In comparison, cocaine's half-life is a approximately 1 hour, which accounts for shorter psychostimulant effects than amphetamine and methamphetamine. Studies find a 1.5-hour half-life for cathinone, although we need pharmacokinetic information on the rapidly emerging synthetic cathinones (Toennes et al., 2003). Methylphenidate's half-life is approximately

2 hours, requiring additional administrations during a day for a steady drug effect. Given this, a physician may prescribe amphetamine (Adderall) for ADHD to school-aged children in order to avoid having the medication wear off during a school day. Researchers are also developing new formulations of the methylphenidate to prolong its effects (Childress, Sallee, & Berry, 2011).

Stop & Check

1. Why might a user prefer to inhale psychostimulant drugs compared to other administration methods?
2. Why are knowing a drug's metabolites important for learning about psychostimulant effects?

1. The inhalation route offers quicker absorption than insufflation or even intravenous administration. 2. Many psychostimulant drugs alone or in combination with alcohol produce active metabolites, including those acting as psychostimulant drugs.

Psychostimulants and Monoamine Neurotransmitters

Amphetamines

Amphetamines cause an increase in synaptic dopamine levels through two mechanisms of action (**figure 6.8**). First, amphetamine and methamphetamine expel dopamine from the neuron through dopamine membrane transporters. Amphetamine and methamphetamine do this by causing a reversal in the direction of the dopamine transporter. Second, at high doses, amphetamine drugs prevent dopamine storage. Amphetamine and methamphetamine do this by entering dopamine storage vesicles through the vesicular transporter and displacing dopamine from the vesicle.

REVIEW! Dopamine enters vesicles through a vesicular transporter. After release, dopamine molecules reenter the terminal through dopamine membrane transporters. Chapter 3 (pg. 75).

Amphetamine and methamphetamine also enhance, to a lesser extent than dopamine, serotonin and norepinephrine levels through acting at axonal terminals. Like dopamine, amphetamine and methamphetamine both prevent serotonin and norepinephrine storage, and they reverse the direction of the membrane transporter for these neurotransmitters (Seidel et al., 2005).

Methylphenidate and Cathinones

The pharmacological actions of methylphenidate resemble those of amphetamine. These drugs prevent reuptake of dopamine, serotonin, and norepinephrine but do so with less efficacy than amphetamine. Also like amphetamine, methylphenidate prevents the storage of dopamine in synaptic vesicles (Pan et al., 1994).

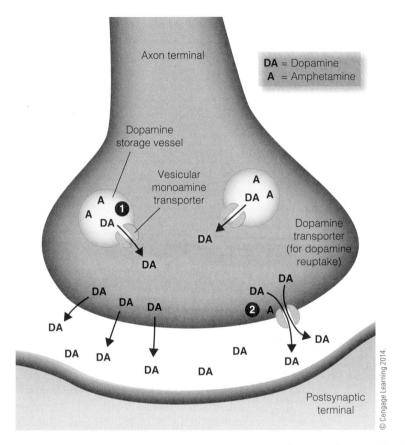

Amphetamine and methamphetamine cause an increase in synaptic dopamine levels through (1) displacing dopamine from dopamine storage vesicles and (2) reversing the direction of the dopamine transporter.

figure **6.8**

Cathinone and synthetic cathinones remain to be fully characterized, but evidence so far suggests pharmacological actions similar to amphetamine for membrane transporters (Kalix, 1981). Baumann and colleagues (2012) recently conducted an evaluation of two synthetic cathinones, mephedrone and methylone, on neurotransmission of monoamine neurotransmitters (**figure 6.9**). They found that both compounds reduced reuptake of dopamine, norepinephrine, and serotonin. By accompanying these findings with microdialysis procedures, they found that elevated concentrations of these neurotransmitters occurred in the nucleus accumbens in laboratory rats. The researchers also tested methamphetamine for comparison, revealing that both compounds exhibited weaker potency than methamphetamine on dopamine and norepinephrine reuptake as well as weaker effects on dopamine and norepinephrine release. Methamphetamine and mephedrone exhibited similar potency for effects on serotonin transporters and serotonin release.

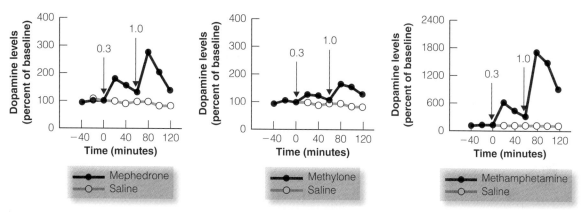

Mephedrone (left), methylone (center), and methamphetamine (right) increase dopamine concentrations in the nucleus accumbens. The *y*-axis refers to dopamine concentrations expressed as a percentage of predrug injection levels (i.e., baseline), and the *x*-axis represents the time course for the experimental session. The dose and injection times appear with arrows on the graph. The filled symbols represent the test drug, whereas empty circles represent a placebo condition (i.e., saline injections). (Adapted by permission from Macmillan Publishers Ltd: *Neuropsychopharmacology* (2012) 37, 1192–1203; Baumann, et al. Copyright © 2012.)

figure 6.9

Cocaine

The primary mechanisms of action for cocaine involve prevention of monoamine reuptake by blocking the membrane transporters for dopamine, norepinephrine, and serotonin (Chen, Sachpatzidis, & Rudnick, 1997; Jones, Garris, & Wightman, 1995; Ritz, Cone, & Kuhar, 1990) (**figure 6.10**). The active metabolite cocaethylene, produced after ingesting both cocaine and alcohol, also functions as a dopamine reuptake inhibitor (McCance et al., 1995). Cocaine also acts as a Na^+ channel blocker when delivered in a high concentration. This concentration far exceeds those necessary for producing the psychoactive effects just described, and actually will cause serious adverse effects and possibly death. However, these adverse effects can be avoided by applying cocaine locally; in doing so, cocaine serves as a local anesthetic. In fact, the discovery of these properties revolutionized ophthalmic surgery, because cocaine not only numbs the eye but also temporarily stops bleeding during surgery because of its vasoconstricting properties (dos Reis, 2009).

Cocaine- and Amphetamine-Regulated Transcript

cocaine- and amphetamine-regulated transcript (CART) Peptide neurotransmitter that is produced after psychostimulant administration.

The cocaine- and amphetamine-regulated transcript (CART), is a peptide neurotransmitter that is produced after psychostimulant administration. Acute administration of a psychostimulant drug causes the activation of the gene for CART, leading to the synthesis of the CART peptide, which is then stored in vesicles within axon terminals. CART peptides are found in the hypothalamus and mesolimbic dopamine system, where they increase dopamine release, although the precise mechanisms responsible for these actions remain unknown. CART peptides produce psychostimulant-like increases

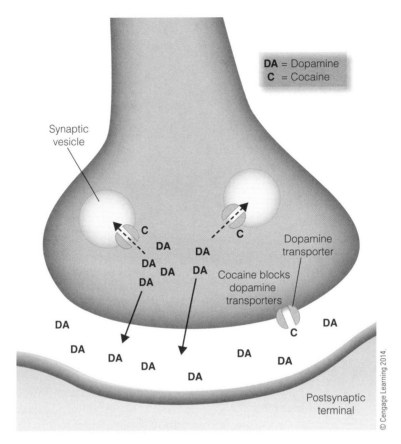

© Cengage Learning 2014.

figure 6.10 Cocaine causes an increase in synaptic dopamine levels by blocking the dopamine transporter and thus reducing reuptake. Cocaine also inhibits dopamine's entry into vesicles.

in locomotor activity, yet CART peptides prevent psychostimulant-induced increases in locomotor activity. Thus, CART appears to alter the effects of psychostimulant drugs, but the exact mechanisms and effects are largely unknown (Hubert, Jones, Moffett, Rogge, & Kuhar, 2008).

Stop & Check

1. Through similar mechanisms, the amphetamines, methylphenidate, cathinones, and cocaine all enhance synaptic levels of the neurotransmitters _____, _____, and _____.

2. Unlike the other psychostimulants, what other actions does cocaine have?

3. What peptide neurotransmitter is released on acute administration of certain psychostimulant drugs?

1. dopamine, norepinephrine, serotonin **2.** At high doses, cocaine acts as a Na⁺ channel blocker, which accounts for its local anesthetizing properties. **3.** CART, which stands for *cocaine- and amphetamine-regulated transcript.*

Pharmacological Effects of Psychostimulants

Physiological Effects

Psychostimulant drugs produce most of their physiological effects by activating the sympathetic nervous system. Activation of the sympathetic nervous system increases heart rate, constricts blood vessels, relaxes airways, dilates pupils, inhibits salivation, inhibits digestion, and produces various other effects described in Chapter 2 (see **table 6.2** here). Sigmund Freud described many of these sympathetic nervous system effects in *Über Coca*. Freud, who tested cocaine on himself, described a moderate increase in pulse rate that was "often accompanied by a rumbling . . . from high up in the intestine," an effect observed in two other individuals. These two individuals had also experienced "an intense feeling of heat in the head," and Freud added, "I noticed this in myself" (Freud, 1974).

Activation of the sympathetic nervous system accounts for many of the uses and risks associated with psychostimulants. Psychostimulants ease nasal congestion by constricting swollen blood vessels in the sinuses and nasal passages. They also open airways in the lungs. These actions explain why ephedra is an effective herbal remedy for colds and why its main constituents, ephedrine and pseudoephedrine, serve as effective ingredients in cold medications. Psychostimulants can cause hyperthermia, especially when used during strenuous physical exertion. Indeed, amphetamines contributed to the hyperthermia-related deaths of several athletes in the 1960s and 1970s (Wyndham 1977). Wide public attention was given to ephedra after it contributed to the heat-stroke–related death of Baltimore Orioles pitcher Steve Bechler in 2003.

Psychostimulants also reduce appetite. As stated previously, psychostimulants served as appetite suppressant drugs called **anorectics** during the 1950s and 1960s. In the 1990s, a combination therapy of the amphetamines

anorectics Appetite-suppressant drugs.

table **6.2**

Selected Objective and Subjective Psychostimulant Effects		
Objective effects		
Physiological effects	**Behavioral effects**	**Subjective effects**
Increased heart rate	Psychosis, including hallucinations	Increased energy
Blood-vessel constriction (high blood pressure)	Increased motor activity	Increased alertness
Airway relaxation		Improved sense of well-being
Pupil dilation		Euphoria
Dry mouth (reduced salivation)		Anxiousness
Inhibited digestion		Agitation
Increased body temperature		
Tooth decay with chronic use		

© Cengage Learning 2014

fenfluramine and phentermine, together referred to as *fen-phen*, proved remarkably effective for weight loss. Another amphetamine, dexfenfluramine (Redux), was also used in combination with phentermine. Severe adverse cardiovascular effects resulting in heart valve damage and some deaths led to an abrupt decline of fen-phen treatments for obesity.

Psychostimulants reduce hunger through actions in the hypothalamus, a key structure for the regulation of appetite. Within this structure, enhanced dopamine release contributes to appetite suppression. CART also plays a role in hunger. In the hypothalamus, CART is activated by the appetite-suppressing hormone leptin. Correlational studies suggest that impaired CART functioning, because of polymorphisms of the CART gene, is associated with obesity (Vicentic & Jones, 2007).

Behavioral Effects

Increased behavioral activity is a key feature of psychostimulant drugs. These effects are dose dependent and affect both purposeful and purposeless behavior. At lower doses, psychostimulants produce an increase in *purposeful* behavior—that is, it appears to be goal directed. For example, a laboratory rat pressing a lever to receive food reinforcers is engaging in purposeful behavior. Relatively low doses of psychostimulants can cause *faster* lever pressing, an increase in this purposeful behavior. In humans, an increase in purposeful behavior may result in fast speech or faster completion of tasks. A review of scientific studies on this topic suggests that increased purposeful behavior occurs from increased dopamine concentrations in the nucleus accumbens (Ellinwood, King, & Lee, 2000).

These activity changes in purposeful behavior also have rate-dependent effects. For drugs, **rate dependent effects** reflect differences in a drug's behavioral effects as a function of predrug administration response rates (Ginsburg, Pinkston, & Lamb, 2011). Psychostimulant drugs increase low rates of baseline behavioral activity. On the other hand, psychostimulant drugs decrease high rates of baseline behavioral activity. As shown in **figure 6.11**, for example, amphetamine increased activity in rats that had relatively low rates of lever pressing. However, amphetamine *decreased* activity in rats that had a relatively high rate of lever pressing (MacPhail & Gollub, 1975). These properties may explain why amphetamine and methylphenidate are effective for treating ADHD.

At higher doses, psychostimulants produce an increase in *purposeless* behavior. In nonhuman animals, this increase in purposeless behavior is called **stereotypy**. Stereotypy in rodents is characterized by repetitive grooming, head swaying, gnawing, or licking. In humans, we refer to stereotypic effects as **punding**. Punding may consist of repetitive teeth grinding, tapping, skin picking, or nail biting. Increased dopamine concentrations in dorsal portions of the basal ganglia, particularly the caudate nucleus, appear most associated with purposeless behavior (Ellinwood et al., 2000).

rate dependent effects
Differences in a drug's behavioral effects as a function of predrug administration response rates.

stereotypy
Psychostimulant-produced purposeless behavior.

punding
Psychostimulant-induced stereotypy in humans.

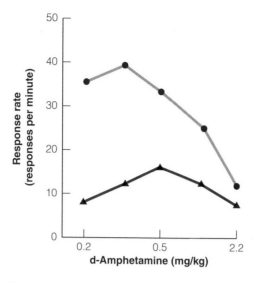

figure **6.11**   D-amphetamine reduces high response rates (circles) and increases low response rates (triangles) at an appropriate dose—0.5 mg/kg—in rats. (Data from MacPhail & Gollub, 1975.)

Subjective Effects

In humans, low doses of psychostimulants provide feelings of increased energy, alertness, a sense of well-being, enthusiasm, and other positive emotional effects (Smith & Davis, 1977). Such doses are used to combat fatigue and reduce the symptoms of narcolepsy. Higher doses of psychostimulants, when administered through a route that offers rapid absorption, also produce a "rush" and euphoria. Active metabolites that function as psychostimulants enhance these effects. Recreational users administer these higher doses.

REVIEW! Subjective effects are uniquely experienced by the individual and cannot be directly observed by others. Objective effects can be measured by recording overt behavior or physiological events. Chapter 1 (pg. 11).

Drug discrimination procedures measure the subjective effects of psychostimulants (**see box 6.1**). For example, Johanson and colleagues (2006) used a drug-discrimination procedure to determine if human participants experienced the same subjective effects for cocaine as they do for methamphetamine. During training, the participants were reinforced with money for correctly identifying a cocaine like effect or non-cocaine like effect. After training was completed, the participants were administered methamphetamine instead of cocaine. Most of the participants, however, indicated that they had received cocaine. Based on these results, the subjective effects of cocaine and methamphetamine appear to be similar.

box **6.1** Drug Discrimination

A **drug-discrimination procedure** trains an organism to recognize or discriminate between the subjective effects of a particular drug when compared to noticeably different effects. This procedure is used in other animals and humans to assess the subjective effects of both recreational and therapeutic drugs.

Drug-discrimination procedures often are conducted in rats, pigeons, or monkeys using operant chambers. In a typical design, researchers select a **training drug**, which is a psychoactive of interest for the study. The training drug is also called a **discriminative stimulus**. After administration of the training drug, the animal is placed into the operant chamber containing two levers—buttons (often referred to as *keys*) or some other type of operandi. Only responses on one operandum will be reinforced, usually by delivery of a food pellet or small water cup. On a different day, the organism is administered the training drug vehicle, the inert solution in which the drug was dissolved, and only responses on the other operandum will be reinforced. After extensive training, an organism learns to associate one operandum with the training drug's subjective effects and the other operandum with the absence of the training drug's effects.

Note that *drug discrimination* and *self-administration* procedures are different. In a self-administration procedure, which is used for break-point studies, animals produce a behavioral response to *receive a drug injection*. In a drug-discrimination procedure, animals must

attend to a drug's subjective effects in order to receive food, water, or other type of reinforcer.

To place the drug discrimination procedure into context, consider the following study by de la Garza and Johanson (1985) using pigeons. The operandi used in this study were two response keys. One key was associated with cocaine and other was associated with *saline*—that is, the absence of cocaine's stimulus effects. These cocaine or saline training conditions alternated in daily sessions until the pigeons correctly responded to each condition with greater than 90-percent accuracy.

After training, the pigeons were administered different drugs to determine if the pigeons responded on the cocaine key, indicating cocaine-like stimulus effects, or the saline key, indicating *non*-cocaine like stimulus effects. Box 6.1 figure 1 shows these study results.

These figures show the percentage of pecking that occurred on the cocaine key during test sessions for each drug and dose tested. At 1.0 mg/kg and 2.0 mg/kg doses, d-amphetamine caused almost all of the key pecks to occur on the cocaine lever. Similarly, the highest dose of cathinone produced nearly all pecks on the cocaine key. Both d-amphetamine and cathinone are psychostimulant drugs that have similar subjective effects as cocaine and may represent the stimulus effects of cocaine in this task. However, pentobarbital, a barbiturate that exhibits very different subjective effects than cocaine, resulted in few pecks on the cocaine key.

As presented in Chapter 5 (box 5.1), break points also assess the strength of positive mood effects of psychostimulant drugs. For example, **figure 6.12** shows the results of break-point studies conducted in rats using d-amphetamine, methamphetamine, cocaine, and other psychostimulants. In these studies, the break points for the highest doses of d-amphetamine and methamphetamine are both found at 268 responses per reinforcer. The break point for cocaine was 178 responses, lower than either d-amphetamine or methamphetamine. Thus, rats were willing to work harder for d-amphetamine and methamphetamine than for cocaine (Richardson & Roberts, 1996).

REVIEW! A break point is the maximum level of responding a subject is willing to do in order to receive a drug injection. Chapter 5 (pg. 140).

Adverse Effects

Psychostimulants produce many adverse physiological effects on the body. Among the most prominent are cardiovascular dysfunction, pulmonary dysfunction, abnormal fetal development, and tooth decay. Adverse effects also

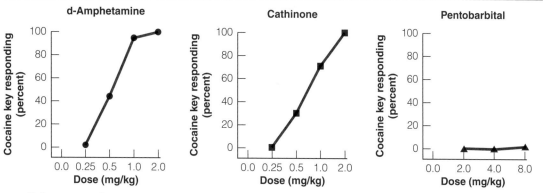

box 6.1, figure 1

The psychostimulant drugs d-amphetamine (left) and cathinone (middle), but not the barbiturate pentobarbital (right), engendered cocaine key responding in a cocaine drug-discrimination task. The y-axis refers to the percentage of key pecks occurring on the cocaine key, and the x-axis refers to the dose of the drug. (Data from de la Garza & Johanson, 1985.)

Human drug-discrimination procedures are similar to animal drug-discrimination procedures. In place of an operant chamber, human participants emit responses on a computer mouse; clicks usually substitute for key pecks or lever presses. Money usually serves in place of food pellets.

drug-discrimination procedure Procedure that trains an organism to recognize or discriminate between the subjective effects of a particular drug when compared to noticeably different effects.

There are many variations on the typical drug-discrimination design. For example, two or more training drugs may be used in the same procedure, or there may be more than two operandi used in an operant chamber. These design variations can provide a further resolution of the biological actions supporting a drug's subjective effects.

training drug Psychoactive drug of interest for certain kinds of behavior studies, such as drug discrimination.
discriminative stimulus A stimulus that signals an opportunity for reinforcement.

occur from the conditions of drug use. Drug administration in unclean environments or through shared needles exposes users to a high risk of infection. Among the most common diseases associated with abuse of intravenously administered drugs are the human immunodeficiency virus (HIV), hepatitis, and tuberculosis (Brecher, 1972; Cadet & Krasnova, 2007; Ellinwood et al., 2000).

Cardiovascular effects represent the greatest risk of psychostimulant use. Enhanced sympathetic nervous system activation taxes the cardiovascular system by constricting blood vessels and increasing heart rate. These actions lead to an increased risk of hypertension, stroke, aortic rupture, and heart attack. Hypertension during psychostimulant use is an important cause of abnormal fetal development. Through blood-vessel constriction, total blood flow to the fetus is reduced, causing limited oxygen availability and nutrient delivery. These effects, in turn, contribute to lower fetal growth and the risk of severe injury to the fetus, including hemorrhage, ischemia, and neuronal death.

The adverse effects on pulmonary function include injury during inhalation, hemorrhaging, edema, and tissue inflammation. Normal pulmonary

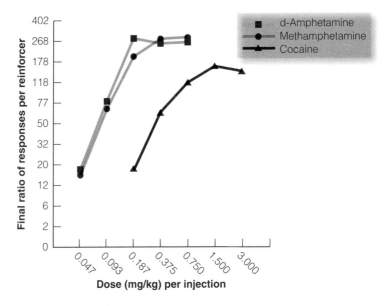

figure 6.12 The break point for three psychostimulant drugs is shown as the highest "final ratio" completed. On the bottom (*x*-axis) is the amount of drug delivered per injection. Cocaine, shown by the triangles, had a lower break point than both d-amphetamine (squares) and methamphetamine (circles). (Richardson & Roberts, 1996. By permission.)

meth mouth Tooth decay caused by methamphetamine use.

function is compromised when sympathetic nervous system activity is significantly enhanced as well as when the lungs are exposed to vapor from inhaled methamphetamine or crack cocaine. Smoking these drugs exposes the lungs to the drug as well as any harmful byproducts produced during the drug's synthesis (Ellinwood et al., 2000; Lineberry & Bostwick, 2006).

Among the psychostimulant drugs, methamphetamine use is most associated with tooth decay, a condition referred to as **meth mouth**. The American Dental Association describes these teeth as "blackened, stained, rotting, crumbling, or falling apart" (American Dental Association, 2005). Meth mouth occurs even when methamphetamine does not contact the teeth.

Important contributing factors for meth mouth include poor dental hygiene, such as brushing and flossing, as well as damaged gums due to contact with inhaled chemicals during drug use. Two other contributing factors for meth mouth occur from activation of the sympathetic nervous system. First, methamphetamine's activation of the sympathetic nervous system reduces salivation, which has important protective properties for preventing tooth decay. Second, reduced saliva causes *dry mouth*, which motivates a methamphetamine user to drink fluids. Methamphetamine users tend to consume sugary soft drinks, and exposing teeth to sugar, particularly in the absence of saliva's tooth protective properties, leads to cavities and tooth decay (Klasser & Epstein, 2005).

psychostimulant-induced psychosis Psychotic behavior caused by psychostimulant use.

Psychostimulants also produce psychosis at high doses. **Psychostimulant-induced psychosis** is similar to symptoms of schizophrenia, including paranoia,

formication Sensation of insects or worms crawling under the skin.

agitation, and auditory hallucinations. Given that psychostimulants enhance brain dopamine levels, psychostimulant-induced psychosis suggests that abnormally high dopamine levels exist in schizophrenia. Yet psychostimulant-induced psychosis also differs from psychosis in schizophrenia. First, many psychostimulant hallucinations are tactile. High psychostimulant doses cause **formication**, a sensation of insects or worms crawling under the skin. Such tactile hallucinations are less common for schizophrenia. Second, psychostimulant-induced psychosis often includes visual hallucinations and occasional olfactory hallucinations. Psychosis in schizophrenia mainly includes auditory hallucinations.

Stop & Check

1. Activation of the _____ nervous system accounts for many of the physiological objective effects of psychostimulant drugs.

2. Appetite-suppressant effects are the reason why psychostimulant drugs have been used to treat _____.

3. Although low psychostimulant doses may increase purposeful behavior, high psychostimulant doses may increase _____ behavior.

4. How do subjective effects of cocaine compare to methamphetamine?

1. sympathetic **2.** obesity **3.** purposeless **4.** Both drugs produce euphoria and other positive mood effects. Moreover, humans trained to recognize the subjective effects of cocaine misidentify methamphetamine as cocaine.

Psychostimulant Drugs Produce Sensitization and Tolerance

Either sensitization or tolerance can occur during chronic psychostimulant administration. Sensitization tends to occur for *purposeless* behavior. In rats, sensitization presents as an increase in stereotypic behaviors such as sniffing and head movements (Robinson & Becker, 1986). Repeated administration of psychostimulant drugs may also lead to incentive sensitization, which may play an important role in the development of psychostimulant addiction (Robinson & Berridge, 2003). Tolerance occurs to the positive subjective effects of psychostimulants by creating a need to use higher doses of a psychostimulant drug to achieve these effects. However, the initial "high" first felt from a psychostimulant drug can be hard to achieve. Cocaine users, for example, seldom experience the same rush they felt on first using cocaine, and the search for this rush is a driving force in cocaine addiction.

REVIEW! Incentive salience describes the heightened neurobiological and behavioral responses to stimuli associated with drug use. Chapter 5 (pg. 138).

We find that a key form of psychostimulant tolerance is *pharmacodynamic tolerance*. Although many pharmacological actions may play a role, pharmacodynamic tolerance relies in part on changes in dopamine D_2 receptor sensitivity. Barrett and colleagues (1992) demonstrated a link between D_2 receptors and repeated psychostimulant administration using a drug-discrimination procedure (**figure 6.13**). In this study, rats learned to discriminate

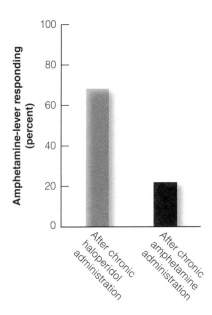

In rats trained to discriminate haloperidol versus amphetamine in a two-lever drug-discrimination task, a test session conducted after chronic administration of haloperidol (left) led to increased amphetamine-lever responding, whereas a test session conducted after chronic administration of amphetamine (right) led to decreased amphetamine-lever responding (see text for further details). The y-axis refers to percent of responses occurring on the amphetamine lever. (Data from Barrett et al., 1992.)

figure 6.13

the D_2 receptor antagonist and antipsychotic drug haloperidol versus the psychostimulant drug d-amphetamine. The latter causes D_2 receptor activation by enhancing synaptic dopamine levels. After learning this discrimination, a chronic treatment regimen was employed. During this regimen, animals were either treated with haloperidol or with d-amphetamine for 10 consecutive days. On the day after treatment ended, the rats were placed in the operant chamber without a drug injection and were free to choose the appropriate lever, either haloperidol or amphetamine.

Rats chronically treated with haloperidol chose the amphetamine lever, whereas chronically treated d-amphetamine rats chose the haloperidol lever. This happened because pharmacodynamic tolerance developed over the course of the treatment regimen. The study authors speculated that synaptic sites adapted to haloperidol's repeated blockade of D_2 receptors by increasing the sensitivity of D_2 receptors. Similarly, the synaptic sites adapted to repeated activation of D_2 receptors by d-amphetamine by decreasing the sensitivity of D_2 receptors. When they returned the rats to the operant chamber for a drug-discrimination test, chronically treated haloperidol rats had an oversensitive dopamine state; these effects resembled d-amphetamine–like stimulus effects. Similarly, the chronically treated d-amphetamine rats had an undersensitive dopamine state; these effects resembled haloperidol-like stimulus effects.

Cross tolerance also occurs between psychostimulant drugs. In an early characterization of psychostimulant cross tolerance, Woolverton and colleagues (1978) demonstrated that rats tolerant to cocaine-induced reductions in milk intake exhibit this same tolerance when treated with amphetamine. The same was true when amphetamine-tolerant rats were treated with cocaine.

A psychostimulant drug's dosing frequency plays an important determining role for sensitization or tolerance. Sensitization occurs after a period of intermittent dosing of psychostimulants, whereas tolerance occurs after continuous dosing of psychostimulants. Researchers best demonstrate these frequency differences in animals. In rats, which exhibit much shorter elimination half-lives for psychostimulants compared to humans, intermittent dosing might consist of one or more injections per day, occurring at times when the primary effects of a drug have worn off. In humans, intermittent drug administration might consist of less-frequent drug administrations per week. Given the half-life of amphetamine in humans, two or three amphetamine administrations per week might qualify as intermittent drug administration. Continuous dosing consists of a steady and constant infusion of drug. In humans, continuous dosing consists of drug administrations given when drug molecules remain in the body from the previous administration. Depending on the particular drug, continuous administration might consist of one or multiple administrations per day (Ellinwood et al., 2000).

Stop & Check	1. In addition to sensitization for purposeless behavior, what other type of sensitization occurs during long-term use of psychostimulant drugs?
	2. Reduced D_2 receptor sensitivity after prolonged administration of a psychostimulant drug is an important mechanism of _____ tolerance.
	3. Cross tolerance implies that an individual who tolerates high doses of cocaine would tolerate _____ doses of amphetamine.

1. In addition to sensitization to purposeless behavior, incentive sensitization may also occur. **2.** pharmacodynamic **3.** high

FROM ACTIONS TO EFFECTS
Psychostimulant Addiction

Linking Pharmacological Actions to Reinforcing Effects

Increased dopamine neurotransmission in the nucleus accumbens mostly accounts for the reinforcing features of psychostimulant drugs. In particular, these actions rely on dopamine D_2 receptors. The positive subjective effects of d-amphetamine, for example, can be blocked by D_2 receptor antagonists such as the antipsychotic drug haloperidol.

For cocaine, reinforcing effects also depend on the activation of dopamine D_1 receptors and serotonin neurotransmission. Greater activation of D_1 receptors occurs because of cocaine-induced elevations in dopamine levels. Caine and colleagues (2007) demonstrated the importance of D_1 receptors using self-administration procedures in dopamine D_1 receptor knock-out mice and wild-type mice. The wild-type mice readily learned to self-administer cocaine in this procedure, but none of the D_1 receptor knock-out mice learned to self-administer cocaine. Serotonin transporter blockade also contributes to cocaine's subjective effects. For example, serotonin transporter knock-out rats exhibit enhanced cocaine self-administration, hyperactivity, and conditioned place preference compared to wild-type rats (Homberg et al., 2008).

REVIEW! Receptor knock-out mice lack certain receptors as a result of genetic modification. Wild-type mice are not genetically modified. Chapter 2 (pg. 56).

The withdrawal symptoms associated with psychostimulants primarily occur from psychological dependence rather than physical dependence. Just as psychostimulants produce increases in activity, enjoyment, and euphoria, withdrawal from psychostimulants produces lethargy, lack of joy, and *dysphoria*, which is characterized as feelings of hopeless, unhappiness, and discomfort. During Sigmund Freud's era, this withdrawal state was called *cocaine blues*.

Genetics Influence the Susceptibility to Psychostimulant Addiction

Genetic animal studies provide a framework for identifying possible links between human genetic differences and susceptibility to psychostimulant addiction. There are three primary ways that genetic differences alter psychostimulant drug effects.

First, genetic differences can alter the rate of drug metabolism. If an individual's genetic expression of P450 enzymes leads to a quicker metabolism of a psychostimulant drug, this will shorten the duration of the drug's effects. Shorter drug effects may lead to more-frequent drug use. Second, a genetic predisposition can enhance the subjective effects of psychostimulant drugs. Individuals have a greater risk of drug addiction if they experience powerful reinforcing effects. Third, genetic predisposition can alter the negative effects of psychostimulant drugs. Drug addiction is unlikely to develop for an individual who experiences adverse effects or negative subjective effects (Haile, Kosten, & Kosten, 2009).

C-1021T polymorphism
Polymorphism that causes low expression of dopamine β-hydroxylase, the enzyme that converts dopamine to norepinerphrine.

The **C-1021T polymorphism** has received much attention by psychostimulant addiction researchers. This polymorphism causes low expression of dopamine β-hydroxylase, the enzyme that converts dopamine to norepinerphrine. Based on animal research that evaluated inhibitors of dopamine β-hydroxylase, psychostimulants likely exhibit lower norepinephrine release for those with lower dopamine β-hydroxylase expression compared to those exhibiting normal dopamine β-hydroxylase expression (Schroeder et al., 2010).

Through these actions, the C-1021T polymorphism may increase the negative subjective effects of psychostimulants. Kalayasiri and colleagues (2007) studied the relationship between the C-1021T polymorphism and cocaine's subjective effects. This study used a cocaine self-administration experiment in humans with the C-1021T polymorphism. A greater degree of paranoia was observed in participants homozygous for the C-1021T polymorphism compared to other study participants. Cocaine users consider paranoia an aversive effect; some individuals experience and report paranoia and other features of psychosis and cite these as reasons for seeking addiction treatment (Brady, Lydiard, Malcolm, & Ballenger, 1991).

Treatments for Psychostimulant Addiction

The therapies for psychostimulant addiction address two primary phases of recovery: abstinence and relapse. Abstinence consists of detoxification from a drug. During detoxification (*detox*), the withdrawal effects of psychostimulant use are most prominent. Treatment for detoxification involves hospitalization and medical treatment.

disulfiram Medication used for treating alcohol addiction that inhibits aldehyde dehydrogenase.

One treatment is **disulfiram**, a medication used to treat alcohol addiction. Disulfiram is an inhibitor of aldehyde dehydrogenase, an enzyme involved in alcohol metabolism, as well as an inhibitor of dopamine β-hydroxylase, an enzyme that converts dopamine to norepinephrine. Several clinical studies have evaluated disulfiram after cocaine administration, generally finding reduced positive subjective effects, including a reduced high or rush, and enhanced negative subjective effects, including paranoia, agitation, and nervousness (Baker, Jatlow, & McCance-Katz, 2007; Hameedi et al., 1995). Individuals with a C-1021T polymorphism described previously are even more susceptible to negative subjective effects from disulfiram and cocaine administration (Haile et al., 2009). However, the ability of disulfiram to reduce positive subjects may depend on dose. For example, Oliveto and colleagues (2011) found that lower doses of disulfiram actually increased the frequency of cocaine use over several weeks of treatment in cocaine-addicted users.

Many studies have evaluated modafinil (Provigil) for aiding psychostimulant detoxification. Modafinil engenders mild psychostimulant effects and has approved therapeutic uses for narcolepsy. Like other psychostimulants, modafinil elevates dopamine levels in the nucleus accumbens, yet these elevations are lower and longer lasting compared to other psychostimulant drugs. Perhaps for these weaker effects, modafinil may provide a safe substitute for abused psychostimulant drugs.

To investigate modafinil as a treatment for psychostimulant addiction, Dackis and colleagues (2004) evaluated 8 weeks of modafinil treatment, combined with psychotherapy, in cocaine-addicted individuals enrolled in an outpatient treatment program. Researchers collected and tested urine samples each week to determine abstinence from cocaine. During the course of the study, modafinil significantly increased the number of patients remaining abstinent from cocaine (**figure 6.14**). Although these study results show promise, another study using modafinil failed to show changes in the frequency of cocaine use in addicted users (Anderson et al., 2009). Thus, modafinil for psychostimulant addiction requires further investigation.

Tricyclic antidepressant drugs such as imipramine effectively reduce craving, depression, and other withdrawal symptoms during psychostimulant detoxification. Chronic tricyclic antidepressant treatment elevates dopamine, norepinephrine, and serotonin levels, which may address a deficiency in these neurotransmitters during psychostimulant withdrawal. Addressing these deficiencies can aid in relapse prevention. For example, in an assessment of methamphetamine relapse rates, imipramine treatment was associated with significantly longer stays in a free drug-addiction clinic (Galloway, Newmeyer, Knapp, Stalcup, & Smith, 1996).

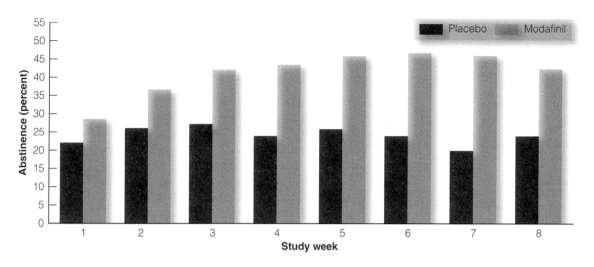

Modafinil reduced the number of relapses in cocaine-dependent patients over the course of 8 weeks. (Adapted by permission from Macmillan Publishers Ltd: Dackis, C. A., Kampman, K. M., Lynch, K. G., Pettinati, H. M., & O'Brien, C. P. (2004). A Double-Blind, Placebo-Controlled Trial of Modafinil for Cocaine Dependence. *Neuropsychopharmacology*, 30(1), 205–211., copyright 2004.)

figure 6.14

Drugs that facilitate GABA neurotransmission also demonstrate clinically efficacy for preventing psychostimulant relapse. For example, the anticonvulsant drug topiramate (Topamax) is commonly used for cocaine relapse prevention. In one clinical study, 60 percent of former cocaine-dependent patients treated with topiramate were completely abstinent for more than 3 weeks, compared to 26 percent of those treated with placebo (Kampman et al., 2004). Another anticonvulsant drug, vigabatrin (Sabril), provided similar improvements in treatment outcomes for cocaine-addicted patients (Kampman, 2010). Drugs that facilitate GABA neurotransmission may interrupt associative learning processes important during the preoccupation and anticipation stage of addiction. By interrupting these processes, these treatments may weaken sensitized incentive processes for drug seeking and use (Koob & Volkow, 2009).

Finally, researchers have recently developed approaches for vaccinating against psychostimulant effects as a way to prevent or eliminate abuse (Shen, Orson, & Kosten, 2012). The general approach consists of the production of antibodies that bind to a psychostimulant drug and prevent the drug from crossing the blood–brain barrier. Martell and colleagues (2009) evaluated the utility of a cocaine vaccine for relapse prevention in cocaine-addicted patients. After waiting 8 weeks for the antibodies to reach sufficient levels, researchers evaluated patients for cocaine abstinence by analyzing urine samples. Cocaine-free urine samples were more frequent for those with high antibody levels than compared to those with low antibody levels. Yet, even in the high antibody group, researchers found that less than 50 percent of patients were ultimately cocaine free. Thus, although this approach has appeal, further vaccine development is needed. Indeed, the vaccine strategy for preventing or eliminating psychostimulant continues as an important line in addiction treatment (Moreno, Mayorov, & Janda, 2011; Wee et al., 2012).

Stop & Check

1. What are the two primary aims of pharmacological treatment for psychostimulant addiction?

2. For the treatment of psychostimulant addiction, how might disulfiram drug therapy be related to the C-1021T polymorphism?

3. What are the shared pharmacological mechanisms for modafinil and tricyclic antidepressants that may be important for treating psychostimulant addiction?

1. To treat withdrawal symptoms during abstinence and prevent relapse. 2. Like individuals with the C-1021T polymorphism, disulfiram lowers the expression of dopamine β-hydroxylase, causing unpleasant subjective effects to occur when a psychostimulant is administered. 3. Modafinil and tricyclic antidepressants increase dopamine, norepinephrine, and serotonin concentrations just as amphetamine and cocaine do. In this way, these drugs may provide a replacement of these elevated neurotransmitters during psychostimulant use.

▶ CHAPTER SUMMARY

Psychostimulant drugs, also called *sympathomimetics*, increase psychomotor and sympathetic nervous system activity and promote alertness and positive mood. Common psychostimulant drugs include amphetamine drugs, cathinones, and cocaine. Many psychostimulant drugs are derived from plants and are produced legally or illegally. Traditionally, the plants containing psychostimulants were used by humans, often through chewing leaves. Psychostimulants such as methamphetamine and cocaine also are prepared in a base form that can be smoked. Psychostimulant drugs are administered in many forms, including insufflation, intravenous injection, and inhalation. Among these administration routes, inhalation provides the quickest drug effects. Many psychostimulant drugs have active metabolites that also exhibit psychostimulant effects.

Elevated dopamine levels in the nucleus accumbens account for the reinforcing effects of psychostimulant drugs, and elevated peripheral dopamine and norepinephrine levels account for increased sympathetic nervous system activity. Psychostimulants increase heart rate, blood pressure, body temperature, and other sympathetic nervous system functions. Behaviorally, psychostimulants increase purposeful activity at lower doses and purposeless activity at higher doses. High doses can produce psychotic behavior that resembles positive symptoms in schizophrenia. The subjective effects of psychostimulants include positive mood effects such as increased energy, alertness, and euphoria—and negative mood effects such as anxiousness, agitation, and paranoia. Sensitization occurs for purposeless behavior and for the incentive value of conditioned stimuli during prolonged use of psychostimulants, whereas tolerance occurs for the subjective effects of psychostimulants.

Pharmacological treatments for psychostimulant addiction either address withdrawal symptoms during abstinence or attempt to prevent relapse. These treatments act on the same sites of actions as psychostimulants such as the tricyclic antidepressant drugs or act through other mechanisms such as the anticonvulsant drug topiramate. Researchers have also investigated vaccination strategies for preventing psychostimulant effects.

KEY TERMS

Psychostimulant

Amphetamines

Cathinone

Cocaine

Coca paste

Freebasing

Methylecgonidine

Cocaine- and
  amphetamine-
  regulated transcript
  (CART)

Anoretics

Rate dependent effects

Stereotypy

Punding

Drug-discrimination
  procedure

Training drug

Discriminative stimulus

Meth mouth

Psychostimulant-induced
  psychosis

Formication

C-1021T polymorphism

Disulfiram

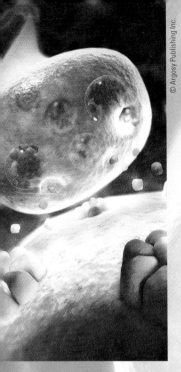

© Argosy Publishing Inc.

CHAPTER **7**

Nicotine and Caffeine

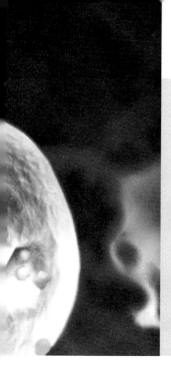

Is Nicotine Not Addictive?

On April 14, 1994, a House subcommittee met to discuss the health concerns of tobacco use. Before the committee were seven corporate executive officers of large U.S.-based tobacco companies. In his opening remarks, the subcommittee chair reviewed the risks of tobacco use: high mortality rate, cancer, heart disease, and lung disease. Then Rep. Ron Wyden (D.–Oregon) asked the first question: "Yes or no, do you believe nicotine is not addictive?"

The executives' responses made this hearing famous. Down the line, every CEO made a clear, simple answer to Wyden's answer: Nicotine is not addictive.

Did these CEOs have a defensible position? As presented later in this chapter, the CEOs' answers depend on how addiction is defined.

In Chapter 6, we considered the most powerful psychostimulants: amphetamines, cathinones, and cocaine. The current chapter covers two less-powerful but more-often-used psychostimulant drugs: nicotine and caffeine.

Nicotine: Key Psychoactive Ingredient in Tobacco

tar Particles released from tobacco that contain nicotine and other tobacco chemicals.

Nicotine is the central psychoactive ingredient in tobacco. Tobacco consists of leaves from plants in the genus *Nicotiana*, of which the primary nicotine-containing species grow in South and North America (**figure 7.1**). Traditional forms of tobacco consisted of rolled tobacco leaves, and modern versions consist of cigars and cigarettes. When tobacco is chewed or smoked, small nicotine-containing tobacco particles called **tar** and other tobacco chemicals enter the body.

Cigarettes are the most commonly used tobacco product. A typical cigarette user consumes 13 cigarettes per day. A cigarette is composed of a tobacco blend rolled in a thin sheet of paper. Many cigarettes contain a filter of cellulose acetate that reduces the amount of tobacco tar inhaled. The tobacco portion of a regular cigarette is approximately 60 mm (2.25 in.) in length, and filtered cigarettes have a 25 mm (~1 in.) filter and usually shorter length of tobacco. Depending on the size and blend, a cigarette contains 1–2 mg of nicotine.

Cigars vary widely in diameter, length, and nicotine content. For example, a Winchester Little Cigar is 8 mm (~⅓ in.) in diameter and 60 mm (2⅓ in.) long, whereas a CuestaRey No. 1 is 20 mm (~¾ in.) in diameter and 211 mm (8⅓ in.) in length. A Winchester Little Cigar contains 5.9 mg of nicotine, and a CuestaRey No. 1 cigar contains 335.2 mg of nicotine (Henningfield, Fant, Radzius, & Frost,

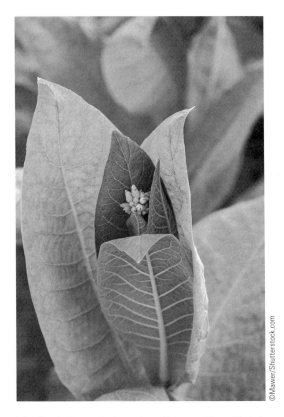

©Mawer/Shutterstock.com

figure **7.1** Nicotine is the central psychoactive constituent in tobacco plants. (From www.marvistavet.com /html/body_nicotine_poisoning_in_pets.html.)

1999). Water pipe or *hookah* smoking is increasingly prevalent among younger Western adults, although it has been a standard method of smoking in the Middle East for centuries. With this form, inhaled tobacco smoke first passes through a bowl of water (**figure 7.2**). Many users believe that this method reduces the harmful effects of tobacco, although studies of water-pipe tobacco exposure fail to support this belief (Ahmed, Jacob, Allen, & Benowitz, 2011; Jacob et al., 2011).

Smokeless tobacco products consist of any tobacco form intended for absorption in the mouth. Products called *chew*, *snuff*, and *dipping tobacco* consist of a tobacco blend that a user either chews or pockets in his or her cheek. When the product is spent, users spit the tobacco out. *Dissolvable tobacco* is another type of smokeless tobacco. These products come in the form of sweetened strips, sticks, or pellets that dissolve in the mouth. Dissolvable tobacco products contain amounts of nicotine similar to those found in cigarettes. For example, a strip contains 0.6 mg of nicotine, and a stick contains 3.1 mg of nicotine. The resemblance of these products to candy recently led to redesigning the appearance of these products (Connolly et al., 2010).

Tobacco use is widespread. In 2009, 70 million Americans ages 12 and older—a little less than 25 percent of the U.S. population—had used tobacco

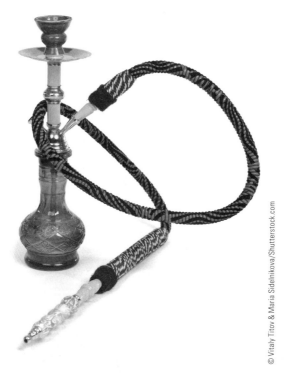

figure 7.2 A water pipe or *hookah* is traditionally used for smoking tobacco and is increasingly used among young Western adults.

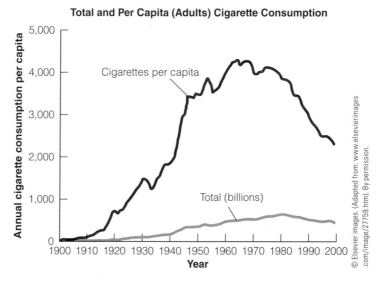

figure 7.3 Cigarettes are widely consumed, but their use has declined since the 1960s as tobacco's adverse health effects have become more publicly known in the U.S.

products within the preceding month. However, tobacco use is declining in the United States. Cigarette use in the United States peaked during the 1960s and has steadily decreased since (**figure 7.3**). This trend is not found for all tobacco products, however. In particular, cigar use is increasing (Nyman, Taylor, & Biener, 2002).

U.S. cigar use has risen dramatically since the 1990s. Between 1998 and 2004, cigar use increased more than 70 percent. Baker and colleagues (2000) offer two important reasons for this trend. First, the cigar industry aggressively marketed cigars during the 1990s. In particular, advertisements used celebrities to glamorize cigar smoking. Second, many tobacco users perceive cigars as safer alternatives to cigarettes. Among cigar smokers, fewer than half believed that cigars increase cancer risk, and few consider themselves to be at a high risk for cancer.

According to the World Health Organization, tobacco use is high in many parts of Europe and Asia and throughout Central and South America (**figure 7.4**). Asia includes the highest rates. More than 60 percent of males

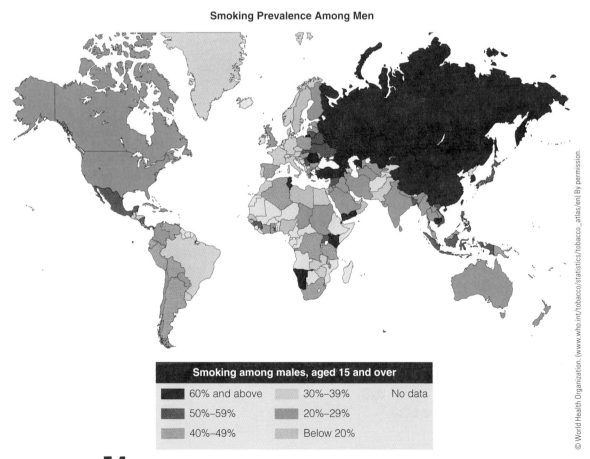

Smoking Prevalence Among Men

Smoking among males, aged 15 and over		
60% and above	30%–39%	No data
50%–59%	20%–29%	
40%–49%	Below 20%	

© World Health Organization. (www.who.int/tobacco/statistics/tobacco_atlas/en) By permission.

figure 7.4   The highest rates of tobacco use are found in many parts of Europe and Asia.

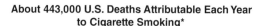

About 443,000 U.S. Deaths Attributable Each Year to Cigarette Smoking*

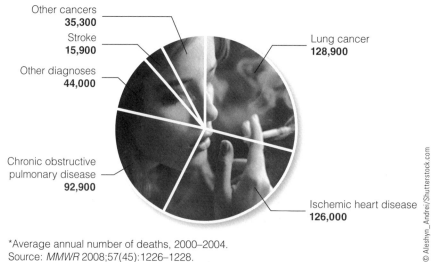

Other cancers **35,300**

Stroke **15,900**

Other diagnoses **44,000**

Chronic obstructive pulmonary disease **92,900**

Lung cancer **128,900**

Ischemic heart disease **126,000**

*Average annual number of deaths, 2000–2004.
Source: *MMWR* 2008;57(45):1226–1228.

figure 7.5 Lung cancer, chronic obstructive pulmonary disease such as emphysema, and heart disease are the greatest causes of death associated with tobacco use.

in the Russian Federation and China use tobacco products. Males generally use tobacco products more than females, but these differences vary between countries. For example, equal smoking rates occur among males and females in Norway and Sweden, whereas less than 10 percent of females smoke in the Russian Federation and China.

Tobacco use has serious health effects. The three primary causes of tobacco-related death each year are cancer, pulmonary disease, and cardiovascular disease. According to the U.S. Centers for Disease Control and Prevention, 443,000 tobacco-related deaths occurred each year between 2000 and 2004. Of those deaths, more than 75 percent resulted from at least one of these three conditions, with lung cancer being the leading cause of tobacco-related deaths (**figure 7.5**).

Secondhand smoking also increases the health risks of those exposed to it. In 2005, this form of tobacco exposure accounted for 3,000 deaths from lung cancer and 46,000 deaths related to coronary heart disease. Secondhand smoke exposure also accounted for 430 sudden infant death syndrome incidents in that same year (CDC, 2008).

Discovery of Tobacco

The discovery of fossilized leaves of *Nicotiana tabacum* in Peru suggest that tobacco existed at least 2.5 million years ago. Indigenous peoples in the Americas, including the Mayas, Incans, Toltecs, and Aztecs, smoked tobacco

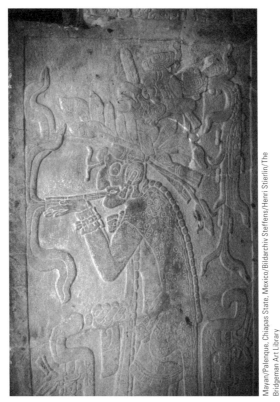

Mayan/Palenque, Chiapas State, Mexico/Bildarchiv Steffens/Henri Stierlin/The Bridgeman Art Library

figure **7.6**   Tobacco was smoked by ancient Mayan priests for ceremonial purposes.

as part of their religious practices. In religious ceremonies, tobacco was smoked to achieve a trancelike state (**figure 7.6**).

Religious practices remained the primary use of tobacco until European discovered tobacco during Columbus's 1492 expedition. After Columbus landed in the Bahamas, the native Arawak gave dried tobacco leaves as a gift to the explorer. Not realizing the significance of the tobacco leaves to the Arawak, Columbus simply discarded them. A few days later, however, Columbus noted that the leaves had "high value among [the Arawak]."

Rodrigo de Jerez, a member of Columbus's expedition, participated in the native practice of rolling tobacco leaves and smoking them. Thus, Jerez became the first European to smoke tobacco. In fact, he became a habitual user and brought back a large personal tobacco supply to Spain. Yet the frightening site of tobacco smoke coming from his mouth and nose brought him to judgment by the holy inquisitors, who imprisoned him for 7 years.

Use of tobacco in Europe soon grew. By the mid-16th century, tobacco was a widely traded commodity. Complaints against tobacco also grew. The first medical concern against using tobacco was published in the early 17th century, which compared the deleterious health effects of chimneysweeps to those of tobacco smokers. In 1610, Sir Francis Bacon noted the difficulty in quitting tobacco use. In 1634, Russian Tsar Michael I decreed that a first offense for tobacco use was punishment by whipping and transport to Siberia; the second offense was death (Brecher, 1972).

In 1612 Jamestown, John Rolfe raised the first European tobacco crop for commercial use, marking the beginning of a thriving American industry that remains active today. Nearly 200 years later, in 1809, Louis Nicolas Vanquelin isolated nicotine as a key ingredient in tobacco.

The beginning of the 20th century marked a renewed study of tobacco's health effects. Early in this century, scientists studied the effects of tobacco and cancer in animals, and biologist Davis Jordan publicly stated, "[T]he boy who smokes cigarettes need not be anxious about his future—he has none." In 1938, a study by Raymond Pearl reported that heavy smokers lived a shorter life than nonsmokers (Borio, 2011).

By the 1990s, the health risks of tobacco were well characterized and widely publicized. As presented at the beginning of this chapter, the 1994 tobacco hearings included the testimony of seven tobacco company CEOs who denied any knowledge of tobacco's adverse effects. Today, tobacco products must include special health warning labels, but the product is still sold legally throughout the world.

Stop & Check

1. What is the key psychoactive ingredient in tobacco?
2. Among the many forms of tobacco, which product remains the most used?
3. What is the greatest cause of death from smoking?
4. In which American colony was the first tobacco crop grown?

1. Nicotine 2. Cigarettes 3. Lung cancer 4. Jamestown

Pharmacokinetic Properties and Tobacco Use

Nicotine Absorption Through Lung and Oral Tissues

Nicotine is absorbable through many forms of administration. Smoking tobacco is the most common administration route for nicotine. On entry into the body, tar, the particulate matter produced from burning tobacco, adheres to tissues in the mouth, nose, throat, and lungs. When exhaled, tar also adheres to the skin. Through contact with tissue, nicotine and many other chemicals found in tar are absorbed into the bloodstream. Given the large surface area of the lungs, smoked tobacco provides the most effective route of nicotine administration.

The freebase form of nicotine best absorbs through mucous membranes in the mouth. The greatest amount of freebase nicotine that can be absorbed is 50 percent, which occurs at a pH of 8.02. As pH levels deviate from 8.02, the percentage of freebase nicotine decreases, as shown for dissolvable

table **7.1**

pH and % Free Nicotine in Selected Dissolvable Camel Tobacco Products		
Camel brand	**pH**	**% Free nicotine**
Mellow Orb	7.82	38.5
Fresh Orb	7.1	28.0
Mellow Stick	7.51	23.5
Fresh Strip	8.02	50.2

Adapted from Rainey et al., 2011.

nicotine products in **table 7.1**. Many smokeless and dissolvable tobacco products offer pH values close to 8.02 (Djordjevic, Hoffman, Glynn, & Connolly, 1995; Henningfield, Radzius, & Cone, 1995; Rainey, Conder, & Goodpaster, 2011).

When inhaling tobacco smoke, the acidity of smoke from a cigarette reduces saliva to a pH less than 6.0, substantially reducing the amount of freebase nicotine available for absorption in the mouth (Armitage & Turner, 1970). On the other hand, smoke from cigars tends to have pH levels closer to 7.0, although the pH levels vary considerably, depending on the size of the cigar and part of the cigar smoked (Henningfield et al., 1999).

Most tobacco products result in blood nicotine concentrations of 12 to 16 nanograms* per milliliter, although absorption times vary. Peak absorption for nicotine from cigarettes occurs after approximately 7 minutes. Nicotine absorption times for smokeless tobacco products tend to peak between 20 and 30 minutes after introduction (Henningfield & Keenan, 1993). In addition to the speed of nicotine delivery, tobacco smoking provides users the ability to adjust the amount of nicotine absorbed. A smoker accomplishes these adjustments by varying the number of inhalations, duration of an inhalation, completeness of inhalation, and the number of cigarettes smoked (Frederiksen, Martin, & Webster, 1979).

Liver Enzyme Differences and the Metabolism of Nicotine

Once absorbed, nicotine readily passes through the blood–brain barrier. In the liver, CYP-2A6 enzymes metabolize 80 percent to 90 percent of nicotine, producing the active metabolite **cotinine**, which exhibits pharmacological actions similar to nicotine. Genetic polymorphisms influence CYP-2A6 activity levels. CYP-2A6*4, *7 and *9 polymorphisms exhibit reduced CYP-2A6 activity, causing slower metabolism of nicotine to cotinine. In other words, nicotine levels remain higher in body because of reduced metabolism. These polymorphisms are prevalent within Asian populations. Individuals who exhibit homogenous

cotinine Metabolite of nicotine.

*A nanogram is one billionth, or 10^{-9}, of a gram.

mutant forms of these gene polymorphisms or heterogeneous mutant forms that have a combination of the *4, 7*, or *9 polymorphisms, tend to be light smokers and have a lower risk of tobacco-related health effects (Ariyoshi et al., 2002; Minematsu et al., 2006; Yusof & Gan, 2009).

The half-life for nicotine is approximately 2 hours, but this clearance time depends on a smoker's status. Chronic smokers have a 30-percent faster elimination rate of nicotine than nonsmokers. These findings suggest that chronic tobacco use sensitizes pharmacokinetic processes for nicotine (Perkins et al., 1994). The half-life for cotinine is approximately 17 hours (Pérez-Stable, Herrera, Jacob, & Benowitz, 1998). Both nicotine and cotinine are primarily eliminated from the body through urine, and so a simple urine analysis for cotinine can reveal tobacco use more than a day later.

Stop & Check

1. Why is inhalation the most effective route for absorbing nicotine from tobacco tar?
2. What is the active metabolite for nicotine?

1. The lungs have a large surface area that helps speed delivery of nicotine to the brain after blood absorption. The large surface area also overcomes the poor absorption of nicotine when delivered in tobacco smoke, which has a less-than-ideal pH of approximately 6. 2. Cotinine

Nicotine and Nervous System Functioning

Nicotine functions as an agonist for cholinergic nicotinic receptors (**figure 7.7**), one of the two major cholinergic receptor families. Cotinine, the active metabolite of nicotine, serves as a weak agonist for nicotine receptors. As shown in **figure 7.8**, agonists for nicotinic receptors such as acetylcholine and nicotine cause the receptor channels to open. When nicotine activates channels, the drug elicits its acute drug effects, which are described later in this chapter.

REVIEW! Nicotinic receptors are ionotropic and comprised of α and β subunits. Nicotinic receptors can include other subunit types as well, which are denoted by different Greek symbols. The configuration of these subunits defines each receptor's name. Chapter 3 (pg. 89).

After a short period of time, however, the receptors enter a desensitized state, which limits the duration of action for nicotine's acute pharmacological effects. During the desensitized state, the channels close and the receptors cannot be activated. These receptors enter this desensitized state even when the receptors remain bound by an agonist. After a period of time, the desensitized state ends and the receptors can again be activated by an agonist.

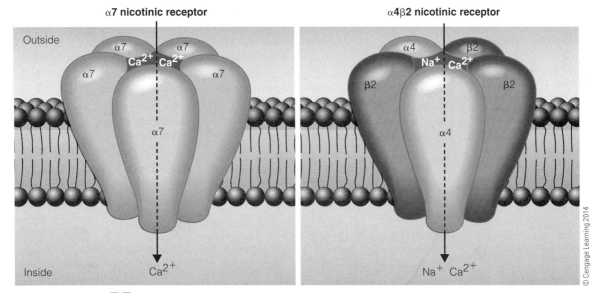

figure 7.7   Each nicotinic ionotropic receptor is comprised of a configuration of α and β subunits.

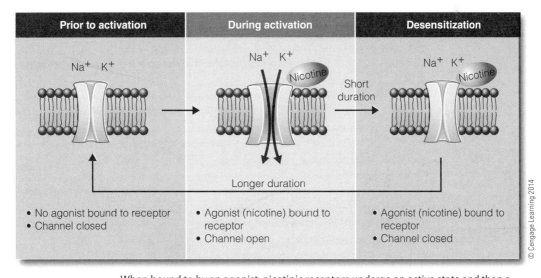

figure 7.8   When bound to by an agonist, nicotinic receptors undergo an active state and then a desensitized state. The receptor cannot be activated during the desensitized state, and the desensitized state occurs for a longer period of time than the active state.

functional antagonism
An indirect or atypical means of inhibiting a receptor's activity, such as when the net effects of a receptor agonist consists of a longer inactivated receptor state and a shorter activated receptor state.

upregulation Increased production of proteins.

Because of desensitization, agonists cause nicotinic-receptor channels to remain closed *longer* than they are open. In this way, nicotinic-receptor agonists also produce **functional antagonism**, meaning that nicotine causes these receptors to have a longer inactivated state than an activated state. Thinking of nicotine as a *functional antagonist* is useful for understanding changes in nicotinic receptors during chronic nicotine administration. During such administration, the brain compensates for the repeated closing of nicotinic-receptor channels by *upregulating* nicotinic receptors. **Upregulation** refers to an increased production of proteins.

Both the central and peripheral nervous systems contain nicotinic receptors. Peripherally, nicotinic receptors are located postsynaptically on neuromuscular junctions in the somatic nervous system. Within neuromuscular junctions, the activation of $\alpha_1 \beta_1 \delta \gamma$ nicotinic receptors** on muscle fibers causes muscles to contract.

Nicotinic receptors are located in ganglia of the autonomic system, including both the sympathetic and the parasympathetic nervous systems. Of these two systems, the activation of nicotinic receptors primarily increases sympathetic nervous system activity (Li, LaCroix, & Freeling, 2009). Different subtypes of nicotinic receptors are likely involved in the sympathetic and parasympathetic systems. For cardiovascular effects, Li and colleagues (2009) discovered that α_7 receptors activate the parasympathetic nervous system, whereas $\alpha_4 \beta_2$ receptors activate the sympathetic nervous system.

REVIEW! The autonomic nervous system includes the sympathetic nervous system, which increases physiological activity, and the parasympathetic nervous system, which decreases physiological activity. Chapter 2 (pg. 37).

Nicotinic receptors are found throughout the central nervous system and play an important role in many nervous system processes. The cerebral cortex and hippocampus, two brain areas important for cognitive functioning, highly express both $\alpha_4 \beta_2$ and α_7 nicotinic receptors. High amounts of $\alpha_4 \beta_2$ nicotinic receptors are also found in the basal ganglia, an area important for regulating movement, and the substantia nigra, the source of dopamine neurons that terminate in the basal ganglia. In the dopamine reward pathway, the ventral tegmental area contains $\alpha_4 \beta_2$ and $\alpha_4 \alpha_6$[†] receptors, and the nucleus accumbens also contains $\alpha_4 \beta_2$ receptors (Yang et al., 2011; Zhao-Shea et al., 2011).

The activation of nicotinic receptors in either the ventral tegmental area or the nucleus accumbens increases dopamine release in the nucleus accumbens. Researchers discovered these effects using microdialysis techniques in animals (see box 3.1). For example, Nisell and colleagues (1994) infused nicotine into either the ventral tegmental area or the nucleus accumbens in rats. Microdialysis probes in these structures collected cerebrospinal fluid samples for dopamine analysis. The infusion of nicotine in the ventral

---

**During embryonic development, the γ is replaced by an ε subunit.
[†]There is another subunit on this receptor that is currently unknown.

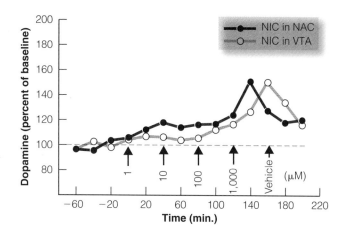

Infusion of nicotine into either the ventral tegmental area (empty circles) or the nucleus accumbens (filled circles) increases dopamine release in the nucleus accumbens. (Nisell, M., Nomikos, G. G. and Svensson, T. H. (1994), Infusion of Nicotine in the Ventral Tegmental Area or the Nucleus Accumbens of the Rat Differentially Affects Accumbal Dopamine Release. *Pharmacology & Toxicology*, 75: 348352. doi: 10.1111/j.1600-0773.1994.tb00373.x. Reproduced with permission of John Wiley & Sons Ltd.)

figure 7.9

tegmental area produced a large, sustained increase in dopamine levels in the nucleus accumbens. When infused into the nucleus accumbens, nicotine produced a much shorter increase in dopamine levels in the nucleus accumbens (**figure 7.9**). Based on these findings, nicotine acts in both areas to elevate dopamine levels in the nucleus accumbens, but nicotine's actions in the ventral tegmental area are especially effective for inducing dopamine release in the nucleus accumbens.

In addition to enhancing the release of dopamine in the brain, the activation of nicotinic receptors influences many other neurotransmitters in the brain, including acetylcholine, glutamate, GABA, norepinephrine, serotonin, and the hormone vasopressin. These widespread interactions preclude identifying highly specific roles that nicotinic receptors have on behavior. Clearly, by acting on nicotinic receptors, nicotine and other nicotinic-receptor agonists have global effects on the central nervous system.

Beyond nicotine, other compounds in tobacco may act in the nervous system, possibly enhancing nicotine's effects (Khalil, Steyn, & Castagnoli, 1999). In particular, many chemicals in tobacco inhibit MAO_A and MAO_B activities. These actions may explain why long-term smokers exhibit a 40-percent decrease in MAO_B levels (Fowler et al., 1996).

REVIEW! Monoamine oxidase (MAO) is an enzyme that breaks down, or catabolizes, dopamine, norepinephrine, and serotonin. Chapter 3 (pg. 86).

MAO inhibition enhances the effects of nicotine on dopamine levels in the nucleus accumbens. In a microdialysis study conducted by Lotfipour

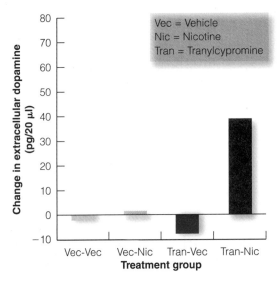

figure **7.10** Rats treated with both nicotine and tranylcypromine, an MAO reuptake inhibitor, exhibited a substantially greater increase in nucleus accumbens dopamine levels than rats treated with either drug alone. (Data from Lotfipour et al., 2011.)

and colleagues (2011), rats treated with both nicotine and tranylcypromine, an $MAO_{A/B}$ reuptake inhibitor, exhibited a substantially greater increase in nucleus accumbens dopamine levels than rats treated with either drug alone (**figure 7.10**).

Stop & Check

1. At nicotinic cholinergic receptors, nicotine functions as a(n) _____.

2. Nicotine causes an increase in dopamine release in the nucleus accumbens by acting on nicotinic receptors in the nucleus accumbens and the _____.

3. What is another compound in tobacco that may facilitate nicotine's effects?

1. agonist **2.** ventral tegmental area **3.** An MAO inhibitor

Nicotine's Potent Pharmacological Effects

Nicotine produces substantial physiological, behavioral, and subjective effects, and tobacco, the main source of nicotine, produces a host of adverse effects. When characterizing the pharmacological effects of nicotine, the length of nicotine use is important. Because upregulation of nicotinic receptors occurs during repeated administration, the acute effects of nicotine can differ from the chronic effects of nicotine. Thus, the effects of nicotine in a first-time smoker can differ greatly from the effects of nicotine in a long-time smoker.

Nicotine's Effects on Cardiovascular Function and Appetite

Nicotine produces widespread physiological effects. The two most notable are on the cardiovascular system and appetite. In both smokers and nonsmokers, nicotine produces significant cardiovascular effects consisting of increases in heart rate and blood pressure. Because these effects are observed in smokers, a tolerance to these effects does not occur during chronic nicotine administration. However, acute tolerance differs from chronic tolerance. Acute tolerance to nicotine's effects on heart rate and blood pressure happens when nicotine is administered soon after the previous administration (Perkins et al., 1994) (**figure 7.11**). Acute tolerance occurs partly because the subsequent nicotine administration occurs while many nicotinic receptors remain in a desensitized state.

Acute tolerance occurs each morning for most smokers. Nicotine delivered from the first cigarette of the day causes an increase in heart rate and blood pressure. The next cigarette exhibits weaker effects on heart rate and blood pressure. Because of acute tolerance, heart rate and blood pressure tend to return to normal levels.

Nicotine reduces appetite in both non-tobacco users and long-term smokers. These effects were demonstrated by Perkins and colleagues (1991). In this study, nicotine was administered to either non-tobacco users or smokers, who had not smoked since the night before. In both groups of participants, nicotine reduced self-reported hunger and the number of snack foods consumed

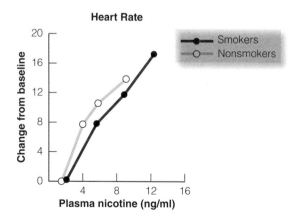

figure 7.11 Nicotine administered to nonsmokers (empty symbols) and smokers (solid symbols) who had abstained from smoking since the evening before assessment increased heart rate (left figure). During the course of several trials, the effects of nicotine on heart rate are reduced (right figure). (Data from Perkins et al., 1994.)

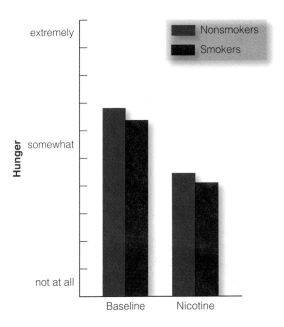

figure **7.12** After test subjects fasted overnight, administration of nicotine significantly reduced feelings of hunger in both smokers and nonsmokers compared to placebo. (Data from Perkins et al., 1991.)

during the testing sessions (**figure 7.12**). The appetite-suppressing effects of nicotine contribute to weight loss in many tobacco users, and tobacco users often cite potential weight gain as a reason not to quit.

Nicotine Affects Movement and Cognitive Functioning

Nicotine's behavioral effects include alterations in movement and cognitive function. These effects differ between naïve and chronic tobacco users. Nicotine produces effects on motor stability. These changes are particularly noticeable in the hands. Reduced hand steadiness and hand tremor occur after nicotine administration to non-tobacco users. Tolerance occurs with these effects in tobacco users (Perkins et al., 1994).

Nicotine's effects on psychomotor function also differ between acute and chronic administration. Acute administration of nicotine in nicotine-naïve users causes a decrease in psychomotor activity. However, sensitization to these effects occurs during chronic administration. Thus, in chronic tobacco users, nicotine increases psychomotor function. For example, Perkins and colleagues (1994) reported that nicotine administration increases the rate of finger tapping in chronic smokers, but decreases the rate of finger tapping in nonsmokers.

Animal studies also find differences between acute and chronic nicotine administration. For example, Pehrson and colleagues (2008) studied locomotor activity in rats during 14 days of nicotine administration (**figure 7.13**). On the first day of treatment, nicotine suppressed locomotor

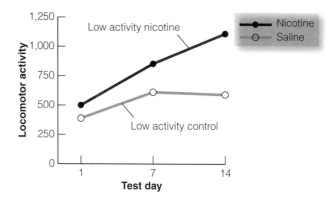

figure **7.13**

Nicotine-treated rats (solid symbols) exhibited increased locomotor activity on the 7th and 14th days of treatment compared to saline-treated rats. The y-axis shows locomotor activity as an expression of number of photobeams rats crossed within a test chamber. The x-axis refers to the number of days of treatment. (Data from Pehrson et al., 2008.)

activity as indicated by fewer photobeam breaks in an open-field apparatus. However, on the 7th and 14th days of treatment, nicotine enhanced locomotor activity.

Although public attitudes toward nicotine are generally negative, nicotine may show some benefits for cognitive functioning. Studies show that nicotine improves attention, particularly when reorienting attention toward another stimulus (Thiel, Zilles, & Fink, 2005), and improves information processing (Juliano, Fucito, & Harrell, 2011; Wesnes & Warburton, 1984).

In attention tasks, nicotine improves information processing by shortening times to detect stimuli. Wesnes and Warburton (1983) first demonstrated these effects, finding that nicotine improved the detection of targets during an 80-minute task in nicotine-naïve users. David Warburton later reflected that this seminal study was first rejected from a journal because the editor refused to publish "anything good about nicotine" (Warburton, 2002).

stroop test Standard attention test used for neuropsychological assessments that evaluates reaction times to mismatched stimulus presentations.

Nicotine's improvements in attention occur after chronic administration as well. For example, Perkins and colleagues (1994) used a **Stroop test**—a standard attention test used for neuropsychological assessments that evaluates reaction times to mismatched stimulus presentations—to assess attention after nicotine administration in both nonsmokers and smokers. Nicotine improved reaction times in both test subjects, both nonsmokers and smokers.

Aside from information processing and attention, the effects of nicotine on memory are unclear. In the study by Perkins and colleagues (1994), nicotine also improved memory in a word list recall test, which required participants to remember words presented to them in a list. Nicotine's memory improvements were greater in nonsmokers than in smokers, suggesting that smoker's develop a tolerance to these effects. Yet many studies also fail to show improvements in memory after nicotine treatment, and some studies show that nicotine worsens memory in chronic smokers (Ernst et al., 2001; Myers, Taylor, Moolchan, & Heishman, 2007; Park, Knopick, McGurk, & Meltzer, 2000).

Many studies have evaluated nicotine for the treatment of Alzheimer's disease. Biologically, nicotine reduces the destructive effects of amyloidbeta proteins in the hippocampus, an important characteristic of this disease. However, Deng and colleagues (2010) demonstrated that nicotine worsens the memory-inducing impairments caused by amyloidbeta proteins in rats. In humans, some studies report a decreased risk of Alzheimer's disease in smokers, whereas other studies report an increased risk. Heavy smoking, at least, is not beneficial for Alzheimer's disease; in fact, Rusanen and colleagues (2011) found that heavy smoking increases the risk of Alzheimer's disease by 157 percent.

box 7.1 Conditioned Taste Aversion

A **conditioned taste aversion** is the result of a pairing process between a noxious stimulus and a novel-tasting substance. This procedure also is called the *Garcia effect* in recognition of a discovery by John Garcia in 1955 (Garcia, Kimeldorf, & Koellino, 1955). Garcia discovered that rats ingested less of a saccharin solution after an occasion in which prior consumption of the solution was followed by gastrointestinal pain. Conditioned taste aversion is a process resembling classical, or Pavlovian, conditioning procedures.

Many psychoactive drugs function as noxious stimuli, allowing them to be studied in a conditioned taste-aversion procedure. In a typical procedure, researchers give water-deprived rats access to two water bottles. One bottle contains the usual tap water, whereas the other bottle contains a novel, and often sweet-tasting, solution. After overcoming a *neophobic reaction*—that is, a rat's natural fear response to ingesting novel substances—rats consume the novel solution.

After a session in which rats consume the novel-tasting substance, researchers conduct one or multiple pairing sessions with a drug or its placebo. The timing of a drug injection is set to produce noxious effects after a session when subjects consume the novel substance. We refer to this type of session as a *pairing session*. A conditioned taste aversion is demonstrated if significantly less solution is consumed during subsequent sessions.

For example, nicotine produces a robust conditioned taste aversion. In one of the earliest characterizations of nicotine in this procedure, Stolerman (1983) conducted repeated pairings over several sessions with nicotine and a flavored solution consisting of either saccharin or sodium chloride. Selected results from this study are shown in box 7.1, figure 1. Over the course of several trials, the nicotine-paired solutions were consumed less, whereas saline-paired solutions were consumed at the normal level.

Although conditioned taste aversion appears to be only a measure of adverse effects, this is not necessarily the case. For many recreational drugs, the doses used to achieve positive subjective effects are the same doses effective for producing conditioned taste aversions (Wise, Yokel, & Wit, 1976).

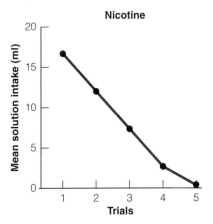

box 7.1, figure 1

Less consumption of a flavored solution occurred after pairing the solution with the effects of nicotine in rats. The x-axis represents the number of consecutive pairing sessions, and the y-axis represents the volume of solution consumed. (Data adapted from Stolerman et al., 1983.)

Conditioned taste aversion Result of a pairing process between a noxious stimulus and a novel tasting substance.

Nicotine's Positive and Negative Subjective Effects

Nicotine's subjective effects vary greatly between acute and chronic administration. In non-tobacco users, nicotine produces negative subjective effects, including nausea and disequilibrium. In addition, as described in the study by Perkins and colleagues (1994), nicotine produces feelings of jitteriness, tension, and confusion in nonsmokers. Yet acute tolerance to these negative subjective effects occurs after subsequent nicotine administrations.

A conditioned taste-aversion procedure can demonstrate nicotine's aversive effects as well as acute tolerance to these aversive effects. The conditioned taste-aversion procedure is described in **box 7.1**. Prus and colleagues (2007) used this procedure to link the timing of nicotine administration with the time course of nicotinic-receptor changes (**figure 7.14**). For rats treated with nicotine 5 minutes before a pairing session with saccharin, less saccharin was consumed on the following day. This pairing session took place during the activated nicotinic-receptor state.

In this same study, another group of rats was treated with nicotine 90 minutes before the pairing session and given a second treatment of nicotine 5 minutes before the session. These rats drank more of the saccharin solution on the following day. For these rats, the second injection of nicotine occurred when the nicotinic receptors were desensitized, thus reducing aversive effects from occurring during or after the pairing session.

Long-term treatment with nicotine also causes tolerance to these negative subjective effects. Without negative subjective effects, chronic tobacco users only experience positive subjective effects from nicotine. In chronic smokers, nicotine administration produces feelings of vigor, arousal, and reduced fatigue (Perkins et al., 1994). Chronic smokers report that the effects of nicotine are pleasant and enjoyed and produce a positive mood (Myers et al., 2007). These smokers can detect a distinct rewarding effect with each puff of cigarette smoke.

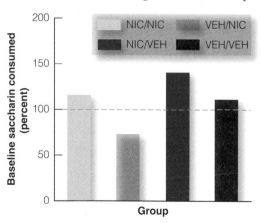

Nicotine failed to exhibit a conditioned taste aversion (NIC/NIC group) when nicotine was administered during the nicotine receptor desensitized state. See text for further details.
(Prus, A. J., Maxwell, A. T., Baker, K. M., Rosecrans, J. A., & James, J. R. (2007). Acute behavioral tolerance to nicotine in the conditioned taste aversion paradigm. *Drug Development Research*, 68(8), 522–528. doi: 10.1002/ddr.20219. Reproduced with permission of Wiley Inc.)

figure 7.14

The positive subjective effects of nicotine can be difficult to establish in animals. In a standard self-administration procedure (see box 5.1), rats will not learn to self-administer nicotine because of the initial adverse effects experienced on first exposure to nicotine. In other words, if the effects are negative, an animal will avoid those effects rather than seek to achieve them. To observe the reinforcing effects of nicotine in this procedure, researchers use a variation on the standard self-administration design.

For example, Boules and colleagues (2011) used a common design variation to study nicotine self-administration in rats. First, these researchers trained rats to press a lever for sucrose food pellets. Then the researchers changed the consequence for pressing a lever from the sucrose food pellet to an intravenous nicotine injection. Because the rats had learned to repeatedly press the lever for sucrose pellets in the past, they persisted in pressing the lever, resulting in further nicotine injections. Through this process, tolerance quickly developed to nicotine's negative effects. After a tolerance developed to the negative effects, the reinforcing effects of nicotine administration were sufficient to maintain lever pressing.

Other components in tobacco may contribute to the reinforcing effects of nicotine. In particular, MAO inhibitors found in tobacco enhance nicotine-induced effects on nucleus accumbens dopamine levels. Self-administration of nicotine is enhanced by MAO inhibition (Guillem et al., 2005; Villégier, Lotfipour, McQuown, Belluzzi, & Leslie, 2007). For example, in a study by Villégier and colleagues (2007), the MAO inhibitor tranylcypromine facilitated self-administration for nicotine in rats. This facilitation avoided the need to have a prior training history, allowing the researchers to use a standard self-administration procedure. Rats that did not receive the MAO inhibitor were unable to self-administer nicotine without altering the standard procedure. These findings suggest that an addiction to tobacco may develop more rapidly than an addiction to only nicotine.

The Serious Adverse Effects of Tobacco Use

Many of the severely adverse effects associated with nicotine are the result of its vehicle of administration: tobacco. Tobacco contains thousands of chemicals, including carcinogens such as nitrosamines. **Nitrosamines** are chemicals shown to produce cancerous tumor growth. The release and inhalation of tar from smoked tobacco provides direct contact of these carcinogens with tissue in the mouth, throat, esophagus, and lungs.

nitrosamines Chemicals shown to produce cancerous tumor growth.

Tobacco is a cause of pulmonary diseases such as **emphysema**, a type of chronic obstructive pulmonary disorder caused by irreversible lung damage (**figure 7.15**). The symptoms of emphysema include shortness of breath, wheezing, chronic cough, and fatigue. Emphysema patients are treated with a bronchodilator inhaler such as albuterol to open lung passages.

emphysema Type of chronic obstructive pulmonary disorder caused by irreversible lung damage.

Tobacco use also increases the risk of cardiovascular disease. Nicotine in tobacco causes arteries and blood vessels to narrow and constrict, increasing heartrate. Together, these effects increase the risk of heart attack, ischemia, stroke, and diseases associated with impoverished blood to flow to other organs.

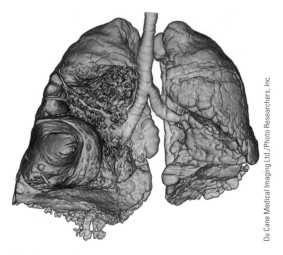

Du Cane Medical Imaging Ltd./Photo Researchers, Inc.

figure 7.15   Emphysema, shown in the lung on the right, is a smoking-related irreversible lung damage. A healthy lung is shown on the left.

REVIEW! Ischemia consists of damaged and dysfunctional tissue from restricted blood supply. Stroke is an interruption in blood supply in the brain. Chapter 2 (pg. 49).

During pregnancy, tobacco causes slower gestational development, preterm births, and low birth weight. Any number of chemicals in smoked tobacco can interfere with prenatal development, but reduced oxygen to the fetus is an important contributor.

Nicotine and Psychological Dependence

As noted at the beginning of this chapter, seven tobacco company CEOs famously testified that nicotine is nonaddictive. This opinion, of course, lies in the best interest of tobacco companies, which seek to minimize tobacco regulation. Beyond this conflict of interest, the basis for their opinion depends on the different ways drug addiction has been defined.

As described in Chapter 5, traditional notions of drug addiction were largely based on opioids and alcohol. For drugs like these, addiction appears as intense motivation to seek and use a substance, often at the expense losing one's career or jeopardizing relationships with friends or family. When considering addiction as only this, the CEOs likely felt comfortable asserting the nonaddictive nature of nicotine.

The American Psychiatric Association's *Diagnostic and Statistical Manual* (DSM-IV), however, offers other features of *substance dependence*—namely, that individuals express difficulty quitting or reducing use. When nicotine use discontinues, chronic users may experience a collection of psychological withdrawal symptoms called the **nicotine abstinence syndrome**, which is characterized by craving, irritability, anxiety, hostility, concentration difficulties, impatience, and insomnia. Avoidance of nicotine's withdrawal

nicotine abstinence syndrome Nicotine withdrawal symptoms characterized by craving, irritability, anxiety, hostility, concentration difficulties, impatience, and insomnia.

effects is an important contributor to tobacco usage. Based on the dependence criteria described in the DSM, nicotine is an addictive substance. Further, as described previously in this chapter, nicotine exhibits a rapid tolerance to both physical and psychological effects during chronic use. Given our modern conceptions of substance dependence, few people would agree with a tobacco company's claims that their products do not cause addiction.

Stop & Check

1. During sustained use, nicotine produces a(n) _____ in locomotor activity.
2. Nicotine improves two particular aspects of attention: orientation to a stimulus and _____.
3. On first using nicotine, the positive subjective effects are blocked by _____ effects.
4. How might the reinforcing effects of tobacco differ in magnitude from the reinforcing effects of nicotine?
5. Many of the adverse effects associated with nicotine actually result from _____, the nicotine vehicle.
6. Repeated nicotine use causes an upregulation of nicotinic receptors, which is the result of_____ of nicotinic receptors

1. increase. However, the first administration of nicotine causes a decrease in locomotor activity. The increase in locomotor activity during sustained nicotine use is described as *sensitization*. **2.** information processing. **3.** aversive. **4.** Tobacco smoke contains many chemicals that may enhance nicotine's reinforcing effects. Therefore, smoking may produce a greater reinforcing effect than nicotine alone. **5.** tobacco **6.** desensitization

Environmental, Genetic, and Receptor Differences Between Light and Heavy Tobacco Users

chippers Smokers who fail to develop an addiction to tobacco.

Humans vary in their susceptibility to nicotine addiction. People who are the most resistant to nicotine addiction are called **chippers**. These are light smokers who fail to develop an addiction to tobacco. Chippers are long-term smokers, but they typically only smoke just a few cigarettes a day. They comprise approximately one-third of all smokers (Shiffman, 1989).

Chippers smoke cigarettes the same way as normal smokers—that is, they fully inhale tobacco smoke, have the same puff duration, and have the same interval times between each puff (Brauer, Hatsukami, Hanson, & Shiffman, 1996). Chippers and regular smokers have similar abilities to absorb and metabolize nicotine. However, chippers fail to show significant pharmacological effects from tobacco, and they fail to exhibit withdrawal symptoms when deprived of tobacco.

Exactly how chippers resist nicotine addiction is unknown. Two possible explanations concern environmental and genetic factors. For an environmental explanation, Shiffman (1989) found that chippers, more often than smokers, had greater coping skills, less stress, and better social support structures. These psychosocial factors may reduce an individual's risk of developing a substance addiction.

Genetically, chippers and chronic smokers differ in gene expression for α_5, α_3, and β_4 receptor subunits, which are found on chromosome 15 (Saccone et al., 2007). Of these, the single nucleotide polymorphism Chrna4 for the α_5 unit is particularly associated with greater risk of nicotine dependence. Although this subunit has not been directly implicated in the reinforcing effects of nicotine, this subunit alters state changes from active to desensitized in α_4 subunit nicotinic receptors (Ramirez-Latorre et al., 1996). As noted already in this chapter, $\alpha_4\beta_2$ receptors facilitate the reinforcing effects of nicotine.

These genetic variations suggest that differences in nicotinic receptors may facilitate the resistance of chippers for nicotine addiction. In particular, chippers may have weaker acute tolerance to the effects of nicotine because of diminished desensitization of nicotinic receptors. Reduced acute tolerance to nicotine would produce longer-lasting effects (Rosecrans, 1995).

To better understand nicotine tolerance in chippers, animal studies have assessed the association between nicotinic receptor desensitization and acute tolerance. For example, rats that differed in nicotinic receptor desensitization were studied in the conditioned taste-aversion procedure study by Prus and colleagues (2007) described previously. Like the earlier experiment, rats were injected with nicotine both 90 minutes and 5 minutes before a pairing session. The rats used for this experiment were either normal or had diminished nicotinic receptor desensitization. In the normal rats, saccharin consumption increased the following day because the injection of nicotine 5 minutes before the pairing session occurred during the nicotine receptors' desensitized state, preventing aversive effects. However, in the rats with diminished nicotinic receptor desensitization, saccharin consumption decreased the following day because the receptors were not desensitized and thus did not prevent aversive effects (**figure 7.16**).

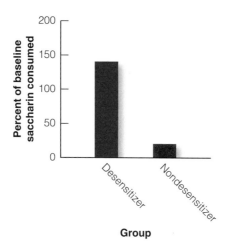

Nicotine administered during the desensitized nicotinic-receptor state produces a conditioned taste aversion in rats that exhibit reduced nicotinic-receptor desensitization. See text for further details. (Prus, A. J., Maxwell, A. T., Baker, K. M., Rosecrans, J. A., & James, J. R. (2007). Acute behavioral tolerance to nicotine in the conditioned taste aversion paradigm. Drug Development Research, 68(8), 522-528. doi: 10.1002/ddr.20219. Reproduced with permission of Wiley Inc.)

figure 7.16

These data suggest that differences in nicotinic receptor desensitization differ between individuals and that these differences significantly alter acute tolerance to nicotine.

FROM ACTIONS TO EFFECTS
Why People Smoke and How They Quit

Humans learn to use tobacco for many reasons. Many people begin smoking because their friends smoke. Smoking may also be common in an individual's family or culture. Tobacco advertisers market cigarettes as fun, cool, sexy, and rebellious. Not too long ago, workers who smoked were allowed frequent short smoke breaks, whereas nonsmokers had to continue working.

As smoking persists, an addiction to nicotine develops, serving as the primary reason for tobacco use. For frequent smokers, the effects of nicotine become associated with routine, everyday activities such as talking on a phone, watching TV, or working on a computer. Associative learning processes incentivize these conditioned responses, leading to the preoccupation and anticipation features of addiction as described in Chapter 5. Without having a cigarette, these stimuli lead to craving tobacco, which makes quitting difficult.

Although many people succeed in quitting tobacco "cold turkey," others need to develop a treatment plan. Many psychotherapeutic approaches address the behavioral cues that trigger a craving to smoke. Smokers learn to identify the causes of these cravings and make attempts to diminish the influence of these cravings. Many treatment plans also employ pharmacological strategies that address changes in the nicotinic receptor system resulting from chronic nicotine administration.

As described previously, nicotinic receptors are upregulated during chronic nicotine administration, creating a need for nicotine to maintain this sensitized state. An abrupt drop in nicotine levels leaves these extra receptors inactivated, leading to withdrawal symptoms. To address the absence of nicotine, treatments mostly fall into one of three categories: nicotine-replacement therapy, nicotinic-receptor agonism, and antidepressant drugs (Polosa & Benowitz, 2011).

nicotine-replacement therapy Therapy that consists of using a nontobacco nicotine product to minimize or prevent withdrawal symptoms.

Nicotine-replacement therapy consists of using a non-tobacco nicotine product to minimize or prevent withdrawal symptoms. To reduce their dependence on nicotine, users gradually reduce the dose of nicotine used until they reach a point where few withdrawal symptoms occur in the absence of nicotine. This approach may take weeks or months. Nicotine-replacement therapy products include nicotine skin patches, gum, nasal spray, and inhalers.

varenicline (Chantix) Partial agonist for nicotinic receptors.

Nicotinic-receptor agonist medications also reduce withdrawal symptoms. The first drug approved from this class approved by the Food and Drug Administration is **varenicline (Chantix)**, a partial agonist for nicotinic receptors (Coe et al., 2005). By acting as a partial agonist, less activation of nicotinic receptors occur. When varenicline is taken, smoking becomes less enjoyable and overall produces weaker pharmacological effects (Gonzales et al., 2006; Polosa & Benowitz, 2011). However, these pharmacological actions tend to reduce smoking in fewer than half of all smokers (Gonzales et al., 2006).

Antidepressant drugs reduce smoking by addressing nicotine's effects on dopamine. The most commonly prescribed antidepressant drug for nicotine cessation is bupropion (Zyban or Wellbutrin). By blocking reuptake of dopamine, bupropion elevates dopamine levels within synapses. Researchers hypothesize that when this occurs in the nucleus accumbens, the elevated dopamine levels make up for the lack of nicotine-induced dopamine elevations. Although this drug produces pharmacological actions suggestive of reducing smoking, fewer than one-third of patients in clinical studies have successfully abstained from smoking when taking bupropion (Gonzales et al., 2006).

Stop & Check

1. Given that the first use of nicotine causes aversive effects, why does tobacco use continue?
2. Chippers smoke without developing a nicotine addiction, possibly because they exhibit weaker _____ tolerance to nicotine.
3. Why are nicotine-replacement therapies helpful for tobacco-cessation programs?

1. Behavioral reasons account for the persistent use of tobacco until tolerance to adverse effects develop. **2.** acute **3.** Nicotine-replacement therapies address changes that chronic nicotine use causes to the nicotinic-receptor system. A nicotine-replacement therapy provides a gradual reduction in physiological nicotine levels, allowing this receptor system to slowly adapt to a nicotine-free state, thereby reducing withdrawal symptoms.

Caffeine

caffeine Psychostimulant compound and a member of the xanthine chemical class.

Caffeine is a psychostimulant compound and a member of the xanthine chemical class. Other xanthines, including theobromine and theophylline, also exhibit psychostimulant effects. However, caffeine is by far the most used and is the main topic for this section. Approximately 90 percent of Americans consume caffeine on a regular basis and average about 227mg of caffeine per person each day (Frary, Johnson, & Wang, 2005). Best estimates indicate that children consume about half the caffeine as adults, although data on young children are generally lacking (Temple, 2009). In one study, average caffeine intake consisted of 52 mg in 5–7 year olds and 109 mg in 8–12 year olds (Warzak, Evans, Floress, Gross, & Stoolman, 2011).

Caffeine and Related Compounds in Plants

Caffeine, and to a lesser extent other xanthine compounds, exist in many plants grown naturally in the environment. Caffeine, theobromine, and theophylline are found in kola nuts and cocoa tree nuts, which we find in cola soft drinks and chocolate, respectively. Colas contain caffeine from kola nuts, and chocolate has caffeine from cocoa nuts. A large variety of tea leaves also contain caffeine, theobromine, and theophylline. Coffee beans, which are brewed for coffee drinks, are a significant source of caffeine. Because caffeine represents the most-used and strongest-acting compound among naturally occurring xanthines, this chapter will focus on the use and properties of caffeine.

The caffeine content among products varies. A 10-ounce (oz.) cup of regular coffee contains approximately 200 mg of caffeine, and a 16-oz. coffee, the "grande" size at Starbucks, contains approximately 320 mg of caffeine. For coffee, the caffeine content varies, in part, with roasting time. Darker-roast coffees, which are roasted longer, tend to have less caffeine content than lighter-roast coffees.

A 10-oz. cup of tea contains approximately 100 mg of caffeine, or half as much caffeine as coffee. A 1-oz. piece of chocolate contains approximately 25 mg of caffeine. **Figure 7.17** lists the caffeine content of other popular substances (Mayo Foundation, 2011).

Energy drinks are rapidly growing in popularity for their invigorating properties. They contain a large amount of caffeine, often around 200 mg. Beyond describing energy-enhancing effects, advertisers also promote energy drinks for weight loss, physical stamina, and athletic performance. Individuals 25 years and younger, including a significant portion of children 12 and younger, consume nearly half of all energy drinks. College students report that between 39 percent and 57 percent of them had consumed energy drinks within the previous month (Malinauskas, Aeby, Overton, Carpenter-Aeby, &

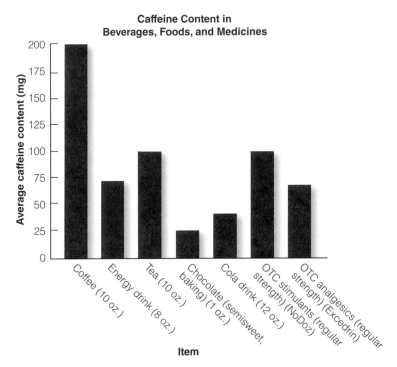

figure **7.17** Caffeine content in selected beverages, foods, and medicines. (From Mayo Foundation, 2011; Reissig et al. 2009.)

Barber-Heidal, 2007; Miller, 2008). Energy drinks are the fastest-growing beverage in the United States, accounting for $9 billion in sales in the United States in 2011 (Arria & O'Brien, 2011).

Energy drinks not only include caffeine as a direct ingredient but also may include caffeinated products such as kola nut, yerba maté, and cocoa. They often include other xanthines such as theobromine and theophylline. Many other chemicals in energy drinks also promote energy-enhancing effects, including sugar and a variety of herbs, amino acids, and plant extracts (Arria & O'Brien, 2011).

Alcoholic beverages have also become a popular source of caffeine. These beverages, referred to as a **caffeinated alcoholic beverages**, consist of mixing energy drinks such as Red Bull with alcohols such as vodka. Many concoctions are now sold this way, including Four Loko, a popular alcohol and energy-drink beverage now banned in many states. The energy-drink component of these beverages can temporarily counter alcohol's intoxicating effects, thus facilitating excessive drinking and an increased risk of alcohol poisoning.

caffeinated alcoholic beverages Beverage made by mixing energy drinks with alcohol.

Caffeine Has an Ancient History

The plant products just listed were consumed long before the Europeans discovered them. Teas were used in China for thousands of years, and coffee beans were brewed in Arabia since at least 1000 A.D. In South and Central America, the Olmec, Maya, Toltec, and Aztec cultures consumed cocoa beans. European explorers subsequently brought cocoa seeds to Europe, and Europeans harvested the seeds and commonly prepared cocoa with sugars and milk to make chocolate drinks and candies.

The very first human discoveries of the invigorating properties of these plants are shrouded in stories passed through an oral history, as reviewed by Fredholm (2011). For example, scholars often report a story about an Ethiopian named Kaldi as the discoverer of coffee. Kaldi observed that his goats became excited after consuming berries from a coffee bush, which he confirmed on trying the berries himself.

Before 1000 A.D., people normally consumed coffee by eating coffee beans, but around 1000 A.D., brewed coffee became popular. Brewed coffee became a social drink in Arabia, and students and scholars consumed coffee in intellectual centers. In fact, a type of coffee bar consumed in intellectual centers in Turkey was given the name *mekteb-i-irfan*, meaning "the school of the wise."

Coffee was not immediately accepted in Europe, and an attempt to persuade Pope Clement VIII (reign 1592 to 1605) to officially ban this "Muslim drink" led him to state: "This satanic drink is in truth so good that it would be a pity if only nonbelievers were allowed to drink it. We will fool Satan and baptize it so that it becomes a Christian drink, with no danger for the soul."

Thus, social barriers to coffee consumption in Europe soon fell. The first European cafés appeared in the early 1700s. These cafés were male-only establishments that not only served coffee but also sold newspapers and cultural reviews. The British, however, preferred tea, possibly because of the influence of the British East India Company, which facilitated a strong tea trade with India. Russia also preferred tea over coffee, possibly because of that nation's ties with China.

Friedlieb Runge first extracted caffeine in 1819, and Emil Fischer identified caffeine's chemical properties in 1881. Other xanthene discoveries came later. Theobromine was first extracted in 1841, and Fischer discovered its chemical structures in 1882. Soon after this, Fischer discovered theophylline, another xanthine.

Stop & Check

1. In addition to coffee, teas, and soda, energy drinks are a major source of _____.

2. Coffee beans have been brewed since at least 1000 A.D. in _____.

1. caffeine 2. Arabia

Caffeine Absorption, Duration, and Interaction with Other Psychoactive Drugs

Caffeine is readily absorbed through oral administration, reaching peak blood levels after 30 minutes (Blanchard & Sawers, 1983). Peak plasma caffeine levels are reached after 2 hours. Caffeine penetrates both brain and placental blood barriers.

The liver metabolizes caffeine primarily by the enzyme CYP-1A2 and, to a lesser extent, by the enzyme CYP-2E1. Most individuals metabolize approximately 90 percent of caffeine, although the amount of caffeine metabolized depends on the activity of these enzymes. For example, individuals with reduced CYP-1A2 enzymatic activity metabolize less caffeine, subsequently prolonging caffeine's pharmacological effects.

Enzymatic involvement with other drugs also may alter the metabolism rate for caffeine. For example, many antidepressant drugs are CYP-1A2 enzyme inhibitors. Thus, individuals who take these antidepressant drugs metabolize less caffeine. Given that caffeine can produce anxiousness (see pharmacological effects below), this interaction effect may weaken an antidepressant drug's effectiveness if caffeine intake is not monitored (Fredholm & Arnaud, 2011). On the other hand, smoking enhances CYP-1A2 activity, resulting in increased metabolism of caffeine (Begas, Kouvaras, Tsakalof, Papakosta, & Asprodini, 2007; Joeres et al., 1988).

The metabolism of caffeine produces active metabolites that, like caffeine, belong to the xanthene class of drugs (**figure 7.18**). In particular, these metabolites include theophylline, theobromine, and another xanthine compound with related psychoactive effects, paraxanthine. Unlike theophylline and theobromine—which, as stated earlier, occur naturally in plants—paraxanthine only occurs when metabolically converted from caffeine. The relative distribution of metabolites produced from caffeine consists of 70–80 percent paraxanthine, 7–8 percent theophylline, and 7–8 percent theobromine (Begas et al., 2007).

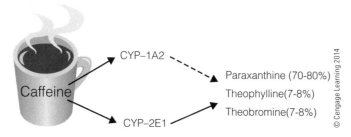

The liver enzymes CYP-1A2 and CYP-2E1 convert caffeine into xanthine metabolites, including theophylline and theobromine. The dashed arrow indicates that less conversion occurs from CYP-1A2 to theophylline and theobromine.

figure 7.18

The body primarily eliminates caffeine through the kidneys. The rate of elimination varies widely from approximately 3 to 10 hours (Blanchard & Sawers, 1983). The range in elimination rates may explain why some individuals have difficulty sleeping at night if they drink coffee in the afternoon, whereas other individuals have no difficulty sleeping at night after drinking coffee in the evening. Cigar or cigarette smoking doubles the rate of caffeine elimination because of the above-mentioned increased metabolic activity (Joeres et al., 1988). Because of this increased elimination rate, smokers may drink more coffee to maintain caffeine's effects.

Caffeine: Antagonist for Adenosine Receptors

Caffeine's primary mechanism of action is antagonism of adenosine A1 and A2 receptors. Adenosine is a neurochemical that has inhibitory effects on neurons throughout the central and peripheral nervous system. In particular, adenosine has inhibitory effects on cholinergic neurons in the cerebral cortex and on dopamine neurons in the basal ganglia. By blocking adenosine receptors, caffeine prevents the inhibitory influence of adenosine within these parts of the brain (Fisone, Borgkvist, & Usiello, 2004).

Stop & Check

1. How can enzymatic activity in the liver influence caffeine's effects?
2. Caffeine is an antagonist for _____ receptors.
3. In the peripheral nervous system, caffeine facilitates dopamine receptor activation by preventing adenosine from decreasing the binding _____ of dopamine receptors.

1. The behavioral effects of caffeine will persist longer in individuals who are slower metabolizers of caffeine. In a slow metabolizer, caffeine's effects may persist into nighttime and interfere with sleep. In addition, drugs may interact with CYP-1A2 enzymes, potentially slowing the metabolism of caffeine. 2. adenosine 3. affinity

Caffeine: Mild Psychostimulant Effects

Caffeine exhibits many physiological, behavioral and subjective effects, including increased heart rate, blood-vessel constriction, breathing rate, reduced appetite, attention, alertness, and positive mood. Caffeinated products usually are consumed for their fatigue-fighting properties and are commonly consumed by people in the morning after waking up (Brecher, 1972) and when attempting to stay alert at work (Ker, Edwards, Felix, Blackhall, & Roberts, 2010).

caffeinism Condition characterized by agitation, anxiety, insomnia, and negative mood as well as rapid heart rate and high blood pressure.

Consuming high doses of caffeine leads to **caffeinism,** a condition characterized by agitation, anxiety, insomnia, and negative mood as well as rapid heart rate and high blood pressure. This condition can occur at doses of 500 to 1,000 mg of caffeine, although tolerance to caffeine may require even higher doses before a person exhibits caffeinism.

Based on the high caffeine content and the presence of other stimulant chemicals, the risk of adverse effects for energy drinks may be greater than for coffee, tea, and other traditional caffeinated products. In addition to caffeine's adverse effects, energy-drink ingredients can cause hypertension, abdominal pain, and seizures when administered at high enough quantities. Moreover, the chemical ingredients in energy drinks can interact with psychoactive medications. For example, two ingredients found in many energy drinks—5-hydroxytryptophan and yohimbine—can strengthen the adverse effects of antidepressant drugs (Arria & O'Brien, 2011).

Tolerance and Dependence During Sustained Caffeine Use

Tolerance occurs with many of caffeine's acute subjective effects, including positive mood, improved alertness, and anxiousness, whereas tolerance may not occur with caffeine's physiological effects, including changes in cardiovascular activity and blood-vessel constriction (Hughes, Oliveto, Liguori, Carpenter, & Howard, 1998; Sigmon, Herning, Better, Cadet, & Griffiths, 2009). Daily consumption also leads to features of dependence, as demonstrated by the occurrence of withdrawal symptoms when first discontinuing use. In a recent survey, Juliano and colleagues (2012) recorded the prevalence of withdrawal symptoms among adult respondents who expressed interest in reducing or quitting caffeine use (**figure 7.19**). These individuals reported an average of 548 mg of caffeine per day, approximately double the normal daily average intake for U.S. adults (Frary et al., 2005). Nearly 90 percent experienced a headache, and approximately 85 percent experienced cravings for caffeine. Other common withdrawal symptoms included difficulty in concentrating, fatigue, irritability, and anxious or depressed mood. The study authors also noted that more than 40 percent of participants felt functionally impaired without caffeine.

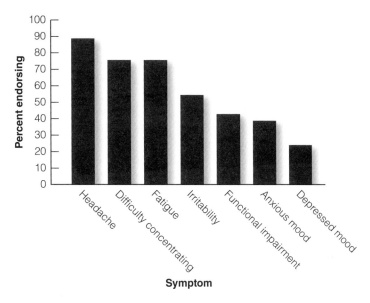

figure 7.19 Many study respondents who reported a desire to reduce and quit caffeine reported withdrawal symptoms. (Data from Juliano et al., 2012.)

Stop & Check

1. An increase in positive mood is one of the many _____ effects of caffeine.
2. Excessive doses of caffeine can produce _____, which is characterized by agitation, anxiety, insomnia, and other symptoms.
3. Other chemicals in energy drinks by interact with _____ drugs, causing an increase in adverse effects.
4. In the absence of caffeine, hostility, fatigue, and negative mood are indications of _____ on caffeine.

1. psychostimulant **2.** caffeinism **3.** antidepressant **4.** dependence

FROM ACTIONS TO EFFECTS
Why People Consume Caffeinated Products

Improvements in mood and alertness are important reasons for seeking caffeinated products such as coffee, tea, and other caffeinated beverages. Moreover, these and other products such as chocolate taste good, which adds to their appeal. Yet during the course of repeated use, a dependence on caffeine, as indicated by withdrawal symptoms, may facilitate consumption of caffeinated products.

Given the prevalence of caffeine use, most readers of this text probably consume caffeinated products on a daily basis. In particular, you may use coffee, a soft drink, or an energy drink to help wake up in the morning. If this describes you, then consider this: Is the tiredness you feel in the morning natural—or is it caffeine withdrawal?

Assuming that you do not consume a caffeinated product within several hours before bedtime, sleeping 6–8 hours may provide for a total caffeine abstinence period of about 10–12 hours. This abstinence period exceeds caffeine's elimination half-life, suggesting that your body's caffeine levels will be low or absent by morning. Indeed, many studies describe morning as an early withdrawal state for chronic caffeine users (James & Rogers, 2005). Thus, for most people, caffeine's ability to fight morning sleepiness may have a lot to do with removing caffeine's withdrawal symptoms.

Although the DSM-IV does not consider caffeine as generating a substance-dependence disorder, the American Psychiatric Association plans to include *caffeine use disorder* in the upcoming DSM-V, which is due out in 2013 (American Psychiatric Association, 2012). This decision supports clinical studies that have sought to adopt general features of substance dependence toward characterizing the problem use of caffeine (Bernstein, Carroll, Thuras, Cosgrove, & Roth, 2002; Griffiths & Chausmer, 2000). In an assessment of caffeine dependence, Bernstein and colleagues (2002) evaluated caffeine use among a sample of U.S. teenagers. Among the 36 teenagers assessed, 22.2 percent exhibited a sufficient number of symptoms to meet the DSM diagnostic criteria for substance dependence. The most commonly observed symptoms included tolerance, withdrawal symptoms, desire to quit or unsuccessful efforts to control use, and continued use despite physical or psychological problems. The total group of teenagers studied reported 244 mg of caffeine per day, with values ranging from as little as 49 mg to as much as 767 mg of caffeine per day. This study came out before the popularity of energy drinks, and currently no published studies exist on the prevalence of substance dependence among energy-drink users.

Although many researchers support applying substance-dependence criteria to caffeine use, others are unconvinced. In a review of scientific studies that assessed caffeine use, Satel (2006) concluded that caffeine does not meet substance-dependence criteria. Key points in Satel's study consist of weak or inconsistent reporting of withdrawal effects, a failure to demonstrate strong compulsions to use caffeine. Given that caffeine appearsneither irresistible nor a cause of social disruption, Satel argues that caffeine fails a common-sense test as an addictive substance. Thus, the inclusion of caffeine use disorder in the DSM-V is expected to be a point of debate among experts on addictive drugs.

▶ **CHAPTER** SUMMARY

This chapter has covered two widely used psychostimulant drugs: nicotine and caffeine. Tobacco products are the key source of nicotine.

Cigarette smoking is the most common form of nicotine administration, but other forms of tobacco such as smokeless tobacco and dissolvable tobacco are popular as well. Tobacco use has a long history, dating back to the ancient uses in the Americas and then reaching Europe after Columbus's expedition to the New World.

Nicotine is delivered to the body in tobacco tar and is absorbed through tissues in the lungs, throat, mouth, and skin. Inhalation is the most efficient route for nicotine delivery. Nicotine is metabolized in the liver, producing cotinine, an active metabolite.

Nicotine produces an increase in nucleus accumbens dopamine levels by activating nicotinic cholinergic receptors in the nucleus accumbens and ventral tegmental area. Continine also is an agonist for these receptors, but it has a much weaker affinity than nicotine. Nicotine increases sympathetic nervous activity and increases locomotor activity during repeated administration.Nicotine also improves attention. Subjectively, nicotine produces adverse effects on first usage, but tolerance to the effects soon subsides to reveal positive subjective effects. Most of nicotine's adverse effects are the result of tobacco, which contains many known cancer-causing agents. In addition to cancer, tobacco increases the risk of cardiovascular disease and lung disease. Because of desensitization at nicotinic receptors, upregulation of nicotinic receptors occurs during chronic use. Upregulation leads to a sensitized behavioral state.

Nicotine addiction accounts for chronic, habitual tobacco use. Quitting nicotine is difficult in part because of the association of tobacco use with everyday activities. Further, upregulation of nicotinic receptors facilitates a physiological dependent state, requiring sustained elevated nicotine levels for normal functioning.

Caffeine is a xanthine psychostimulant drug found naturally in kola nuts, cocoa tree nuts, and tea leaves. The most common caffeine sources include coffee, tea, and energy drinks. Caffeine-containing leaves and nuts were long used in China and Arabia, and teas and coffee were used throughout Europe beginning in the 1700s.

Caffeine is orally administered and is metabolized in the liver. Caffeine's elimination rate varies, depending on liver enzymatic activity. Caffeine's effects are derived through antagonism of adenosine receptors, not only producing an improvement in alertness, mood, and energy, but also a facilitation of dopamine's effects on the sympathetic nervous system. Excessive caffeine intake produces caffeinism, which is characterized by agitation, anxiety, and negative mood. Tolerance soon develops to caffeine's effects during chronic use, and continued caffeine use is mostly maintained by avoidance of caffeine-withdrawal symptoms.

KEY TERMS

Tar

Cotinine

Functional antagonism

Upregulation

Stroop test

Conditioned taste aversion

Nitrosamines

Emphysema

Nicotine abstinence syndrome

Chippers

Nicotine-replacement therapy

Varenicline (Chantix)

Caffeine

Caffeinated alcoholic beverages

Caffeinism

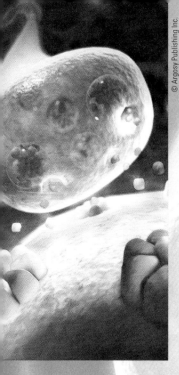

CHAPTER **8**

Alcohol

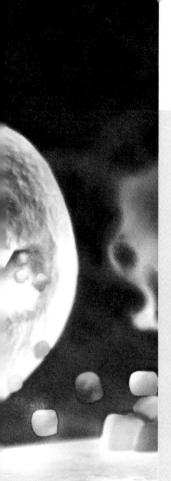

"Halfway to Concord" and "Taking Hippocrates' Grand Elixir"

We all know colloquial phrases for overdrinking alcohol such as "getting drunk." Such terms are nothing new, as evidenced by a letter, titled "The Drinker's Dictionary," which appeared in *The Pennsylvania Gazette* on January 13, 1737. As the author of that letter noted, drunkenness "bears no kind of similitude with any sort of virtue, from which it might possibly borrow a name; and is therefore reduc'd to the wretched necessity of being express'd by distant round-about phrases as they come to be well understood to signify plainly that A MAN IS DRUNK." The letter included a comprehensive alphabetized listing of terms and phrases for drunkenness. A couple of the terms are still used today such as *tipsy*. Most seem obscure, though, such as "He sees the bears," "loaded his cart," and "He's eat a toad & half for breakfast." Although this compilation provides an amusing perspective on terms and phrases for drunkenness in the 16th century, we also regard this letter as an interesting work in American history, one of the many early American writings by author Benjamin Franklin.

Alcohol: The Most Commonly Used Depressant Substance

ethyl alcohol An alcohol that functions as a central nervous system depressant.

Beverage alcohol consists of any drink containing **ethyl alcohol**, also known as ethanol, a central nervous system (CNS) depressant. We regularly contact other forms of alcohol, but these types are not safe to drink. One of these types is *isopropyl alcohol*, or *isopropanol*, which is commonly known as *rubbing alcohol*. Another type is *methyl alcohol*, or *methanol*. Methyl alcohol is an industrial solvent used in many products, including antifreeze. Methanol acts as a toxin for optic nerves; if consumed, it causes blindness.

Beverage alcohol is widely consumed across the world, second only to caffeine. According to the World Health Organization, approximately 2 billion people a year consume alcoholic beverages, and approximately 76 million individuals have an alcohol use disorder such as alcohol addiction. As shown in **figure 8.1**, alcohol consumption per capita varies between countries. The highest alcohol consumptions levels occur in Europe, the Russian Federation and former Soviet states, North America, South America, and Australia. The Middle East reports the lowest levels of alcohol consumption (World Health Organization, 2012).

World Alcohol Consumption

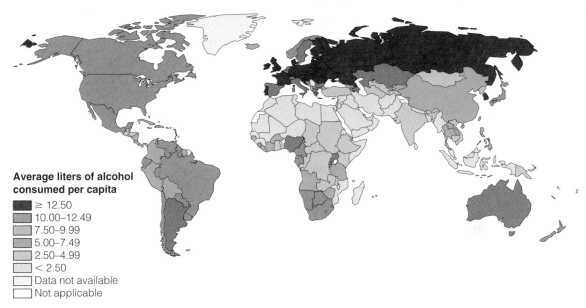

Average liters of alcohol consumed per capita

- ≥ 12.50
- 10.00–12.49
- 7.50–9.99
- 5.00–7.49
- 2.50–4.99
- < 2.50
- Data not available
- Not applicable

figure 8.1   Alcohol Consumption per Capita per Year in Liters of Pure Alcohol. (© World Health Organization (http://gamapserver.who. int/gho/static_graphs/gisah/Global_adult_percapita_consumption_2005.png) By permission.)

According to a 2009 survey conducted by the Substance Abuse and Mental Health Services Administration (SAMHSA), more than half of all U.S. individuals 12 and older have consumed alcohol within the last 30 days. The youngest of those surveyed, 12- to 17-year-olds, represent approximately 15 percent of alcohol consumers. Seven percent of those surveyed reported heavy drinking. In a separate study, 18 percent of U.S. individuals 12 and older had an alcohol use disorder (Hasin, Stinson, Ogburn, & Grant, 2007).

Alcohol Production Through Fermentation and Distillation

Beer, wine, and spirits serve as the primary sources of beverage alcohol. As presented in Chapter 7, certain energy drink mixes such as Four Loko also contain alcohol. Small amounts of alcohol are also found in vinegar and certain liquid medications such as cough syrups.

The amount of alcohol in a beverage is labeled in two ways: by percentage and by proof. **Percentage alcohol** refers to the number of grams of alcohol found in 100 milliliters of solution. For example, 50 g of alcohol in 100 ml of solution equates to 50 percent. The **proof of alcohol** is a numerical value that is double the actual percentage of alcohol. For example, a beverage with 50 percent alcohol is 100 proof.

percentage alcohol
Number of grams of alcohol found in 100 milliliters of solution.

proof of alcohol
Numerical value that is double the percentage of alcohol.

fermentation Alcohol production using yeast cells and some type of starch such as grains or fruit.

Recreational alcoholic beverages vary in percent alcohol content, depending on whether brewers used a fermentation method or a distillation method. **Fermentation** is a process of alcohol production using yeast cells and some type of starch such as grain or fruit. During fermentation, yeast interacts with sugars from starches, creating alcohol. The longer that yeasts have to metabolize these sugars, the greater the percentage of alcohol produced. The approximate upper limit for alcohol production using fermentation is 15 percent. Higher alcohol percentages kill yeast cells, causing fermentation to end.

Most beers and wines contain less than 15 percent alcohol. Beer is made by exposing yeast cells to a certain type of starch such as malted barely, wheat, or rice. During the fermentation process, brewers add other ingredients such as hops and fruit to further promote fermentation and provide flavoring. Most commercial domestic beers are made from barley and hops and contain about 5 percent alcohol. Some countries are known for unique varieties of beer. Belgium, for example, produces fruitier beers, and Japan produces rice beers.

Wine is made from fermented fruit. Most wine makers use grapes, which provide a sugar source, along with certain acids, enzymes, and nutrients during the fermentation process. Beyond grapes, some winemakers use other fruits such as strawberries or cherries. Wines made from fruits other than grapes are called *fruit wines*. In general, wines contain approximately 12–15 percent alcohol.

distilled alcoholic beverages (spirits) Alcoholic beverages produced through distillation; have a higher alcohol content than beer and wine.

Distilled alcoholic beverages, or **spirits**, are produced through distillation and have a higher alcohol content than beers and wines. Distillation is a method that separates alcohol from a fermented mixture. During this process, distillers heat a fermented mixture until it exceeds alcohol's boiling point. At this boiling point, alcohol evaporates; the alcohol vapors are routed through tubes into a cooler compartment where the alcohol returns to a liquid form, making a highly concentrated alcoholic solution.

Distilled alcoholic beverages are referred to as *liquors* or *spirits*. These alcoholic beverages contain at least 20 percent alcohol and come in many different varieties such as brandy, gin, rum, tequila, vodka, and whiskey. The different flavors born from distillation depend on the starch used in fermentation, the filtration methods used to purify the alcohol collected during distillation, and the method of storage. In other words, along with the distilled alcohol, other chemicals collect in the fermented brew, and the desired flavor in part depends on the filtration of these chemicals from the distilled solution and the type of container in which the end product is aged or stored.

One of the purest distilled spirits is a grain-based alcohol marketed as Everclear. Everclear is highly filtered so that it contains a high concentration of alcohol with few other chemicals. The varieties of Everclear vary from 75 percent to 95 percent alcohol. The highest concentration version is illegal to sell in some U.S. states. Vodka consists of another highly filtered distilled spirit that may be based on grains or other starch sources. Although many vodkas contain around 50 percent alcohol, other varieties may contain as much as

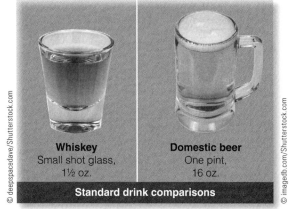

© deepspacedave/Shutterstock.com

Whiskey
Small shot glass,
1½ oz.

Domestic beer
One pint,
16 oz.

© imagedb.com/Shutterstock.com

Standard drink comparisons

figure **8.2**   Standard Drink Comparisons Between Whiskey and Domestic Beer.

95 percent. Brandy, whiskey, and rum typically contain 40–60 percent alcohol and vary in bitterness and flavor.

Home distillation is illegal in most U.S. states. These methods produce a beverage often referred to as *moonshine*. Home-distillation methods, however, are notorious for dangerous impurities, including methanol.

Given the enormous variety of alcohol concentrations among beverages, health officials compare beverages according to standard drink units. A **standard drink** contains 14 grams of 100-percent alcohol, which is equivalent to about 2/3 fluid ounce. To put this in perspective, a small shot glass holds about 1½ fluid ounces. A standard drink equivalent of 190-proof Everclear (95 percent alcohol) fills about half of a small shot glass. A standard drink equivalent of whisky is approximately 1½ fluid ounces and fills a small shot glass. For a typical domestic beer, the standard drink equivalent consists of 16 ounces or one pint (National Institute on Alcohol Abuse and Alcoholism, 2012) (**figure 8.2**).

standard drink Drink that contains 14 grams of 100-percent alcohol; equivalent to about 2/3 fluid ounce.

Stop & Check

1. Of the many types of alcohol, which is safe to drink (in moderation)?
2. If an alcoholic drink is 40 percent alcohol, what is the proof?
3. Although fermentation can produce as much as 15 percent alcohol, higher concentrations can be achieved using _____.
4. Alcoholic beverages are compared for alcohol content by referring to _____ drinks, which are equivalent to 14 grams of 100-percent alcohol.

1. Ethyl alcohol, also known as *ethanol* **2.** The proof of an alcoholic beverage is double the percentage of alcohol. A 40-percent alcoholic drink is 80 proof. **3.** distillation **4.** standard

The History of Alcohol Consumption

Scholars hypothesize that early neolithic peoples raised and fermented grapes as early as 6000 B.C. The recorded history of alcohol dates to Sumerian writings in 3200 B.C. During this period, early taverns in Samaria and Egypt sold alcohol, and traders transported alcohol throughout the known world.

Both wine and beers were described during this age. Wine was a limited commodity and considered a drink of luxury for consumption by ruling figures. Sumerian writings describe a beer made from barley. Egyptian writings describe many types of beers made from barley as well as a beer called *hek* made from honey. In both Samaria and Egypt, beer making was common in households, and the recreational use of beer was a normal part of everyday life.

Opposition to alcohol also existed during this time. In 2000 B.C., an Egyptian priest wrote a letter to one of his pupils, stating "I forbid thee to go to the taverns . . . thou are degraded like the beasts." The Code of Hammurabi, written around 1750 B.C., regulated drinking establishments called "wine shops" to prevent riotous gatherings.

Aside from recreational purposes, the Sumerians also used alcohol as a vehicle for many medicines. Around 800 B.C., Greeks used wine in religious ceremonies and to treat pain. Moderate drinking occurred soon after Rome's founding around 750 B.C. However, rampant drinking occurred around 200 B.C. and was a hallmark of Roman culture through its fall around 200 A.D. By this time, alcohol consumption was a normal part of European life.

Distilled alcohol arrived around 1250 A.D., mostly as an expensive medicine, and its lauded benefits led to the term *aqua vitae*, the water of life. The sense of youth, vitality, and physical well-being led to describing distilled alcohol as a *spirit*. Brandy was the primary spirit consumed until around the late 1400s, when a Scottish publication described a recipe for whiskey made from malted barley rather than wine. In 1550, a publication in Holland described the first recipe for gin. Rum was popular in colonial America because of its low production cost and the triangle trade that brought inexpensive sugar cane to the colonies.

Many alcohol-related adages have their origins in this period. In England, public houses—*pubs*—served alcoholic drinks in pints and quarts. The oldest pub in English history is Ye Olde Fighting Cocks, which was established sometime in the 12th century and still operates today. The phrase "Mind your p's and q's," meaning "Be careful of your behavior," was derived from the practice of publicans (pubkeepers) who recorded the number drinks in pints or quarts served to each customer. A publican "minded his p's and q's" if he didn't lose money, and a customer "minded his p's and q's" if he did not get drunk (Austin, 1985; Carson-Dewitt, 2003).

In the early 1800s, a powerful alcohol prohibition movement began in the United States. Many groups contributed to this movement including the American Temperance Union and the Washingtonians. Joining them were Protestants, Catholics, and other religious organizations.

These political forces achieved many local and state bans on alcohol sales and consumption. After overcoming a pause in these efforts during the

18th Amendment
Amendment to U.S. Constitution that banned the sale and distribution of alcohol.

American Civil War, they eventually were influential enough to help pass the National Prohibition Act, which became the **18th Amendment** to the U.S. Constitution in 1920. This amendment did not ban alcohol consumption, but it did ban the sale and distribution of alcohol. The 18th Amendment failed to eliminate alcohol use. In many communities, the ban on sale of alcohol was virtually ignored, and *bootleggers*, those that illegally transported alcohol in the United States, were often regarded as celebrities. In 1933, the 21st Amendment repealed the 18th Amendment. Still, although the federal government no longer prohibits the sale of alcohol, some towns and counties remain "dry" to this day. One of the most famous dry counties is Moore County, Tennessee—ironically, the home of Jack Daniel's distillery, a well-known whiskey producer (Carson-Dewitt, 2003; Hall, 2010).

Stop & Check

1. The _____ provided the first written evidence of alcoholic beverages.
2. Other than recreational use, what were the first spirits used for?
3. Which U.S. constitutional amendment prohibited the sale and distribution of alcohol?

1. Sumerians 2. Dating back to 1250 A.D., the first spirits were used as medicines. 3. The 18th Amendment

Pharmacokinetic Factors and Alcohol's Effects

Alcohol is highly soluble in water and fat, allowing for easy absorption in tissue. Users consume alcohol orally, and after ingestion alcohol absorbs into the bloodstream through the gastrointestinal tract. Most alcohol absorbs through the upper intestine because of its large surface area. In the intestine, alcohol also impairs thiamine transporter function, also known as Vitamin B1, reducing thiamine availability for critical cellular functions in the body (Subramanya, Subramanian, & Said, 2010).

blood alcohol concentration (BAC)
Number of grams of alcohol in a 100-ml volume of blood.

We measure the amount of alcohol in the body as a **blood alcohol concentration (BAC)**. A BAC calculation indicates the number of grams of alcohol in a 100-ml volume of blood. For example, 1 gram of alcohol in 100 ml of blood equates to a BAC of 1.0. This is an extremely high and fatal concentration of alcohol. A drink or two may only produce a BAC of 0.04. The maximum BAC from an alcoholic drink occurs after approximately 45 minutes (Dubowski, 1985).

alcohol dehydrogenase
Enzyme that metabolizes alcohol.

acetaldehyde Metabolite produced from enzymatic conversion of alcohol with alcohol dehydrogenase.

Enzymes in the stomach, liver, and other parts of the body metabolize alcohol. The enzyme **alcohol dehydrogenase** metabolizes 95 percent of alcohol. It converts it to **acetaldehyde**, a chemical that produces noxious effects (Zimatkin, Liopo, & Deitrich, 1998). In addition to alcohol dehydrogenase, other metabolic processes in tissues throughout the body, including the brain,

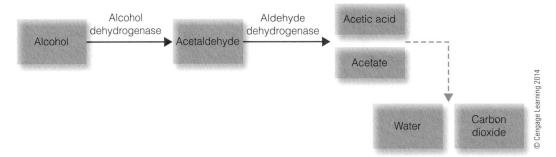

© Cengage Learning 2014

figure **8.3**   The metabolic process for alcohol consists of conversion to acetaldehyde and then conversion of acetaldehyde to acetic and acetate. Other metabolic process cause acetic acid and acetate to convert to water and carbon dioxide.

convert alcohol to acetalhyde. Acetaldehyde converts to acetic acid and acetate by different forms of the enzyme aldehyde dehydrogenase (Chinnawirotpisan et al., 2003). Another process converts acetic acid and acetate to carbon dioxide and water (**figure 8.3**).

Both the stomach and liver contain alcohol dehydrogenase enzymes. Little alcohol metabolism takes place in an empty stomach because alcohol is quickly digested to the intestines in the absence of food. However, on a full stomach, alcohol remains in the stomach longer, giving alcohol greater exposures to alcohol dehydrogenase enzymes. In this case, some of the alcohol metabolizes before reaching the intestines for absorption. After absorption, alcohol dehydrogenase enzymes in the liver metabolize most of the remaining alcohol.

As described in Chapter 4, the rate of alcohol elimination follows zero-order kinetics. Most individuals eliminate approximately 10 to 14 mL, or about ½ ounce, of 100-percent alcohol per hour. The general concept for alcohol elimination indicates that this elimination rate remains the same regardless of the amount of alcohol consumed. However, a truer picture of alcohol elimination presents a mix of zero-order and first-order kinetics, depending on the dose of alcohol ingested and the amount of enzymes available for metabolizing alcohol. Zero-order kinetics apply to alcohol's elimination rate until all available enzymes for metabolizing alcohol become saturated or completely occupied. This can occur from attaining and maintaining high BACs. After saturating alcohol metabolic enzymes, the elimination rate of alcohol approximates reductions in half-lives, which resembles first-order kinetics (Dubowski, 1985).

REVIEW! Zero-order kinetics refers to drug-elimination rates that do not occur in half-lives. Chapter 4 (pg. 110).

Although 95 percent of alcohol is metabolized, the body eliminates the remaining 5 percent percent of alcohol, unchanged, from the lungs. The ratio of alcohol concentration in expelled air to blood is 1:2,300 (Dubowski, 1985). Breathalyzer tests use this ratio to accurately determine the amount of alcohol in blood. The amounts of alcohol analyzed are expressed as BAC. For example, saying someone "blew a 0.11" means that the individual had a

BAC of 0.11. Researchers correlate blood alcohol's pharmacological effects, and law enforcement uses BACs to determine if someone is legally intoxicated.

Stop & Check

1. The percentage of alcohol in blood is referred to as the _____.
2. The enzyme alcohol dehydrogenase converts alcohol to _____.
3. Because a set rate of 10 to 14 ml of alcohol are eliminated per hour, alcohol is eliminated following _____ kinetics.

1. blood alcohol concentration **2.** acetaldehyde **3.** zero-order

Alcohol and Central Nervous System Functioning

The pharmacological actions of alcohol in the body involve many different neurotransmitter systems and depend on the amount of alcohol consumed. These pharmacological actions involve GABA, glutamate, endogenous opioid, dopamine, serotonin, and endocannabinoid systems.

Alcohol and GABA$_A$ Receptors

Alcohol acts directly on ionotropic GABA$_A$ receptors, which produce inhibitory effects on neurons (Mihic et al., 1997). When GABA activates GABA$_A$ receptors, the associated channels open and cause negatively charged chloride ions to enter the neuron. Negatively charged ions in turn hyperpolarize the neuron, inhibiting the neuron's activity.

Alcohol binds to and functions as a positive modulator for GABA$_A$ receptors (Ticku, Burch, & Davis, 1983). Positive modulation of GABA$_A$ receptors increases the length of receptor activation and increases the flow of chloride ions into the neuron. These two actions enhance the inhibitory effects of GABA$_A$ receptors.

REVIEW! Positive modulators facilitate neurotransmitter effects at a receptor. Chapter 4 (pg. 120).

The location of GABA$_A$ receptors determines the effects of alcohol. Although many brain structures contain GABA$_A$ receptors, those most relevant to alcohol's CNS depressing effects include the cerebral cortex, hippocampus, and thalamus. These three structures are important for information processing, memory, and other cognitive activities.

GABA$_A$ receptors also mediate alcohol's reinforcing effects (**figure 8.4**). First, alcohol facilitates GABA$_A$ receptor activation in the nucleus accumbens, a known receptor action that produces reinforcing effects. Second, alcohol activates GABA$_A$ receptors located on GABA neurons in the ventral tegmental area. The activation of these receptors causes reduced GABA release, in turn decreasing the inhibition of dopamine neurons (Xiao, Zhou, Li, & Ye, 2007). Reduced inhibition of dopamine neurons results in enhanced dopamine release in the nucleus accumbens, a known rewarding action (Yoshimoto, McBride, Lumeng, & Li, 1992).

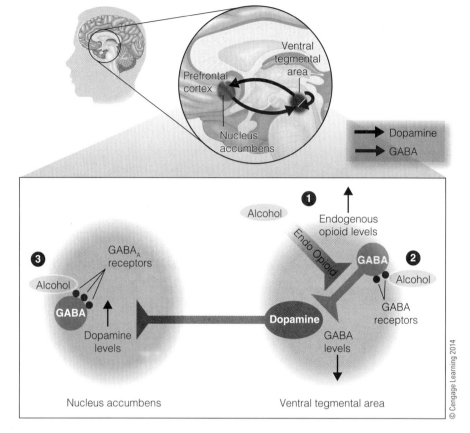

Alcohol produces reinforcing effects through GABA neurotransmission in three ways:
(1) Alcohol enhances endogenous opioid release (β-endorphin), which inhibits GABA neuron
activity. (2) Alcohol enhances the inhibitory effects of GABA$_A$ receptors on ventral tegmental
GABA neurons. These two mechanisms prevent GABA's inhibition of dopamine neurons and
cause increased nucleus accumbens dopamine release. (3) Alcohol also produces reinforcing
effect by facilitating GABA$_A$ inhibition of GABA neurons in the nucleus accumbens.

figure 8.4

In addition to acting on GABA$_A$ receptors in the ventral tegmental
area, alcohol indirectly inhibits GABA neurons by increasing levels of the
endogenous opioid β-endorphin (Schulz, Wüster, Duka, & Herz, 1980). In
the ventral tegmental area, β-endorphin activates inhibitory opioid receptors
on these GABA neurons, further contributing to diminished GABA release
(Xiao & Ye, 2008).

Chronic administration of alcohol causes several changes in alcohol's
effects on GABA neurons. First, chronic administration reduces the number
of GABA$_A$ receptors. Second, GABA$_A$ receptors become less affected by
alcohol (Montpied et al., 1991). Third, alcohol produces a lower increase
in β-endorphin levels, resulting in less inhibition of GABA neurons (Schulz
et al., 1980).

Glutamate NMDA* Receptors and Alcohol's Pharmacological Effects

Alcohol also produces depressant effects by inhibiting excitatory glutamate NMDA receptors. NMDA receptors produce excitatory effects and facilitate learning and memory processes. Like GABA$_A$ receptors, alcohol binds noncompetitively to NMDA receptors, but not at a clearly identified site (Krystal, Petrakis, Mason, Trevisan, & D'Souza, 2003). After binding to the receptor, alcohol inhibits ion passage through the NMDA receptor channel.

Chronic alcohol administration increases the number of NMDA receptors. During withdrawal from alcohol, the enhanced levels of NMDA receptors allow glutamate to exhibit greater excitatory effects on neurons. These greater excitatory effects increase the risk of seizures, a serious alcohol withdrawal symptom (Grant, Valverius, Hudspith, & Tabakoff, 1990; Hillbom, Pieninkeroinen, & Leone, 2003).

Alcohol: Inhibited Neurotransmission

Voltage-gated calcium channels facilitate neurotransmitter release and many other functions, including gene expression and enzyme regulation. Not only does the nervous system contain voltage-gated calcium channels, but also so does the heart, smooth muscle, kidneys, and pancreas. There are six known types of voltage-gated calcium channels; these are classified by the letters L, N, P, Q, R, and T. Among these, alcohol inhibits the L-type calcium channel.

Because of the widespread expression of L-type calcium channels in the brain, alcohol's inhibitory actions through these channels cause generalized effects. Overall, acute administration of alcohol reduces neurotransmitter release from axon terminals containing these channels. However, alcohol inhibition of L-type calcium channels specifically inhibits vasopressin release. By inhibiting vasopressin levels, alcohol causes an increase in urination. In addition, diminished vasopressin activity impairs cognition, disrupts circadian rhythm, lowers blood pressure, and enhances aggression (Walter & Messing, 1999).

REVIEW! Vasopressin is an antidiuretic hormone, meaning that it causes the kidneys to absorb more water from the bloodstream. Chapter 3 (pg. 94).

Alcohol and Serotonin Receptors

In addition to the other mechanisms described so far, alcohol also increases serotonin concentrations in the nucleus accumbens (Yoshimoto et al., 1992). As reviewed in Chapter 6, increased serotonin concentrations in the nucleus accumbens contribute to the reinforcing effects of cocaine and amphetamine, suggesting that increased serotonin levels may contribute to alcohol's reinforcing effects as well. Alcohol also appears to exhibit specific actions on serotonin ionotropic 5-HT$_3$ receptors and metabotropic 5-HT$_{2A}$ receptors.

---

*N-methyl-D-aspartate

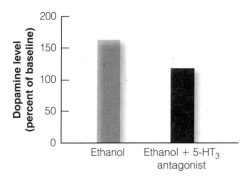

figure 8.5 The serotonin-3 receptor antagonist ICS 205-930 prevented alcohol from increasing nucleus accumbens dopamine levels in rats. (Campbell & McBride, 1995. By permission.)

REVIEW! An ionotropic receptor contains an ion channel, and a metabotropic receptor uses a G-protein to carry out intracellular effects Chapter 3 (pg. 76).

Alcohol causes the activation of $5HT_3$ receptors through either of two ways. First, alcohol enhances serotonin levels, leading to greater activation of $5HT_3$ receptors. In the nucleus accumbens, for example, alcohol-induced increases in serotonin levels causes the activation of $5\text{-}HT_3$ receptors, as well as any other serotonin receptors in the vicinity. Second, alcohol increases the flow of positively charged ions through the $5\text{-}HT_3$ ion channel (Machu & Harris, 1994).

The involvement of $5HT_3$ receptors in alcohol-induced dopamine release can be assessed pharmacologically. Campbell and McBride (1995) used a microdialysis procedure in rats to assess alcohol administration with a $5\text{-}HT_3$ receptor antagonist on dopamine release in the nucleus accumbens (**figure 8.5**). In rats treated only with alcohol, dopamine levels significantly increased. Yet in rats administered the $5HT_3$ receptor antagonist ICS 205-930 into the nucleus accumbens, alcohol failed to increase dopamine levels (Ding et al., 2011). These findings suggest that $5\text{-}HT_3$ may be important for alcohol's ability to increase dopamine concentration in the nucleus accumbens.

In addition to $5\text{-}HT_3$ receptors, $5\text{-}HT_{2A}$ receptors in the ventral tegmental area also contribute to alcohol effects on nucleus accumbens dopamine levels. As demonstrated in a study by Ding and colleagues (2009), the direct infusion of a $5\text{-}HT_{2A}$ receptor antagonist into the ventral tegmental area reduced self-administration of alcohol in rats. The researchers attributed reduced self-administration to diminished dopamine release in the nucleus accumbens.

Alcohol and the Endocannabinoid System

The endocannabinoid system may contribute to alcohol's reinforcing and other pharmacological effects. These interactions may depend partly on the role of the cannabinoid CB_1 receptor, which, as described in Chapter 11, influences the activity of dopamine neurons within the reward circuit. In a microdialysis study by Cohen and colleagues (2002), administration of the CB_1 receptor antagonist rimonabant prevented alcohol from increasing dopamine levels in the nucleus accumbens of rats. In another microdialysis study, alcohol failed to increase nucleus accumbens dopamine levels in CB_1 receptor knock-out mice (Hungund, Szakall, Adam, Basavarajappa, & Vadasz, 2003).

Stop & Check

1. Alcohol functions as a positive modulator for _____ receptors.
2. Alcohol inhibits ion passage through glutamate _____ receptors.
3. Alcohol's actions on L-type calcium channels have specific effects on the hormone _____.
4. Alcohol acts on the serotonin receptors 5-HT$_{2A}$ and _____.

1. GABA$_A$, **2.** NMDA **3.** vasopressin **4.** 5-HT$_3$

Pharmacological Effects of Alcohol

Alcohol's pharmacological effects vary, depending on alcohol's concentration in the body. In general, higher concentrations yield depressant effects on physiological and psychological functions, whereas lower concentrations yield excitatory effects for certain physiological and psychological functions. In addition, some of alcohol's effects change during chronic usage.

Types of Drinking and Number of Drinks Consumed

Health officials apply certain terms to describe amounts of alcohol consumed. Studies use these terms to relate alcohol consumption to pharmacological effects. Moderate drinking consists of about two standard drinks per day for men and one standard drink per day for women (**table 8.1**). By this definition, light drinking is less than these amounts. Heavy drinking consists of more than four drinks per day for men and three drinks per day for women (Dufour, 1999). Further, heavy drinking can also consist of at least 14 drinks per week for men and 7 drinks per week for women.

table **8.1**

Different Types of Drinking	
Type of drinking	**Standard drinks consumed**
Light drinking	Less than 2 drinks per day for men; less than 1 drink per day for women
Moderate drinking	Two drinks per day for men; one drink per day for women
Heavy drinking	At least 4 drinks per day for men; at least 3 drinks per day for women
Binge drinking	Drinking occurs in short time period consisting of at least 5 drinks per day for men and at least 4 drinks per day for women.
Extreme drinking	Two or three times the number of drinks considered as binge drinking

© Cengage Learning 2014

Heavy drinking during a short period of time is given a unique term: **binge drinking**. It consists of drinking at least five standard drinks for men and four standard drinks for women during one occasion. This definition is also called the "5/4 rule," referring to the drink definitions for men and women, respectively (Wechsler et al., 2002). These sessions can achieve BACs of 0.08 and higher.

Extreme drinking consists of consuming two to three times more alcohol than in binge drinking. It is not uncommon among young adults. In a survey conducted among freshman after their first two weeks in college, White and colleagues (2006) found that nearly 30 percent of men and 10 percent of women had already engaged in extreme drinking.

Extreme drinking is especially prominent during 21st birthday celebrations in the United States. According to surveys conducted by Rutledge and colleagues (2008), most individuals at their 21st birthday reported binge drinking. Approximately 12 percent engaged in a type of extreme drinking called "21 for 21," meaning drinking 21 drinks on their 21st birthday. The involvement in 21 for 21 was similar between men and women in this survey. The estimated BAC levels among these drinkers exceeded 0.26.

Acute Alcohol Consumption and Cardiovascular and Respiratory Functioning

Light to moderate alcohol consumption primarily affects the respiratory and cardiovascular systems. Heavy drinking causes a variety of adverse physiological effects, as discussed later in this chapter. Alcohol's respiratory effects depend on the concentration level. At lower alcohol concentrations, such as a BAC around 0.03, alcohol increases respiration. Beyond these concentrations, alcohol inhibits respiration, and this inhibition increases as the alcohol concentration increases. Respiratory inhibition is a key factor in alcohol poisoning.

Alcohol produces concentration-related effects on the cardiovascular system. Alcohol causes blood vessels to dilate, improving blood flow throughout the body. By increasing blood flow in the skin and extremities, alcohol provides feelings of warmth and contributes to a false but common belief that alcohol warms the body. In truth, the diversion of blood flow to the skin and extremities diminishes blood flow to core body organs. This actually makes the body colder (Oscar-Berman & Marinković, 2007).

Alcohol's cardiovascular effects at low alcohol concentrations are not only safe but also can promote cardiovascular health. Some of these health benefits include a reduced risk of ischemia, stroke, and vascular-related dementias. The health benefits of daily low alcohol use result from four primary effects (see **table 8.2**).

REVIEW! Ischemia is a reduced blood supply, and it often results from constricted blood vessels Chapter 2 (pg. 49).

First, chronic light daily alcohol use increases high-density lipoprotein (HDL) levels, also referred to as "good cholesterol." HDLs reduce other cholesterols in the circulatory system.

Second, chronic light daily use of alcohol reduces pro-inflammatory cellular signaling that contributes to the thickening of artery walls.

table **8.2**

Effects of Light and Heavy Alcohol Consumption on Cardiovascular Health	
Light chronic consumption (1–2 drinks per day)	**Heavy chronic consumption (several drinks per day)**
Decreased risk of ischemia	Increased risk of ischemia
Decreased risk of heart disorders	Increased risk of heart disorders
Decreased risk of heart attack	Increased risk of heart attack
Decreased risk of stroke	Increased risk of stroke

© Cengage Learning 2014

Third, acute alcohol administration disrupts blood platelets from bonding together to form clots, the immediate cause of heart attacks and stroke.

Fourth, acute alcohol administration causes blood clots to separate by causing the activation of *plasmin*, the enzyme responsible for degrading the bonding components between platelets in blood clots (Zakhari, 1997).

Although we find that light alcohol consumption provides health benefits for cardiovascular functioning, individuals with certain genetic traits may experience harm to the cardiovascular system from light or moderate consumption. For example, individuals with a polymorphism for the alcohol dehydrogenase type 3 enzyme may exhibit a reduced rate of alcohol metabolism and subsequently have an increased risk of heart attack associated with moderate alcohol consumption (Hines et al., 2001).

Alcohol's Depressive Effects on Behavior and Cognitive Functioning

Alcohol's depressant effects affect behavior and cognitive processing. Beginning at low BACs, alcohol impairs balance and equilibrium (**figure 8.6**). Impaired equilibrium occurs at BACs as low as 0.05 (Liguori, D'Agostino, Dworkin, Edwards, & Robinson, 1999). This BAC falls below the legal limit for U.S. states, but it serves as the legal driving limit for many European countries. During field sobriety testing, which is conducted when a police officer suspects an individual is driving intoxicated, equilibrium is assessed by having an individual walk on a straight line, walk and then turn, or attempt to balance on one leg.

disinhibition
Weakening of behavioral control

Alcohol use also causes poor judgment as a result of **disinhibition**, a weakening of behavioral control that manifests as poor risk assessment, engagement in dangerous behavior, and impulsivity. Disinhibition with alcohol use can cause socially unconventional behavior such as loud outbursts or aggressive behavior (Oscar-Berman & Marinković, 2007).

impulsivity Decision making without reflecting adequately on the consequences of those decisions

A specific disinhibition trait in alcohol use is **impulsivity,** or decision making without reflecting adequately on the consequences of those decisions. Researchers use delay-discounting designs to measure impulsivity. These procedures present a participant with a choice between an immediate small reward or a delayed larger reward. Both acutely alcohol-treated participants and former alcohol-addicted participants exhibit impulsivity deficits in such tasks (Bjork, Hommer, Grant, & Danube, 2004).

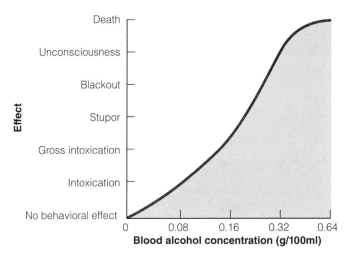

figure **8.6** Relationship between blood alcohol concentration (BAC, *x*-axis) and pharmacological effects. The legal limit for operating a motor vehicle in most states is 0.08. (Adapted from the Center for Disease Control (2011) and Loyola Marymount University (2006).)

alcohol priming
Tendency of users to develop an urge to consume more alcohol after have one or two drinks of alcohol.

After consuming one or two drinks of alcohol, users develop an urge to consume more alcohol, a phenomenon described as **alcohol priming**. The phenomenon may be partly the result of alcohol's ability to disinhibit behavior and to increase impulsive decision making. Priming occurs in nonaddicted alcohol users, irrespective of drinking patterns, as shown in **figure 8.7** (Rose & Grunsell, 2008).

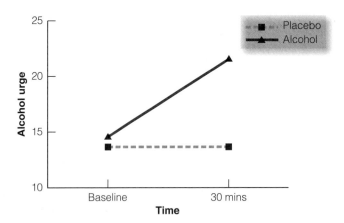

figure **8.7** An urge to consume more alcohol occurred 30 minutes after consuming an alcoholic drink, as shown by the triangles. Baseline represents the urge to drink before consuming the first alcoholic drink. The *y*-axis represents the level of urge to consume alcohol. (Rose, A. K., & Grunsell, L. (2008). The Subjective, Rather Than the Disinhibiting, Effects of Alcohol Are Related to Binge Drinking. *Alcoholism: Clinical and Experimental Research*, 32(6), 1096–1104. doi: 10.1111/j.1530–0277.2008.00672.x. Reproduced with permission of John Wiley & Sons Ltd.)

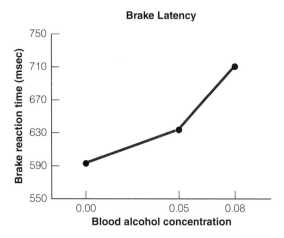

Brake Latency

BACs as low as 0.05, shown on the *x*-axis, significantly impair brake reaction time (*y*-axis) in a driving simulator. (Liguori, A., D'Agostino, R. B., Dworkin, S. I., Edwards, D., & Robinson, J. H. (1999). Alcohol Effects on Mood, Equilibrium, and Simulated Driving. *Alcoholism: Clinical and Experimental Research*, 23(5), 815–821. doi: 10.1111/j.1530-0277.1999.tb04188.x. Reproduced with permission of John Wiley & Sons Ltd.)

figure 8.8

Alcohol markedly reduces reaction time. These slower reaction times can occur at relatively low BACs and are especially dangerous when driving. Researchers use simulators to measures alcohol's effects on driving. In a study conducted by Liguori and colleagues (1999), placebo- and alcohol-treated participants operated a simulator to drive on a straight road at 50 miles per hour. During the simulation, yellow barricades appeared a random intervals, requiring participants to immediately press on the brake pedal. The reaction time consisted of the time between the presentation of the barricade and the pressing of the brake pedal.

Figure 8.8 shows the results from this driving simulator study. Compared to placebo-treated participants, alcohol-treated participants reacted slower to the yellow barricades. These reaction deficits occurred for BACs as low as 0.05, and they were especially pronounced at a 0.08 BAC, a legal limit for operating motor vehicles in most states.

Reductions in reaction time extend to prenatally exposed infants as well. Jacobson and colleagues (1994) tested the reaction time of infants from mothers who reportedly consumed small amounts of alcohol throughout their pregnancy. None of the infants was diagnosed with fetal alcohol syndrome. Despite this, these infants exhibited significantly reduced reaction times compared to those whose mothers did not consume alcohol during pregnancy.

divided attention
Sustained attention on a stimulus despite the presence of distracters.

In addition to reaction time, alcohol significantly impairs **divided attention**, or sustaining attention on a stimulus despite the presence of distracters. Schulte and colleagues (2001) demonstrated alcohol-associated deficits in divided attention. Using the grid shown in **figure 8.9**, the researchers asked individuals to identify square patterns formed by X's in a rapid series of differently patterned screens. On this task, alcohol-treated participants who had a BAC of 0.05 or higher produced more errors than placebo-treated patients.

One type of divided attention task requires participants to identify square patterns with X's in an array such as this. Each array is shown only briefly. (With kind permission from Springer Science+Business Media: Schulte, T., Müller-Oehring, E. M., Strasburger, H., Warzel, H., & Sabel, B. A. (2001). Acute effects of alcohol on divided and covert attention in men. *Psychopharmacology*, 154(1), 61–69. doi: 10.1007/s002130000603, Fig 1.)

figure **8.9**

Divided attention deficits, in particular, may help explain some of the characteristics of alcohol-related vehicle crashes. Johnston (1982) suggested that most crashes occur during obstructed road conditions such as maneuvering a vehicle around a tight curve. Such conditions rely on focused divided attention in order to successfully steer the vehicle amid a variety of other road conditions.

However, alcohol does not affect all types of attention equally. Light to moderate alcohol consumption does not affect *vigilance*, or the state of readiness for detecting and responding to unpredictable events. Nor does light to moderate alcohol consumption disrupt sustained attention, which is demonstrated by having someone focus intently on a single stimulus.

Alcohol produces deficits in memory, particularly at BACs of approximately 0.08 and higher. In a study of human volunteers with BACs of 0.04 and 0.08, those with BACs of 0.08 exhibited significant deficits in *episodic memory*, the conscious memory of a personally experienced event, and *semantic memory*, the memory of verbal or written information (Kleykamp, Griffiths, & Mintzer, 2010). However, BACs of 0.08 do not significantly affect working memory unless the working memory task is especially difficult (Grattan-Miscio & Vogel-Sprott, 2005; Gundersen, Specht, Grüner, Ersland, & Hugdahl, 2008; Kleykamp et al., 2010). Deficits in memory appear worse during inclining BACs than during declining BACs (Schweizer & Vogel-Sprott, 2008).

Alcohol and Positive Subjective Effects

After consuming alcohol, individuals usually report an improvement in mood. These effects increase as alcohol concentrations increase. Human study participants can detect clear drug effects at BACs of 0.05: a high and mild dizziness (Liguori et al., 1999). Alcohol users with BACs of 0.08 and higher report feelings of intense well-being.

Alcohol also produces relaxing effects, and many users consume alcohol to reduce anxiety. In fact, Conger (1956) developed a *tension reduction hypothesis* to explain habitual alcohol use. An important part of this hypothesis is that anxiety sufferers have a greater likelihood to drink. Although this hypothesis is difficult to confirm in humans, animals identified with anxious traits have a greater likelihood to self-administer alcohol compared to nonanxious animals (Primeaux, Wilson, Gray, York, & Wilson, 2006; Spanagel et al., 1995). Moreover, stress and anxiety serve as predictors for alcohol addiction, as noted later in this chapter.

Stop & Check

1. The game 21 for 21 is an example of _____ drinking.
2. How does alcohol produce feelings of warmth?
3. A specific disinhibitory effect of alcohol is _____, which can be measured using delay-discounting tasks.
4. Alcohol also impairs _____, which may explain why alcohol-related crashes occur during obstructed driving conditions.
5. Two key subjective effects of alcohol are an improvement in mood and a reduction in _____.

1. extreme 2. Alcohol dilates blood vessels, increasing blood flow to the skin and extremities. This provides a feeling of warmth. 3. impulsivity 4. divided attention 5. anxiety

Severe Adverse Effects of High BAC

alcohol stupor Dulled senses and poor cognitive function caused by overconsumption of alcohol; also known as drunken stupor.

Acute alcohol consumption generates severe adverse effects above a 0.20 BAC (see figure 8.6). At these BACs, drinkers develop an **alcohol stupor**, or *drunken stupor*, that is characterized by disorientation, dulled senses, and poor cognitive function. Someone described as *drunk*, *smashed*, or *hammered* exhibits many of the signs of stupor.

blackout Reversible drug-induced dementia characterized by stupor and anterograde amnesia.

At BACs of 0.25 and higher, drinkers can develop a reversible drug-induced dementia. Reversible drug-induced dementia is characterized by stupor and anterograde amnesia, better known as **blackout**. Anterograde amnesia is the inability to form new memories. Thus, when drinkers blackout, they cannot remember the events that occurred after reaching those high BACs. This type of dementia is called *reversible* because the effects subside as BAC levels decline (Oscar-Berman & Marinković, 2007).

At higher BACs, drinkers may pass out. Unconsciousness occurs when alcohol in the brain reaches sufficient concentrations to dampen cortical functioning and cortical arousal areas in the forebrain and brainstem. As BACs rise further, so does the inhibition of CNS functioning.

alcohol poisoning Alcohol-induced inhibition of autonomic system functions, including breathing, heart functioning, and the gag reflex.

A particular risk of high BACs is the suppression of function in the hindbrain, which includes the medulla, a structure critical for autonomic processes such as breathing. BACs of approximately 0.25 and higher can cause **alcohol poisoning**, an alcohol-induced inhibition of autonomic system functions, including breathing, heart functioning, and the gag reflex. During alcohol poisoning, most deaths occur from depressed respiration (Adinoff, Bone, & Linnoila, 1988).

Binge and extreme drinking carry a significant risk of alcohol poisoning. The number of drinks consumed during these forms of drinking reach these high BACs, yet the speed of alcohol consumption is the most critical determinant for alcohol poisoning. As stated previously, although users feel alcohol's effects within minutes, the maximum absorption of alcohol occurs after 30 minutes. This means that a quick succession of alcoholic drinks, like drinking a line of shots, during a binge causes a dramatic increase in BAC levels.

Chronic Heavy Alcohol Consumption and Adverse Cardiovascular and CNS Effects

Although chronic light alcohol consumption may provide positive benefits for the cardiovascular system, chronic heavy alcohol consumption causes many negative effects: increased risks of ischemia, stroke, and heart attack. One of these adverse effects is cardiomyopathy, which consists of any number of specific disorders that affect the heart muscle. Chronic heavy alcohol use can cause **alcoholic cardiomyopathy**, which is characterized by low cardiac output because of enlargement of the heart and dilation of the heart chambers. This disorder leads to congestive heart failure, the inability to adequately supply blood to the body.

alcoholic cardiomyopathy Low cardiac output from enlargement of the heart and dilation of heart chambers caused by heavy and chronic alcohol use.

Heavy acute or chronic alcohol consumption can cause cardiac arrhythmias, which are characterized by abnormal or rapid heartbeats. Cardiac arrhythmias that occur after an acute heavy drinking episode constitute what is referred to as a *holiday heart syndrome.* These effects range in severity and account for approximately 5 percent of alcohol-related deaths (Zakhari, 1997).

Unlike the dilating effects of light alcohol consumption, heavy alcohol consumption constricts blood vessels. This hypertensive state is particularly dangerous for individuals suffering from cardiomyopathy, because the ability to pump blood is already diminished. Hypertension requires increased heart output to deliver blood through the high-pressure system (Zakhari, 1997).

Chronic alcohol consumption also taxes the liver. The alcohol metabolic process causes oxidation of liver cells over time, resulting in cellular damage and the development of **cirrhosis**, a chronic liver disease characterized by tissue scarring and poor liver functioning. Poor liver functioning impairs metabolism of nutrients from foods, protein synthesis, and other vital processes (Lieber, 1997).

cirrhosis Chronic liver disease characterized by tissue scarring and poor liver function.

fetal alcohol syndrome Disorder characterized by physical and neurological abnormal development.

Alcohol use during pregnancy can cause **fetal alcohol syndrome**, a disorder characterized by physical and neurological abnormal development. Babies with fetal alcohol syndrome have characteristic facial abnormalities, such as a widened distance between the eyes, and risk of a variety of other physiological effects, such as congenital heart defects and abnormal development of the eyes and ears (**figure 8.10**). These babies develop more slowly intellectually and cognitively and maintain deficiencies in these areas.

The full onset of fetal alcohol syndrome is most associated with heavy alcohol use, particularly from pregnant mothers who engaged in binge drinking. Lesser amounts of alcohol consumed during pregnancy can produce a weaker fetal alcohol syndrome, referred to as *alcohol-related neurodevelopmental disorder.* A child born without the full spectrum of fetal alcohol disorder

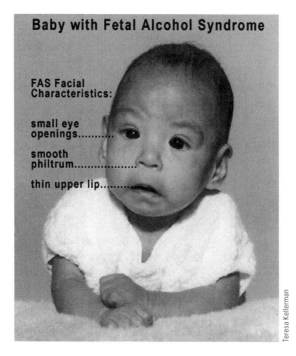

Baby with Fetal Alcohol Syndrome

FAS Facial Characteristics:

small eye openings...........

smooth philtrum....................

thin upper lip.........

Teresa Kellerman

figure 8.10 Alcohol use during pregnancy can cause fetal alcohol syndrome, a disorder noted for physical facial abnormalities, as shown in the photograph, and other physical and neurological abnormalities.

symptoms will have fewer physiological, behavior, and cognitive deficits (Sokol, Delaney-Black, & Nordstrom, 2003).

How much alcohol is safe to drink during pregnancy? The specific limit of alcohol consumption during pregnancy is a moving target. Most physicians recommend no consumption during pregnancy, whereas some advise only occasional consumption (Anderson et al., 2010). In 2005, U.S. Surgeon General Richard Carmona stated in an advisory on fetal alcohol syndrome risk that "it is now clear that no amount of alcohol can be considered safe [during pregnancy]" (Carmona, 2005). This remains the recommendation from the U.S. surgeon general as well as the Centers for Disease Control and Prevention and the National Institute on Alcohol Abuse and Alcoholism.

Long-term, heavy use of alcohol may cause a serious central nervous system disorder called **Korsakoff's syndrome**, a condition characterized by memory loss, false memories, poor insight, apathy, and tremor. Coma can also occur in Korsakoff's syndrome. This disorder manifests from the destruction of nervous system tissue resulting from thiamine, or vitamin B1, deficiency. Thiamine is deficient because alcohol inhibits thiamine absorption from the intestinal tract, as described previously (Kopelman, Thomson, Guerrini, & Marshall, 2009). A less severe form of Korsakoff's syndrome is called *alcohol dementia*, which consists primarily of deficits in cognitive functioning (Moriyama, Mimura, Kato, & Kashima, 2006).

Korsakoff's syndrome Condition caused by heavy, long-term alcohol use resulting in memory loss, false memories, poor insight, apathy, and tremor.

Stop & Check

1. Chronic heavy alcohol use can produce _____, an enlargement of the heart and dilation of heart chambers.

2. Alcohol use during pregnancy can cause _____.

3. Chronic heavy alcohol use diminishes absorption of thiamine, which can cause a central nervous system disorder called _____.

1. alcoholic cardiomyopathy **2.** fetal alcohol syndrome **3.** Korsakoff's syndrome

Alcohol: Tolerance and Sensitization

acute tolerance to alcohol Tolerance that occurs when alcohol's behavioral effects are weaker for declining blood alcohol concentrations than for inclining blood alcohol concentrations.

metabolic tolerance to alcohol Increase in liver alcohol dehydrogenase enzymes resulting in an increased rate of alcohol metabolism.

pharmacodynamic tolerance to alcohol Reduced physiological responsiveness to alcohol's pharmacological actions.

Acute tolerance to alcohol occurs when alcohol's behavioral effects are weaker for declining BACs than for inclining BACs. The term *acute tolerance* refers to the development of tolerance during the same session (Fillmore, Marczinski, & Bowman, 2005). The chart in **figure 8.11** illustrates this condition.

In figure 8.11, alcohol administration caused BACs to steadily increase until a maximum BAC of 0.12 was reached. Behavior was significantly impaired when BACs first reached 0.08. After the peak BAC, a BAC of 0.08 was again reached as BACs were declining later in the session. The second 0.08 BAC on the *declining* BAC curve, however, was less impairing than the first 0.08 BAC on the *inclining* BAC curve. In other words, tolerance developed to the effects of a 0.08 BAC.

Other forms of tolerance develop through chronic administration. One of these forms is **metabolic tolerance to alcohol,** which consists of an increase in liver alcohol dehydrogenase enzymes and results in an increased rate of alcohol metabolism. The increased rate of alcohol metabolism diminishes BAC levels (Israel et al., 1979).

Another form of chronic tolerance is **pharmacodynamic tolerance to alcohol,** or reduced physiological responsiveness to alcohol's pharmacological actions. Pharmacodynamic tolerance is known to occur with glutamate NMDA receptors. As described previously, alcohol inhibits the function of NMDA receptors. During chronic administration, NMDA receptors are

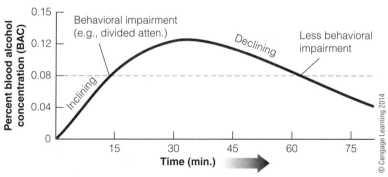

figure **8.11** Acute tolerance occurs when behavioral impairment is less during declining BACs than during inclining BACs.

upregulated in order to compensate for alcohol's inhibitory actions at NMDA receptors (Gulya, Grant, Valverius, Hoffman, & Tabakoff, 1991).

Chronic alcohol administration also produces **behavioral tolerance to alcohol**, which is defined as a reduced behavioral impairment to alcohol. For example, Goodwin and colleagues (1971) demonstrated that experienced drinkers performed better on a simple motor task than novice drinkers after the administration of alcohol.

In addition to tolerance, sensitization also occurs to some of alcohol's pharmacological effects. **Sensitization to alcohol** consists of an increase in alcohol's efficacy. In particular, sensitization occurs to alcohol's reinforcing effects. In animals, chronic alcohol administration produces increases in alcohol self-administration, locomotor activity, and sexual behavior. Chronic alcohol administration also produces greater increases in dopamine levels in the nucleus accumbens compared to acute alcohol administration (for review, see Fish, DeBold, & Miczek, 2002).

Alcohol Addiction and Withdrawal

Chronic heavy alcohol use often leads to an alcohol use disorder. The *Diagnostic and Statistical Manual* (fourth edition) (DSM-IV) identifies two primary types of alcohol use disorders: alcohol abuse and alcohol dependence. Alcohol dependence is generally synonymous with the term *alcoholism*, although alcoholism lends itself more to a disease concept of alcohol dependence. An individual diagnosed with alcohol dependence may meet all of the general DSM criteria for substance dependence as described in Chapter 5.

Alcohol abuse is a chronic disorder characterized by persistent alcohol use despite causing social, occupational, or legal problems. Alcohol abuse can cause someone to repeatedly miss work or to be late for a child's school activities. Moreover, someone may routinely consume alcohol during physically dangerous situations such as driving. As described in Chapter 5, DSM criteria for abuse is similar to dependence, except that abuse fails to show evidence of tolerance and withdrawal.

Experts generally agree there are two subtypes of alcohol addiction—type I and type II—although neither is included in the DSM-IV. In 1987, Claude Cloninger first described the characteristics of these two types of alcohol addiction (Cloninger, 1987). Cloninger characterized **Type I alcohol addiction** as occurring with those 25 and older and having low genetic risk but high psychosocial risk. Environmental variables such as stressful interpersonal situations or psychological disorders primarily account for type I alcohol addiction. Cloninger characterized **type II alcohol addiction** as occurring with those younger than 25 and exhibiting high genetic risk and traits associated with poor impulse control. Type II alcohol-addicted individuals often have a parent who was a chronic alcohol user, and they tend to engage in heavy drinking at a young adult age (**table 8.3**).

A physiological dependence develops during alcohol addiction and leads to severe and potentially life-threatening withdrawal symptoms. Seizures are the primary withdrawal symptom of concern. Seizure risk develops as the

behavioral tolerance to alcohol Reduced behavioral impairment to alcohol.

sensitization to alcohol Increase in alcohol's efficacy, especially its reinforcing effects.

type I alcohol addiction Alcohol addiction that occurs at age 25 or older, has low genetic risk, and exhibits high psychosocial risk.

type II alcohol addiction Alcohol addiction that occurs before age 25, exhibits high genetic risk, and has traits associated with poor impulse control.

table **8.3**

Types of Alcohol Addiction	
Types of alcohol addiction	**Description**
Type I	Occurs at age 25 and older; has low genetic risk and high psychosocial risk
Type II	Occurs at less than age 25; has high genetic risk and poor impulse control

© Cengage Learning 2014

brain adapts to alcohol's chronic actions in the brain. In particular, chronic alcohol use is associated with increased levels of glutamate NMDA receptors and decreased levels of $GABA_A$ receptors. The result of having more excitatory receptors and fewer inhibitory receptors, respectively, is a hyperactivated state in many brain regions. This state sets the occasion for seizures. Because of this, anticonvulsant drugs should be provided during the first days of alcohol-cessation therapy (Hall & Zador, 1997).

Repeated alcohol withdrawals, which may occur with someone who repeatedly quits and relapses, can increase the risk and severity of withdrawal seizures. An increased seizure risk from repeated withdrawals is called *kindling* (Ballenger & Post, 1978). Beyond seizure risk, alcohol withdrawal can produce an **alcohol withdrawal syndrome**, also referred to as **delirium tremens**, that is characterized by hallucinations, trembling, confusion, disorientation, and agitation (Hall & Zador, 1997).

alcohol withdrawal syndrome (delirium tremens) Alcohol withdrawal syndrome characterized by hallucinations, trembling, confusion, disorientation, and agitation.

Stop & Check

1. How is acute alcohol tolerance shown?
2. Between the two types of alcohol addiction, which has the greatest genetic risk?
3. Which alcohol withdrawal symptom is the greatest concern?

1. Acute alcohol tolerance is shown when declining BACs exhibit weaker effects than inclining BACs. **2.** Type II alcohol addiction **3.** seizures

Psychosocial Interventions, Therapeutic Drugs, and Alcohol Use Disorders

A variety of therapeutic strategies exist for treating alcohol addiction. The ultimate goal of alcohol abuse and addiction treatment is to eliminate the behavioral, social, and physical harm caused by alcohol use. To achieve this goal, most therapeutic approaches seek complete abstention from alcohol use. However, some therapeutic approaches seek to transform problem alcohol use into controllable alcohol use.

alcoholics anonymous A 12-step therapeutic program for alcohol addiction that encourages drinking abstinence for its anonymous members.

The 12-step recovery program **Alcoholics Anonymous (AA)** represents the most recognized therapy for alcohol addiction. Although numbers are difficult to determine because of the protected identities of participants, AA estimates it has approximately 1.2 million members in the United States and 800,000 members elsewhere in the world (Alcoholics Anonymous, 2012). During AA meetings, a member shares personal stories about his or her struggles with alcohol use and connects with a sponsor who is normally a long-time AA member in recovery from alcohol addiction. AA programs provide extensive social support to encourage abstinence from drinking. Those who optimally respond to AA therapy have frequent meeting attendance, actively seek advice from AA sources, and strongly adhere to 12-step beliefs (Morgenstern, Kahler, Frey, & Labouvie, 1996).

Cognitive–behavioral therapies for alcohol dependence seek to improve an individual's cognitive and behavioral skills in changing problem alcohol use. This approach views alcohol dependence as a maladaptive learning pattern that can be adjusted by replacing maladaptive responses with adaptive responses. These approaches have users learn to identify and cope with conditions that facilitate problem alcohol use such as stress and alcohol-related stimuli. By addressing alcohol use as maladaptive behavior, complete cessation of alcohol use is not the ultimate therapeutic goal per se. Rather, therapists seek to eliminate the problems associated with alcohol use, which may or may not require abstinence. These therapies are sometimes referred to as *controlled drinking therapies* because a user may learn to avoid excessive alcohol use and accompanying problems without completely abstaining from alcohol (Longabaugh & Morgenstern, 1999).

Pharmacological treatments for alcohol addiction attempt to reduce alcohol intake by (1) producing aversive effects, (2) weakening effects, or (3) reducing cravings (**table 8.4**). Disulfiram (Antabuse) has been used since 1949 to treat alcohol addiction. Disulfiram discourages alcohol use by generating aversive effects through disrupting alcohol's metabolic process in the body. **Disulfiram** inhibits acetaldehyde dehydrogenase enzyme activity, the enzyme that breaks acetaldehyde down into inactive metabolites. After consuming alcohol,

Disulfiram Treatment for alcohol addiction that inhibits acetaldehyde dehydrogenase enzyme activity, causing noxious effects.

table 8.4

Pharmacological Treatments for Alcohol Addiction		
Pharmacological treatment	Approach	How it works
Disulfiram	Aversive effects when alcohol consumed	Causes acetaldehyde buildup during alcohol consumption
Naltrexone	Weakens alcohol's reinforcing effects	Blocks opioid receptors, preventing disinhibition of ventral tegmental dopamine neurons
Acamprosate	Weakens alcohol's reinforcing effects and reduces cravings for alcohol	Substitutes for alcohol's pharmacological actions by activating GABA receptors and blocking glutamate NMDA receptors

© Cengage Learning 2014

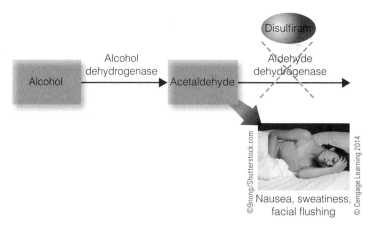

Nausea, sweatiness, facial flushing

figure **8.12** Disulfiram inhibits the metabolism of acetaldehyde, causing acetaldehyde buildup and aversive effects after alcohol consumption.

disulfiram, through inhibiting this enzyme, causes a buildup of acetaldehyde. Acetaldehyde, in turn, causes a number of adverse physiological effects, including nausea, sweatiness, and facial flushing (**figure 8.12**). By producing these adverse effects, disulfiram deters alcohol consumption (Heather, 1989).

Disulfiram appears most effective at reducing alcohol consumption when patients are willing to participate in cessation programs and when disulfiram compliance is supervised. Otherwise, alcohol-addicted individuals who are coerced, often through court-mandated treatment, into taking disulfiram either fail to take the medications regularly or switch to alternative drugs of abuse (Heather, 1989). Only one in five patients treated with disulfiram remain abstinent one year later (Miller, Walters, & Bennett, 2001).

Although disulfiram treatment generates aversive effects, naltrexone treatment may reduce alcohol's reinforcing effects. **Naltrexone** is an opioid receptor antagonist approved in Canada, Europe, and the United States for treating alcohol addiction. By blocking opioid receptors, naltrexone may interfere with endogenous opioid mediation of alcohol's reinforcing effects, as described previously in this chapter (Volpicelli, Sarin-Krishnan, & O'Malley, 2002).

Gonzales and Weiss (1998) demonstrated naltrexone's reduction of alcohol's reinforcing effects in rats using both self-administration and microdialysis procedures. In this study, rats self-administered less alcohol after naltrexone administration. Moreover, naltrexone caused a weaker elevation of nucleus accumbens dopamine levels after alcohol administration (**figure 8.13**). In humans, naltrexone prevents alcohol-addicted individuals from consuming alcohol to dangerously high BACs (Volpicelli, Alterman, Hayashida, & O'Brien, 1992). Beyond this, however, naltrexone provides less than promising results for alcohol addiction. In a one-year clinical study conducted by Krystal and colleagues (2001), naltrexone, in combination with psychosocial therapy, failed to increase the number of alcohol-free days compared to placebo.

naltrexone Opioid receptor antagonist approved for treating alcohol addiction.

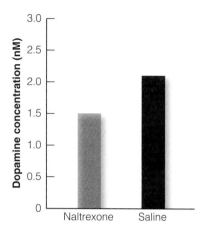

figure 8.13 The opioid receptor antagonist naltrexone reduces alcohol's elevation of nucleus accumbens dopamine concentrations. The y-axis shows the amount of dopamine contained in each collected sample, as measured in nanomolar concentrations. (Data from Gonzales & Weiss, 1998)

Acamprosate (Campral) is a treatment approved by the Food and Drug Administration for alcohol addiction. It acts on GABA and NMDA receptors. Research suggests that acamprosate may treat alcohol addiction by reducing cravings for alcohol (Littleton, 1995). Acamprosate may achieve these results by substituting for two primary mechanisms of action for alcohol. First, acamprosate exhibits agonist actions at GABA receptors. Second, acamprosate functions as an antagonist for glutamate NMDA receptors. In clinical trials, acamprosate modestly reduces craving and increases the number of alcohol-abstinent days (Volpicelli et al., 2002). However, a collection of more recent studies has found that at 6- and 12-month follow-ups with patients taking acamprosate, generally 20–40 percent of patients report alcohol abstinence (Mason, 2001).

Stop & Check

1. Among the psychotherapies for alcohol addiction, which approach may not have alcohol abstinence as a goal?

2. How does disulfiram cause aversive effects after alcohol consumption?

1. Cognitive–behavioral strategies seek to reduce maladaptive behavior associated with alcohol. These strategies may succeed in reducing such maladaptive behavior without alcohol abstinence. For this reason, these approaches are often referred to as *controlled-drinking therapies*. 2. Disulfiram inhibits breakdown of the alcohol metabolite acetylaldehyde, a noxious chemical.

FROM ACTIONS TO EFFECTS
Hangover

||

hangover Unpleasant experience that may occur after alcohol consumption.

Hangover is an unpleasant experience that occurs after alcohol consumption. Its symptoms include headache, a poor sense of overall well-being, diarrhea, fatigue, and nausea. Headache is the most common symptom (Harburg, 1981) (**figure 8.14**). There is no set limit of drinks that will trigger hangover symptoms. The risk of hangover varies from individual to individual because of such factors as alcohol tolerance, enzymatic breakdown, medication interactions, and overall physical health. Other factors are addressed in the following text (Prat, Adan, & Sanchez-Turet, 2009).

Hangovers not only are unpleasant but also are associated with cognitive deficits. These deficits occur even when BAC reaches zero. In a study by Howland and colleagues (2010), those experiencing hangover with no BAC levels exhibited significant deficits in reaction time and attention. The severity of the hangover relates to the magnitude of these deficits.

Hangover is highly prevalent in the general population. Based on survey information, nearly 75 percent of those drinking to intoxication have experienced a hangover, and about half of these drinkers experienced hangover within the last year. The prevalence of these debilitating effects present a high economic burden from worker absenteeism, low productivity, and accidents. Absenteeism, in particular, accounts for billions in lost wages each year (Wiese, Shlipak, & Browner, 2000).

Hangover symptoms appear around 6–8 hours after drinking ceases. These symptoms begin to occur as the BAC approaches 0, and they worsen when the BAC reaches 0. Once hangover symptoms occur, they remain for as long as 14–16 hours. The cause of hangover is not entirely understood. Currently, there are thought to be five possible contributors to hangover.

The first contributor to hangover may be acute alcohol withdrawal. Many of the features of hangover match the DSM-IV characteristics for alcohol withdrawal. Moreover, alcohol consumption reduces hangover symptoms (Swift & Davidson, 1998). Unlike alcohol addiction, however, hangover symptoms do not develop into further stages of alcohol withdrawal such as seizures.

A second possible contributor to hangover is the buildup of acetaldehyde after alcohol consumption. As previously described, alcohol dehydrogenase converts alcohol to acetaldehyde. Acetaldehyde produces aversive hangover-like effects. However, alcohol consumption must be very high to produce sufficient buildup of acetaldehyde

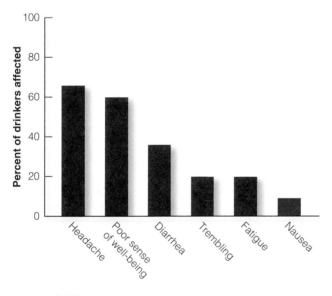

figure **8.14**
Percentage of drinkers suffering from hangover symptoms after an evening of drinking. (Data from Harburg et al., 1981.)

to produce aversive symptoms. Further, hangover symptoms occur when the body no longer contains acetaldehyde.

A third possible contributor for hangover may be acetate accumulation. A metabolite of acetaldehyde, acetate accumulates to much greater levels in the body than acetaldehyde and may be present in the body when hangover symptoms begin. Acetate causes other effects in the body, such as increased levels of adenosine, and causes headaches in humans and laboratory animals. Adenosine produces increased pain sensitivity and fatigue. Thus, acetate together with its production of adenosine may contribute to many hangover symptoms. In a demonstration of acetate's effects, Maxwell and colleagues (2010) assessed the effects of acetate on headache in laboratory animals. The resulting headache from acetate was substantially reduced with treatment by caffeine, an adenosine receptor antagonist.

A fourth possible contributor to hangover is direct action by alcohol. Alcohol consumption causes dehydration, electrolyte imbalance, low blood sugar, vasodilatation, and gastric irritation. All of these effects could support the symptoms of hangover. However, studies indicate that these specific effects are most related to *severe* hangover.

The fifth possible contributor for hangover is overconsumption of other chemicals in alcoholic drinks. These other chemicals can include acetones, polyphenols, and methanol. Methanol, in particular, is known to produce aversive effects similar to hangover. Moreover, hangover symptoms are worse for drinks with a high number of fermentation byproducts, referred to as *congeners*, than those with less congener content. In a study conducted by Chapman (1970), more participants exhibited hangover after consuming bourbon, a drink with high congener content, than those who consumed vodka, a drink with low congener content.

Is there a treatment for hangover? All of the possible explanations for hangover just given are suggestive for potential treatment avenues. In practice, however, research addressing these explanations has yet to provide scientifically proven treatments. There still remains only one way to completely prevent hangover: Do not overindulge.

Stop & Check

1. What is the most common hangover symptom?
2. Hangover symptoms worsen as the BAC approaches _____.
3. One of the possible explanations for hangover is that there is a buildup of _____, similar to how disulfiram reduces alcohol consumption.
4. Why might coffee reduce hangover symptoms?

1. Headache **2.** zero **3.** acetaldehyde **4.** Coffee contains caffeine, an adenosine receptor antagonist. Adenosine antagonism can counteract elevated adenosine levels, which cause elevated pain sensitivity and fatigue.

▶CHAPTER SUMMARY

Central nervous system depressants produce reinforcing and relaxing effects. By far the most used CNS depressant is alcohol, chemically known as *ethyl alcohol*. Although alcohol has been used for thousands of years, U.S. alcohol sales were prohibited during the 1920s.

Alcohol drink concentrations are measured as percentages or by proof, and we compare alcoholic drinks according to *standard drink* units. We also relate alcohol pharmacological effects to blood alcohol concentrations (BACs). Multiple steps occur for alcohol metabolism, and the alcohol elimination rate follows zero-order kinetics. Alcohol exhibits diverse pharmacological actions involving facilitation of GABA receptors, inhibition of NMDA receptors, activation of serotonin receptors,

inhibition of calcium channels, and indirect actions involving endogenous opioids and endocannabinoids. These actions lead to reinforcing effects as well as impairing effects on cognition and behavior-reinforcing effects. Acute alcohol use can produce hangover, an overall sense of poor well-being marked by symptoms such as headache and nausea. Other adverse alcohol effects relate to long-term chronic usage, including damage to the heart and central nervous system. Several forms of tolerance develop for alcohol, and heavy chronic alcohol usage elicits severe withdrawal symptoms, including seizures. Alcohol is highly addictive and is addressed by both psycho-therapeutic and pharmacological treatment strategies.

KEY TERMS

Ethyl alcohol

Percentage alcohol

Proof of alcohol

Fermentation

Distilled alcoholic beverages (spirits)

Standard drink

18th Amendment

Blood alcohol concentration

Alcohol dehydrogenase

Acetaldehyde

Binge drinking

Extreme Drinking

Disinhibition

Impulsivity

Alcohol priming

Divided attention

Alcohol stupor

Blackout

Alcohol poisoning

Alcoholic cardiomyopathy

Cirrhosis

Fetal alcohol syndrome

Korsakoff's syndrome

Acute tolerance to alcohol

Metabolic tolerance to alcohol

Pharmacodynamic tolerance to alcohol

Behavioral tolerance to alcohol

Sensitization to alcohol

Type I alcohol addiction

Type II alcohol addiction

Alcohol withdrawal syndrome (delirium tremens)

Alcoholics Anonymous

Disulfiram

Naltrexone

Hangover

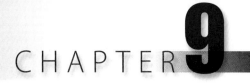

CHAPTER **9**

GHB, Inhalants, and Anesthetics

- ► Gamma-Hydroxybutyrate
- ► Inhalants
- ► From Actions to Effects: Stimulus Properties of GHB and Toluene
- ► Chapter Summary

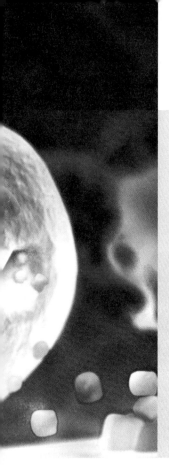

Did Ancient Greek Oracles Come from Chemical Inhalants?

On the slope of Mount Parnassus, ancient Greeks sought the advice of their gods through communicating with the Pythia at the Temple of Apollo. The Pythia, local women who served as mediums for the gods, received their oracles by entering a small, enclosed basement chamber filled with a vapor arising from exposed chasms or springs of water in the temple floor.

Most modern scholars, having failed to verify any such gas emissions, long considered such stories about the Pythia as either mistaken or fraudulent. Yet in 2001, de Beor and colleagues (2001) discovered that the temple's small chasms and springs contained minerals capable of producing ethylene, a known intoxicating agent that causes delirium, disinhibition, euphoria, and even feelings of disembodiment. Yet to the Pythia of ancient Greece, this mind-altering experience served as their connection with the gods.

From de Boer, Hale, and Chanton, 2001.

Chapter 8 dealt with alcohol, the most widely consumed depressant substance. This chapter will consider other depressant substances found within our society: the substance GHB and agents administered in vaporous form called *inhalants*.

Gamma-Hydroxybutyrate

gamma-hydroxybutyrate (GHB) Substance that serves as both a drug and a neurotransmitter that produces CNS depressant effects.

Gamma-hydroxybutyrate (GHB) is both a drug and a neurotransmitter that has depressant effects on the central nervous system (CNS). GHB is a white, tasteless powder that dissolves easily in water. Depending on the formulation, GHB has both recreational and instrumental uses. As a club drug, GHB goes by many street names, including "Gamma-OH," "Georgia Home Boy," and "Liquid E" (Drug Enforcement Administration, 2012a). GHB earned a negative reputation in the late 1990s as a substance used in sexual assault (ElSohly & Salamone, 1999). The media most often refers to GHB-associated sexual assault as *date rape*, although many of these assaults do not occur during a date and often the victim fails to even recall meeting the assailant. Because of its use as a club drug and in sexual assaults, the Drug Enforcement

Administration (DEA) categorized GHB as a schedule I controlled substance in 2000 (Drug Enforcement Administration, 2012b).

Physicians use another formulation of GHB, *sodium gamma-hydroxybutyrate*, as a treatment approved by the Food and Drug Administration (FDA) for narcolepsy, a disorder characterized by extensive daytime sleepiness ("FDA-approved labeling," 2005). This formulation, which the DEA assigns as schedule III, goes by the generic name *sodium oxybate* and the trade name *Xyrem*. Although prescribing a depressant to relieve daytime sleepiness may seem strange, researchers find that GHB addresses some of the neuropathological features of narcolepsy, leading to a reduction in its symptoms. More on this later in the chapter.

Recreational users obtain GHB either from illicit sources or by synthesizing GHB from gamma-butyrolactone (GBL). Because GBL serves as an immediate precursor to GHB, the DEA categorizes GBL as a schedule I controlled substance. However, given the legitimate uses of GBL in many household products, such as in stain and paint removers, the DEA exempts products containing less than 70 percent of GBL (Drug Enforcement Administration, 2010). GHB and GBL also occurs in small amounts in red and white wines, vinegar, beer, and coffee (Elliott & Burgess, 2005). As described later in the chapter, GBL serves as a prodrug by metabolically converting to GHB in the body.

Approximately 1 percent or less of U.S. individuals 12 and older abuse GHB (Substance Abuse and Mental Health Services Administration, 2010). Although this rate seems low overall, some areas of the country see more prevalent use. Twenty percent of local and state law enforcement agencies report moderate to high GHB availability (National Drug Intelligence Center, 2004). Together, these data suggest that either users underreport GHB abuse or that GHB is being used for nonrecreational uses such as drug-facilitated sexual assaults.

Uses for GHB

Researchers first synthesized GHB in 1960 as part of an effort to develop compounds with a similar chemical structure to the neurotransmitter GABA. After its discovery, physicians used GHB as an anesthetic agent. In the late 1970s, researchers discovered that the body naturally synthesizes GHB in the central nervous system. In the 1980s, GHB was widely available as a potential supplement for enhancing muscle growth among weight lifters, although no evidence supports the beneficial use of GHB for this purpose (Andresen, Aydin, Mueller, & Iwersen-Bergmann, 2011; Volpi et al., 1997). Because of concerns over GHB-induced adverse effects, including intoxication and deep unconsciousness, the FDA banned the over-the-counter sale of GHB in 1990 (Woodworth, 1999).

During the 1990s, GHB began to be used in clubs and at parties for its euphoric effects. Along with the recreational use of GHB, law enforcement agencies began investigating increasing charges of GHB use in sexual assault. In particular, reports stated that assailants secretly added GHB to alcoholic drinks, strengthening alcohol and GHB's depressant effects.

As the association of GHB with clubs and sexual assaults strengthened, local and state governments passed laws regulating and banning GHB possession and use. During this period, the U.S. Drug Enforcement Agency monitored GHB as a substance of concern; in 2000, the DEA placed GHB on the controlled substances schedule (Drug Enforcement Administration, 2012a). According to law enforcement agencies, the availability and use of GHB has declined significantly since these regulations went into effect (**figure 9.1**) (Carter, Griffiths, & Mintzer, 2009).

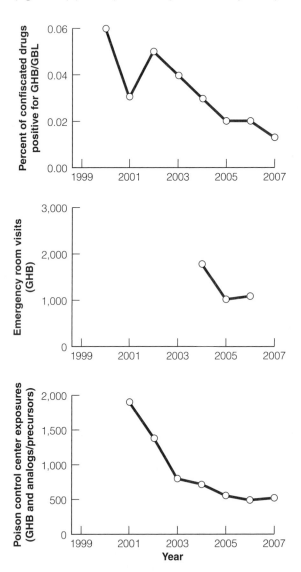

GHB use has declined sharply since its schedule I categorization in 2000, according to measures of illicit GHB seizure, emergency room visits, and poison control reports. (With kind permission from Springer Science+Business Media: Carter, L., Griffiths, R., & Mintzer, M. (2009). Cognitive, psychomotor, and subjective effects of sodium oxybate and triazolam in healthy volunteers. *Psychopharmacology* (Berl), 206(1), 141–154. doi: 10.1007/s00213-009-1589-1, p. 14.)

figure 9.1

Stop & Check

1. GHB, gamma-hydroxybutyrate, is not only a drug but also a _____.

2. To obtain GHB for recreational purposes, what other substances might a user seek?

3. What factors led to the banning of GHB possession and use?

1. neurotransmitter **2.** Because GHB is a controlled substance, users may seek compounds such as GBL that serve as prodrugs for GHB. **3.** GHB became known for its adverse effects and its use in sexual assaults.

GHB: Natural and Synthetic

GHB is both a naturally occurring substance in the CNS and a synthetically produced drug. In the body, naturally occurring GHB is a metabolite of the inhibitory neurotransmitter GABA. The metabolic process begins when the enzyme GABA transaminase converts GABA to its metabolite succinic semialdehyde. The enzyme succinic semialdehyde reductase transforms succinic semialdehyde to GHB (**figure 9.2**) (Andresen et al., 2011).

As previously stated, certain substances serve as prodrugs for GHB. Figure 9.2 shows the process of these metabolic reactions for producing GHB. Its primary prodrugs consist of the chemicals GBL and another substance named *1,4-butanediol*. These chemicals use the alcohol metabolic pathway to produce GHB. First, when 1,4-butanediol enters the liver or the stomach, alcohol dehydrogenase converts 1,4-butanediol to GBL. Second, in the liver, the enzyme aldehyde dehydrogenase converts GBL to GHB (**figure 9.3**).

REVIEW! The enzyme alcohol dehydrogenase converts alcohol to acetaldehyde, which is in turn converted to acetic acid by the enzyme aldehyde dehydrogenase. Chapter 8 (pg. 231).

As a salt, the drug GHB easily dissolves in liquid. The liquid form of GHB, or GHB's chemical precursors, are colorless and tasteless. The oral delivery of GHB is most common for recreational use and for assaults such as date rape. Although GHB can be delivered intravenously, this administration route is seldom used. GHB readily penetrates the blood–brain barrier after absorption from the gastrointestinal tract (Andresen et al., 2011). After oral administration in humans, GHB reaches peak levels in blood after 15–45 minutes, and pharmacological effects first occur within 15–20 minutes and last approximately 2 hours (Carter et al., 2009; Mason & Kerns, 2002).

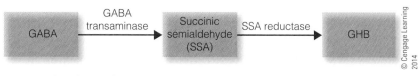

figure **9.2** GHB is produced naturally in the body through a metabolic process starting with the neurotransmitter GABA.

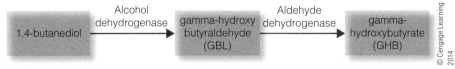

figure 9.3 The precursor chemicals 1,4-butanediol and GBL can produce GHB through the alcohol metabolic pathway.

In the liver and brain, the enzyme GHB dehydrogenase transforms GHB into its own precursor chemical, succinic semialdehyde, which then converts to the neurotransmitter GABA. The elimination half-life for GHB from the body is only 30 minutes, and it can remain at detectable levels in blood for only 4–8 hours and in urine for only 8–12 hours. These short elimination periods make determining GHB's use in sexual assault difficult (LeBeau et al., 1999). Although tests confirm GHB use in 1–5 percent of sexual assaults, the majority of suspected drug-facilitated sexual assault victims present themselves to authorities too late for GHB detection (Zvosec & Smith, 2009). Moreover, standard blood tests conducted after sexual assault do not detect GHB. Instead, victims must notify health professionals that they suspect the use of GHB so that proper tests will be conducted (National Drug Intelligence Center, 2004).

GHB Pharmacological Action

As stated previously, GHB is not only a drug but also a neurotransmitter. The neurotransmitter GHB is found throughout the brain. After synthesis, GHB accumulates within vesicles used for storing GABA. Given that GABA facilitates GHB synthesis and that the same vesicles store both GABA and GHB, many GABA neurons likely release both GABA and GHB (**figure 9.4**) (Muller et al., 2002).

Currently, researchers have confirmed only one type of GHB receptor, but evidence suggests the existence of a second GHB receptor. The GHB receptor is a G-protein–coupled receptor that causes inhibitory effects on neurons. The GHB receptor is found throughout the brain, but is highly concentrated in the hippocampus. The cerebral cortex and basal ganglia also exhibit high GHB receptor concentrations (**figure 9.5**) (Maitre, 1997). Beyond the GHB receptor, studies indicate that GHB functions as an agonist for the $GABA_B$ receptor (Diana et al., 1991; Pistis et al., 2005).

GHB reenters neurons through a sodium-coupled monocarboxylate transporter (figure 9.4) and then rapidly degrades to form GABA, as described previously (Cui & Morris, 2009; Roiko, Felmlee, & Morris, 2012). In fact, although GHB eliminates from the body in 30-minute half-lives, GHB degrades in the brain in 5-minute half-lives (Doherty, Stout, & Roth, 1975). Thus, given the rapid degradation to GABA, many of GHB's pharmacological effects may be accounted for by GABA neurotransmission (Wu et al., 2003).

GHB has complex effects on the regulation of dopamine. At low doses in animals, GHB inhibits the firing of dopamine neurons and the release of

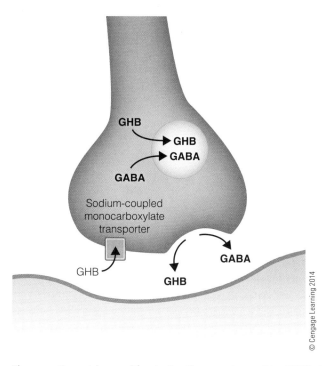

© Cengage Learning 2014

figure 9.4   The synaptic vesicles used for storing the neurotransmitter GABA also store GHB. Subsequently, many GABA neurons may release both GABA and GHB. GHB reenters neurons through a sodium-coupled monocarboxylate transporter.

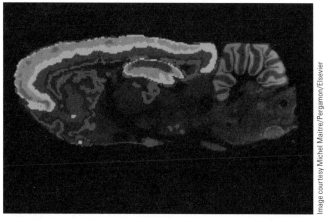

Image courtesy Michel Maitre/Pergamon/Elsevier

figure 9.5   GHB receptors are found throughout the brain, particularly in the hippocampus, cerebral cortex, and basal ganglia. Darker areas represent dense GHB receptor concentrations. (From Maitre, 1997.)

dopamine from these neurons. High doses of GHB in animals initially produce this same effect, but afterward we find increased dopamine concentrations in the nucleus accumbens and other parts of the basal ganglia (Maitre, 1997). Thus, high doses of GHB exhibit changes in dopamine levels predictive of generating reinforcing effects.

Stop & Check

1. GHB is synthesized from the neurotransmitter _____.
2. GHB is an endogenous neurotransmitter that activates GHB and _____ receptors.

1. GABA 2. GABA

GHB's Depressant Pharmacological Effects

Studies find that GHB has a complex series of pharmacological effects. Early pharmacological studies found that GHB elicits a unique sleeping pattern that is characterized by growth-hormone release during the first two hours of sleep and longer periods of deep sleep (**Box 9.1**). The combination of enhanced growth-hormone release and deep sleep made GHB an attractive substance for many bodybuilders seeking a substance to enhance muscle repair and growth as well as enhancing restorative sleep. However, these purported benefits have never been substantiated (Okun, Boothby, Bartfield, & Doering, 2001).

GHB's effects on growth hormones and deep sleep may have important benefits for narcolepsy. Although narcolepsy is generally considered a disorder of daytime sleepiness, it also consists of fragmented and nonrestorative sleep. These disruptions to nighttime sleeping also lead to deficiencies in growth hormone, which researchers speculate could contribute to this disorder. When given at nighttime, sodium oxybate, the FDA-approved form of GHB, restores growth-hormone deficits and increases the length of nighttime sleeping in narcolepsy patients. As a result of improved nighttime sleeping, patients have reduced episodes of sleeping during the day (Donjacour et al., 2011; Okun et al., 2001).

Recreational users characterize three general ranges for orally used GHB doses: *light* doses ranging from 6 to 17 mg/kg, *common* doses ranging from 11 to 28 mg/kg, and *strong* doses ranging from 22 to 51 mg/kg (Oliveto et al., 2010).* Studies in controlled laboratory conditions report that GHB increases blood pressure at strong doses; no other appreciable physiological effects occur within these dose ranges (Abanades et al., 2006; Oliveto et al., 2010).

Many of GHB's behavioral and subjective effects depend not only on the dose but also on the time course. Studies find that strong doses of GHB cause confusion and induce drowsiness (Oliveto et al., 2010). Survey data among GHB users and anecdotal reports suggest that memory loss most often occurs after GHB use, as opposed to during GHB use, for about half of GHB users.

---

*Amounts converted to mg/kg based on mean weight for U.S. male adults.

Anecdotal reports describe memory-impairing effects seldom occurring for doses as low as 10 mg/kg (Mamelak, 1989; Miotto et al., 2001). Strong doses produce significant impairments in balance as demonstrated when study participants attempt to stand on one foot or perform other motor tasks. Peak effects for these motor effects occur 1 hour after administration (Abanades et al., 2006). Sexual predators use GHB, particularly in combination with alcohol, to make a victim appear inebriated and induce memory loss from an assault (Varela, Nogue, Oros, & Miro, 2004).

GHB users report positive subjective experiences that contribute to GHB use. In a survey conducted by Miotto and colleagues (2001), the majority of regular GHB users reporting experiencing euphoria, happiness, increased sexuality, optimism, and other positive subjective effects during GHB use. However, this study did not identify the doses used or provide information on the time course for these effects.

GHB studies conducted in laboratory conditions have attempted to relate subjective effects to doses and time course. Stimulant-like subjective effects tend to occur for common doses early in GHB's time course, peaking around 45 minutes. During this stimulant phase, study participants report feeling stimulated, experiencing amphetamine-like effects, and having feelings of greater energy. They also reported liking the drug's effects. Depressant-like subjective effects tend to occur later in GHB's time course for common and strong doses, peaking at around 1.5 hours. During the depressant phase of this time course, participants report feeling drunk, dizzy, drowsy, confused, and sedated (Abanades et al., 2006; Oliveto et al., 2010) (**table 9.1**).

GHB Overdose and Risk for Addiction

Many of GHB's adverse effects arise from overdose or GHB withdrawal. GHB overdose presents as nausea, unconsciousness, reduced blood pressure, and lowered heart rate. However, most emergency room visits related to GHB, particularly those involving cardiovascular effects, involve the use of other substances, including alcohol or other depressant drugs (Chin, Sporer, Cullison, Dyer, & Wu, 1998).

table **9.1**

Time-Dependent Subjective Effects of GHB	
~45 minutes	**1½ hours**
Stimulated	Drunk
Amphetamine-like effects	Dizzy
Greater energy	Drowsy
Enjoy the drug effects	Confused
	Sedated

© Cengage Learning 2014.

box **9.1** Electroencephalography

Electroencephalography (EEG) is a method for recording the electrical activity of brain areas through electrodes placed on the scalp. Brain electrical activity is recorded when electrons on the metal of the scalp electrodes are moved by electrical changes occurring beneath the electrode. These electrical changes occur because of exchanges of ions within neurons, particularly ion passage in neuronal axons. Ion passage occurs on neuronal axons during the resting potential when potassium (K^+) ions enter and sodium (Na^+) ions exit a neuron, during action potentials when Na^+ ions rapidly enter a neuron, and during refractory periods when K^+ ions exit a neuron. When these electrical events occur among thousands of neurons in a part of the brain at the same time, then these overall electrical changes are detected on EEG electrodes.

EEG electrodes detect several types of electrical frequencies presented in hertz (Hz), a value that represents the number of waves produced within on second. The alpha frequency consists of 8–12 Hz (box 9.1 figure 1). Alpha waves become larger—that is, have greater amplitude—during relaxation and when eyes are closed. They are prominent during the early stages of sleep. The beta frequency is characterized by 12–30 Hz and is low amplitude and irregular during thinking, concentration, movement, and when eyes

are opened. Other frequencies, which include delta and theta, are most often studied during the stages of sleep. Deep sleep, in particular, consists of slow delta and theta waves.

During research or clinical assessment, EEGs recordings are made when participants are exposed to some type of stimulus or engaging in a task. An **evoked potential** is an EEG recording during a specific stimulus presentation. An **event-related potential** is an EEG recording during a behavioral or cognitive activity.

Researchers use EEG to study drug effects such as CNS depressant drugs. For example, in a study conducted by Metcalf and colleagues (1966), GHB produced a synchronized, slow wave that is characteristic of a deep sleep. Yet these slow wave patterns were seen in awake participants. These findings suggest that GHB inhibits cortical arousal centers such as the reticular formation.

electroencephalography (EEG) Method for recording the electrical activity of brain areas through electrodes placed on the scalp.

evoked potential EEG recording during a specific stimulus presentation.

event-related potential EEG recording during a behavioral or cognitive activity.

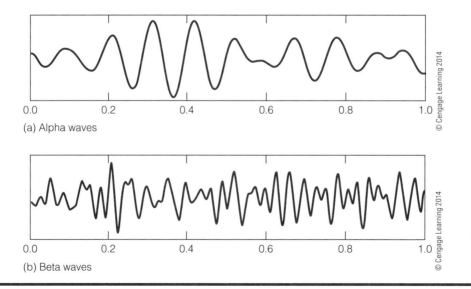

0.0   0.2   0.4   0.6   0.8   1.0
(a) Alpha waves   © Cengage Learning 2014

0.0   0.2   0.4   0.6   0.8   1.0
(b) Beta waves   © Cengage Learning 2014

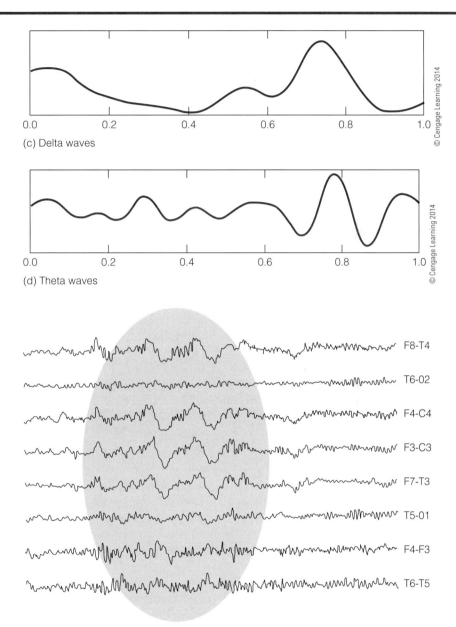

(c) Delta waves

(d) Theta waves

F8-T4

T6-02

F4-C4

F3-C3

F7-T3

T5-01

F4-F3

T6-T5

box **9.1**, figure **1**

In awake participants, GHB produced slow wave bursts characteristic of delta and theta waves (circled). Delta and theta waves normally occur during deep sleep. (Metcalf et. al., 1966. By permission.)

An acute withdrawal period follows an episode of GHB use. Most regular users report exhaustion, memory loss, confusion, and clumsiness after GHB use. Some users also report anxiety, insomnia, depression, and dizziness (Miotto et al., 2001).

GHB use seldom meets the *Diagnostic and Statistical Manual* (DSM) criteria for substance dependence. When use appears to meet these general criteria, the use pattern consists of individuals taking GHB around the clock, about every 1–3 hours. This manner of use creates a physical dependency that results in the appearance of severe withdrawal symptoms occurring within 2–6 hours after using GHB. These symptoms include tremor, seizures, memory loss, anxiety, and confusion (Andresen et al., 2011).

Stop & Check

1. Why have some weight lifters used GHB?
2. During GHB use, when might a user experience stimulant or depressant effects?
3. Why might it be difficult to isolate GHB's overdose effects during an emergency room visit?

1. GHB elicits increases in growth hormone and increased deep sleep, leading weight lifters to believe that GHB may promote muscle repair and growth as well as enhance restorative sleep. **2.** Some of GHB's subjective effects depend on time course. Studies show that stimulant effects occur earlier in GHB's time course than do depressant effects. **3.** Users seldom take GHB alone. When overdose occurs, physicians often suspect an interaction between GHB and another substance such as alcohol, which, in particular, may interact with GHB to impair cardiovascular function.

Inhalants

inhalants Vaporous chemicals that elicit psychoactive effects.

Inhalants refer to vaporous chemicals that elicit psychoactive effects. Inhalants represent a large class of compounds that include volatile alkyl nitrites, nitrous oxide, and volatile solvents, fuels, and anesthetics (Balster, 1998; Williams & Storck, 2007). The most representative alkyl nitrite consists of *amyl nitrite*, a compound abused in the 1960s and 1970s for its ability to provide feelings of warmth, throbbing sensations, light headedness, and enhanced sexual experiences (Balster, 1998; Everett, 1972). Users also refer to amyl nitrite as *poppers* in reference to the sound made when users broke open the small glass ampoules, or vials, containing this compound.

Nitrous oxide, also known as *laughing gas*, represents another abused inhalant largely because of its exhibiting euphoric effects, along with a mixture of depressant and hallucinogenic effects (Balster, 1998). The most common source for abuse of nitrous oxide consists of aerosol sprays. In particular, many users inhale nitrous oxide from aerosolized whipped cream containers,

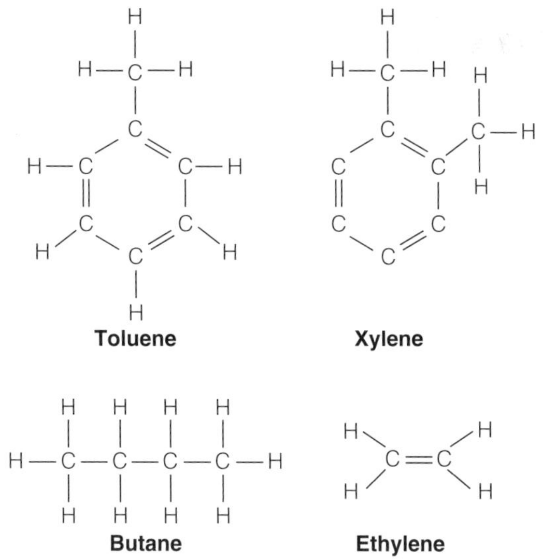

figure 9.6 Many inhalants are hydrocarbon chemicals, which consist entirely of carbon (C) and hydrogen (H) atoms.

which release a puff of nitrous oxide just before releasing whipped cream; users refer to these containers as *whippets* (Howard & Perron, 2009).

By far, the majority of abused inhalants consists of volatile solvents, fuels, and anesthetics. The most frequently used compound in this category is toluene, but others include gasoline, butane, xylene and acetone. Many of these chemicals are hydrocarbons, referring to their composition of entirely carbon and hydrogen atoms (**figure 9.6**). These chemicals exist among many household products or in products readily available at hardware stores. Many glues such as model airplane cement contain toluene, and aerosol cans and cigarette lighters contain butane. We find xylene in certain cleaning solutions and in solvents for dissolving oil-based paints. Solutions for dissolving nail polish and paint often contain acetone (Lubman, Hides, & Yucel, 2006). Mentioned at the beginning of this chapter, researchers discovered that another hydrocarbon compound, ethylene, may have been emitted from beneath the Temple of Apollo, possibly accounting for the experiences of the Pythia when in small, enclosed spaces (de Boer et al., 2001).

Adolescents represent the largest portion of inhalant users. Approximately 2 million adolescents use inhalants, with most inhalant use occurring at age 14. They are the most widely abused drugs for U.S. adolescents below 8th grade, and 12th graders report lower rates of inhalant use, suggesting that inhalant use decreases as adolescents grow up (Johnston, O'Malley, & Bachman, 2003). Researchers find that geographical isolation, poverty, and unemployment represent important risk factors for inhalant abuse, although inhalant abuse is less likely to occur with African American children, children from two-parent households, and children with strong academic performance (Cairney, Maruff, Burns, & Currie, 2002; Nonnemaker, Crankshaw, Shive, Hussin, & Farrelly, 2011).

Beyond the pharmacological effects of inhalants, users find two important practical aspects that make inhalant abuse relatively easy. First, none of the products containing commonly abused inhalants are illegal to purchase. Second, the intoxication users achieve from inhalants wears off quickly, allowing an inhalant to be used after school and then letting the user go home sober soon afterward (Cohen, 1977; Kurtzman, Otsuka, & Wahl, 2001).

History of Inhalants

The opening of this chapter provided an intriguing finding about ethylene gases likely contributing to the spiritual experiences of ancient Greek oracles (de Boer et al., 2001). Even though ancient human history has scattered tales of ritualistic inhalation of vapors, most of our history of inhalant use comes during the age of modern chemistry. Two of the oldest known psychoactive inhalants include nitrous oxide and ether. After Joseph Priestley discovered nitrous oxide in 1776, Sir Humphrey Davy in the same year discovered that it produced an excited state, hence the name *laughing gas*. Davy gathered together many people for nitrous oxide parties. We attribute the discovery of nitrous oxide's anesthetic effects to Horace Wells, who observed an individual's apparent lack of pain while intoxicated with nitrous oxide and decided to try it out for pulling teeth, albeit with limited success. However, other dentists and physicians perfected its use, and nitrous oxide remains a common anesthetic gas today (Brecher, 1972).

Some of the first reports of inhalant sniffing occurred immediately after World War II (Kerner, 1988). The first scientific report on glue sniffing came out in the *Journal of the American Medical Association* in 1959, which reported on arrests for glue sniffing made in Arizona and Colorado (Glaser & Massengale, 1962). The first major indication of an epidemic came from a

Stop & Check

1. What is the most commonly abused inhalant?
2. In addition to ease of access, what is another practical reason why adolescents abuse toluene?
3. Although nitrous oxide first gained notoriety as laughing gas, what was an important therapeutic use of this inhalant?

1. Toluene, which is found in many types of glue. **2.** The effects of toluene wear off quickly, allowing for an adolescent, for example, to sniff glue after school and then go home sober soon after. **3.** Nitrous oxide exhibits anesthetic effects and eventually became an important anesthetic gas for dental procedures.

report by Bass (1970), who reported 110 cases of sudden death occurring from inhalant abuse. Today, although these remain legal substances because of their use in everyday products, many states and localities have laws banning glue sniffing and the abuse of other inhalants (Brecher, 1972; Williams & Storck, 2007).

Inhalants: Rapid Absorption and Elimination

Users generally administer inhalants by taking a series of inhalations over 15–20 minutes, briefly achieving inhalant concentrations of more than 6,000 parts per million. Three common approaches to inhaling solvents are called *sniffing*, *huffing*, and *bagging*. Sniffing involves directly inhaling vapors emitted from a small container or a soaked cloth. Huffing involves placing a soaked cloth directly over the mouth or nose, usually to increase the amount of compound inhaled. Bagging consists of a user placing a compound in a small paper or plastic bag and then inhaling the contained vapors (Kurtzman et al., 2001; Lubman, Yucel, & Lawrence, 2008).

Most inhalants offer high lipid solubility, making for rapid absorption and penetration through tissues, including the brain. In animals, intravenous delivery of toluene achieves peak levels in the brain within 1–3 minutes, and these brain levels of toluene reduce by half after approximately 20 minutes. However, toluene eliminates more slowly from white matter in the brain and reduces by half after 30 minutes (Gerasimov, 2004). As described previously, the rapid elimination of inhalants offers an important practical appeal to adolescents who seek to sober up before going home after school.

Actions of Inhalable Solvents

As already noted, inhalants represent a large class of diverse compounds that lead to a variety of different pharmacological actions. This chapter focuses on the actions of toluene and related inhalable chemicals because these are the most commonly abused inhalants. Toluene and most other inhalants elicit depressant effects through mechanisms shared with alcohol, including antagonism of NMDA* receptors and positive modulation of GABA$_A$ receptors.

REVIEW! Positive modulators increase the ability of a neurotransmitter to bind to and activate a receptor. Chapter 4 (pg. 120).

Like alcohol, acute toluene administration acts as a noncompetitive antagonist for NMDA receptors, eliminating the flow of ions through the NMDA channel (Cruz, Mirshahi, Thomas, Balster, & Woodward, 1998). Several days of repeated toluene exposure leads to an increase in NMDA receptors, suggesting a potential mechanism for pharmacodynamic tolerance (Bale, Tu, Carpenter-Hyland, Chandler, & Woodward, 2005). Also like alcohol, acute toluene administration increases the activation of GABA$_A$ receptors by serving as a positive modulator, and repeated toluene administration results in decreased activation of GABA$_A$ receptors (Bale, Tu,

---

*NMDA = N-methyl-D-aspartate.

Carpenter-Hyland, Chandler, & Woodward, 2005; Beckstead, Weiner, Eger, Gong, & Mihic, 2000). Beyond NMDA and GABA$_A$ receptors, toluene may also function as an antagonist for serotonin (5-HT$_3$) receptors and nicotinic receptors (Lopreato, Phelan, Borghese, Beckstead, & Mihic, 2003).

Microdialysis studies evaluating toluene's ability to enhance nucleus accumbens dopamine levels, an action usually predictive of a drug's reinforcing effects, provide mixed results. Gerasimov and colleagues (2002) failed to find changes in dopamine concentrations in the nucleus accumbens in rats exposed to 3,000 parts per million toluene. On the other hand Riegel and colleagues (2007) found increased dopamine concentrations in the nucleus accumbens in rats after administration of toluene directly into the ventral tegmental area. Yet these authors found that dopamine occurred at a specific dose of toluene; above or below this level, doses failed to increase dopamine concentrations in the nucleus accumbens.

Inhalants: Pharmacological Effects and Interference with Oxygen Intake

Like many other depressant drugs, toluene and other inhalants initially exhibit stimulant-like effects and later exhibit depressant-like effects. From reviewing numerous clinical studies on acute inhalant effects, Kurtzman and colleagues (2001) describe four general stages of inhalant effects (**table 9.2**). The first stage begins within a few minutes after inhalation. During the first stage, an inhalant elicits stimulant-like positive subjective effects, including excitation, euphoria, and exhilaration. As these researchers report, this stage resembles the initial effects of alcohol for most users.

The second stage consists of many behavioral effects that resemble alcohol intoxication. The behavioral effects include disorientation, slurred speech, and confusion. However, unlike general alcohol intoxication, toluene may also produce hallucinations, particularly during frequent use (Cruz & Dominguez, 2011). The third stage of inhalant intoxication consists of further depressant effects, including a blunting of sensations and poor motor coordination.

table **9.2**

Stages of Inhalant Effects	
Stage	**Effects**
1	Stimulant-like positive subjective effects, including excitation, euphoria, and exhilaration.
2	Behavioral effects resembling alcohol intoxication, including disorientation, slurred speech, and confusion. Hallucinations may occur.
3	Enhanced depressant effects, including blunted sensations and impaired motor coordination.
4	Overdose consisting of stupor, unconsciousness, seizures, breathing cessation, and cardiac arrest.

© Cengage Learning 2014.

Depending on the amount of inhalant administered, users may also experience a fourth stage of intoxication that consists of an overdose condition characterized by a series of adverse effects including stupor, seizure, unconsciousness, cessation of breathing, and cardiac arrest. Adverse effects during the fourth stage serve as the primary features of **sudden sniffing death syndrome**. Poor oxygen availability is another important contributor to sudden sniffing death syndrome. Oxygen impoverishment occurs when inhalant vapors compete with the inhalation and absorption of oxygen. Low oxygen levels significantly impair brain and cardiovascular function. Sudden sniffing death syndrome can occur when someone is startled while highly intoxicated with an inhalant. In particular, this may occur if an adolescent sniffing glue is caught by a parent. Oxygen delivery serves as the primary treatment for treating inhalant overdose (Alper et al., 2008; Kurtzman et al., 2001).

Chronic heavy use of inhalants can produce severe neural damage, including cortical white matter degeneration and ventricle enlargement, an indicator of brain tissue loss (Rosenberg, Grigsby, Dreisbach, Busenbark, & Grigsby, 2002). This damage is consistent with a study conducted by Hormes and colleagues (1986) in inhalant users. These researchers assessed individuals who used high concentration of toluene chronically for more than 2 years. Most of these individuals exhibited severe cognitive impairment, muscle weakness, tremor, poor eye tracking, poor hearing, and a poor sense of smell.

According to the DSM-IV, chronic inhalant use may also develop into an inhalant dependence. During dependence, a user may exhibit tolerance as defined by requiring greater amounts of an inhalant to achieve the same effect. Although the DSM defines inhalant dependence as being similar to most substance dependence disorders, it states that withdrawal symptoms either do not occur or are generally mild and not clinically significant (American Psychiatric Association, 2012). In a study by Ridenour and colleagues (2007), however, 11 percent of inhalant-dependent users described experiencing headaches, nausea, hallucinations, craving for an inhalant, depressed mood, and fast heartbeat as time passed after inhalant use. However, these authors did note that unlike most substance dependencies, withdrawal symptoms most likely occur after a binge with inhalants and tend to occur for only one or two days.

sudden sniffing death syndrome Inhalant overdose characterized by a series of adverse effects including stupor, seizure, unconsciousness, cessation of breathing, and cardiac arrest.

Stop & Check

1. What is the primary pharmacological action of inhalable solvents?
2. The primary adverse physiological effects of inhalable solvents result from competition with _____.
3. What types of brain damage occur during long-term inhalant use?

1. Inhalable solvents facilitate activation of GABA receptors. **2.** oxygen **3.** Researchers find degeneration of cortical white matter and enlarged ventricles.

FROM ACTIONS TO EFFECTS
Stimulus Properties of GHB and Toluene

As first presented in Chapter 6, box 6.1, drug-discrimination procedures provide the ability to determine similarities among the subjective effects of different drugs. Researchers also use this procedure to determine the role different receptor actions may play in a drug's subjective effects. Drug-discrimination procedures provide important information on the receptor actions for depressant drugs, as illustrated in the section on the discriminative stimulus properties of GHB and toluene.

Cook and colleagues (2006) conducted a drug-discrimination study using mice trained to discriminate a dose of GHB versus saline—that is, a placebo. After the mice learned to perform this discrimination accurately, the researchers gave the mice doses of alcohol to determine which lever the mice would choose. When given alcohol, some mice responded on the GHB lever but others responded on the saline lever, suggesting to these researchers that alcohol's subjective effects do not closely resemble GHB's subjective effects.

As an important next step in this research area, Baker and colleagues (2008) conducted a three-lever drug-discrimination procedure that required rats to discriminate alcohol for one lever, versus GHB for another lever, versus saline for the third lever. In this way, rats had to attend to the different subjective effects between alcohol and GHB to accurately learn this procedure. After the rats achieved a high accuracy of performance, these researchers conducted a series of tests to determine the receptors important for the discriminative stimulus effects for these compounds.

The study by Baker and colleagues (2008) provided several interesting findings about the discriminative stimulus effects of GHB (**figure 9.7**). First, both GBL and 1,4-butanediol led animals to respond on the GHB-appropriate lever, probably because GBL and 1,4-butanediol convert to GHB in the body through metabolic processes. Second, a benzodiazepine drug, which functions as a $GABA_A$ positive modulator, led to more responses on the alcohol lever and few responses on the GHB lever, suggesting that, consistent with GHB's known pharmacological actions, $GABA_A$ receptor actions do not contribute to GHB's subjective effects.

Third, administration of the $GABA_B$ receptor agonist baclofen led animals to press the GHB lever, which supports pharmacological evidence that GHB acts as a $GABA_B$ receptor agonist. Finally, when the researchers administered the NMDA receptor antagonist ketamine, rats mostly responded on the alcohol lever rather than the GHB lever. This also supports known pharmacological evidence, because alcohol serves as an antagonist at NMDA receptors, whereas GHB appears devoid of NMDA receptor effects.

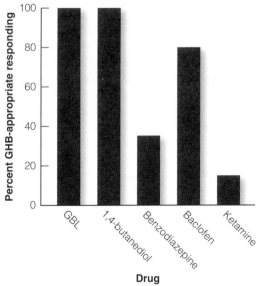

figure 9.7
Drug-discrimination experiments reveal receptor actions important for GHB's subjective effects. For simplicity, this figure only shows the percentage of responses occurring on the GHB-appropriate lever. See text for further details on this study. (Data from Baker et al., 2008.)

Drug-discrimination findings also correspond with the pharmacological actions of toluene. For example, Rees and colleagues (1987) trained mice to discriminate toluene, which was injected as a liquid solution, from the drug's vehicle. They first verified that mice would press the toluene lever and administered toluene via inhalation. After verifying this, they found that administration of the GABA$_A$ receptor positive modulator pentobarbital led to toluene lever responding. This finding coincides with toluene's positive modulation of GABA$_A$ receptors.

In a separate study, Shelton and Balster (2004) trained mice to discriminate an NMDA receptor antagonist, dizocilpine, from saline in a drug-discrimination task. Although toluene exhibits antagonism of NMDA receptors, the mice failed to choose the dizocilpine lever after toluene administration. The researchers concluded that NMDA receptor antagonism may not be important for toluene's subjective effects, as far as this model can identify.

|||||||||||||||||||||||||||||||||||||||||||||||||||||||||||||||||||||||||||||||||||||||||||||||||||||||||||||||||||||||||||||||||||||||||||||||||||||||||||||||

Stop & Check

1. What do drug-discrimination procedures tell us about the subjective effects of GHB?

2. What mediates the stimulus properties of toluene?

1. Although pharmacological procedures determine the receptor actions of psychoactive drugs, drug-discrimination procedures link these receptor actions to a drug's subjective effects. For GHB, we learn that activation of GABA$_B$ receptors contribute to its subjective effects. We also learn that the prodrugs GBL and 1,4-butanediol also produce GHB-like subjective effects, likely by producing GHB through metabolism. 2. Based on drug-discrimination procedures, positive modulation GABA$_A$ receptors elicit toluene-like stimulus properties.

▶ CHAPTER SUMMARY

Gamma-hydroxybutyrate (GHB) is both a drug and a neurotransmitter that produces depressant effects. The drug is colorless and tasteless and used as a recreational substance, sexual assault drug, and therapeutically to treat narcolepsy. Because GHB is a controlled substance, many users instead seek one of GHB's prodrugs, GBL or 1,4-butanediol. Neurotransmitter synthesis of GHB begins with the inhibitory neurotransmitter GABA. GHB is stored in vesicles with GABA; when released, it binds to GHB receptors and GABA$_B$ receptors. The pharmacological effects of GHB include prolonged deep sleep, confusion, drowsiness, memory impairment as well as positive subjective effects such as euphoria and optimism.

Inhalants include volatile alkyl nitrites, nitrous oxide and volatile solvents, fuels, and anesthetics, among which toluene is the most used. Adolescents serve as the greatest majority of inhalant users. Inhalants absorb rapidly, readily penetrate tissues, and then have short-lasting effects. Their pharmacological actions depend on antagonism of NMDA receptors and positive modulation of GABA$_A$ receptors. Inhalants produce a time-dependent course of stimulant and depressant effects. Inhalant overdose may lead to sudden sniffing death syndrome, and long-term inhalant abuse may damage parts of the brain.

KEY TERMS

Gamma-hydroxybutyrate (GHB)

Inhalants

Sudden sniffing death

syndrome

Electroencephalography

Evoked potential

Event-related potential

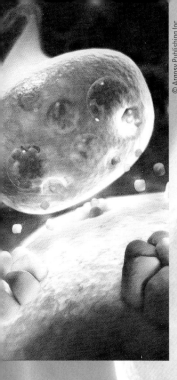

© Argosy Publishing Inc.

CHAPTER **10**

Opioids

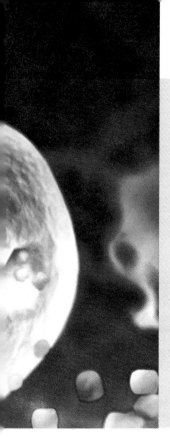

A "Treatment" for Morphine Addiction?

At the turn of the 19th century, Americans had an epidemic of morphine use. The drug's powerful analgesic effects made it popular medicine for a variety of ailments, but around this time morphine's withdrawal effects became a concern. This led to a medical dilemma: Maintaining morphine treatment led to tolerance and the emergence of withdrawal symptoms if physicians did not increase the dose. On the other hand, removing morphine not only led to withdrawal symptoms but also the natural reemergence of symptoms the drug was meant to treat. Searching for answers, physicians took an unfortunate turn toward a "treatment" that was said to prevent morphine withdrawal and any subsequent problems emerging from removing morphine. Unfortunately the cure— heroin—was worse, a problem not fully realized until scientists discovered heroin's chemical relationship to morphine years later.

From Duarte (2005).

opioids Psychoactive substances that elicit pharmacological effects by acting on opioid receptors in the CNS and other parts of the body.

Opioids consist of psychoactive substances that elicit pharmacological effects by acting on opioid receptors in the central nervous system (CNS) and other parts of the body. They are among the most effective pain-relieving medications today and among the most sought after substances for abuse. The term *narcotic*, from Latin for "sleep-inducing," generally serves as a synonymous term for an opioid compound, although narcotic is used imprecisely to describe many other types of controlled substances, including psychostimulant drugs such as cocaine.

Opioids serve as major drugs of abuse in the United States. The prevalence of opioid abuse is not only due because of its reinforcing effects but also because of its ease of access. In 2008, there were 213,000 reported heroin users in the United States, up from 153,000 only a year before. Prescription opioid drugs such as hydrocodone (Vicodin) and oxycodone (OxyContin) are also popular because they produce powerful reinforcing effects and are easy to obtain. In 2010, 8 percent of all 12th-grade high school students had abused Vicodin within the past year.

Many individuals obtain opioids by drinking over-the-counter cough syrups that contain the opioid drug dextromethorphan. Dextromethorphan represents the "DM" in the brand name cough syrup Robitussin DM. The slang term *robo-tripping* refers to drinking large quantities of cough syrups for recreational opioid use. Recreational cough syrup use was reported in 6.3 percent of 12th-grade high school students in 2009 (Substance Abuse and Mental Health Services Administration, 2010).

Opioids: Natural and Synthetic

There are two main types of opioid compounds: those produced naturally in the environment and those produced through chemical synthesis in a laboratory. Natural opioids are found in opium exudant from poppy plants, *Paver somniferum. Paver somniferum* is an annual flowering plant that stands 3 to 4 feet high and has a vibrant pink, red, white, or violet flower (**figure 10.1**).

A large seedpod, as shown in figure 10.1, is revealed after the flower petals fall off only 2–4 days after flowering. After scoring the pod with a knife, a white substance emerges that turns red when exposed to air. This reddish resin is raw opium, and the opium is scraped from the seedpod to be used as is or for further refinement and processing (Booth, 1998). Most opium production occurs in Afghanistan, with production also found in Pakistan, Myanmar, Colombia, and Mexico (United Nations Office of Drugs and Crime, 2010).

The primary **naturally occurring opioids** found in opium are morphine and codeine (Wu & Wittick, 1977). The U.S. Drug Enforcement Administration (DEA) categorizes morphine and codeine as controlled substances, but they are

naturally occurring opioids Opioids found in opium, including morphine and codeine.

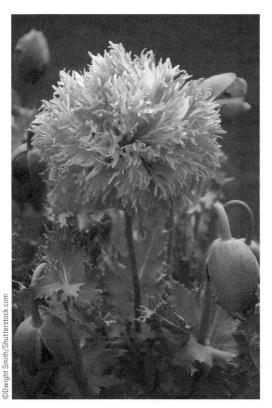

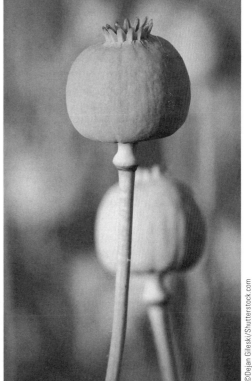

figure **10.1** *Paver somniferum* is an annual flowering plant that reveals an opium-containing seedpod after its petals fall off.

table **10.1**

DEA Schedules for Selected Opioids	
Drug	**Schedule**
Buprenorphine	III
Codeine for cough syrup preparations	V
Diacetylmorphine (heroin)	I
Fentanyl	I
Hydrocodone	II
Morphine	II
Inhalation	II
Opium extract	II
Thebaine	II

Adapted from the DEA Controlled Substances Schedules. (http://www. deadiversion.usdoj.gov /schedules/index.html)

not schedule I substances because of their legitimate medical uses. Morphine is a schedule II drug and is only available in hospitals, and codeine is a schedule III or IV product, depending on the quantity, and is used in prescription cough suppressants (Drug Enforcement Administration, 2012b) (**table 10.1**). Thebaine is another component of opium but is a relatively minor component and exhibits different pharmacological effects (Wu & Wittick, 1977).

All other opioids are synthetically produced (**table 10.2**). Semisynthetic opioids are synthesized from morphine or codeine. Semisynthetic opioids include diacetylmorphine (heroin), buprenorphine (Subutex), hydrocodone, and oxycodone (OxyContin). Percoset is a combination of oxycodone and acetaminophen (Tylenol), and Vicodin is a combination of hydrocodone and acetaminophen. **Fully synthetic opioids** are not derived from morphine, codeine, or any other naturally occurring opioids. Fully synthetic opioids include fentanyl (Duragesic), methadone (Dolophine), and levacetylmethadyl (LAAM).

Naturally occurring opioids and synthetic opioids were developed for medicinal purposes. However, many opioids such as heroin offer powerful reinforcing effects, precluding their medical use because of their addiction risk.

fully synthetic opioids Opioids not derived from morphine, codeine, or any other naturally occurring opioid.

table **10.2**

Opioids		
Naturally occurring	Morphine	Codeine
Semisynthetic	Buprenorphine (Subutex) Diacetylmorphine (Heroin)	Hydrocodone (Vicodin) Oxycodone (Oxycontin)
Fully synthetic	Fentanyl (Duragesic) Levacetylmethadyl (LAAM)	Methadone (Dolophine)

Producers illegally synthesize heroin from morphine through a process that begins with extracting morphine from opium and then applying industrial chemical agents to synthesize heroin. After synthesis in clandestine laboratories, heroin is packed and illegally shipped throughout the world (Hosztafi, 2001).

Stop & Check

1. Why are opioid drugs easy to access?
2. What are the two primary opioids in poppy plants?
3. Morphine is used in the clandestine production of _____, a common recreationally used opioid drug.

1. Although known illicit drugs such as heroin remain available, many users abuse prescription and over-the-counter medications that contain opioids. 2. Morphine and codeine 3. heroin

History of Opium Use

Opium has been used since prehistoric times. Archeological research revealed evidence of *Paver somniferum* plants in neolithic villages in Switzerland. Historical records indicate opium cultivation in Egypt and Asia Minor in 3000 B.C., and ancient medical texts throughout Europe, the Middle East, and northern Africa list numerous medical uses for opium. Greek physician Hippocrates (460–357 B.C.) detailed the sleep-inducing and pain-relieving effects of opium and dismissed the magical interpretation of these effects by priests. Theophrastus (371–287 B.C.), a philosopher, referred to poppy juices as *opion*, which is now translated as *opium* (Duarte, 2005).

After Rome conquered Greece, opium soon became intertwined with Roman culture and became a treatment for a virtual endless list of maladies, including deafness, poisoning, and leprosy. The Romans regarded the poppy plant as a symbol of pain and death and regarded it as a convenient lethal poison. Arabs during this time cultivated and sold opium as a trading commodity. Moreover, they advanced the medical study of opium. Arab physician Avicenna (980–1037 A.D.) medically used opium for dysentery, diarrhea, and eye diseases as part of his 14-volume *Canon of Medicine*.

In the 16th century, Europeans developed and popularized a number of opium-containing medical potions, including laudanum. In the 1660s, English physician Thomas Sydenham developed the most common variety of laudanum. In this version, Sydenham comprised a drink containing opium, cinnamon, saffron, and fortified wine from the Canary Islands.

During the 19th century, drug stores legally sold opium products such as morphine. In addition to selling morphine or another opioid as is, various elixirs for treating illnesses and pain contained morphine or a similar substance. Near the end of the 19th century, the addictive effects of opioids received greater focus, and the beginning of the 20th century marks the religious and political movements leading up to the Harrison Act of 1914 (Booth, 1998; Duarte, 2005).

The Harrison Act did not directly ban opioid use, but rather limited the prescribing and sale of opioids for medical uses. Law enforcement interpreted this law as a means to prevent physicians from prescribing opioids to reduce opioid withdrawal symptoms. The enforcement of this law triggered an epidemic of addicted individuals who, according to a New York Medical Journal editorial on May 15, 1915, led to "crimes of violence . . . due usually to desperate effects by addicts to obtain drugs, but occasionally to a delirious state induced by sudden withdrawal" (Brecher, 1972). Many other controlled substances acts followed. Today, opioids are among the most highly regulated medicines.

The terminology for opioids has changed over the years. Originally, the term *opiate* referred only to opium-derived compounds. The term *opioids* referred to other opioid drugs. For example, under this distinction, morphine is an *opiate*, whereas heroin is an *opioid* (Steinberg & Sykes, 1985). However, these conventions are seldom followed, and in general the term *opioid* describes all types of opioid and opiate compounds. Thus, *opioid* is the term used throughout this chapter.

Stop & Check

1. What was the primary use of opium in ancient human history?
2. What was the first major U.S. law enacted to regulate opioid drug sales?

1. Opium was primarily used as a medicine in ancient history. Even though opioids are still used medicinally, their addictive properties have garnered much attention in modern history. 2. The Harrison Act of 1914

Pharmacokinetic Properties and Opioid Abuse

In general, users administer opioids through inhalation, oral administration, or intravenous administration. The preferred routes of opioid administration depend on the particular drug and the purpose for using it. To achieve reinforcing effects, users prefer intravenous injection or inhalation for a rapid speed of onset. The intravenous route also provides immediate relief from pain. Physicians prescribe codeine for oral administration to suppress coughing (Farré & Camí, 1991). After absorption, opioids permeate the blood–brain barrier and enter the brain. Opioids differ in lipid solubility, affecting the time it takes them to reach the brain. For example, heroin crosses through the blood–brain barrier faster than morphine, which may explain why users prefer heroin over morphine for achieving reinforcing effects (Oldendorf, Hyman, Braun, & Oldendorf, 1972) (**figure 10.2**).

Opioids are primarily metabolized in the liver, often producing metabolites that have biological effects. Morphine, for example, produces the biologically active metabolite morphine-6-glucoronide, a potent analgesic that may account for many of morphine's analgesic effects (Christrup, 1997). Opioid metabolites provide key indicators of opioid use and are detectable in urine samples. However, the presence of opioid metabolites may not identify

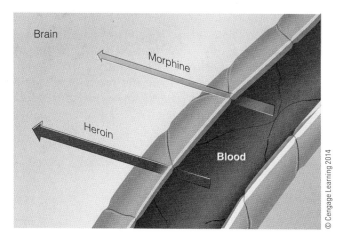

figure 10.2   Because of its greater lipid solubility, heroin enters the brain more readily than morphine.

the exact opioid used. For example, morphine is a metabolite of codeine and a secondary metabolite of heroin (Rook, Hillebrand, Rosing, van Ree, & Beijnen, 2005; Yeh & Woods, 1970) (**figure 10.3**). Thus, the presence of morphine in a urine sample could suggest morphine, codeine, or heroin use, but not the exact drug used.

If a technician needs to identify the precise opioid used, then other metabolites must be tested for. For example, heroin is metabolized to monoacetylmorphine, which is then converted to morphine. The presence of both monoacetylmorphine and morphine might suggest heroin use. In addition, street heroin often includes acetylcodeine, which is metabolized to codeine. The added presence of codeine in a urine analysis would further indicate heroin use.

The elimination rate of opioids varies from drug to drug. Many heroin-cessation programs prescribe patients methadone, partly because of methadone's long elimination rate. Methadone levels peak in the body several hours

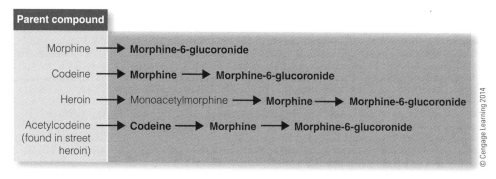

figure 10.3   Many opioid drugs have active metabolites, often including morphine. The active metabolites appear in bold.

after administration and remain at biologically active levels 24 hours after administration (Vos, Ufkes, Wilgenburg, Geerlings, & Brink, 1995). Although methadone remains in the body, it functions to prevent heroin withdrawal symptoms from occurring. The semisynthetic opioid buprenorphine also exhibits a weak euphoric effect and offers long elimination rate. Given these traits, opioid-cessation programs also use buprenorphine as a substitute for an addictive opioid drug (Comer, Collins, & Fischman, 2001).

Stop & Check

1. Opioids are usually administered orally, intravenously, or through _____.
2. What is a common active metabolite of many opioid drugs?

1. inhalation 2. Morphine and morphine-6-glucuronide

Opioid Drug Interactions with the Endogenous Opioid System

The endogenous opioid system includes opioid neurotransmitters and receptors. These endogenous neurotransmitters are neuropeptides and are produced from three propeptides: proopiomelanocortin, proenkephalin, and prodynorphin. Cleavage of proopiomelanocortin produces β-endorphin (**figures 10.4 and 10.5**). Cleavage of proenkephalin produces met-enkephalin and leu-enkephalin, and cleavage of prodynorphin produces dynorphin A, dynorphin B, and neoendorphin (Chavkin, James, & Goldstein, 1982; Comb, Seeburg, Adelman, Eiden, & Herbert, 1982; Hughes, Smith, Morgan, & Fothergill, 1975).

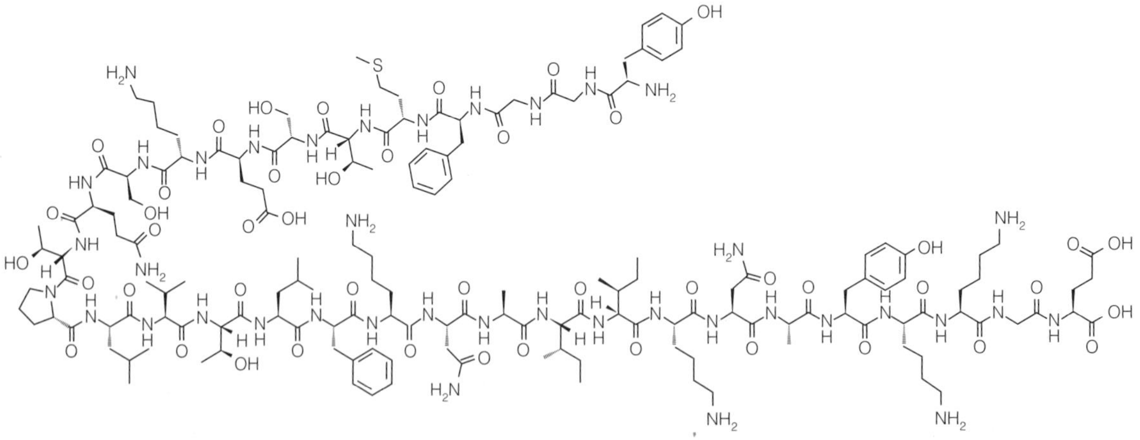

figure 10.4 The endogenous opioid β-endorphin is comprised of 31 amino acids. A strand of amino acids is called a *peptide*, and shorter peptides such as β-endorphin are "cleaved" from longer peptides called *propeptides*. To better illustrate the origin of opioid peptides, the schematics shown in figure 10.5 are used.

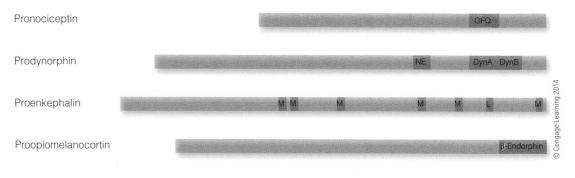

These schematics illustrate propeptides and constituent peptides. The dynorphin A and B peptides are represented as a segment of the propeptide prodynorphin. There are multiple leu- and met-enkaphalin peptides found on proenkephalin, and β-endorphin is a peptide found on proopiomelanocortin. OFQ=orphanin FQ, NE =neoendorphin, DynA = dynorphin A, DynB=Dynorphin B, and M=met-enkephalin, L=leu-enkephalin.

figure **10.5**

REVIEW! Neuropeptides are synthesized within a neuron's soma. They are often a segment of a longer peptide known as a *propeptide*. *Cleavage* refers to the separation of this segment from a longer peptide. Chapter 3 (pg. 92).

The endogenous opioids bind to three types of opioid receptors: β-endorphin, met-enkephalin, and leu-enkephalin bind to μ (pronounced "mu") opioid receptors and δ ("delta") opioid receptors. The dynorphin neurotransmitters selectively bind to κ ("kappa") receptors (**table 10.3**). Most of the pharmacological effects associated with opioids are derived through activating μ and δ receptors (Trigo, Martin-García, Berrendero, Robledo, & Maldonado, 2010). Kappa receptors, on the other hand, elicit hallucinogenic effects (Roth et al., 2002). A kappa receptor drug called *salvinorin A* is presented in Chapter 12.

The endogenous opioid system may also include the neuropeptide nociceptin. Nociceptin, also known as *orphanin FQ*, is produced from pre-pronociceptin and binds to the opioid receptorlike-1 (ORL-1) receptor. The ORL-1 receptor is also called the *nociceptin receptor*. The structure of the

table **10.3**

Endogenous Opioid Neurotransmitters and Their Matching Receptors	
Endogenous opioid neurotransmitter	**Receptor activated**
β-endorphin	μ (mu) δ (delta)
Met-enkephalin and leu-enkephalin	μ δ
Dynorphin	κ (kappa)
Nociceptin	ORL-1

© Cengage Learning 2014

ORL-1 receptor is similar to other opioid receptors, supporting the case that nociceptin is another opioid neurotransmitter.

Beyond these structural similarities, the ORL-1 receptor exhibits pharmacological effects that oppose those of other opioid receptors. In particular, the activation of ORL-1 receptors can limit the analgesic effects produced by μ opioid receptor agonists such as morphine. The location of ORL-1 receptors may account for these and other opposing effects. ORL-1 receptors are either located on different neurons than other opioid receptors or found on a different part of the neuron where other opioid receptors are located (Meunier, 1997).

Opioid receptors, including the ORL-1 receptor, are G-protein–coupled metabotropic receptors. Through activation of G proteins, these receptors reduce metabolic activity within neurons. The internal neuronal mechanisms involved in these inhibitory effects are complex and not entirely identified. One known inhibitory mechanism consists of the activation of inwardly rectifying K^+ channels. A **G-protein–coupled inwardly rectifying K^+ channel (GIRK)**, causes the influx of K^+ when a neuron is hyperpolarized and diminished K^+ influx when a neuron is depolarized. Through these properties, GIRKs help maintain a neuron's resting potential. When these membrane channels are activated, which happens from activation of ORL-1 receptors, a neuron's membrane potential approaches a resting potential (Meunier, 1997; Trigo et al., 2010).

G-protein–coupled inwardly rectifying K^+ channel (GIRK) A K^+ channel that causes the influx of K^+ when a neuron is hyperpolarized and less K^+ influx when a neuron is depolarized.

REVIEW! A resting potential describes a negatively charged local potential that precedes an action potential. Chapter 3 (pg. 67).

Adaptation occurs to opioids during repeated administration. One of these adaptive processes involves a reduction in sodium–potassium pump activity. By reducing this activity, a neuron membrane adapts to the inhibitory effects of opioids by depolarizing the membrane. This adaptive process increases the excitability of a neuron, which serves to counteract an opioid drug's inhibitory effects. When an opioid drug is not present, this state of depolarization increases a neuron's activity (Trigo et al., 2010).

REVIEW! The sodium–potassium pump maintains a negative resting state potential by expelling three Na^+ ions for every two K^+ ions brought into a neuron. Chapter 3 (pg. 69).

Opioid Drugs: Classification by Receptor Action

pure opioid receptor agonists Drugs that act as full receptor antagonists at μ opioid receptors.

Opioids differ in opioid receptor actions, and this in turn accounts for different pharmacological effects between opioids. Given this, opioids also are classified by their receptor actions. In particular, these receptor actions mostly refer to drugs acting on μ opioid receptors. **Pure opioid receptor agonists** produce full agonist actions at μ opioid receptors. Many of these drugs also act as full agonists at other opioid receptors. Morphine is an example of a pure opioid receptor agonist (Hughes, Kosterlitz, & Leslie, 1975).

partial opioid receptor agonists Drugs that produce partial agonist actions at μ opioid receptors and therefore do not produce the same magnitude of pharmacological effects achieved by pure opioid receptor agonists.

Many opioid drugs serve as **partial opioid receptor agonists**, producing partial agonist actions at μ opioid receptors and therefore not producing the same magnitude of pharmacological effects achieved by pure opioid receptor agonists. Buprenorphine is classified as a partial opioid receptor agonist and exhibits weaker pharmacological effects compared to a pure opioid receptor agonist such as morphine (Virk, Arttamangkul, Birdsong, & Williams, 2009). For example, Dahan and colleagues (2006) found that even though buprenorphine exhibited gains in pain-relieving effects as they raised the dose in human volunteers, a ceiling effect was reached for respiratory depressant effects. Thus, they concluded that buprenorphine serves as an analgesic opioid drug that fails to cause significant impairments in breathing. Other unique actions of buprenorphine are presented in the following text.

REVIEW! Partial agonists have a lower efficacy for activating receptors than full agonists do. Chapter 4 (pg. 120).

pure opioid receptor antagonists Drugs that act as full receptor antagonists at μ opioid receptors.

Pure opioid receptor antagonists act as full receptor antagonists at μ opioid receptors. These drugs not only fail to produce opioid pharmacological effects but also inhibit opioid system activity by preventing endogenous opioids from binding to opioid receptors. Physicians prescribe pure opioid receptor antagonists for treating opioid addiction (Fudala & Woody, 2002). The "From Actions to Effects" section describes this and other approaches for treating opioid addition.

mixed opioid receptor agonist–antagonists Drugs that exhibit agonist actions at some opioid receptors while exhibiting antagonist actions at other opioid receptors.

The final type of an opioid drug is a mixed opioid receptor agonist–antagonist. **Mixed opioid receptor agonist–antagonists** exhibit agonist actions at some opioid receptors while exhibiting antagonist actions at other opioid receptors. Together, these actions limit the magnitude of opioid pharmacological effects. For example, the mixed opioid receptor agonist–antagonist pentazocine (Talwin) exhibits a ceiling effect for reducing pain (Shu et al., 2011). Many opioids were once classified as mixed receptor agonist–antagonists but have since been found to act through other mechanisms such as partial agonism or through other receptors such as the recently discovered ORL-1 opioid receptor.

Buprenorphine is an opioid drug found to act through many mechanisms. First, as stated earlier, buprenorphine acts as a partial agonist at μ opioid receptors. Second, buprenorphine is an antagonist for δ receptors. Third, it has as an active metabolite, norbuprenorphine, which acts as a full agonist at both μ and δ receptors.

A fourth mechanism may contribute to buprenorphine's ceiling effects for pain. Buprenorphine is an agonist for the ORL-1 receptor. Activation of the ORL-1 receptor counteracts the pharmacological effects produced by the activation of other opioid receptor types. Thus, ORL-1 receptor activation opposes the effects produced through μ and δ receptor activation, accounting for buprenorphine's limiting effects for pain (Lutfy & Cowan, 2004).

Different mechanisms of action produced by opioid receptors produce different discriminative stimulus effects (see box 6.1 to review the drug-discrimination procedure). This was demonstrated in a study by Platt and

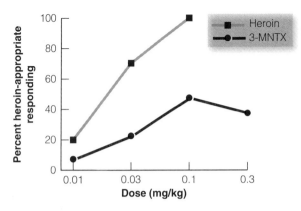

figure 10.6 In monkeys trained to discriminate the stimulus effects of heroin, heroin produced 100-percent heroin-appropriate responding, whereas the μ opioid receptor partial agonist 3-MNTX produced fewer heroin-appropriate responses. The y-axis shows the percentage of heroine-appropriate responses made, and the x-axis shows the dose of 3-MNTX or heroin tested. (Data from Platt et al., 2004.)

colleagues (2004) using rhesus monkeys trained to discriminate the stimulus effects of heroin, a pure opioid receptor agonist (**figure 10.6**). In these monkeys, full opioid receptor agonists produced heroin-like stimulus effects, whereas an experimental μ opioid receptor partial agonist called 3-MNTX produced weak heroin-like stimulus effects.

Stop & Check

1. Endogenous opioids are cleaved from four different _____.
2. Opioid receptors are G-protein–coupled receptors that produce _____ effects on neurons.
3. Should buprenorphine still be considered a representative drug for partial opioid receptor agonists?

1. propeptides **2.** inhibitory **3.** Although buprenorphine is still classified as a representative of the partial opioid receptor agonist class of drugs, it exhibits many other actions that may alternatively account for its pharmacological effects. In particular, buprenorphine's ceiling effect can be accounted for not only through partial opioid receptor agonism but also through antagonism of δ receptors and activation of ORL-1 receptors.

Opioid System Interactions with Reward, Pain, and Stress Systems

Endogenous and exogenous opioids produce reinforcing effects by affecting dopamine and GABA neurotransmission. Opioids increase dopamine release primarily by binding to μ opioid receptors on GABA neurons in the ventral tegmental area. **Figure 10.7** shows the series of actions involved in this reward circuitry.

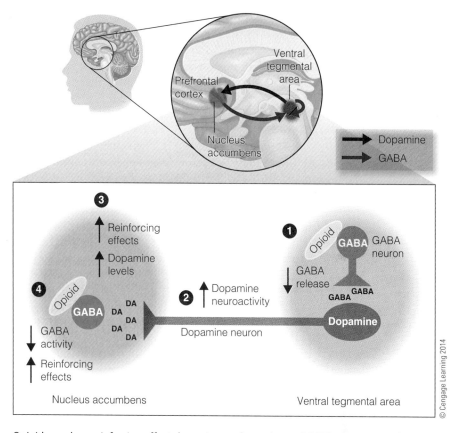

Opioids produce reinforcing effects by acting on dopamine and GABA neurons in either the ventral tegmental area or the nucleus accumbens. (1) This occurs through an opioid's activation of opioid receptors on GABA neurons in the ventral tegmental area, causing reduced GABA release and reduced activation of GABA receptors on dopamine neurons. (2) This in turn increases the activity of dopamine neurons. (3) This causes increased dopamine release in the nucleus accumbens, an action that increases reinforcing effects. (4) An opioid's activation of opioid receptors on nucleus accumbens GABA neurons causes a reduction in GABA neuron activity, an action associated with increased reinforcing effects.

figure 10.7

REVIEW! The ventral tegmental area contains dopamine neurons, which send axons to the nucleus accumbens, other parts of the limbic system, and the cerebral cortex. Chapter 3 (pg. 86).

First, opioids inhibit the activity of GABA neurons in the ventral tegmental area. In this structure, GABA activates inhibitory GABA receptors on dopamine neurons, causing a reduction in neuronal activity. Reduced dopamine neuronal activity causes less dopamine release in the nucleus accumbens and a subsequent reduction in reinforcing effects. Opioids prevent these inhibitory effects by reducing GABA release from GABA neurons. By removing this inhibition, the activity of dopamine neurons increases, leading to greater dopamine release in the nucleus accumbens (McBride, Murphy, & Ikemoto, 1999; Omelchenko & Sesack, 2010; Wise, 1989).

Second, opioids produce reinforcing effects through acting on μ opioid receptors in the nucleus accumbens. The majority of μ opioid receptors in the nucleus accumbens are found on GABA neurons. Many of these GABA neurons send axons to the ventral tegmental area, where they may contribute to the inhibition of dopamine neurons as just described. Here, too, opioids reduce the activity of GABA neurons, and this in turn disinhibits dopamine neuronal activity (Kalivas, Churchill, & Klitenick, 1993; McBride et al., 1999; Svingos, Moriwaki, Wang, Uhl, & Pickel, 1997; Wise, 1989).

Opioids also closely interact with pain afferents to the brain, as shown in **figure 10.8**. We can think of the communication of pain sensation, called *nociception*, to the brain as a relay involving two pathways. The first pathway includes two types of axons, referred to as Aδ and C fibers, that communicate nociceptive information from the source of a painful stimulus to the dorsal horn of the spinal cord. Within the dorsal horn, these pathways release the neurotransmitters glutamate and substance P at postsynaptic terminals on spinothalamic neurons. During inflammation or after suffering a trauma, enhanced pain sensitivity—called *hyperalgesia*—may occur because of a process of synaptic strengthening called *long-term potentiation* (described in detail in Chapter 12) (Ikeda et al., 2006). This process results in greater pain signaling between the first pain fibers and the spinothalamic neurons. Spinothalamic neurons send nociceptive information to the thalamus, which distributes it to the somatosensory cortex and two structures in the limbic system, the cingulate cortex and the amygdala. The somatosensory

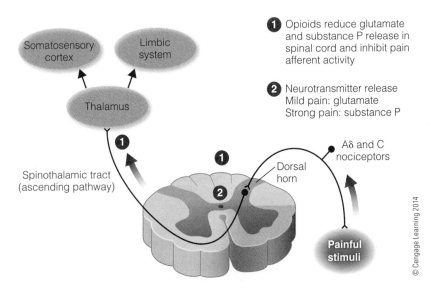

Opioids inhibit nociception by inhibiting glutamate and substance P release in the dorsal horn of the spinal cord and by decreasing the activity of neurons communicating pain information to the brain.

figure **10.8**

cortex processes the nociceptive information while the cingulate cortex and amygdala lead to emotional responses to pain and play a role in approach and avoidance behavior (Watkins, Milligan, & Maier, 2001; Willis & Westlund, 1997).

REVIEW! The peripheral nervous system sends sensory information to the dorsal horn of the spinal cord, whereas motor information comes from the ventral horn of the spinal cord. Chapter 2 (pg. 36).

Opioids weaken neurotransmission within these pain pathways. First, all four types of opioid receptors reside on C and Aδ axon terminals. The activation of these opioid receptors causes a reduction in glutamate and substance P release, thereby reducing pain signaling (Chen & Sommer, 2006; Ossipov et al., 2004). Chronic administration of opioids appears to produce long-term potentiation as a compensatory action for these inhibitory effects. Just as seen with inflammation and trauma, opioid withdrawal-induced long-term potentiation causes enhanced pain sensitivity (Drdla, Gassner, Gingl, & Sandkuhler, 2009). Second, neurons from parts of the periaqueductal gray release endogenous opioids in the medulla, which contains a high density of μ opioid receptors. Activating opioid receptors in the medulla inhibits the activity of spinothalamic neurons passing through the medulla, thus reducing nociceptive information flow to the thalamus (Ossipov et al., 2004).

Opioid receptors are found outside the nervous system as well, including the immune, cardiovascular, respiratory, and digestive systems (Stein, Schafer, & Hassan, 1995). These peripheral actions contribute to inhibition of respiration, cardiovascular function, and digestion by opioid receptor agonists. Chronic administration of an opioid agonist also suppresses immune system functioning by reducing the reproduction of immune system cells (Roy & Loh, 1996).

Opioid Reinforcing and Analgesic Effects

Opioid Receptor Agonists and Reinforcing Effects

The subjective effects of an opioid receptor agonist occur during four phases. The *rush* phase is the initial and rapid onset of euphoria that occurs within seconds of the injection of heroin or other opioid agonist. The rush is a key achievement for opioid recreational use. As the rush subsides, a second phase called the *high* sets in, which is generally characterized by feelings of joy and ease. A third phase is occasionally referred to as a *nod* and is characterized by calm, disinterest, and unawareness of surroundings. During the nod phase, anxiety is lifted and users may doze in a light sleep. Although the nod is different from euphoria, many users find this relaxed state to be quite enjoyable. Finally, the fourth phase is referred to as *straight* and consists of a period of normalcy between craving an opioid and feeling the euphoric or other positive effects of an opioid (Agar, 1974).

Based on surveys in humans, users report positive subjective effects from opioid receptor agonists. In one such study, Preston and colleagues (1988) assessed the subjective effects of the opioid receptor agonist hydromorphone by using questionnaires to rate the degree of *liking*, *high*, *good effects*, and other terms associated with a positive subjective experience. When asked to rate these effects some minutes after hydromorphone administration, all participants rated hydromorphone as highly enjoyable, according to these scales. The participants also were surveyed after receiving an injection of hydromorphone and the opioid receptor antagonist naloxone. After this treatment combination, the participants no longer recorded increases in liking, high, or good effects.

Self-administration procedures also indicate that opioid receptor agonists produce potent reinforcing effects. Further, the duration of these reinforcing effects alters drug-seeking behavior. A self-administration study conducted by Panlilio and Schindler (2000) demonstrated these properties (**figure 10.9**). In this study, rats were assessed on a progressive ratio schedule for opioid injections. In one group of rats, the opioid was heroin; in another group of rats, the opioid was remifentanil (Ultiva). Remifentanil exhibits similar actions to heroin, except that remifentanil has an elimination half-life of only 40 seconds!

Both heroin and remifentanil achieved similar break points in this study, but the remifentanil rats reached the break point much sooner than the heroin rats because of a much shorter postreinforcement during responding for remifentanil. Because the reinforcing effect of remifentanil was short lived, the rats quickly returned to lever pressing after every injection, thus shortening

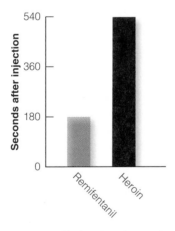

During a self-administration study, rats resumed responding more quickly after receiving an injection of the short action opioid agonist remifentanil than rats after receiving an administration of heroin. The y-axis shows the number of seconds between an injection and a following response. (Data from Panlilio & Schindler, 2000.)

figure 10.9

the postreinforcement pause. Heroin-treated rats had longer periods of time between receiving an injection and when they resumed lever pressing.

The subjective effects of opioids readily pair with environmental stimuli, which researchers demonstrate using a conditioned place preference procedure (see **box 10.1**). This procedure is often used to study the reinforcing effects of opioids such as heroin. For example, Spyraki and colleagues (1983) used a conditioned place preference procedure to study the effects of heroin administration in rats. A single dose of heroin was paired with one compartment of a shuttle box, and the heroin vehicle was paired with the opposite compartment for 4 days each. After pairing, rats spent significantly more time in the heroin-paired environment than the vehicle-paired environment (**figure 10.10**). A preference for the drug compartment implies an association between the compartment and heroin's reinforcing effects.

REVIEW! A *vehicle* is the solvent in which a drug is dissolved. Functionally, a vehicle is a placebo. Chapter 1 (pg. 13).

Researchers have also found a role for glutamate NMDA receptors in opioid reinforcing effects using the conditioned place preference procedure. In a study conducted by Popik and Kolasiewicz (1999) a conditioned place

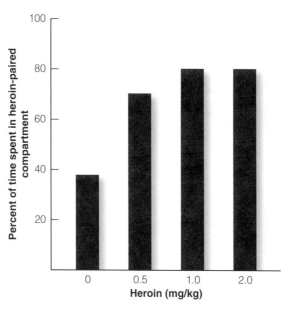

After pairing sessions were completed in a conditioned place preference procedure, rats preferred the shuttle-box compartment associated with heroin's pharmacological effects compared to the compartment not associated with these effects. The *y*-axis shows the percentage of time spent in the heroin-paired compartment. The *x*-axis shows the doses of heroin tested; a zero (0) dose refers to vehicle. (With kind permission from Springer Science+Business Media: Spyraki, C., Fibiger, H. C., & Phillips, A. G. (1983). Attenuation of heroin reward in rats by disruption of the mesolimbic dopamine system. *Psychopharmacology*, 79(2), 278–283. doi: 10.1007/bf00427827, p. 6.)

figure **10.10**

box **10.1** Conditioned Place Preference

During a **conditioned place preference** procedure, an organism associates a unique environment with a drug's reinforcing effects. Researcher's typically conduct this procedure with rats or mice using a shuttle box. Most shuttle boxes have two or three connected compartments with doorways between each compartment, as shown box 10.1 figure 1. Researchers design each compartment to have a different appearance (e.g., white walls versus black walls), floor texture (e.g., horizontal bars versus a wire grid), and odor in the compartment waste pans (e.g., pine shavings versus cellulose bedding).

A conditioned place preference develops over the course of several pairings with a reinforcing drug. Generally, researchers devote three to five pairing sessions with a drug's reinforcing effects and a specific shuttle-box

compartment. Other pairing sessions occur with the drug's vehicle and the opposite compartment. After drug- and vehicle-pairing sessions, researchers place a trained animal into the shuttle box with all compartment doors raised, allowing the animal free access to any compartment. A conditioned place preference is shown when rats spend significantly more time in the drug-paired compartment than in the vehicle-paired compartment.

To demonstrate the process of conditioned place preference, Mucha and colleagues (1982)

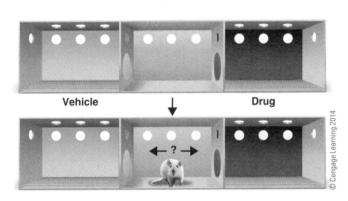

Vehicle   ↓   Drug

© Cengage Learning 2014

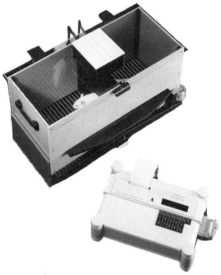

Ugo Basile Italy

box **10.1**, figure **1**

After pairing different parts of a shuttle box with either drug or vehicle (top row), researchers test for a conditioned place preference by placing a subject in a neutral part of the box and allowing the subject to freely explore the shuttle-box chambers.

preference for morphine was established in rats (**figure 10.11**). In the test session, where rats were given the choice to move freely between the morphine- and vehicle-paired compartments, these researchers treated rats with a glutamate NMDA receptor antagonist, called NPC17742. NPC17742 caused rats to have a significantly lower preference for the morphine-paired compartment. This reduction in preference for the morphine-paired compartment also occurred when NPC17742 was directly injected into the ventral tegmental area or the nucleus accumbens. Since this compound functioned as an antagonist for NMDA receptors, these researchers concluded that NMDA receptor agonism may, therefore, facilitate morphine's reinforcing effects.

conducted four pairing sessions with an intravenous morphine or saline injection given 4 minutes before the session. Each compartment contained different environment stimuli. After conducting four daily sessions each with morphine and saline, rats were placed in the chamber without an injection and allowed to explore both compartments. Rats spent significantly more time in the morphine-associated compartment than the saline-associated compartment.

Next, Mucha and colleagues (1982) conducted the same procedure with the noxious substance lithium chloride. After several pairings, rats spent significantly

more time in the saline-paired compartment. In this case, the researchers demonstrated a conditioned place aversion. During a **conditioned place aversion** procedure, an organism associates a unique environment with a drug's aversive effects. In this case, animals avoid the drug-paired side.

conditioned place preference Behavioral procedure in which an organism associates a unique environment with a drug's reinforcing effects.

conditioned place aversion Behavioral procedure in which an organism associates a unique environment with a drug's aversive effects.

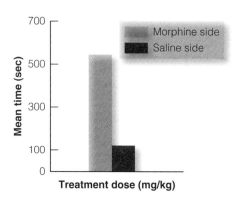

box 10.1, figure 2
Rats spent significantly more time in a morphine-paired compartment than a saline-paired compartment, demonstrating a conditioned place preference. The y-axis represents time spent in a compartment, and the x-axis represents the dose of morphine administered. Light blue bars refer to the morphine compartment. (Mucha et al., 1982. By permission.)

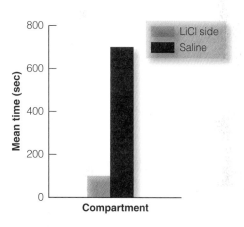

box 10.1, figure 3
Rats spent significantly more time in a saline-paired compartment than a lithium-chloride–paired compartment, demonstrating a conditioned place aversion. The y-axis represents time spent in a compartment. Light blue bars refer to the lithium-chloride compartment. (Mucha et al., 1982. By permission.)

REVIEW! During drug addiction, glutamate levels are elevated in mesolimbic dopamine structures, including the nucleus accumbens and ventral tegmental area. Increased glutamate levels lead to increased activation of glutamate NMDA receptors. Chapter 5 (pg. 146).

Self-administration studies also reveal a role for glutamate in an opioid drug's reinforcing effects. For example, LaLumiere and Kalivas (2008) conducted a reinstatement in period in rats that learned to self-administer heroin. After initiating reinstatement with an administration of heroin, microdialysis procedures revealed that nucleus accumbens concentrations of

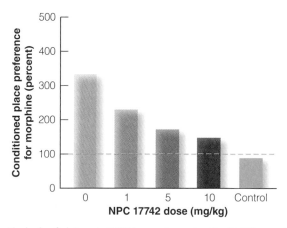

Blockade of glutamate NMDA receptors using the NMDA receptor antagonist NPC 17742 prevents the recall of the morphine preference for one side of a shuttle-box compartment. Glutamate release is an important contributor to opioid addiction. (With kind permission from Springer Science+Business Media: Popik, P., & Kolasiewicz, W. (1999). Mesolimbic NMDA receptors are implicated in the expression of conditioned morphine reward. *Naunyn-Schmiedeberg's Archives of Pharmacology*, 359(4), 288–294. doi: 10.1007/pl00005354, p. 7.)

figure 10.11

glutamate increased. After finding these changes in glutamate levels, these researchers found that they could prevent heroin reinstatement by inhibiting glutamate neurons that innervate the nucleus accumbens. From these findings, reducing glutamate neurotransmission may reduce a wanting state for heroin.

REVIEW! Reinstatement consists of a return to drug self-administration responding that usually occurs after an administration of the drug, presentation of a stimulus associated with the drug, or the causation of stress. Chapter 5 (pg. 141).

REVIEW! Wanting occurs when stimuli associated with drug use command attention and elicit a salient motivational state toward pursuing the drug. Chapter 5 (pg. 142).

Opioid Analgesic Effects

As noted previously, opioids have a traditional use for treating pain, and today they remain the most effective medications for this purpose. Morphine, the key constituent in opium, as described previously, represents the gold standard for opioid analgesics, although physicians frequently prescribe other μ opioid receptor agonists, including oxycodone and fentanyl, for severe pain management (Gomes et al., 2011). However, studies find that opioid analgesics lack significant efficacy for neuropathic pain, which is derived from damage to pain-signaling neurons, or idiopathic pain, which consists of pain derived from an unknown organic cause (Arnér & Meyerson, 1988).

Opioid Drugs and Other Therapeutic Effects

Beyond analgesia, the medicinal value of opioids is derived from other effects in the body. The inhibitory effects of opioid receptors in the intestinal tract produce constipation and provide an effective and important treatment for diarrhea. This has long been a key therapeutic use of opium, and opioid drugs are still used for this purpose today. For example, morphine is used in hospitals to reduce diarrhea associated with severe flu or other diseases (De Schepper, Cremonini, Park, & Camilleri, 2004; Shook, Lemcke, Gehrig, Hruby, & Burks, 1989).

Through activating inhibitory opioid receptors in the medulla, opioids also suppress the cough reflex. Therapeutically, opioids remain a highly effective cough suppressant. The natural opioid codeine is still used in prescription-strength cough syrups (Bolser, 2006). Opioids also constrict pupils, which occurs even in low light conditions. This effect, called **miosis**, is a direct effect of opioid receptor activation and occurs at analgesic doses (Ravnborg, Jensen, Jensen, & Holk, 1987).

miosis Pupil constriction that can occur after opioid administration.

Opioid Drugs and Respiratory Function

Opioids impair breathing, and respiratory depression is the primary cause of death from overdose. Respiratory depression occurs at therapeutically effective doses, but is not dangerous unless an individual suffers from a respiratory disorder such as emphysema. The respiratory inhibition is magnified by other drugs such as alcohol and benzodiazepines (Horlocker et al., 2009). Respiratory depression results from inhibitory effects in the medulla, the same area responsible for cough suppression (Etches, Sandler, & Daley, 1989).

User Tolerance and Dependence with Chronic Opioid Administration

Tolerance occurs to all opioid pharmacological effects during repeated opioid use. During chronic administration, users develop a physiological dependence that arises from compensatory actions that counteract an opioid drug's acute effects. These compensatory effects account for the physical withdrawal symptoms from opioids. For example, because opioids produce constipation, the related withdrawal effect is diarrhea. Opioids reduce pain, so the related withdrawal effect is increased pain sensitivity (Gossop, Bradley, & Phillips, 1987; Ossipov et al., 2004). Users also develop a tolerance for the reinforcing effects of opioids, resulting in the use of escalating doses to achieve desirable effects. Psychological withdrawal effects can include drug cravings and depressed mood (Gossop et al., 1987). **Table 10.4** lists these and other withdrawal effects from opioid use.

table **10.4**

| Opioid Pharmacological Effects and Withdrawal Symptoms ||
Acute pharmacological effect	Withdrawal symptom
Analgesia	Pain sensitivity
Constipation	Diarrhea
Decreased blood pressure	Increased blood pressure
Euphoria	Dysphoria and depression
Hypothermia	Hyperthermia
Relaxation	Restlessness
Respiratory depression	Hyperventilation

Based on Brecher, 1972.

Stop & Check

1. Opioids cause an increase in dopamine levels in the _____.
2. An advantage of using opioids is that they can reduce pain without inducing _____.
3. In ancient times, opium was considered effective for many different ailments. Why was this the case?

1. nucleus accumbens 2. sleep 3. Opium improved many symptoms associated with severe illness, including pain relief, diarrhea, and cough.

FROM ACTIONS TO EFFECTS
Pharmacological Approaches for Treating Opioid Addiction

detoxification Process that uses an opioid agonist or antagonist to reduce withdrawal symptoms.

long-term opioid detoxification
Detoxification process that lasts approximately 180 days and occurs by prescribing an opioid receptor agonist or a partial opioid receptor agonist to replace the illicit opioid drug.

Pharmacological treatments for opioid addiction include detoxification and the management of cormorbid disorders. **Detoxification** is the first step of an opioid-cessation program. Detoxification uses an opioid agonist or antagonist to reduce withdrawal symptoms. Detoxification procedures vary in time course, ranging from long-term detoxification to ultrarapid detoxification (**table 10.5**).

Long-term detoxification lasts approximately 180 days and occurs by prescribing an opioid receptor agonist (such as methadone or LAAM) or a partial opioid receptor agonist (such as buprenorphine) to replace the illicit opioid drug. These therapeutic opioid drugs prevent serious withdrawal symptoms, have long-lasting effects, and engender weak or no euphoria and other positive subjective effects (Gossop et al., 1987).

Long-term detoxification occurs outside of hospital settings. Instead, medications can be prescribed in a normal doctor's office or in *methadone clinics*. Methadone clinics must abide by regulations the FDA and the DEA for handling and dispensing methadone.

table 10.5

Detoxification Programs				
Detoxification type	Opioid receptor treatment	Approximate length	Facility	Withdrawal symptoms
Long-term	Agonist or partial agonist	180 days	Outpatient clinic; methadone clinic	Mild
Short-term	Agonist or partial agonist	30 days	Inpatient	Moderate. May require treatment.
Rapid	Antagonist	10 days	Inpatient	Severe. Requires treatment.
Ultrarapid	Antagonist	2 days	Inpatient hospital setting	Severe. Requires anesthesia.

short-term opioid detoxification
Detoxification process that lasts as long as 30 days and usually uses opioid receptor agonists.

rapid detoxification
Detoxification process lasting as long as 10 days and using opioid antagonist administration in a treatment facility.

ultrarapid opioid detoxification
Detoxification process lasting as long as 2 days and using opioid antagonist administration in a hospital setting.

These regulations include drug testing clients for illicit substance use and requiring that clients have frequent contact with medical staff, counselors, and social workers.

Short-term detoxification programs last as long as 30 days and usually use opioid receptor agonists such as methadone and LAAM. Short-term detoxification is more aggressive than long-term detoxification and includes moderate withdrawal symptoms. These programs may be entirely conducted in an in-patient treatment facility.

Rapid detoxification lasts as long as 10 days, and **ultrarapid detoxification** lasts as many as 2 days. Rapid detoxification is conducted in hospital or in-patient treatment facilities, and ultrarapid detoxification is conducted in hospital settings. Both programs utilize an opioid receptor antagonist such as naltrexone or naloxone. Naltrexone and naloxone provide long-lasting occupancy of μ opioid receptors, preventing activation of these receptors by opioid receptor agonists such as heroin. These antagonist actions increase the severity of withdrawal symptoms but also shorten the total duration of withdrawal symptoms (Loimer, Schmid, Presslich, & Lenz, 1989).

Ultrarapid detoxification uses high doses of an opioid receptor antagonist, which further worsens and shortens withdrawal symptoms. Patients must be anesthetized during the most severe withdrawal effects, which occur during the first several hours of treatment. After this, the withdrawal symptoms taper off over the course of 1–2 days.

By blocking opioid receptors, the body quickly adapts to the lack of opioid receptor activation. Thus, even though withdrawal symptoms are severe during rapid or ultrarapid detoxification, they do not last as long as normal withdrawal symptoms. Moreover, many withdrawal symptoms such as diarrhea and pain sensitization are treated by non-opioid medications such as Imodium, an antidiarrhea medication, or acetaminophen, an analgesic. Drugs that act as α_2 adrenoceptor agonists, such as clonidine, can be used to reduce hypertension, restlessness, insomnia, hostility, and other peripheral withdrawal symptoms. Benzodiazepine drugs can also reduce anxiety, hostility, and restlessness during opioid detoxification.

Individuals addicted to opioids may have other psychological disorders to treat, including an addiction or depression. In particular, 20-50 percent of individuals addicted to opioids have an antisocial personality disorder. Other common comorbid conditions include HIV infection, AIDS, hepatitis B and other medical conditions related to shared needle use or unprotected sex. The risk of these medical conditions is a major rationale for "harm reduction" programs, which provide safe alternatives to risky health choices associated with illicit opioid use, including clean needle access, medical testing and medical treatment.

As described in previous chapters, opioid and other drug-addiction treatment programs offer limited success. During detoxification, many patients either discontinue treatment or return to drug use after treatment ends. As presented in Chapter 5, follow-ups 5 years later of patients who underwent methadone treatment revealed that most patients had resumed regular use of an opioid drug (Hubbard, Craddock, & Anderson, 2003). Other follow-up studies reveal that those who remain drug free tend to be married, better employed, better educated, and psychologically healthy (Simpson & Marsh, 1986). Although a pharmacological treatment may weaken withdrawal symptoms, medications alone may be insufficient for providing improvements in these areas of social adjustment.

1. Two important reasons for opioid addiction are reinforcing effects and _____ on opioids.

2. During opioid detoxification programs, medications are provided into order to reduce the severity of _____ symptoms.

1. dependency 2. withdrawal

▶ CHAPTER SUMMARY

Opioid drugs are powerful pain-relieving and reinforcing substances used for medical and recreational purposes. Opioids are found naturally in poppy plants and are synthesized in laboratories. Opioids drugs can be inhaled, ingested orally, or injected intravenously. Endogenous opioid neurotransmitters are peptides that bind to μ, δ, κ, and nociceptin receptors.

The reinforcing effects of opioids derive from elevating dopamine levels and reducing GABA neuron activity in the nucleus accumbens. Opioids inhibit pain sensation by reducing glutamate and substance P neurotransmitter release in the spinal cord and by inhibiting

pain afferents to the brain. Tolerance develops quickly to opioid pharmacological effects, preventing long-term therapeutic use and requiring greater doses for recreational use.

Opioid addiction is maintained by avoiding withdrawal symptoms and achieving reinforcing effects. Detoxification programs address these components of addiction by reducing withdrawal symptoms. Long-term detoxification programs utilize a safer replacement for the illicit opioid drug, whereas rapid detoxification programs shorten withdrawal symptoms by using an opioid receptor antagonist. Treatment programs also address comorbid medical conditions.

KEY TERMS

Opioids

Naturally occurring opioids

Semisynthetic opioids

Fully synthetic opioids

G-protein–coupled inwardly rectifying K+ channel (GIRK)

Pure opioid receptor agonists

Partial opioid receptor agonists

Pure opioid receptor antagonists

Mixed opioid receptor agonist-antagonists

Miosis

Detoxification

Long-term opioid detoxification

Short-term opioid detoxification

Rapid detoxification

Ultrarapid opioid detoxification

Conditioned place preference

Conditioned place aversion

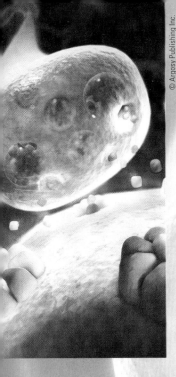
© Argosy Publishing Inc.

CHAPTER **11**

Cannabinoids

Should Medical Marijuana Be Legal?

Both opponents and proponents of legalized medical marijuana have strong opinions. Those who favor medical marijuana argue that, as an herbal remedy, marijuana offers therapeutic benefits for many chronic conditions, including pain, glaucoma, and even cancer. On the other hand, opponents argue that patients should instead take medications approved by the Food and Drug Administration, such as Marinol, that act like key pharmacologically active compounds found in marijuana.

Most patients prefer marijuana to drugs such as Marinol, suggesting that marijuana may be more effective and better tolerated. However, opponents argue that medical marijuana is just a means of getting high. Given the increasing trend by U.S. states to legalize medical marijuana, this debate will not likely end anytime soon. This chapter considers both the recreational and medical uses of marijuana, including considerations about the tolerability of marijuana-like drugs such as Marinol.

From Marmor (1998) and Clark, Capuzzi, and Fick (2011).

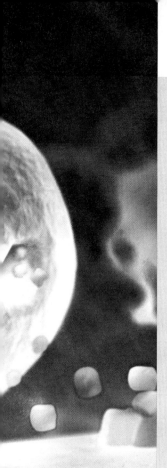

cannabis Three varieties of plants that contain naturally occurring psychoactive cannabinoids.

phytocannabinoids Biologically active substances found in cannabis plants.

Δ^9-tetrahydrocannabinol (Δ^9-THC) Key psychoactive substance in cannabis.

Cannabinoid drugs consist of psychoactive substances that act on cannabinoid receptors in nervous system. The term *cannabinoid* comes from cannabis plants, which contain the naturally occurring types of cannabinoid compounds. **Cannabis** plants come in three varieties: (1) *Cannabis sativa*, the most commonly used; (2) *Cannabis indica*; and (3) *Cannabis ruderalis*. These plants are also referred to as *hemp*, although the name refers technically to fibers of a plant and thus can describe many different types of plants.

The flowers and leaves of cannabis plants contain *trichomes*, small hairlike structures with glands that release a resin containing a number of biologically active substances referred to as **phytocannabinoids**. Phytocannabinoids include cannabis's key psychoactive ingredient, Δ^9-tetrahydrocannabinol (Δ^9-THC), as well as other compounds such as Δ^8-tetrahydrocannabinol (Δ^8-THC), cannabidiol, cannabinol, N-alklamide, and B-caryophyllene (Gertsch, Pertwee, & Di Marzo, 2010). The composition of the compounds in cannabis varies, depending on the variety of cannabis, the region in which it is grown, the plant's level of maturation, and the part of the plant sampled. *Cannabis sativa* plants can contain the greatest concentrations of Δ^9-THC relative to other varieties, and *Cannabis indica* tends to have a relatively greater concentration of cannabidiol

table **11.1**

Phytocannabinoid Composition of *Cannabis Sativa* Leaves at Different Stages of Maturation			
Phytocannabinoid	**Δ^9-THC (%)**	**Cannabidiol (%)**	**Cannabinol (%)**
June	0.2	0.1	0.1
August	7.1	1.0	0.7

Data from Bruci et al., 2012.

compared to Δ^9-THC, although Δ^9-THC concentrations can vary considerably (Hillig & Mahlberg, 2004). Trichomes appear mostly on the leaves and flowers of cannabis plants, yielding relatively higher concentrations of Δ^9-THC than other phytocannabinoids. As shown in **table 11.1**, the concentration of Δ^9-THC in *Cannabis sativa* increases with the maturation of the plant (Bruci et al., 2012).

Marijuana consists of dried cannabis flowers, leaves, and stems compressed and rolled for smoking. Slang terms for marijuana include *weed*, *pot*, *reefer*, and *grass*. The most commonly known term for cannabis, *pot*, may derive from a Mexican slang term for marijuana, *potiguaya* (Booth, 2005). **Hashish** consists of a condensed preparation of cannabis that primarily contains the trichome resins from the plant. Hashish and hashish oils contain greater concentrations of Δ^9-THC than other preparations (Ashton, 2001).

In addition to the forms of cannabis just described, we find a recent emergence of herbal marijuana alternatives, which are commonly referred to as *synthetic marijuana*. **Herbal marijuana alternatives** such as K2 and Spice contain laboratory-synthesized cannabinoid receptor agonists such as the compound WIN52212-2. The term also applies to a substance to which a user adds Δ^9-THC. A popular form of herbal marijuana alternative involves spraying a synthetic cannabinoid compound on herbs that a user then smokes like marijuana (Hu, Primack, Barnett, & Cook, 2011).

Much like bath salts (see Chapter 6), sellers market herbal marijuana alternatives for seemingly benign purposes such as for potpourri or as incense. These compounds emerged from scientific research endeavoring to develop cannabinoid receptor drugs as tools for learning about the brain's endocannabinoid system. Because these are experimental compounds, there remains a paucity of findings about their pharmacological effects, although many reports suggest that herbal marijuana alternatives exhibit different properties, such as psychostimulant or hallucinogenic effects, than traditional cannabis preparations (Rosenbaum, Carreiro, & Babu, 2012).

In the United States, as previously noted, the Drug Enforcement Administration (DEA) has classified cannabis products and herbal marijuana alternatives as schedule I controlled substances. The DEA also classifies Δ^9-THC as a schedule I substance, although it classifies the prescription Δ^9-THC, known as dronabinol (Marinol), as a schedule III controlled substance. The DEA

hashish Condensed preparation of cannabis that primarily contains the trichome resins from the plant.

herbal marijuana alternatives Laboratory-synthesized cannabinoid receptor agonists.

table **11.2**

Controlled Substances Act Codes for Cannabinoid Compounds	
Drug	Controlled substance schedule
Cannabis	I
Dronabinol (Marinol; synthetic Δ⁹-THC)	III
Tetrahydrocannabinol (any form of THC, including Δ⁹-THC and Δ⁸-THC)	I
Herbal marijuana alternatives (e.g., WIN52212-2)	I

Adapted from the Controlled Substances Schedule found at the DEA site. (http://www.deadiversion.usdoj.gov/schedules/index.html)

permanently added herbal marijuana alternatives as schedule I controlled substances in 2012 (**table 11.2**).

Marijuana is one of the most commonly used *illicit* substances in the world. According to the World Health Organization, approximately 2.5 percent of the world's population consumes cannabis on a regular basis. According to data from the 2009 U.S. National Survey on Drug Use and Health, 16.7 million Americans aged 12 and older reported having used marijuana during the preceding month (Substance Abuse and Mental Health Services Administration, 2010). Surveys among U.S. 12th graders in 2010 indicated that 36 percent had used cannabis within the previous year, and 11 percent had used an herbal marijuana alternative (Johnston, O'Malley, Bachman, & Schulenberg, 2011).

Cannabis is also emerging as a medicinal agent. Despite the federal classification as a schedule I controlled substance, 18 states in the United States, as well as Washington, D.C., allow licensed cannabis use for medical purposes (ProCon, 2012). Canada also allows medical marijuana. A review of cannabis's clinical effectiveness for treating medical disorders appears later in this chapter.

Historical Use of Cannabis

Like other psychoactive plants, cannabis has an ancient history. Some of the earliest records find cannabis used for medical purposes in ancient China. In 2737 B.C., Emperor Shen-Nung is attributed as recommending cannabis resin for "female weakness, gout, rheumatism, malaria, beriberi [sic] [a nervous system disorder caused by thiamine deficiency], constipation, and absent-mindedness." Later in China, physician Hua-T'o wrote of a mixture of cannabis resins and wine to use as a surgical anesthetic (Emboden, 1972).

In Arabia, cannabis was commonly smoked for its mood-enhancing effects. Hashish also began to be used in this region in approximately 1100 A.D. Hashish played a critical role in a religious cult formed by Hashishin ibn al-Sabbah, who commonly went by the name al-Hasan ibn al-Sabbah (ca. 1124 A.D.). During his travels, Marco Polo remarked in his journal about the practices al-Hasan used for recruiting men into his sect:

> Now no man was allowed to enter the Garden save those whom he intended to be his ASHISHIN. There was a fortress at the entrance to the Garden, strong enough to resist all the world, and there was no other way to get in. He kept at his Court a number of the youths of the country, from twelve to twenty years of age, such as had a taste for soldiering, and to these he used to tell tales about Paradise, just as Mahommet had been want to do, and they believed in him just as the Saracens believe in Mahommet. Then he would introduce them into his Garden, some four, or six, or ten at a time, having first made them drink a certain potion which cast them into a deep sleep, and then causing them to be lifted and carried in. So when they awoke they found themselves in the Garden.
>
> When therefore they awoke, and found themselves in a place so charming, they deemed that it was Paradise in very truth. And the ladies and damsels dallied with them to their heart's content, so that they had what young men would have; and with their own good will they never would have quitted the place. (Polo, 1871, pp. 132–134)

Marco Polo expanded on his description of al-Hasan's followers and deadly tactics, writing "[W]hen the Old Man would have any prince slain, he would say to such a youth: 'Go thou and slay So and So; and when thou returnest my Angels shall bear thee into Paradise. And shouldst thou die, natheless even so will I send my Angels to carry thee back into Paradise'" (Polo, 1871, p. 135). We better know the term *hashinin* by its Anglicized version *assassin*.

The use of cannabis in modern medicine largely began from the efforts of William O'Shaughnessy, a British physician working as a professor in Calcutta, India, in 1839. During his time in India, O'Shaughnessy experimented with the medical potential of cannabis, discovering that its sedative and anticonvulsant properties improved some of the symptoms of rabies, tetanus, and cholera (Kalant, 2001). This led Western physicians to consider cannabis as a legitimate medicine.

The Pharmacopoeia of the United States of America lists cannabis as a medicine in volumes published from 1851 to 1942. The United States criminalized cannabis for nonmedical purposes in 1937 (Aggarwal et al., 2009). Even though marijuana remained legal for medical use, the Marihuana Tax Act of 1937 required patients to pay $1 per ounce of marijuana, which largely limited its medicinal use. Possibly because of this tax and declining use, later editions of the pharmacopoeia excluded cannabis from its compilation of medicines (Aggarwal et al., 2009; Kalant, 2001).

Cannabis abuse increased in the late 1950s, and by the 1960s millions of Americans had tried smoking cannabis. In 1969, the U.S. government under President Richard Nixon began search and seizure operations at the U.S.–Mexico border primarily aimed at cannabis smugglers (Brecher, 1972). The first controlled substances schedule in the United States in 1970 included cannabis under schedule I. Since then, the DEA has approved lower scheduling for cannabinoid-based medicines such as dronabinol. The lower scheduling of these medications together with the recent emergence of medical marijuana approval in many U.S. states has led to petitions to the DEA to lower the scheduling level of cannabis. The most recent response to a petition came in 2011 when DEA Administrator Michele M. Leonhart rejected the request because of marijuana's "high potential for abuse," "no currently accepted medical use in treatment in the United States," and lack of "accepted safety for use under medical supervision" (Leonhart, 2011).

Stop & Check

1. A preparation of *cannabis sativa* consisting mostly of dried leaves and stems is called _____.
2. The primary psychoactive ingredient in cannabis is _____.
3. _____ is a condensed form of cannabis consisting mainly of trichome resins.
4. What is the connection between cannabis and the term *assassin*?

1. marijuana 2. Δ^9-THC 3. Hashish 4. *Assassin* is the anglicized form of *hashishin*, cult members who used hashish in their religious and recruiting practices.

Methods of Cannabis Preparation

For both recreational and instrumental purposes, users most often administer cannabis orally or by inhaling. Inhalation is the preferred method for using herbal marijuana alternatives (Ashton, 2001; Hu, Primack, Barnett, & Cook, 2011). For oral administration, users prepare cannabis by baking it into some type of dessert, such as brownies or cookies, or heating it with water to make a tea. Pharmaceutical companies sell prescription dronabinol in a capsule for oral administration.

To smoke cannabis, users roll a cannabis preparation in cigarette paper and then light and smoke it like a cigarette. This preparation is referred to as a *joint*. Alternatively, cannabis may be inhaled through a water-pipe device called a *hookah* or through a less-elaborate pipe referred to as a *bong*. As first described in Chapter 7, water pipes entail inhaling smoke from a plant substance through water. Aside from intentionally smoking cannabis, inhaling secondhand cannabis smoke also achieves psychoactive levels of Δ^9-THC in the body, possibly leading to a *contact high* (Cone & Johnson, 1986).

Fifty percent of Δ^9-THC releases into smoke from lit cannabis. Most of the Δ^9-THC absorbs into the bloodstream and reaches the brain after a few minutes. Approximately half of this amount reaches the brain after oral administration, mainly because of first-pass metabolism in the liver (**figure 11.1**). As

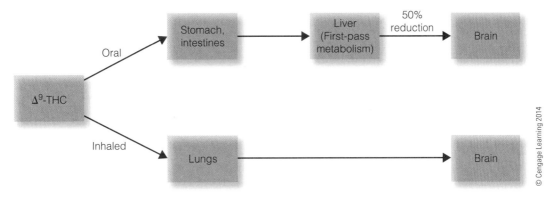

© Cengage Learning 2014

figure 11.1 First-pass metabolism occurring after oral consumption of a Δ⁹-THC product leads to significant reduction in Δ⁹-THC that reaches the brain.

are most compounds, Δ^9-THC is metabolized in the liver by P450 enzymes, and the metabolites themselves produce effects within the body. The primary metabolite of Δ^9-THC is 11-hydroxy-Δ^9-THC, and this metabolite produces psychoactive effects similar to those of Δ^9-THC (Takeda et al., 2010). Δ^9-THC exhibits high lipid solubility, leading to rapid distribution into tissues in the body, including the brain, as well as an accumulation in fat. Δ^9-THC in fat releases slowly over time, leading to long-term pharmacological actions (**figure 11.2**) (Ashton, 2001).

Because of the accumulation of Δ^9-THC in fats, there is a long elimination rate of Δ^9-THC during sustained use. After 4–5 days, Δ^9-THC reaches a peak concentration in fat, which then releases Δ^9-THC slowly with a half-life of 7 days. This half-life makes Δ^9-THC detectable for as long as 30 days after ceasing repeated use (Ashton, 2001).

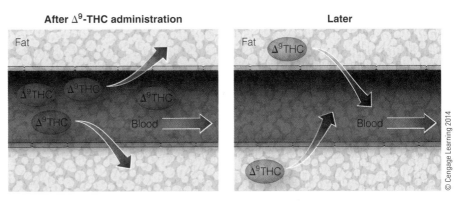

© Cengage Learning 2014

figure 11.2 Δ⁹-THC molecules accumulate in fat after administration (left), leading to a later release of Δ⁹-THC into the bloodstream.

Stop & Check

1. What are the two common administration routes for cannabis?
2. Assuming the same content of Δ^9-THC, why might someone experience greater potency from inhalation than from oral administration?

1. *Inhalation* through smoking and *oral* through eating or drinking. 2. The oral administration routes subjects Δ^9-THC to first-pass metabolism, which limits the amount of Δ^9-THC that reaches the brain.

Cannabinoid Compounds and the Endocannabinoid System

anandamide
Cannabinoid neurotransmitter.

2-arachidonoyl-glycerol (2-AG) Cannabinoid neurotransmitter.

The effects of Δ^9-THC and other psychoactive cannabinoid compounds occur by their actions on the endocannabinoid neurotransmitter system. *Endo* stands for *endogenous* (derived internally), and *cannabinoid* refers to the active compounds found in cannabis plants. Many of their features are still under investigation. Research indicates that two endocannabinoids—**anandamide** and **2-arachidonoyl-glycerol (2-AG)**—serve as the most biologically active neurotransmitters. Several other endocannabinoid neurotransmitters exist but are significantly less active, and their clinical relevance has yet to be evaluated (Battista, Di Tommaso, Bari, & Maccarrone, 2012; Brown, 2007; Felder et al., 1993).

The enzyme phospholipase D acts to convert N-arachidonoyl-phosphatidylethanolamine (NAPE) into anandamide. Unlike other neurotransmitters described in this text, storage vesicles do not store anandamide. The anandamide instead releases from neurons immediately after synthesis. Anandamide returns to a neuron via an anandamide transporter; thereafter, the enzyme fatty acid amide hydrolase (FAAH) breaks anandamide down into inactive components (**figure 11.3**) (Battista, Di Tommaso, Bari, & Maccarrone, 2012; Beltramo et al., 1997).

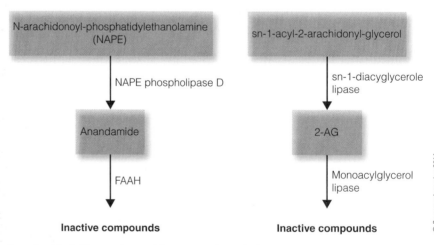

© Cengage Learning 2014

figure 11.3

Anandamide (left) is synthesized from NAPE through a NAPE-phospholipase D enzyme. The enzyme FAAH converts anandamide into inactive components. 2-AG (right) is synthesized from a diaglycerol, such sn-1-acyl-2-arachidonyl-glycerol, by the enzyme sn-1-diacylglycerol lipase. Monoacyglycerol lipase converts 2-AG into inactive components.

The enzyme sn-1-diacylglycerol lipase converts a diacylglycerol containing 2-arachidonate to 2-AG. Just like anandamide, this enzyme is activated by calcium; furthermore, like anandamide, 2-AG is not stored in vesicles. After release, 2-AG returns to the neuron through the same transporters used for anandamide. The enzyme monoacylglycerol lipase breaks down 2-AG into inactive components (figure 11.3) (Blankman, Simon, & Cravatt, 2007; Cravatt et al., 1996).

Cannabinoids and CB₁ and CB₂ Receptors

cannabinoid receptors G-protein-coupled receptors consisting of CB₁ and CB₂ activated by cannabinoids.

The various behavioral and physiological effects described for cannabinoids (e.g., Δ⁹-THC) and endocannabinoids (e.g., anandamide) result from actions at **cannabinoid receptors**. Two such receptors have been confirmed and thoroughly studied: the cannabinoid CB₁ and CB₂ receptors. Both receptors are G-protein–coupled receptors that exhibit inhibitory effects. Researchers have discovered other possible cannabinoid receptors, but these appear less important for explaining the effects of known cannabinoid compounds, so we will not cover these receptors in this text (Brown, 2007).

In the brain, CB₁ receptors densely occur in the basal ganglia, nucleus accumbens, substantia nigra, cerebellum, hippocampus, and cerebral cortex. CB₁ receptors also are found in the hypothalamus, thalamus, and throughout the brainstem (**figure 11.4**) (Herkenham et al., 1990). A dense population of CB₁ receptors also exist in the eye, which may potentially play a role in cannabis-induced reductions of intraocular pressure, discussed later in this chapter

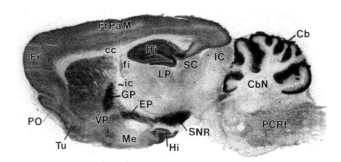

Shown in a sagittal section of a rat brain, the darker portions are the result of higher levels of radioactivity from radiolabeled CB₁ receptors. Thus, the darker portion represents higher densities of CB₁ receptors, and the lighter portion represents lower densities of CB₁ receptors. Key (anterior to posterior): Fr = frontal cortex, FrPaM = motor cortex area , PO = Preoptic area, Tu = olfactory tubercle, cc = corpus callosum, VP = ventral pallidum, fi = fibria of the hippocampus, ic = internal capsule , GP = globus pallidus, EP = exterior pallidus, Me = median eminence , Hi = hippocampus, LP = lateral posterior thalamic nucleus, SC = superior colliculus, SNR = substantia nigra, CbN = cerebellar nuclei, Cb = cerebellum, PCRt = parvicellular reticular nucleus." (Miles Herkenham, NIMH)

figure 11.4

(Porcella, Casellas, Gessa, & Pani, 1998; Porcella, Maxia, Gessa, & Pani, 2000). Outside the brain, CB_1 receptors can be found in the heart, kidneys, liver, spleen, and intestines. With the exception of glial cells, CB_2 receptors reside outside of the brain, particularly in the immune system on macrophages (i.e., white blood cells), leukocytes (including B cells, natural killer cells, and T cells), and mast cells (important for injury response) (Brown, 2007; Munro, Thomas, & Abu-Shaar, 1993).

Cannabinoid compounds vary in their affinity for CB_1 receptors, which can account for their different potencies for eliciting pharmacological effects. **Table 11.3** shows the receptor affinities for selected cannabinoid compounds (see box 2.1 for a review of receptor-binding procedures). Both Δ^9-THC and the endocannabinoid anandamide exhibit high affinities for the CB_1 receptor (Thomas, Gilliam, Burch, Roche, & Seltzman, 1998). The endocannabinoid 2-AG weakly binds to CB_1 receptors (Shoemaker, Joseph, Ruckle, Mayeux, & Prather, 2005). Cannabinol and cannabidiol also have weaker affinities for CB_1 receptors, likely accounting for their weaker potencies compared to Δ^9-THC. The synthetically produced CB_1 agonist WIN55212-2, which users abuse as an herbal marijuana alternative, exhibits at least a 10-fold greater affinity than either Δ^9-THC or anandamide (Thomas, Gilliam, Burch, Roche, & Seltzman, 1998).

Activation of CB_1 receptors leads to increased dopamine concentrations in the nucleus accumbens. In a study by Polissidis and colleagues (2012), administration of the CB_1 receptor agonist WIN55212-2 led to a significant increase in nucleus accumbens dopamine concentrations. Researchers have yet to determine exactly how activation of CB_1 receptors increases dopamine concentrations. The authors of this study speculated that CB_1 receptor agonists

table **11.3**

CB₁ Receptor Binding Affinities for Selected Cannabinoid Compounds		
Compound	**Source**	**Binding affinity expressed as K_i (nM concentration)***
Δ^9-THC (delta-9-tetrahydrocannabinol)	Main psychoactive component in cannabis	37
Cannabinol	Component in cannabis	247
Cannabidiol	Component in cannabis	2283
WIN55212-2	Synthetic CB_1 receptor agonist used for research purposes and abused as an herbal marijuana alternative	2
Anandamide	Endocannabinoid neurotransmitter	30
2-AG	Endocannabinoid neurotransmitter	1750

*Recall that lower values represent high affinities.
Data from Thomas et al., 1998 and Shoemaker et al., 2005.

may act on CB_1 receptors on dopamine neurons in the ventral tegmental area or indirectly influence dopamine neuron activity by acting on CB_1 receptors located on glutamate or GABA neurons.

Stop & Check	
	1. What are the two primary endocannabinoid neurotransmitters?
	2. What effect might a FAAH inhibitor have if someone also was using cannabis?
	3. Activation of CB_1 receptors causes _____ effects on the activity of a neuron.

1. Anandamide and 2-AG. **2.** The FAAH inhibitor would likely enhance the effects of cannabis through increasing levels of the endocannabinoid anandamide. **3.** inhibitory.

Physiological Effects of Cannabinoids

Given the wide reach of the endocannabinoid system, cannabinoid compounds exhibit several physiological effects. Acute administration of a cannabinoid containing Δ^9-THC causes a significant elevation in heart rate, and acute cannabis use is associated with hypotension and heart palpitations (Malit et al., 1975). Cannabis also produces a reddening of conjunctivae, which include the small blood vessels found at the bottom of the eye and membranes around the eye. Δ^9-THC itself appears to exhibit minimal effects on respiration at the usual amounts administered. Much of the respiratory problems associated with cannabinoids occur from smoked preparations, as described later in the chapter (Battista et al., 2012).

Cannabis use produces an increase in appetite, which recreational users refer to as having the "munchies." This is not a uniquely human phenomenon. For example, increased food intake is observed in *Hydra*, a tubular freshwater species that measures only a few millimeters long, after administration of the endocannabinoid anandamide (De Petrocellis, Melck, Bisogno, Milone, & Di Marzo, 1999). Williams and Kirkham (1999) found that anandamide administration led to increases in overnight feeding in rats.

The endogenous cannabinoid system may be important for normal regulation of food intake. This inference is based on the effects that leptin has on anandamide and 2-AG release. After fat cells release leptin, leptin reduces anandamide and 2-AG concentrations in the hypothalamus (**figure 11.5**).

REVIEW! The hypothalamus maintains many physiological processes through motivating an organism's behavior, such as producing hunger to motivate feeding. Chapter 2 (pg. 41).

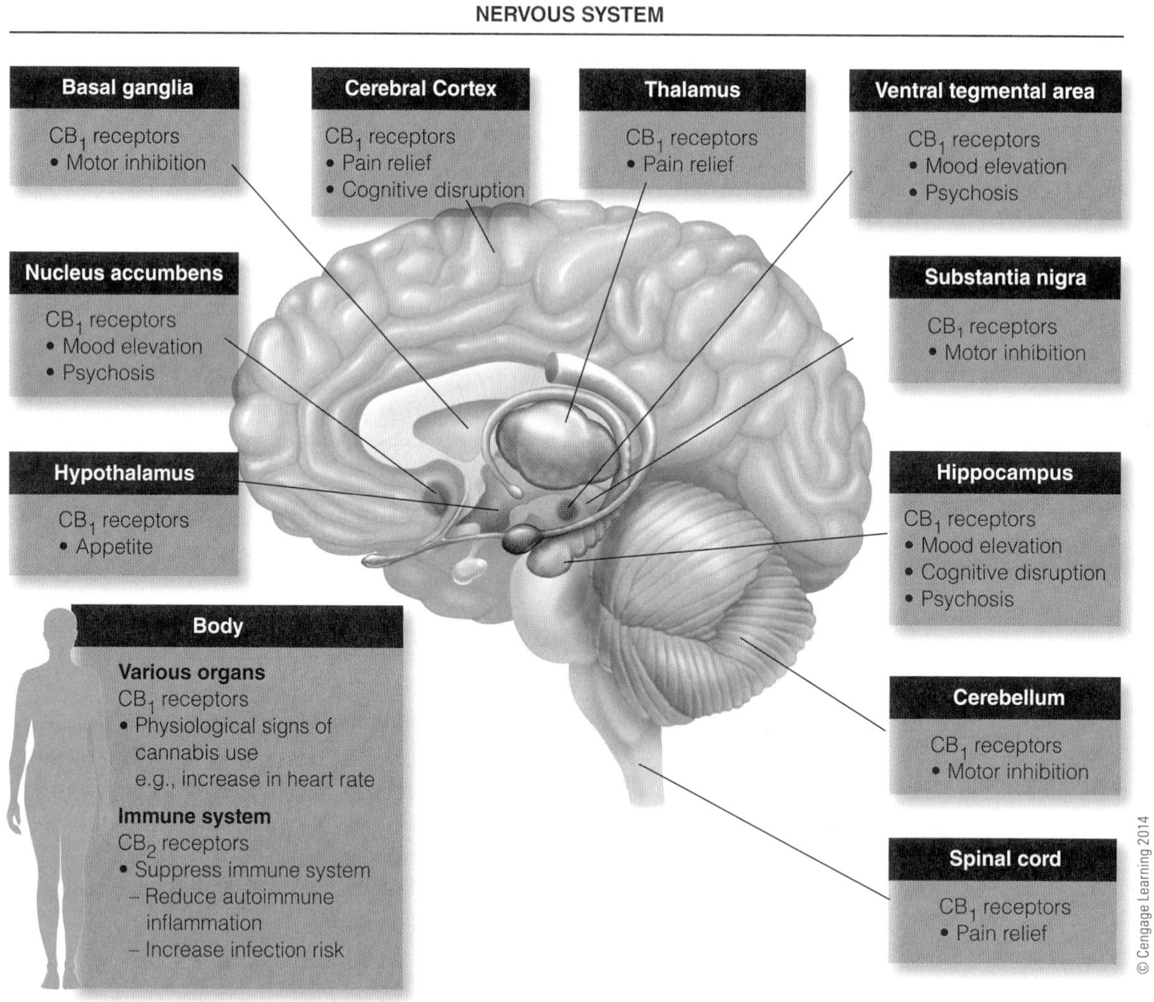

NERVOUS SYSTEM

Basal ganglia

CB_1 receptors
• Motor inhibition

Cerebral Cortex

CB_1 receptors
• Pain relief
• Cognitive disruption

Thalamus

CB_1 receptors
• Pain relief

Ventral tegmental area

CB_1 receptors
• Mood elevation
• Psychosis

Nucleus accumbens

CB_1 receptors
• Mood elevation
• Psychosis

Substantia nigra

CB_1 receptors
• Motor inhibition

Hypothalamus

CB_1 receptors
• Appetite

Hippocampus

CB_1 receptors
• Mood elevation
• Cognitive disruption
• Psychosis

Body

Various organs
CB_1 receptors
• Physiological signs of cannabis use
  e.g., increase in heart rate

Immune system
CB_2 receptors
• Suppress immune system
  – Reduce autoimmune inflammation
  – Increase infection risk

Cerebellum

CB_1 receptors
• Motor inhibition

Spinal cord

CB_1 receptors
• Pain relief

© Cengage Learning 2014

figure 11.5 The psychological and physiological effects of cannabinoids depend on the locations and function impact of CB_1 and CB_2.

Behavioral Effects of Cannabinoids

Many studies find mild memory deficits occurring after acute administration with cannabis or Δ^9-THC. For example, Weil and colleagues (1968) found that, among human volunteers, cannabis use impaired memory performance while failing to impair attention performance. Curran and colleagues (2002) found that a 15-mg/kg dose of Δ^9-THC reduced the number of words that study participants could recall from a list. Like the study by Weil and colleagues (1968), this study failed to find deficits in attention. However, much higher concentrations of Δ^9-THC than those normally seen after oral cannabis use appear to produce impairments in memory, reasoning, and attention (Morrison et al., 2009).

Cannabis tends to impair motor coordination and muscle tone. These effects, coupled with cannabis-induced impairments in reaction, likely contribute to impaired driving ability and an increased incidence of auto accidents (Ramaekers, Berghaus, van Laar, & Drummer, 2004). These effects are directly related to the concentration of Δ^9-THC and coincide with the subjective effects described as being *stoned* (Chesher, Bird, Jackson, Perrignon, & Starmer, 1990). Animal studies suggest that motor effects may change, depending on the dose. In laboratory rats, low doses of CB_1 receptor agonists increase locomotor activity, whereas higher doses decrease locomotor activity (Polissidis et al., 2012).

McGlothlin and West (1968) first proposed an *amotivational syndrome* occurring in cannabis users. They characterized an **amotivational syndrome** as a persisting lack of motivation to engage in productive activities. Individuals with amotivational syndrome exhibit apathy, lethargy, and passivity that are manifest as a failure to follow through on long-term plans, an indulgence in childlike thinking, and an engagement in introversive behavior.

Despite these observations, many researchers have failed to confirm an *amotivational syndrome* in controlled laboratory conditions. Several studies have tested the hypothesis that cannabis use should reduce the effectiveness of reinforcers if it reduces motivation. For example, if an individual loses interest in working, then one may reason that the individual has less motivation to earn money.

Published studies that investigated this hypothesis either reveal no effects on motivation or, in fact, find an increase in motivation. For example, Foltin and colleagues (1990), asked volunteers to live in a laboratory environment for 2 weeks and engage in various activities of low or high effort to earn reinforcers. In this study, a reinforcer was an opportunity to conduct a task an individual preferred more than the one he or she was currently conducting. On certain days, participants smoked cannabis cigarettes, but they smoked placebo cigarettes, which lacked Δ^9-THC, on other days. The researchers reasoned that study participants would express amotivation by choosing less-effortful tasks. Yet when participants smoked the cannabis cigarettes, they actually chose the tasks requiring more effort. Thus, an amotivational syndrome was not apparent. The researchers instead concluded that smoking cannabis made effortful tasks seem less effortful.

amotivational syndrome Lack of motivation to engage in productive activities possibly related to cannabis use.

Subjective Effects of Cannabinoids

The subjective effects of cannabinoids are dose dependent. After a few puffs of marijuana, a user may experience a light-headed, dizzy feeling referred to as a *buzz*. A person with a buzz may also experience tingling sensations in the body. A *high* occurs after additional inhalation and is defined as a euphoric and exhilarating feeling. Increased agitation or anxiety is occasionally reported

accelerated time
Perceived faster passage
of time associated with
cannabis use.

during the buzz and high phases as well. The *stoned* phase occurs with further usage and is described as a calm and relaxed state. This stage is also consistently characterized by **accelerated time**, a perceived faster passage of time, as described previously (Abood & Martin, 1992).

Accelerated time appears to be related to the effects of cannabis on the cerebellum. In a positron emission tomography (PET) imaging study conducted by Mathew and colleagues (1998) used PET to image cerebral blood flow following the administration of Δ^9-THC in human participants. Although findings varied among the participants, those who overestimated time passage exhibited reductions in cerebellar blood flow.

REVIEW! The cerebellum facilitates balance and the timing of movements. Chapter 2 (pg. 45).

To carefully assess the subjective effects of cannabis in humans in a laboratory environment, Curran and colleagues (2002) recruited 50 volunteers who had used cannabis in the past to rate how they felt after oral administration of Δ^9-THC. The investigators chose both a low dose (7.5 mg/kg) and a high dose (15.0 mg/kg) of Δ^9-THC to study, along with a placebo. Researchers employed a double-blind design so that neither the investigators nor the participants knew who received treatments during the study. The participants reported the strongest drug effect when given the highest dose of Δ^9-THC. They liked both the low and high dose of Δ^9-THC equally well, and they liked both more than placebo. Similarly, they also indicated a desire for more of the drug. The highest dose caused the most reports of being stoned, and the participants indicated difficulty remembering things.

Although this study employed oral administration of Δ^9-THC, rather than smoked cannabis, the effects are likely similar. In a study conducted by Hart and colleagues (2002), experienced cannabis smokers reported similar subjective effects, including similar "high" and "stoned" effects between smoked cannabis and oral Δ^9-THC. These findings further implicate Δ^9-THC in the subjective effects of cannabis.

Drug-discrimination studies can be used to study subjective effects in humans as well. In a study conducted by Lile and colleagues (2009), the ability to discriminate between a specific dose of a training drug—in this case, 25 mg of Δ^9-THC—and a compound with no drug effects (i.e., a placebo) were assessed in experienced cannabis users. The participants were given the drug or placebo orally, using pills that were identical in both appearance and taste. In fact, the participants were not even told that the training drug was Δ^9-THC; rather, they were told to closely attend to effects experienced after taking "drug X." The human participants then rated, by repeatedly clicking "drug" or "no drug" on a computer screen, their certainty that they had received drug X. After attaining a high level of accuracy, researchers administered a different test substance to the participants. **Figure 11.6** shows the results from this study. As shown in figure 11.6, although participants responded on drug X after Δ^9-THC administration, they failed to respond on drug X after administration of a benzodiazepine drug, an opioid drug, or a psychostimulant drug. Thus, the stimulus effects of Δ^9-THC appear different from those produced by these other drug classes.

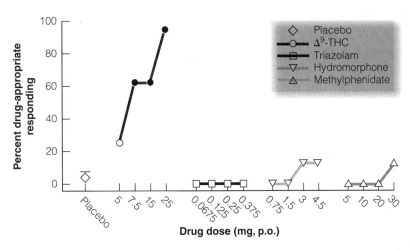

In humans trained to discriminate Δ9-THC versus placebo in a drug-discrimination task, only Δ9-THC produced Δ9-THC-appropriate responding, whereas drugs from other classes did not. (With kind permission from Springer Science+Business Media: Lile, J. A., Kelly, T. H., Pinsky, D. J., & Hays, L. R. (2009). Substitution profile of Delta9-tetrahydrocannabinol, triazolam, hydromorphone, and methylphenidate in humans discriminating Delta9- tetrahydrocannabinol. *Psychopharmacology* (Berl), 203(2), 241, p. 10.)

figure 11.6

Stop & Check

1. What is the hypothesis that many researchers test when investigating a potential amotivation syndrome for cannabis use?

2. Given that cannabis is an appetite enhancer, what therapeutic uses might the cannabinoid receptor antagonist offer?

3. What are the dose-dependent phases of the subjective effects of cannabis?

1. Researchers sometimes assess the effectiveness of reinforcers, reasoning that a user finding a goal less reinforcing would therefore demonstrate reduced motivation. **2.** If cannabis, which acts as an agonist for cannabinoid receptors increases appetite, then a cannabinoid receptor antagonist might decrease appetite. In fact, researchers have assessed cannabinoid receptor antagonists as weight-loss medications. **3.** As the dose increases, an individual will experience buzzed, high, and stoned phases.

Cannabinoid Tolerance and Dependence

Regular cannabis users find tolerance to many of cannabis's behavioral and subjective effects, including memory impairment, motor coordination, and accelerated time passage (Abood & Martin, 1992). A study by Georgotas and Zeidenberg (1979) demonstrated both the development of tolerance and the demonstration of dependence. These researchers recruited 5 healthy male volunteers who agreed to remain in an institutional setting for 8 weeks. During the first 4 weeks, participants had free access to cannabis cigarettes (i.e., joints). **Figure 11.7** shows the frequency of cannabis smoking during this study.

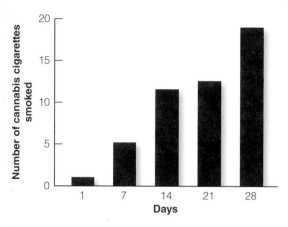

Institutionalized participants with free access to cannabis cigarettes (e.g., joints), steadily increased the number of cigarettes smoked per day during a 4-week study. The participants indicated a need to smoke more cigarettes in order to achieve the same subjective effects. (Data from Georgotas & Zeidenberg, 1976.)

figure 11.7

On the first day of study, each participant smoked one cannabis cigarette of his own choosing. During the last day of these first 4 weeks, each participant smoked an average of 19 cannabis cigarettes (figure 11.7). Over the course of the study, they each smoked an average of 292 cannabis cigarettes. As the amount of cannabis consumed increased, participants became suspicious, paranoid, agitated, apathetic, withdrawn, and depressed.

During these first four weeks, participants complained that the cannabis cigarettes became weak and that the stoned phase was less salient. To overcome this, the participants smoked escalating amounts of cannabis to achieve a desired effect, a classic indication of tolerance. On the day after these 4 weeks, the research team withheld cannabis from study participants. At this point, the participants were described as "very irritable, uncooperative, resistant, and at times hostile." The participants also lacked an appetite and had difficulty sleeping. These withdrawal effects subsided after about a week, and the participants' mood progressively improved during the final three weeks of the study.

Although this study is an extreme example of cannabis use, withdrawal effects were quite apparent and appeared to be countereffects to those elicited by cannabis use. Thus, as cannabis produces a relaxed state, the participants experienced agitation and restlessness. The appetite-enhancing effects of cannabis gave way to appetite suppression during withdrawal.

The fourth edition of the *Diagnostic and Statistical Manual* (DSM-IV) describes a **cannabis dependence** as meeting the general criteria for substance dependence, as presented in Chapter 5. However, the DSM-IV does not include withdrawal symptoms as part of the diagnosing, citing that withdrawal might

cannabis dependence
Cannabis use that meets the general DSM criteria for substance dependence.

occur in some individuals, but with unknown clinical significance (American Psychiatric Association, 2000). Today, many clinicians recognize a series of potential withdrawal symptoms from cannabis, which Beseler and Hasin (2010) describe as "anxiety, insomnia, vivid or unpleasant dreams, hallucinations, restlessness, shaking, depressed mood, hypersomnia, psychomotor retardation, feeling weak or tired, bad headaches, muscle cramps, runny eyes or nose, yawning, nausea, sweating, fever, and seizure." The expected revisions for the DSM-V include a *cannabis withdrawal syndrome* characterized by having any three of a series of possible symptoms, including irritability, anger, aggression, anxiety, difficulty sleeping, decreased appetite, and depressed mood as well as any physical withdrawal symptoms such as stomach pain, tremor, sweating, headache, or fever (American Psychiatric Association, 2012).

Cannabis and Risk of Lung Disease

Although cannabis presents some possible medical benefits for cancer, cannabis cigarettes share a number of carcinogens with tobacco cigarettes. These carcinogens include benzanthracene and benzpyrene compounds. In fact, cannabis cigarettes contain greater amounts of these chemicals than do tobacco cigarettes. Compared to tobacco, cannabis smoking results in greater amounts of tar in the lungs (Ashton, 2001).

Despite sharing similar carcinogen content with tobacco, cannabis smoke also yields different chemicals that may limit a user's risk for lung cancer. This may explain why correlational studies fail to find increased risk of lung cancer among cannabis smokers (Hashibe et al., 2005; Mehra, Moore, Crothers, Tetrault, & Fiellin, 2006). Moreover, cannabis contains compounds shown to reduce cancers of the skin, breast, and prostate, suggesting that these compounds may counteract the carcinogens found in cannabis (Melamede, 2005). Aside from cancer risk, cannabis smoking may increase the risk of respiratory diseases such as bronchitis and emphysema, although this risk increases most for users who smoke both cannabis and tobacco (Ashton, 2001; Tan et al., 2009).

Stop & Check

1. How are the withdrawal effects from cannabis related to the drug effects of cannabis?
2. What is a new feature of the DSM-V for cannabis dependence?

1. The withdrawal effects are compensatory effects of cannabis use. Thus, the withdrawal effect of *reduced appetite* is the result of compensating for the appetite *enhancement* of cannabis. Other withdrawal effects can be linked to the drug effects of cannabis in this way. **2.** Unlike the DSM-IV, the DSM-V will recognize a withdrawal syndrome for cannabis dependence.

FROM ACTIONS TO EFFECTS
Medical Marijuana

IIIIIIIIIIIIIIIIIIIIIIIIIIIIIIIIIIIIIIIIIIIIIIIIIIIIIIIIIIIIIIIIIIIIIIIIIIIIIIIIIIIIIIIIIIIIIIIIIIIIIIIIIIIIIIIIIIIIIIIIIIIIIIIIIIIIIIIIIIIIIIIIIIIIIIIIIIIIIIIIIIIIIIIIIIIIIIIIIIIIIIII

medical cannabis
Use of cannabis for treating medical conditions such as cancer, weight gain, pain, intraocular pressure, and autoimmune diseases.

Although marijuana is a popular drug of abuse, it is also emerging as a medical treatment. When investigating the scientific validity of using marijuana as a medical treatment, researchers study both the effects of smoked or orally consumed cannabis and the effects of phytocannabinoids, including not only Δ^9-THC but also cannabidiol and cannabinol. Amid a number of purported uses, evidence mainly supports **medical cannabis** for potentially treating cancer, unhealthy weight loss, pain, intraocular pressure, and autoimmune diseases (**table 11.4**).

For the treatment of cancer, cannabis may help patients cope with adverse side effects of chemotherapy, the use of medicines that kill rapidly dividing cells. In 1985, the Food and Drug Administration (FDA) approved the prescription of Δ^9-THC, again known as dronabinol (Marinol), for the reduction of nausea and vomiting during chemotherapy. However, with the development of other medications for treating chemotherapy-induced nausea and vomiting, physicians usually do not prescribe dronabinol as a first-line treatment (Todaro, 2012).

Cannabinoids have repeatedly demonstrated appetite-enhancing effects in clinical studies. This property may help promote weight gain conditions that diminish appetite, including cancer, chemotherapy treatment, and HIV infection. Another drug that is chemically similar to THC, nabilone (Cesamet), has been approved for similar uses. Because Δ^9-THC is the central psychoactive ingredient in cannabis, it is likely that cannabis use (e.g., smoking cannabis) has similar benefits (Haney et al., 2007).

Ellis and colleagues (2009) found that smoked cannabis significantly reduces neuropathic pain in HIV-infected patients compared to placebo control. These findings coincided with findings by Ware and colleagues (2010) that smoked cannabis reduces neuropathic pain in patients after suffering a trauma or when recovering from surgery. The pain-relieving properties of cannabinoids may result from activation of CB_1 receptors in the thalamus, brain stem, and cerebral cortex. Moreover, CB_1 receptors are located on neurons within the spinal cord where cannabinoids may reduce pain signaling to the brain (Pertwee, 2001).

Cannabis and phytocannabinoids may offer therapeutic benefits for glaucoma, a disease characterized by damage to the optic nerve from increased fluid pressure in

table 11.4

Medical Uses for Cannabis	
Cancer	Reduces nausea and vomiting associated with chemotherapy
Weight	Promotes weight gain in disorders that diminish appetite
Pain	Reduces neuropathic pain from trauma or surgery
Glaucoma	Relieves intraocular eye pressure
Autoimmune inflammation	Inhibits immune system functioning

© Cengage Learning 2014

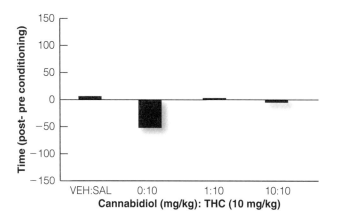

figure **11.8**

In a study by Vann and colleagues (2008), THC (Δ⁹-THC) in the absence of cannabidiol (CBD) (noted by 0:10 in figure) produced a conditioned place aversion in rats. However, when cannabidiol was also administered, noted by the 1:10 and 10:10 ratios, a conditioned place aversion did not occur. The y-axis indicates the amount of time spent in the drug side of the compartment compared to pretraining sessions. Negative time values represent avoidance of the compartment. (Vann et al., 2008. By permission.)

the eye. Hepler and Frank (1971) first reported that smoking cannabis cigarettes led to a significant reduction in intraocular pressure. Several studies reported that Δ⁹-THC engendered similar effects (Merritt, Crawford, Alexander, Anduze, & Gelbart, 1980; Purnell & Gregg, 1975). Porcella and colleagues (2001) also found that a selective CB₁ receptor agonist WIN55212-2 significantly reduced intraocular pressure in patients, concluding that CB₁ receptors play a direct role in mediating fluid pressure in the eye.

Cannabinoids also suppress immune system functioning. These actions are illustrated in a survey of routine cannabis users in Italy and Spain conducted by Pacifici and colleagues (2003). Through analyzing blood drawn from these participants over the course of 6 months, self-reported cannabis use was associated with reduced numbers of natural killer cells as well as general suppressed activity among various immune system cells. This included a reduction in proinflammatory cytokines, as well as an increase in anti-inflammatory cytokines. Thus, cannabis may be effective medicinally for autoimmune inflammation, but cannabis use may also enhance one's risk of infection.

The preceding studies provide evidence for using cannabis and its constituents or synthetic analogs as treatments for certain medical conditions. These findings also suggest that FDA-approved cannabinoid medications may serve in place of using medicinal marijuana. However, medical marijuana may provide greater tolerability than Δ⁹-THC, partly because of variability in absorption and metabolism among different individuals (Joerger et al., 2012). Thus, by smoking cannabis, users can self-regulate the amount used to achieve a desired effect.

Other components in cannabis may limit negative subjective or other behavioral effects of Δ⁹-THC. A study by Vann and colleagues (2008) assessed the effects of Δ⁹-THC in a conditioned place preference model using rats (**figure 11.8**). After completing pairing sessions with Δ⁹-THC or placebo, a test session revealed that rats actually avoided the chamber paired with Δ⁹-THC. In other words, Δ⁹-THC produced a conditioned place *aversion*. In a subsequent experiment, these researchers conducted the same procedure using a combination of Δ⁹-THC and cannabidiol as a treatment condition versus placebo. This time, a test session revealed neither an aversion nor a preference, suggesting that cannabidiol canceled out the aversive effects of Δ⁹-THC.

sativex Cannabinoid medication that consists of a one-to-one ratio of cannabidiol and Δ⁹-THC.

A newer cannabinoid medication called **Sativex** uses a one-to-one ratio of cannabidiol and Δ⁹-THC. This medication is currently approved in the United Kingdom, Spain, and Canada for the treatment of muscle spasms and stiffness in multiple sclerosis. Canada also approved Sativex for the treatment of pain in cancer. Patients indicate that Sativex is generally well tolerated (Barnes, 2006; Wade, 2012).

Stop & Check

1. What is the FDA-approved use for dronabinol?
2. How might cannabis relieve glaucoma?
3. Why might cannabis users prefer smoking cannabis as opposed to taking dronabinol for medicinal purposes?

1. The FDA approved dronabinol for the reduction of nausea and vomiting during chemotherapy. **2.** CB$_1$ receptors in the eye may have a direct role in liquid pressure, a contributor to optic nerve damage in glaucoma. Δ^9-THC in cannabis may relieve this pressure by activating these CB$_1$ receptors. **3.** First, smoking cannabis allows patients to adjust drug levels to achieve and maintain a desired effect. Second, other components in cannabis may counteract some of the negative subjective effects of dronabinol.

▶CHAPTER SUMMARY

Cannabinoids represent a class of drugs that produce psychoactive effects by acting on cannabinoid receptors in the nervous system. Cannabinoids exist in cannabis plants, are produced as synthetic drugs, and occur as endogenous neurotransmitters. Cannabis plants produce psychoactive effects through Δ^9-THC, their main psychoactive constituent. With the exception of prescription Δ^9-THC (dronabinol), the DEA lists cannabinoid compounds as schedule I controlled substances. Users smoke or orally administer cannabinoid compounds. Once in the body, Δ^9-THC has a long elimination rate, which increases during chronic cannabis use. Cannabinoid compounds engender pharmacological actions by acting on the endocannabinoid system, which involves neurotransmitters called *anandamide* and *2-AG* that bind to CB$_1$ and CB$_2$ cannabinoid receptors. Cannabis use increases heart rate, enhances appetite, produces deficits in memory, and impairs motor coordination. The subjective effects include euphoria, relaxation, and overestimation of time passage. Regular use of cannabis results in tolerance to many of its pharmacological effects. There has been extensive research on the use of medical marijuana and cannabinoid compounds. In particular, cannabinoids may reduce adverse effects from chemotherapy, promote weight gain, relieve pain, reduce intraocular pressure, and treat certain autoimmune diseases.

KEY TERMS

Cannabis
Phytocannabinoids
Δ^9-tetrahydrocannabinol (Δ^9-THC)
Hashish
Herbal marijuana alternatives
Anandamide
2-arachidonoyl-glycerol (2-AG)
Cannabinoid receptors
Amotivational syndrome
Accelerated time
Cannabis dependence
Medical cannabis
Sativex

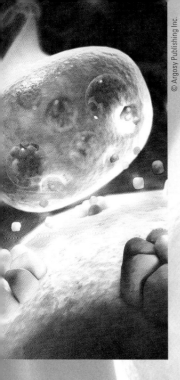

© Argosy Publishing Inc.

Psychedelic Drugs

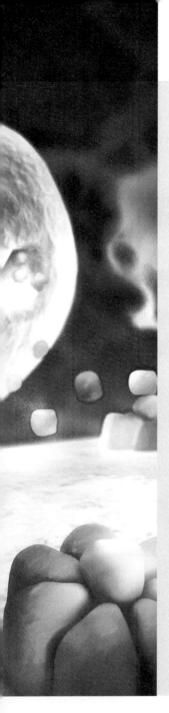

Did Hofmann Take a "Trip?"

While mixing chemicals at Sandoz Laboratories in Switzerland on the afternoon of April 16, 1943, Dr. Albert Hofmann acquired a sudden illness and went home. He recorded his initial symptoms as "great restlessness and mild dizziness." On reaching home, he entered a pleasant delirium containing "extremely excited fantasies" along with "fantastic visions of extraordinary realness and with an intense kaleidoscopic play of colors."

As a seasoned chemist, Hofmann deliberated on the ergot fungi derivatives he made that day and wondered about accidental ingestion. After recovering, Hofmann returned to work and took a tiny amount of one of the derivatives. This led to a similar restlessness and dizziness, but this time he experienced a stronger and different effect. After recovering some hours later, Hofmann wrote of his experience.

> As far as I can remember, the following were the most outstanding symptoms: vertigo, visual disturbances, the faces of those around me appeared as grotesque, colored masks; marked motoric unrest, alternating with paralysis; an intermittent feeling in the head, limbs, and the entire body, as if they were filled with lead; dry, constricted sensation in the throat; feeling of choking; clear recognition of my condition, in which state I sometimes observed, in the manner of an independent neutral observer, that I shouted half insanely or babbled incoherent words. Occasionally I felt as if I were out of my body. . . . Especially noteworthy was the fact that sounds were transposed into visual sensations so that from each tone or noise a comparable colored picture was evoked, changing in form and color kaleidoscopically.

Hofmann provided the first account of a popular recreational substance, the 25th compound of Sandoz Laboratories' lysergic acid series, LSD (Brecher, 1972).

psychedelic drugs
Drugs that induce a reality-altering experience consisting of hallucinations, sensory distortions, or delusions.

Psychedelic drugs induce a reality-altering experience consisting of hallucinations, sensory distortions, or delusions. The term *psychedelic* means "mind expanding." Within this definition, we find a wide variety of pharmacological effects among the psychedelic drugs. Thus, we further classify psychedelic drugs into three general categories: hallucinogens, mixed stimulant–psychedelics, and dissociative anesthetics. This chapter will focus on the representative drugs for each category, including the hallucinogen LSD (*acid*), the mixed stimulant–psychedelic MDMA (*Ecstasy*), and the dissociative anesthetic phencyclidine (*PCP*) (Abraham, McCann, & Ricaurte, 2002).

Hallucinogens

hallucinogens Large class of psychedelic drugs that produce hallucinations as their main pharmacological effects.

lysergic acid diethylamide (LSD) Most representative hallucinogen psychedelic drugs.

Hallucinogens represent a large class of psychedelic drugs that produce hallucinations as their main pharmacological effects. The most representative drug of this class is **lysergic acid diethylamide (LSD)**, which goes by a variety of streets names such as *acid*, *window pane*, and *blotter*, among other street names. Other hallucinogens include psilocybin, mescaline, and dimethyltryptamine. LSD is synthesized from lysergic acid using any number of preparation methods (Soine, 1986). In response to these measures, the Drug Enforcement Administration (DEA) not only classified LSD as a schedule I substance but also classified its precursor, lysergic acid, as a schedule I controlled substance (Drug Enforcement Administration, 2012b).

Psilocybin is the main psychoactive constituent in hallucinogenic mushrooms belonging to the genus *Psilocybe* (Schultes, 1969). User refers to these mushrooms by different street names such as *magic mushrooms* or *shrooms*. After oral administration, psilocybin rapidly converts to its active metabolite psilocin, a hallucinogenic substance that likely accounts for most of psilocybin's effects (Hasler, Bourquin, Brenneisen, Bar, & Vollenweider, 1997).

Mescaline is found in peyote, a small, spineless cactus native to southern North America (**figure 12.1**). Users obtain mescaline by chewing disk-shaped buttons within the cactus crown (Schultes, 1969). Dimethyltryptamine (DMT)

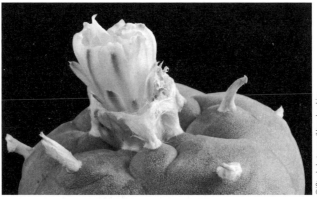

©iStockphoto.com/HansJoachim

figure **12.1**   The peyote cactus contains the hallucinogen mescaline.

is found in *Mimosa hostilis*, *Virola calophylla*, and other hallucinogenic South American plants (Agurell, Holmstedt, Lindgren, & Schultes, 1969). Unlike other hallucinogens, the body produces small amounts of DMT, although the function of endogenous DMT remains largely unknown (Angrist et al., 1976; Axelrod, 1961).

Hallucinogen use is prevalent on college campuses. In surveys conducted in undergraduate college students, approximately 15 percent had used LSD, and nearly 25 percent had used hallucinogenic mushrooms. Among the general U.S. population, fewer than 1.3 million individuals 12 and older had used a hallucinogen within the previous 12 months. LSD was used by fewer than 340,000 U.S. individuals 12 and older (Substance Abuse and Mental Health Services Administration, 2010).

Stop & Check

1. What are the three main types of psychedelic drugs?
2. What is the representative drug for hallucinogens?
3. What is the hallucinogenic compound found in peyote?

1. Hallucinogens, mixed stimulants–psychedelics, and dissociative anesthetics **2.** Lysergic acid diethylamide (LSD) **3.** Mescaline

Origins of LSD and Other Hallucinogens

Primitive cultures used hallucinogenic plants as psychic medicines to treat maladies, communicate with gods, and perform magic (Schultes, 1969). The Aztecs used peyote and similar hallucinogens in religious ceremonies. In addition to rich visual hallucinations, peyote granted perceptions of great insight and altered realities, providing the integral experience of communicating with gods. The Spanish conquistadors banned these practices, but neither the Inquisitors nor military authorities eliminated peyote's ceremonial use.

In the mid-18th century, peyote use was adopted by Native American cultures and was used in religious ceremonies by the Comanche, Kiowa, Cheyenne, and many other tribes. Comanche chief Quanah Parker stated that the Great Spirit Within communicated with him through a peyote experience to make peace with the white man and seek spiritual communion and wisdom.

When Oklahoma outlawed peyote in 1899, Quanah Parker helped persuade the state legislature to overturn the law, which it did in 1908. Peyote's legal status continued largely because of its importance to the Native American Church of North America. As the use of peyote continued in native American tribes, peyote use spread among U.S. college campuses during the 1950s and 1960s (Brecher, 1972). Today, peyote and its primary psychoactive ingredient mescaline are schedule I controlled substances, although this act excludes peyote use for religious purposes by the Native American Church of North America (American Indian Religious Freedom Act Amendments, 1994).

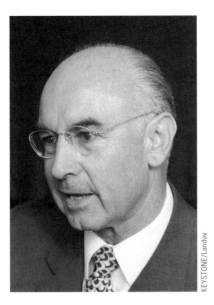

KEYSTONE/Landov

figure 12.2   Swiss chemist Albert Hofmann discovered the hallucinogen LSD.

Although hallucinogenic substances have existed in plants for as long as humans have existed, the popular hallucinogen LSD is a recent invention created in a laboratory. As described in opening of this chapter, Swiss chemist Albert Hofmann accidentally discovered LSD's hallucinogenic effects at Sandoz Laboratories in 1943 (**figure 12.2**). He made this discovery while synthesizing derivatives from ergot, a fungus already known to elicit mild hallucinogenic effects.

Hofmann learned two key things from his self-experiment with LSD. The first was dosage. He took only one-quarter milligram of LSD, which to his surprise produced a strong effect. The second thing was that LSD is a powerful hallucinogenic drug. Hofmann's second "trip" lasted 6 hours, providing the experience described at the beginning of this chapter.

After LSD's hallucinogenic effects were discovered, the substance was tested for a variety of uses. First, the U.S. Army tested LSD as an aid for inducing captured enemy prisoners to talk more freely. The army also tested LSD as a chemical weapon. During the psychoanalysis era, psychiatrists used LSD to gain access to supposedly unconscious thoughts in their patients (Brecher, 1972). Antony Busch and Warren Johnson (1950) published the first paper for LSD use in psychiatric patients, stating that LSD "may offer a means of more readily gaining access to the chronically withdrawn patients" and that its use might shorten psychotherapy. Other studies supported these claims (Chandler & Hartman, 1960; Natale, Kowitt, Dahlberg, & Jaffe, 1978).

In 1960, Sidney Cohen reported on a LSD survey returned by 44 researchers and therapists. These respondents reported administering LSD to nearly

5,000 men and women, equating to more than 25,000 total administrations. The volume of LSD therapeutic use declined, however, as published reports and conference proceedings noted negative psychological experiences, referred to as *bad trips*, emerging in many patients. Many practitioners especially feared producing prolonged bad trips, lasting as long as 48 hours. Occasionally, bad trips led to suicides.

Aside from possible therapeutic benefits, others used LSD to gain insight and achieve deep spiritual experiences. During the 1950s, philosophers, theologians, and even clergy members joined the ranks of LSD users. In the 1960s, LSD became a recreational substance, which in turn facilitated black market LSD production. State and federal regulations for LSD increased as therapeutic use of LSD decreased (Brecher, 1972). Eventually, LSD became a schedule I controlled substance.

Stop & Check

1. Who discovered LSD's hallucinogenic effects?
2. Aside from recreation, what were the other historical uses of LSD?

1. Albert Hofmann, a chemist who worked for Sandoz Laboratories 2. LSD was tested by the U.S. military to aid in prisoner interrogation and to use as a chemical weapon. The drug was also used in psychotherapy.

LSD Ingestion and Effects

LSD and most other hallucinogens are normally orally administered. This was the administration route used by Albert Hofmann's accidental LSD ingestion and self-experimentation described previously. LSD is potent, with effective amounts beginning at only 0.025 mg. Researchers consider 0.075 to 0.15 mg a moderate dose range capable of achieving a significantly altered state of consciousness (Passie, Halpern, Stichtenoth, Emrich, & Hintzen, 2008). Given these doses, an amount of LSD the size of an aspirin tablet would affect 3,000 people.

The high potency of LSD requires a different method for drug preparation. A common preparation method involves applying drops of a solution of LSD onto small squares of blotter paper or the glue sides of postage stamps. In either case, LSD sticks to the paper, and recreational users ingest the drug by licking the paper.

Through the oral administration route, LSD reaches peak absorption after 60 minutes. Cells in the liver metabolize LSD, producing 2-oxo-3-hydroxy-LSD. LSD's elimination half-life is approximately 3 hours, which facilitates pharmacological effects lasting as long as 8 hours (Passie et al., 2008).

LSD and the Serotonin Neurotransmitter System

The chemical structure of LSD resembles serotonin's chemical structure, allowing LSD to act on serotonin receptors (**figure 12.3**). Specifically, LSD functions as a receptor agonist with a high binding affinity for 5-HT_{1A}, 5-HT_{2A}, 5-HT_6, and 5-HT_7 receptors. In particular, LSD activates serotonin receptors located postsynaptically on other neurotransmitter neurons, such as glutamate and GABA neurons (Passie et al., 2008).

$$O = C - N(C_2H_5)_2$$

$$NCH_3$$

$$HO - \quad - CH_2CH_2NH_2$$

Serotonin   **LSD**

figure 12.3   Portions of the LSD molecule resemble the chemical structure of the neurotransmitter serotonin.

modal object completion Perception of object boundaries inferred from incomplete representations of the object.

These neurotransmission effects impact many sensory-processing systems in the brain. First, in the visual cortex, LSD activates both 5-HT$_{1A}$ and 5-HT$_{2A}$ receptors. Hallucinogen activation of serotonin receptors can modify any number of visual processes. For example, these actions can interfere with modal object completion for objects like those shown in **figure 12.4**. **Modal object completion** is a perception of object boundaries inferred from incomplete representations of the object. According to electroencephalogram (EEG)

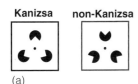

Kanizsa   **non-Kanizsa**

(a)

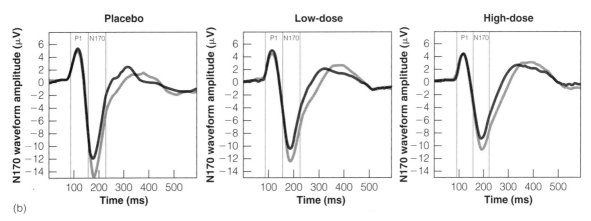

(b)

figure 12.4   LSD and other hallucinogens disrupt the ability to perceive nonexistent borders, a process called *model object completion*, of Kanizsa objects (a). During these tasks, hallucinogens impair the N170 waveform in the occipital lobe on EEG recordings (b). (Kometer et al., 2011. By permission.)

recordings, the N170 waveform is strongly associated with modal object completion. In a study by Kometer et al. (2011) using human volunteers, the LSD-like hallucinogen psilocybin inhibited both modal object completion and weakened N170 waveform amplitudes in specific areas of the visual cortex. Moreover, these reduced N170 waveform amplitudes correlated with overall decreased activity in the occipital lobe (figure 12.4).

Second, hallucinogens alter functioning in the locus coeruleus. In the locus coeruleus, LSD's activation of post synaptic 5-HT$_{2A}$ receptors increases the activity of both glutamate and GABA neurons. Enhanced glutamate release increases sensory signals to the cerebral cortex. At the same time, GABA release decreases spontaneous activity in the locus coeruleus, causing greater refinement of sensory signals sent to the cerebral cortex. In essence, LSD causes normally suppressed sensory information from the locus coeruleus to become more refined and salient.

In the prefrontal cortex, LSD activation of 5-HT$_{2A}$ receptors also causes increased glutamate release. Enhanced glutamate release, in turn, increases activity in the prefrontal cortex, the central integration area for processed sensory information. These findings correlate with human drug imaging data. In a positron emission tomography (PET) imaging study conducted by Vollenweider and colleagues (1997), the LSD-like hallucinogen psilocybin produced a significant increase in the metabolism of labeled glucose, an index of neuronal activity, in the prefrontal cortex. In addition, psilocybin elicited enhanced activity in the temporomedial cortex, a region involved in complex visual processing. These enhanced activity levels in the prefrontal cortex and temporomedial cortex also occurred while participants experienced visual hallucinations.

Stop & Check

1. What is the most common administration route for LSD and other hallucinogens?

2. Although LSD activates many types of serotonin receptors, which receptor is most associated with visual hallucinations?

1. Oral administration **2.** The 5-HT$_{2A}$ receptor

LSD's Mild Physiological Effects and Profound Hallucinogenic Effects

LSD and many other serotonin-like hallucinogens primarily elicit subjective pharmacological effects. Even the LSD megadose taken by Hofmann—0.25 mg—produced few noticeable physiological effects. In his account of the trip, Hofmann said that his physician "found a rather weak pulse, but an otherwise normal circulation," and Hofmann felt fine the next day. At normally used doses, a person may exhibit only modest changes in heart rate, increased pupil diameter, slight dizziness, or mild nausea. The physiological safety of this drug is indicated by a human lethal dose of 14 mg, far above the doses capable of producing hallucinogenic effects (Brecher, 1972).

Although few, if any, physiological effects occur with normally used amounts, LSD and other serotonin-like hallucinogens exhibit pronounced subjective experiences. However, the term *hallucination* needs qualification. A **true hallucination** is a perception of images or sounds that are not real. Drugs such as LSD, on the other hand, alter the perception of things that *are* real. Normal LSD doses cause distorted, waiving, or kaleidoscopic forms of real images in a visual field. These characteristics are called **pseudo-hallucinations** (El-Mallakh & Walker, 2010). True hallucinations *can* occur with LSD, but they are considered rare (Passie et al., 2008).

As previously mentioned, the overall hallucinogenic experience is called a **trip**. A trip can be good or bad. A good trip is characterized by having highly desirable sensory distortions and pseudo-hallucinations. During good trips, users may experience feelings of enhanced perception or insightfulness. A user may also experience **synesthesia**, or experiencing sensory stimuli in an incorrect sensory modality. LSD-elicited synesthesia, for example, often consists of experiencing sounds when seeing colors and vice versa (Brown, McKone, & Ward, 2010). The "From Actions to Effects" section later in this chapter describes synesthesia in greater detail. Hofmann, too, experienced synesthesia, stating that "sounds were transposed into visual sensations so that from each tone or noise a comparable colored picture was evoked, changing in form and color kaleidoscopically" (Brecher, 1972).

A bad trip is associated with disturbing true hallucinations, psychotic episodes, negative emotional states, altered perceptions of time, and out-of-body sensations (Eveloff, 1968). Hofmann experienced a bad trip after intentionally taking LSD. He stated that the faces of those around him "appeared as grotesque, colored masks" and that "I sometimes observed, in the manner of an independent neutral observer, that I shouted half insanely or babbled incoherent words." He reported that this experience was as if "I were out of my body" (Brecher, 1972).

A person's expectations and previous experiences affect LSD's subjective effects. Factors that affect a person's trip can include physical surroundings, current emotional state, comments made by friends, and many other factors. In fact, Eveloff (1968) states that profound skepticism about LSD's effects largely suppress the LSD experience. LSD also causes *hypersuggestibility*, a state that can jeopardize reality testing. Eveloff (1968) reported that during some trips, users have jumped off buildings in the belief they could fly or stepped in front of traveling cars in the belief they lacked material substance.

The nature of hallucinogenic experiences presents an important challenge for hallucinogen research in animals. Even if an animal experienced something like a hallucinogenic trip, how could we tell? Rather than attempt to model such an experience, animal researchers instead study other features of hallucinogens such as their behavioral stimulus properties.

Winter and colleagues (2007) conducted a drug-discrimination study using the hallucinogen mescaline as the training drug in rats. After training

true hallucination
Perception of images or sounds that are not real.

pseudo-hallucinations
Altered perception of things that are real.

trip Hallucinogenic experience.

synesthesia
Experiencing sensory stimuli in an incorrect sensory modality.

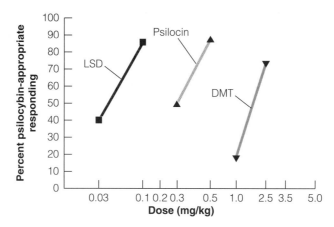

figure 12.5 In a mescaline drug-discrimination study, stimulus generalization occurred from mescaline to the hallucinogenic drugs LSD, psilocybin, and DMT. The *y*-axis shows the percentage of responses occuring on the psilocybin lever, and the *x*-axis shows the doses of each drug tested. (Winter et al., 2007. By permission.)

rats in this task, the researchers conducted tests to determine the similarity between mescaline's stimulus effects and those of other hallucinogenic drugs. As shown in **figure 12.5**, rats exhibited stimulus generalization from mescaline to the hallucinogens LSD, psilocybin, and DMT.

Hallucinogens and Flashbacks

flashback Random, short, and nondistressing memory of a previous hallucinogenic experience.

hallucinogen persisting perception disorder Recurring, lengthy, and unpleasant memory from a previous hallucinogenic experience.

The primary adverse effects of hallucinogens consist of negative subjective experiences, such as those experienced during a bad trip. Occasionally, users may randomly experience a striking memory of the previous trip. Such an experience is referred to as a **flashback** or as a symptom of **hallucinogen persisting perception disorder**. These terms are used somewhat synonymously, but there are key differences in how the terms are applied. *Flashback* usually refers to a short, nondistressing recurrence of a previous trip. On the other hand, hallucinogen persisting perception disorder is characterized by recurring, longer-term, and unpleasant experiences that are difficult to reverse (Lerner et al., 2002).

Stop & Check

1. How does a true hallucination differ from a pseudo-hallucination?
2. How does a good trip differ from a bad trip?

2. A good trip elicits a pleasurable psychedelic drug experience, whereas a bad trip elicits a distressful and disturbing experience.

1. A true hallucination is a perception of something not really there, whereas a pseudo-hallucination is an altered perception of something that really is there.

Mixed Stimulant–Psychedelic Drugs

mixed stimulant–psychedelic drugs
Substances that exhibit both psychostimulant and hallucinatory effects as their primary pharmacological effects.

MDMA (Ecstasy) Mixed stimulant-psychedelic drug; chemically, 3,4-methylenedioxyethamphetamine.

entactogen Term meaning "touching within;" usually in reference to mixed stimulant-psychedelic drugs.

empathogen Term referring to enhanced empathy; usually in reference to mixed stimulant-psychedelic drugs.

rave Large organized party held in a dance club or warehouse where electronic dance music is played with a light show.

Beyond the serotonin-like hallucinogens such as LSD, other psychedelic drugs exhibit broader pharmacological effects. In particular, **mixed stimulant–psychedelic drugs** refers to substances that exhibit both psychostimulant and hallucinations as their primary pharmacological effects. One of these drugs is 3,4-methylenedioxyethamphetamine (**MDMA, or Ecstasy**), although the two terms are not exactly synonymous in use. *Ecstasy* can refer to any number of stimulant or psychedelic preparations that may contain only small amounts, or even no amount, of MDMA. In an analysis of Ecstasy tablets collected by England's Forensic Science Service, a number of tablets contained the MDMA-like drug MDEA (3,4-methylenedioxyethamphetamine) instead of MDMA (Cole, Bailey, Sumnall, Wagstaff, & King, 2002). Other studies report Ecstasy pills containing methamphetamine, dextromethorphan, ketamine, and cocaine.

Although MDMA is best known for its psychedelic and psychostimulant effects, it is also known as an **entactogen**, meaning "touching within," or as an **empathogen**, referring to enhanced empathy. These terms synonymously refer to effects observed in early MDMA studies that users become friendlier, exhibit a closeness with others, and perceive greater insight into their thoughts and emotions (Nichols & Oberlender, 1990). Like LSD, these features made MDMA an attractive adjunctive medication for use in psychoanalysis (Rochester & Kirchner, 1999).

MDMA shares a similar chemical structure with amphetamine and possesses many of amphetamine's psychostimulant effects. Yet MDMA also produces LSD-like hallucinations, so it fits into the mixed psychedelic–stimulant class of drugs. This drug class also includes AMT and 5-MeO-DIPT (Abraham et al., 2002). MDMA is frequently used in **raves**, large organized parties held in dance clubs or warehouses where electronic dance music is played with accompanying light shows. MDMA and other psychedelic drugs enhance this club experience (Miller & Schwartz, 1997).

MDMA users mainly consist of high school and college-aged individuals. According to the National Institute on Drug Abuse, 2.8 million high school students 12 and older used MDMA in 2009. Overall, MDMA prevalence accounted for 4.7 percent of 10th graders and 4.5 percent of 12th graders. MDMA use rises with college-aged students. In a survey conducted among U.S. colleges in the mid-Atlantic region, 9 percent reported using MDMA in their lifetime. For close to half of those college students reporting MDMA use, polydrug use was common, particularly including marijuana, inhalants, LSD, and cocaine (Wish, Fitzelle, O'Grady, Hsu, & Arria, 2006).

MDMA Therapeutic and Recreational Use

MDMA was discovered in 1914 by Merck, the same company that had patented and distributed cocaine during research efforts to develop amphetamine derivatives. Although studied for a time by the U.S. Army, experimental psychopharmacologist Alexander Shulgin popularized the drug for recreational use in the 1970s (McDowell & Kleber, 1994).

Shulgin's career walked a unique path between traditional laboratory scientist and club drug enthusiast. Shulgin was a chemist who had been educated at Harvard and Berkeley and had extensive training in psychopharmacology. He developed industrial chemicals for Bio-Rad Laboratories and Dow Chemical Company. At Dow, Shulgin developed Zectran, the first biodegradable pesticide. Shulgin also had a private laboratory at home, where he developed various psychedelic drugs, which he sampled himself and provided to his friends (Gems, 1999).

Shulgin played an important role in developing and promoting MDMA. After being introduced to the drug, Shulgin developed an easier synthesis method and reported the method to other psychedelic drug enthusiasts. In 1976, Shulgin described MDMA's effects to Leo Zeff, a psychoanalyst who had administered LSD to patients in the 1960s. Intrigued by Shulgin's account, Leo Zeff administered MDMA to several patients. Believing many of MDMA's subjective effects beneficial as a psychoanalytical agent, Zeff reported these accounts to colleagues, spurring an interest in MDMA for psychoanalysis that lasted until the 1980s (Pentney, 2001).

Beginning in the late 1970s, MDMA emerged as a recreational drug. People sought it for spiritual enlightenment, improving sensuality in relationships, and pure enjoyment. In humans, MDMA-related medical problems were rare, with only eight MDMA-related emergency room visits between 1977 and 1981. In laboratory animals, however, the occurrence of both acute and chronic adverse effects led to MDMA being labeled a dangerous drug. In 1985, despite opposition by therapists and recreational MDMA users, the DEA temporarily listed MDMA as a schedule I controlled substance, indicating high abuse potential and no therapeutic usefulness (Pentney, 2001; Rochester & Kirchner, 1999). The schedule I status was made permanent in 1988. Despite nearly two decades of legal therapeutic use, the first clinical trial for MDMA in psychotherapy was published only recently (2011). The study by Mithoefer and colleagues (2011) reported MDMA-assisted improvements in patients with post-traumatic stress disorder (PTSD).

Stop & Check

1. Why is MDMA called an *empathogen*?
2. Although MDMA was developed decades earlier, who popularized MDMA in the 1970s?

2. Psychopharmacologist Alexander Shulgin

1. Empathogen is derived from the tendency of MDMA to induce friendliness, closeness with others, and greater insight into one's thoughts and emotions.

MDMA Metabolism and the Length of Psychedelic Drug Effects

MDMA users prefer to administer MDMA orally, usually through swallowing an MDMA-containing tablet. After swallowing the tablet, MDMA readily absorbs through the gastrointestinal tract, reaching peak blood plasma levels after approximately 2 hours. MDMA's elimination half-life is approximately 9 hours (De La Torre, Farré, Roset, et al., 2000) (see **figure 12.6**).

MDMA is metabolized in the liver primarily by CYP2D6 enzymes and to a lesser extent by other enzymes such as CYP1A2. CYP1A2 converts MDMA to methylenedioxyamphetamine (MDA). Like MDMA, MDA exhibits psychedelic drug effects. Its users thus experience specific MDMA effects and then, after metabolic transformation, effects elicited by MDA as well.

Deficiencies in the CYP2D6 enzyme lead to accumulation of MDMA in the body. Approximately 10 percent of Caucasians exhibit these deficiencies. Accumulated MDMA leads to prolonged drug effects and an increased probability of adverse effects occurring at low to moderate doses. For example, certain *selective serotonin reuptake inhibitors* (SSRIs) such as fluoxetine (Prozac) inhibit CYP2D6 activity. These actions inhibit MDMA metabolism, leading to effects similar to those with inherent CYP2D6 deficiencies (Yang et al., 2006).

Inhibition of MDMA metabolism can occur in people with fully functional CYP2D6 enzymes as well. De la Torre and colleagues studied the blood plasma levels of MDMA to determine MDMA's degradation rate (De La Torre, Farré, Ortuño, et al., 2000). During this study, the researchers found that the MDMA's elimination rate was not constant. Rather, MDMA metabolism slowed down over time. Based on these findings, taking further MDMA doses contributes to stronger and longer-lasting pharmacological effects than may otherwise be expected.

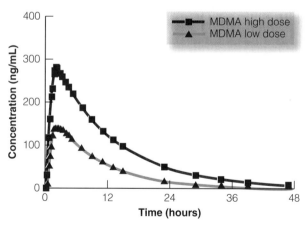

MDMA (Ecstasy) remains in the body well beyond 24 hours, as shown for both a low dose (1.0 mg/kg) and high dose (1.6 mg/kg). The *y*-axis refers to the amount of MDMA in the blood, and the *x*-axis refers to time since MDMA administration. (Kolbrich, E. A., Goodwin, R. S., Gorelick, D. A., Hayes, R. J., Stein, E. A., & Huestis, M. A. (2008). Physiological and subjective responses to controlled oral 3,4- methylenedioxymethamphetamine administration. *J Clin Psychopharmacol*, 28(4), 432–440. doi:, p. 9. By permission.)

figure **12.6**

MDMA and Serotonin and Dopamine Neurotransmission

Acute administration of MDMA alters serotonin neurotransmission at axon terminals through two mechanisms (**figure 12.7**). First, MDMA inhibits serotonin transportation into synaptic storage vesicles. In doing so, MDMA prevents serotonin storage and permits serotonin to escape into the synaptic cleft. Second, MDMA causes the reversal of serotonin reuptake transporters. By reversing serotonin membrane transporters, MDMA expels any unstored serotonin out into the synaptic cleft. Through these two mechanisms, MDMA produces an increase in extracellular brain serotonin levels. These increased serotonin levels lead in turn to increased activation of serotonin receptors (Rudnick & Wall, 1992).

Like amphetamine, MDMA produces similar actions at dopamine axon terminals, leading to enhanced extracellular levels of dopamine in the brain (figure 12.7). However, MDMA's effects on dopamine axonal terminals are weaker than its effects on serotonin axonal terminals. As a result, higher MDMA doses may be necessary to enhance dopamine levels (Abraham et al., 2002; Steele, Nichols, & Yim, 1987).

Chronic administration of MDMA can produce severe damage to serotonin neurons. This damage appears according to every standard measure of serotonin neurons, including loss of brain serotonin, the serotonin metabolite

Low dose

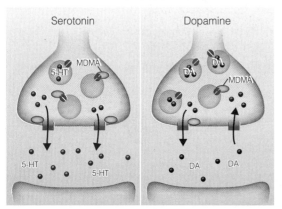

High dose

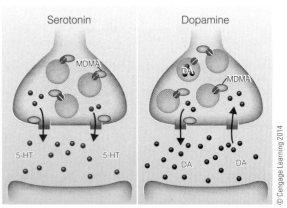

© Cengage Learning 2014

MDMA produces dose-dependent effects on serotonin (5-HT) and dopamine (DA) neurotransmission. At lower doses (left), MDMA effectively inhibits serotonin entry into vesicles and reverses the serotonin reuptake transporter direction. These actions cause large enhancements in serotonin release. Few effects occur at dopamine axon terminals, producing minimal changes in dopamine release. At higher doses, MDMA remains effective at enhancing serotonin levels and also inhibits dopamine entry into vesicles and reverses the dopamine membrane transporter direction. The combination of these actions causes significant enhancements of both serotonin and dopamine levels.

figure **12.7**

5-hydroxyindolacetic acid (5-HIAA), tryptophan hydroxylase, and the serotonin reuptake transporter. Hatzidimitriou and colleagues (1999) provided a striking example of MDMA-induced neuronal loss in monkeys.

In this study, researchers treated monkeys with MDMA daily over 4 days. Two weeks after treatment ended, MDMA-treated monkeys had a dramatic decline in serotonin neuron axons, as shown in the middle panels of **figure 12.8.** Serotonin neuron loss remained low in a monkey assessed 7 years after this

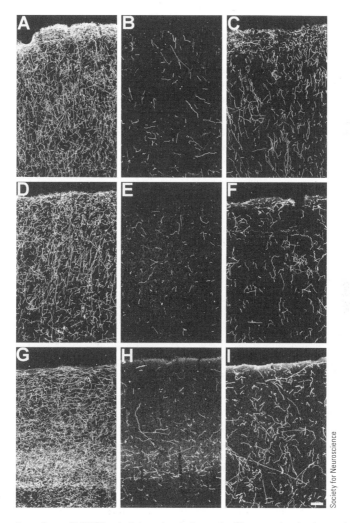

Four days of MDMA administration led to a significant reduction in cortical serotonin neurons 2 weeks after treatment (middle panels) and 7 years after treatment (right panels) compared to a monkey treated with placebo (left panels). The top row of panels (A, B, and C) were dark-field photomicrograph sagittal sections from the frontal cortex. The middle panels (D, E, and H) were taken from the parietal cortex, and the bottom panels (G, H, and I) were taken from the primary visual cortex. (From Hatzidimitriou et al., 1999.)

figure **12.8**

experiment, as shown in the right panel of figure 12.8. This finding suggests a severe neurotoxic effect from repeated MDMA use and a dismal likelihood of neuronal recovery.

Because the cellular techniques used in animals cannot be used in living humans, we lack precise indices of MDMA-induced neurotoxic function in humans. However, the limited data available, in concert with extensive animal data, suggests that serotonin neuron loss occurs in human MDMA users as well. First, heavy MDMA users have less 5-HIAA in cerebrospinal fluid, suggesting less serotonin production in their nervous systems (McCann, Ridenour, Shaham, & Ricaurte, 1994). Second, PET imaging techniques reveal lower levels of serotonin membrane transporters in routine MDMA users. For example, Erritzoe and colleagues (2011) found reduced serotonin reuptake transporter levels in routine MDMA users. Particularly striking, frequent hallucinogen use, such as LSD or mescaline, did not have reductions in serotonin reuptake transporter levels in users. However, MDMA-induced reduction in serotonin reuptake transporter levels may not be permanent. Selvaraj and colleagues (2009) failed to find serotonin reuptake transporter reductions in heavy MDMA users who had refrained from MDMA use for more than 1 year.

Stop & Check

1. How might a drug that inhibits CYP2D6 activity, such as fluoxetine, affect the pharmacokinetics of MDMA?

2. What are the key differences in pharmacological actions between low and high MDMA doses?

3. What effect does sustained MDMA use have on serotonin neurons?

1. The CYP2D6 enzyme metabolizes MDMA. Any drug that inhibits CYP2D6 activity will slow down MDMA metabolism, causing prolonged MDMA effects. 2. Lower MDMA doses primarily enhance serotonin neurotransmission, whereas higher MDMA doses enhance both serotonin and dopamine neurotransmission. 3. Heavy, sustained MDMA use destroys serotonin neurons.

MDMA's Psychedelic and Psychostimulant Effects

The effects that MDMA has in a party setting may differ from those reported under carefully controlled laboratory conditions. These differences occur for multiple reasons. First, as stated earlier in this chapter, the term *Ecstasy* inconsistently refers to MDMA. A so-called Ecstasy tablet may include MDMA, but it also may contain other drugs (Cole et al., 2002). Second, MDMA is seldom taken alone. For example, many club goers take MDMA while consuming alcohol (Mohamed, Hamida, Pereira de Vasconcelos, Cassel, & Jones, 2009). Third, an individual may take MDMA while also taking prescribed psychoactive medications. For example, an individual taking certain antidepressant drugs may have an exaggerated reaction to MDMA's effects (Mohamed,

Ben Hamida, Cassel, de Vasconcelos, & Jones, 2011). Fourth, MDMA's effects vary depending on the dose administered (Abraham et al., 2002).

MDMA's physiological effects resemble those of psychostimulant drugs such as amphetamine at higher doses. For example, Kolbrich and colleagues (2008) assessed the effects of low (1.0 mg/kg) and high (1.6 mg/kg) doses of MDMA in human occasional MDMA users (**figure 12.9**). In these volunteers, only the high MDMA dose produced an increase in heart rate and blood pressure.

REVIEW! Psychostimulant drugs activate the sympathetic nervous system. Chapter 6 (pg. 161).

Low MDMA doses elicit few physiological effects. However, both low and high MDMA doses elicit significant subjective effects. In the same study, Kolbrich and colleagues (2008) found that low MDMA doses produced feelings or sensations of heightened senses, racing thoughts, and euphoric effects. The high MDMA dose included these effects as well as perceptions of increased energy and feelings of closeness to others (figure 12.9).

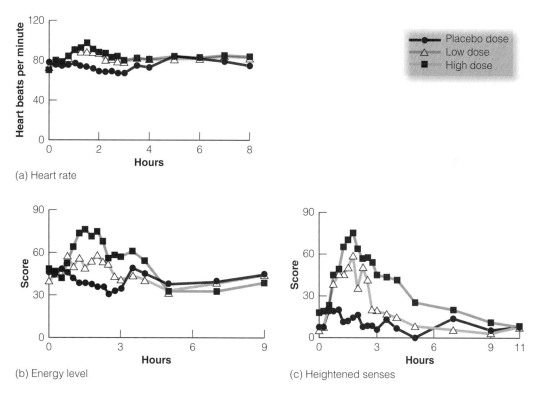

figure 12.9

In human volunteers, a high MDMA dose increases sympathetic nervous system effects such as heart rate (a) and sense of energy (b), whereas low doses create perceptions of heightened senses (c). (Kolbrich, E. A., Goodwin, R. S., Gorelick, D. A., Hayes, R. J., Stein, E. A., & Huestis, M. A. (2008). Physiological and subjective responses to controlled oral 3,4- methylenedioxymethamphetamine administration. *J Clin Psychopharmacol*, 28(4), 432-440. doi: p. 9. By permission.)

The subjective effects of MDMA relate to both psychostimulants and hallucinogenic drugs. Tancer and Johanson (2003) recruited human volunteers to assess the effects of MDMA compared to the psychostimulant d-amphetamine—the hallucinogen metachlorophenylpiperazine (mCPP)—which acts as a serotonin reuptake inhibitor and serotonin receptor agonist mCPP (Bossong et al., 2010). Like d-amphetamine, MDMA produced increases in a scale for drug "liking," an indication of reinforcing effects. Yet, like mCPP, MDMA produced increases in perception and hallucinogen-like effects. There were also shared traits among these drugs. MDMA, d-amphetamine, and mCPP increased ratings of friendliness and talkativeness. Each drug also increased a sense of improved cognition.

Based on animal models, MDMA exhibits reinforcing effects, although in comparison, conventional reinforcing drugs such as methamphetamine produce stronger reinforcing effects. For example, Fantegrossi and colleagues (2002) examined the reinforcing effects of MDMA and methamphetamine in monkeys using a self-administration model. Across a range of doses, subjects self-administered significantly less MDMA compared to methamphetamine (**figure 12.10**).

Beyond reinforcing effects, MDMA is also the representative drug for empathogens, which, as stated previously, refer to enhanced empathy. Women appear more sensitive to MDMA's psychedelic and empathogenic properties than men. In fact, Leicht and colleagues (2001) found women exhibited a greater sensitivity to nearly every measure of MDMA's effects, including overall improved mood, feelings of depersonalization, time-perception changes, and emotional sensitivity. Moreover, women experienced more frequent and profound visual perception changes such as visual hallucinations (pseudo), synesthesia, and memories.

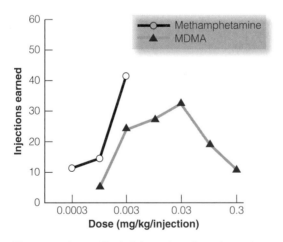

figure **12.10**

Rhesus monkeys self-administered methamphetamine more readily compared to MDMA. The y-axis shows the number of drug injections the monkeys earned during a session, and the x-axis shows the number of doses of self-administered drugs. (With kind permission from Springer Science+Business Media: Fantegrossi, W. E., Ullrich, T., Rice, K. C., Woods, J. H., & Winger, G. (2002). 3,4- Methylenedioxymethamphetamine (MDMA, "ecstasy") and its stereoisomers as reinforcers in rhesus monkeys: serotonergic involvement. Psychopharmacology (Berl), 161(4), 356–3, p. 9.)

As stated previously, animals poorly model the psychedelic effects experienced by humans. However, animal models *can* provide indexes of sociability. Morley and McGregor (2000) used a social interaction test to compare relatively low MDMA doses to placebo. After administration, MDMA-treated rats exhibited fewer aggressive behaviors and greater social interactions with other rats compared to placebo-treated rats (**box 12.1**).

box **12.1** Social Interaction Tests

Social interaction tests assess the effects that drugs have on animal social behavior. These assessments use naturally social species such as rats by placing animals together and observing any of several key social behaviors. Social behaviors in rats, for example, include sniffing, following, and crawling over or under other rats.

In a typical social interaction test in rats, a researcher places two or more rats together in an open field. After placement in the box, researchers score the number of social behaviors, including sniffing, nudging another rats with their snouts, and closely following other rats. To ensure accurate behavioral recording, multiple researchers may score a social interaction test session and compare their scores afterward.

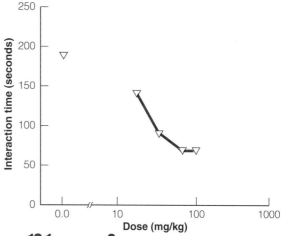

box **12.1**, figure **2**

Phencyclidine-treated rats exhibited significantly reduced social interactions compared to vehicle-treated rats in a social interaction test. The *y*-axis refers to time spent interacting with other rats, and the *x*-axis shows the PCP dose. The zero (0) dose refers to vehicle. (Adapted by permission from Macmillan Publishers Ltd: *Nature*, Sams-Dodd, F. (1998). Effects of continuous D-amphetamine and phencyclidine administration on social behaviour, stereotyped behaviour, and locomotor activity in rats. *Neuropsychopharmacology*, 19(1), 18–25. doi: S0893133X97002005 [pii]. Copyright © 1998.)

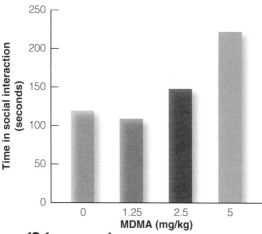

box **12.1**, figure **1**

In a social interaction test, rats treated with the 5.0 mg/kg dose of MDMA spent significantly more time interacting with other rats compared to saline-treated rats. The *y*-axis shows time spent interacting with other rats, and the *x*-axis refers to the dose of MDMA. The zero (0) dose refers to saline. (Morley & McGregor, 2000. By permission.)

Psychedelic drugs affect rodent behavior in social interaction tests. For example, Morley and McGregor (2000) tested the stimulant–psychedelic drug MDMA in rats using this test. This study found that MDMA-treated rats spent significantly more time interacting with other rats compared to saline-treated rats. Using a different psychedelic drug, Sams-Dodd (1998) evaluated the effects of the dissociative anesthetic phencyclidine (PCP) on social behavior in rats. After conducting a social interaction test, PCP-treated rats exhibited reduced social interactions compared to saline-treated rats. In other words, PCP-treated rats appeared socially withdrawn.

MDMA's Psychostimulant Actions

Like the pharmacological effects already described, elevated dopamine and serotonin levels account for MDMA's adverse effects. In particular, MDMA shares adverse effects with many psychostimulant drugs such as methamphetamine. Physiologically, higher doses of MDMA, which are achieved by taking two or more standard MDMA doses, such as 1.6 mg/kg, can substantially activate the sympathetic nervous system, leading to significant increases in heart rate, breathing rate, blood pressure, and body temperature (De La Torre, Farré, Roset, et al., 2000; Kolbrich et al., 2008). This is one of the most common causes of unconsciousness from MDMA use. Other serious problems include brain hemorrhaging and chaotic heartbeat (Kolbrich et al., 2008).

In raves, where dancing occurs in crowded conditions, MDMA use can lead to severe overheating and dehydration, increasing the risk of multiple organ failure. Multiple organ failure from MDMA use is a serious medical event that, in addition to hyperthermia and dehydration, is associated with seizures, muscle breakdown, kidney failure, and blood vessel blockade. Liver damage may also occur because of contaminants produced during MDMA synthesis (Abraham et al., 2002; McDowell & Kleber, 1994).

Psychologically, MDMA doses may cause adverse conditions, including paranoia, true hallucinations, panic, and delirium. Moreover, MDMA overdose can cause impulsive irrational behavior such as walking into the middle of street traffic or attempting to jump from buildings several stories high (Hooft & van de Voorde, 1994; Kaye, Darke, & Duflou, 2009; McDowell & Kleber, 1994).

Rebound effects occur from normal MDMA use. Rebound normally occurs after 24 hours from MDMA use and primarily consists of depression and lethargy. These effects are related to MDMA's pharmacological actions at dopamine and serotonin axon terminals. As described previously, MDMA empties stored serotonin and dopamine from axon terminals and prevents serotonin and dopamine reuptake. These actions leave serotonin and dopamine stores temporarily depleted. Replenishing these stores requires synthesizing new serotonin and dopamine molecules, a process that can take several days for full recovery (**figure 12.11**) (Parrott, 2001).

Cognitive deficits occur from repeated MDMA use. These deficits particularly impact verbal working memory. During verbal working memory tasks, where a participant recalls words given minutes earlier, former heavy MDMA users perform poorer compared to nonrecreational drug users or non-MDMA polydrug users (Schilt et al., 2010). In particular, MDMA users do more poorly on complex verbal memory tasks.

For example, Brown and colleagues (2010) studied verbal working memory in long-term MDMA users and compared their results to those of long-term cannabis users and nonrecreational drug users. The researchers conducted several tasks ranging from simple tasks in which an individual freely recalled words from a list to complex tasks in which an individual recalled words grouped within triplets of associated words. In the associated word triplets, the investigator might have read out loud *frog–chair–apple*, later prompting the participant with the word *frog* and requesting

Acute Administration

Rebound

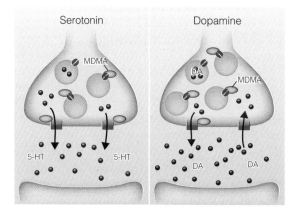

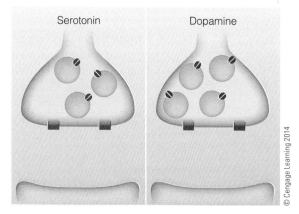

figure **12.11** Acute administration of sufficiently high MDMA doses (left) produces an increase in serotonin and dopamine release. A rebound effect occurs after the stores of dopamine and serotonin have emptied (right), resulting in diminished serotonin and dopamine levels.

the remaining two words. The results? MDMA users performed well on the simple free-word recall task, but not on the difficult triplet-word association task. Given these results, MDMA users appear to have sustained deficits in complex verbal working memory that may fail to improve over time.

Stop & Check

1. How do low-dose MDMA subjective effects differ from high-dose MDMA subjective effects?
2. Why might taking MDMA and dancing at a party be a bad idea?
3. Why do rebound effects occur after MDMA use?

1. Low MDMA doses produce feelings or sensations of heightened senses, racing thoughts, and reinforcing effects. High MDMA doses include these effects—and perceptions of increased energy levels and feelings of closeness to others. **2.** MDMA enhances sympathetic nervous system activity, making an individual prone to hyperthermia, increased heart rate, and hyperventilation. Engaging in physically exerting activities in this state can lead to unconsciousness, brain hemorrhaging, and chaotic heartbeat. **3.** Rebound effects are the result of emptied serotonin and dopamine synaptic pools. The diminished neurotransmitter levels account for depression and lethargy.

MDMA Use in Psychotherapy

As previously noted, psychotherapists administered MDMA to patients during psychoanalysis therapy, providing anecdotal reports of positive results. This continued until the DEA classified MDMA as a schedule I controlled substance in the mid-1980s. The DEA scheduling not only eliminated all therapeutic MDMA use but also precluded clinical studies with MDMA.

The first clinical trial with MDMA was reported in 2011. In this study, Mithoefer and colleagues (2011) assessed low-dose MDMA treatment in conjunction with psychotherapy in patients with PTSD. During the course of the study, patients either received one or two treatments with MDMA or a placebo. Overall, MDMA-treated patients exhibited an 83-percent reduction in PTSD symptoms, whereas placebo-treated PTSD patients only exhibited a 25-percent reduction in PTSD symptoms (**figure 12.12**). The MDMA doses used produced few physiological or adverse effects.

During therapy for PTSD, patients resist thinking about a traumatic experience that led to the disorder. Psychotherapy becomes particularly ineffective for patients unable to tolerate strong feelings or circumvent emotional numbing about the traumatic event. The study authors suggested that MDMA's empathogenic effects may reduce resistance to thinking about an event or facilitate emotions surrounding the effect. In psychotherapy, reducing such barriers provides a therapist access to the root psychic causes of a psychological disorder. Thus, the apparent success of MDMA-assisted psychotherapy for PTSD in this first clinical study supports previous anecdotal claims from therapists who employed MDMA during the years before the DEA's schedule I categorization. However, the clinical study researchers benefited from knowledge of MDMA neurotoxic effects; in response to this evidence, they chose only to administer no more than two low doses of MDMA.

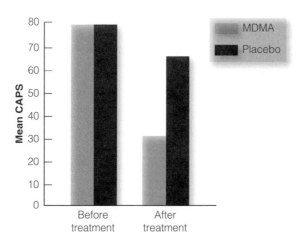

MDMA treatment (solid line) reduced PTSD symptoms according to the Clinician-Administered PTSD Scale (CAPS) to a greater extent than placebo treatment. (Michael C Mithoefer, Mark T Wagner, Ann T Mithoefer, Lisa Jerome, and Rick Doblin The safety and efficacy of ±3,4-methylenedioxymethamphetamine-assisted psychotherapy in subjects with chronic, treatment-resistant posttraumatic stress disorder: the first randomized controlled pilot study *J Psychopharmacol* April 2011 25: 439–452, first published on July 19, 2010 doi: 10.1177/0269881110378371, p. 13. Copyright © 2010 by SAGE. Reprinted by Permisson of SAGE.)

figure **12.12**

Tolerance and Dependence During Chronic MDMA Use

Shulgin, the psychopharmacologist who promoted MDMA, reported that MDMA's positive effects declined after the first seven uses, anecdotally describing tolerance to MDMA's effects. Novice users soon increase the number of MDMA tablets consumed in order to continue achieving positive subjective effects. Experienced MDMA users may take as many as 10–20 tablets in a single occasion. However, a potential confound in this reporting is that, according to MDMA users, MDMA tablets are steadily getting weaker (Parrott, 2001).

A characterization of withdrawal symptoms depends on whether or not to consider *rebound* as a sign of dependence. Rebound fails to meet the classical view on withdrawal symptoms, which normally develop after long-term use. Rebound, instead, could occur after first-time use. When excluding rebound from consideration as withdrawal, researchers seldom find withdrawal symptoms, including any indications of physical dependence or psychological dependence such as drug craving (Parrott, 2001).

Despite a lack of dependence, Cottler and colleagues (2001) found that close to half of MDMA users surveyed met the DSM-IV criteria for substance dependence. Sixty-three percent of those surveyed indicated using MDMA despite having knowledge of its harmful effects. Furthermore, 43 percent reported using MDMA in hazardous situations such as driving a vehicle or having unprotected sex. Thirty-nine percent spent a lot of time trying to obtain and use MDMA.

Stop & Check

1. Why might MDMA aid PTSD therapy?
2. Although somewhat controversial, what are the main arguments that MDMA is an addictive substance?

1. Some therapists contend that MDMA's empathogenic effects enable clients to more readily think about and emotionally engage in events surrounding PTSD's causative traumatic event. 2. First, MDMA exhibits tolerance to subjective effects. Second, many recreational users continue taking MDMA despite knowing the drug is harmful.

Recreational Use of Dissociative Anesthetics

dissociative anesthetics Sedative, pain-relieving drugs that produce feelings of disconnectedness from the body and have depressant and stimulant effects.

Dissociative anesthetics are sedative, pain-relieving drugs that produce feelings of disconnectedness from the body along with depressant and stimulant effects. Not all of these effects occur at the same time but instead depend on the dose taken. There are three primary dissociative anesthetics. **Phencyclidine (PCP)**, also known as *angel dust*, is the most abused dissociative anesthetic. Ketamine, also known as *Special K* or *K*, is another recreationally used dissociative anesthetic. A third dissociative anesthetic, called *dizocilpine* or *MK-801*, is primarily used for research purposes. Beyond these three drugs, dozens of chemical analogues of phencyclidine exhibit similar pharmacological effects (Abraham et al., 2002; Soine, 1986).

phencyclidine (PCP) Most abused drug among the dissociative anesthetics; also known as "angel dust."

Like most psychedelic drugs, phencyclidine and other dissociative anesthetic use occurs in party or club settings. Phencyclidine comes in a variety of forms, including pills, powder, and liquid (Pradhan, 1984). However, just as the term *Ecstasy* applies to more drugs than simply MDMA, the term *phencyclidine* often incorrectly refers to other drugs such as THC, cannabidiol, mescaline, and LSD (Doyon, 2001). Clandestine laboratories provide the main source of phencyclidine and other dissociated anesthetic drugs (Soine, 1986). The U.S. Drug Enforcement Administration lists phencyclidine and ketamine as schedule II substances, reflecting the DEA's view that dissociative anesthetics not only have high abuse potential but also legitimate medical uses (Drug Enforcement Administration, 2012b).

Development of Phencyclidine, Ketamine, and Dizocilpine

Like most psychedelic drugs, phencyclidine, ketamine, and dizocilpine were first developed by pharmaceutical companies. Phencyclidine, the first dissociative anesthetic drug, was discovered in 1926 by Parke, Davis, and Company during a development program for anesthetic drugs. Phencyclidine was used as a veterinary anesthetic and later used as an anesthetic in humans. In humans, however, patients reported experiencing nightmares, severe anxiety, delusional thoughts, and delirium after recovering from anesthesia. Ketamine was also used as an anesthetic drug in humans but was soon discontinued because of similar disturbing effects. However, ketamine remains a common veterinary anesthetic (Abraham et al., 2002; Domino & Luby, 2012).

After abandoning dissociative anesthetics for human anesthetic uses, dissociative anesthetic use continued in two different directions. The first was recreational use. Phencyclidine emerged as a recreational drug during the 1960s. Regarded for relaxing effects, phencyclidine was referred to as the *PeaCe Pill*, leading to the popular street name *PCP*. Users refer to its powder form as *angel dust*. Phencyclidine received a bad street reputation in San Francisco during the mid-1960s, because of the disturbing effects similar to those experienced by phencyclidine anesthesia patients. However, phencyclidine use reappeared in the 1970s and remains a popular recreational substance (Lerner & Burns, 1978).

The second direction for dissociative anesthetic use was psychiatric research. As discussed later in this section, human phencyclidine or ketamine use produces a temporary psychological state remarkably similar to schizophrenia. Phencyclidine-like dissociative anesthetics exhibit hallucinations, paranoia, and other positive schizophrenia symptoms, as well as emotional affect, social withdrawal, and other negative schizophrenia symptoms. Phencyclidine and related dissociative anesthetics also elicit schizophrenia-like cognitive impairments. These pharmacological characteristics led to a new neurological model for understanding schizophrenia, which is described in greater detail in Chapter 15 (Jentsch & Roth, 1999).

Absorption and Elimination of Phencyclidine

Phencyclidine administration includes intravenous injection, inhalation, and insufflation. Phencyclidine was used orally during the 1960s, but users since then have shifted to using the powder form. With the powder form, users insufflate, intravenously inject, or smoke phencyclidine. Further, users may administer phencyclidine with other drugs, such as sprinkling phencyclidine powder onto cannabis joints (Lerner & Burns, 1978).

The administration route affects the onset time for drug effects. Smoking phencyclidine leads to psychoactive effects within 1 to 5 minutes and reaches peak effects within 5 to 30 minutes after administration. Insufflation achieves drug effects within 30 second to 1 minute (Lerner & Burns, 1978). After absorption, phencyclidine's elimination half-life is 18 hours, but it can be as long as 51 hours (Cook, Perez-Reyes, Jeffcoat, & Brine, 1983). Thus, a single administration of phencyclidine produces long-lasting effects.

Stop & Check

1. What is the key psychedelic effect of dissociative anesthetics?
2. How long does phencyclidine remain in the body?

1. Dissociative anesthetic drugs produce feelings of disconnectedness from the body. 2. Phencyclidine, the representative drug for dissociative anesthetics, has an elimination half-life of 18 hours, which accounts for long-lasting pharmacological effects.

Phencyclidine's Dopamine and Serotonin Neurotransmission

Phencyclidine, as well as ketamine and dizocilpine, exhibits a number of pharmacological actions in the nervous system. Overall, phencyclidine affects serotonin, dopamine, acetylcholine, and glutamate neurotransmission (Abraham et al., 2002; Jentsch & Roth, 1999). Phencyclidine causes enhanced serotonin neurotransmission through at least two key mechanisms. First, phencyclidine causes inhibition of the serotonin reuptake transporter. This action prevents serotonin reuptake and causes serotonin levels outside the neuron to increase. Greater serotonin levels cause an increase in serotonin receptor activation. Second, phencyclidine functions as an agonist at 5-HT$_{2A}$ receptors (**figure 12.13**) (Kapur & Seeman, 2002; Smith, Meltzer, Arora, & Davis, 1977).

Phencyclidine has similar actions on the dopamine system. On dopamine axon terminals, the dopamine membrane transporter for reuptake also is inhibited. As with serotonin, this action causes an increase in dopamine levels outside of the neuron, which facilitates activation of dopamine receptors. Phencyclidine is also a partial agonist for dopamine D$_2$ receptors (Kapur & Seeman, 2002; Smith et al., 1977).

REVIEW! A partial agonist is a drug that binds to a receptor but has a weaker ability, compared to full agonists, for activating the receptor. Chapter 4 (pg. 120).

Phencyclidine also acts on other neurotransmitter systems. At higher concentrations, phencyclidine functions as a noncompetitive antagonist for

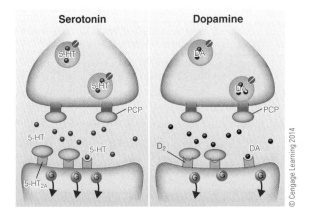

Phencyclidine enhances serotonin neurotransmission (left) by inhibiting serotonin reuptake transporters and activating 5-HT$_{2A}$ receptors. Activating 5-HT$_{2A}$ receptors stimulates associated G proteins. Phencyclidine enhances dopamine neurotransmission (right) through inhibiting dopamine membrane transporters and by functioning as a partial agonist for dopamine D$_2$ receptors. As a partial agonist, phencyclidine activates some D$_2$ receptors while failing to activate others. PCP = phencyclidine, 5-HT = serotonin, DA = dopamine, G = G protein.

figure **12.13**

nicotinic cholinergic receptors at neuromuscular junctions and at ganglia in the peripheral nervous system. Phencyclidine's neuromuscular junction actions cause muscles to contract. At ganglion cells, phencyclidine alters sympathetic and parasympathetic nervous system activity (Fryer & Lukas, 1999). High concentrations of phencyclidine-like drugs also antagonize muscarinic receptors in the central and autonomic nervous systems. Higher concentrations also activate opioid kappa receptors (Hustveit, Maurset, & Oye, 1995).

Dissociative Anesthetics and Glutamate Neurotransmission

In addition to the actions already described, phencyclidine and similar dissociatives function as antagonists for glutamate NMDA* receptors. As described in Chapter 4, NMDA receptors are ionotropic and contain binding sites for many substances on the ion channel's subunits. The NMDA receptor's channel contains a binding site for phencyclidine. When binding to this site, phencyclidine prevents positively charged ions from entering the channel. By preventing NMDA receptor activation, phencyclidine interferes with a process called *long-term potentiation* (Abraham et al., 2002).

long-term potentiation
Form of synaptic plasticity important for learning and memory.

Long-term potentiation is a form of synaptic plasticity important for learning and memory. *Potentiation* means "strengthening," and *plasticity* refers to adaptive change in neural characteristics, often occurring at synapses.

*N-methyl-D-aspartate

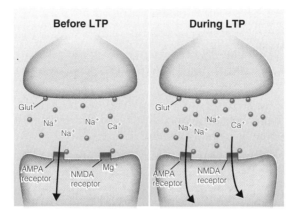
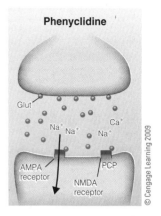

Before long-term potentiation (left synapse), a magnesium ion prevents other ions from entering the NMDA receptor channel. During long-term potentiation (middle synapse), sustained activation of the AMPA receptors elicits sufficient depolarization to expel the magnesium ion from the NMDA receptor channel. The expulsion of magnesium supports a stronger synaptic connection by enabling positively charged ions to the neuron through the NMDA receptor channel. Phencyclidine and other dissociative anesthetic drugs such as magnesium block the NMDA receptor channel. By blocking the NMDA receptor channel, phencyclidine disables long-term potentiation. LTP = long-term potentiation, Glut = glutamate, Na^+ = sodium, Ca^+ = calcium, Mg^+ = magnesium, PCP = phencyclidine.

figure 12.14

Long-term potentiation depends on postsynaptic AMPA** and NMDA glutamate receptors and the neurotransmitter glutamate (**figure 12.14**).

At these synapses, glutamate binds to both AMPA and NMDA receptors. Before long-term potentiation, however, glutamate only successfully activates AMPA receptors. Activation fails to occur at NMDA receptors because a Mg^{+2} ion blocks the NMDA receptor channel, preventing ions from entering the channel. Long-term potentiation occurs when the membrane depolarizes sufficiently to repel the Mg^{+2} ion from the channel. Sufficient membrane depolarization occurs as a result of repeated and sustained AMPA receptor activation.

REVIEW! Both AMPA and NMDA produce excitatory postsynaptic potentials by allowing the entry of positively charged ions such as Na^+. Chapter 3 (pg. 69).

Once depolarization changes dislodge the Mg^{+2} ion from the NMDA channel, Na^+ and Ca_{2+} ions enter the NMDA channel. The entry of additional positively charged ions leads to greater membrane depolarization and facilitates neuronal excitability. Thus, by dislodging the Mg^{+2} ion from the NMDA channel, glutamate becomes more effective in exciting the neuron—that is, by creating excitatory post synaptic potentials. When phencyclidine enters the brain, it acts at NMDA receptors like Mg^+. In doing so, phencyclidine prevents

---

**α-amino-3-hydroxy-5-methyl-4-isoxazole proprionic acid

long-term potentiation from forming or disrupts currently existing long-term potentiated synapses.

REVIEW! *Excitatory postsynaptic potentials* refers to excitatory input from other neurons that result in membrane depolarization. Chapter 3 (pg. 65).

Stop & Check

1. What effects do dissociative anesthetic drugs have on serotonin and dopamine neurotransmission?

2. AMPA and NMDA glutamate receptors are critical for _____, a form of synaptic plasticity important for learning and memory.

3. How does a dissociative anesthetic drug such as phencyclidine interfere with long-term potentiation?

1. Dissociative anesthetics prevent serotonin and dopamine reuptake. They also function as agonists for 5-HT$_{2A}$ receptors and as partial agonists for dopamine D$_2$ receptors. **2.** Long-term potentiation. **3.** Like Mg^{+2}, phencyclidine binds to a site with the NMDA channel, which prevents ions from entering the neuron through the NMDA channel. This action weakens the postsynaptic neurons response to the presynaptic neuron.

The Anesthetic and Psychedelic Effects of Dissociative Anesthetics

Phencyclidine's behavioral effects change by dose. At lower doses, phencyclidine elicits a drunkenlike state. These doses exhibit CNS depressant effects. Moreover, users often report a numbness in fingers and toes, an indication of anesthetic effects. At moderate doses, these drugs produce appreciable numbness throughout the body. These doses relate to an enhanced CNS depressant effect. Moderate doses also elicit psychedelic drug effects.

Phencyclidine offers unique psychedelic effects compared to LSD and MDMA. In particular, phencyclidine elicits a feeling of disconnectedness from the body. Recreational phencyclidine users also report out-of-body experiences, a dissociative effect. This property led to classifying phencyclidine and related drugs as *dissociative* anesthetics.

Moderate doses also impair memory. Thus, dissociative anesthetic users often have a rich psychedelic experience yet cannot remember it later. These memory-impairing effects likely relate to disruption of long-term potentiation. By acting like Mg^{+2} ions that block NMDA receptors, dissociative anesthetics prevent long-term potentiation and, ultimately, the formation of memories (Abraham et al., 2002).

In a study conducted by Morgan and colleagues (2004), human volunteers were assessed on a series of pharmacological measures during intravenous infusion of the phencyclidine-like drug ketamine. When asked to recite a message they heard played from a recorder either 10 or 80 minutes earlier, ketamine-treated patients recalled significantly fewer words compared to placebo-treated patients (**figure 12.15**).

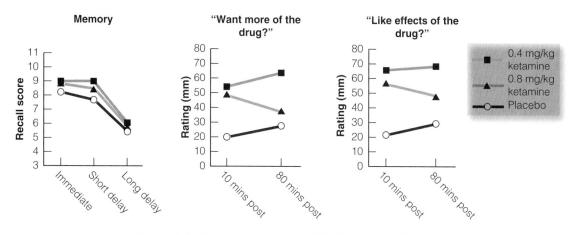

In a study by Morgan and colleagues (2004), both low and high ketamine doses in humans led to significantly poorer recall of a message played either 10 minutes earlier (short delay) or 80 minutes earlier (long delay) (left figure). Ketamine also elicited agreement with the question "Want more of the drug?" (middle) and "Like effects of the drug?" (right). (With kind permission from Springer Science+Business Media: Morgan, C. A., Mofeez, A., Brandner, B., Bromley, L., & Curran, H. V. (2004). Ketamine impairs response inhibition and is positively reinforcing in healthy volunteers: a dose–response study. *Psychopharmacology*, 172(3), 298–308. doi: 10.1007/s00213-003-165, p. 10.)

figure 12.15

Whereas low and moderate doses elicit depressant effects, high phencyclidine doses produce psychostimulant effects. These include an amphetamine-like rush and other increased arousals. Peripherally, high phencyclidine doses elicit sympathetic nervous system activation, leading to increased heart rate, blood pressure, respiration rate, body temperature, and other sympathetic nervous system effects (Siegel, 1978).

Further, phencyclidine psychostimulant effects account for differences in self-administration studies compared to hallucinogens such as LSD. Unlike LSD, animals learn to self-administer phencyclidine. This phencyclidine property was first discovered in 1973 by Robert Balster and colleagues (Balster et al., 1973). In this study, rhesus monkeys initiated lever responding in order to receive intravenous injections of phencyclidine. Data such as these strongly suggest that phencyclidine produces reinforcing effects in human as well.

Morgan and colleagues (2004) also found evidence of reinforcing effects with dissociative anesthetics in humans. During ketamine infusion, participants gave positive responses to reinforcer-related questions posed by the researchers, including "Want more of the drug?" and "Like effects of the drug?" Placebo-treated participants reported none of these positive responses (figure 12.15).

Dissociative Anesthetics and Schizophrenia-Like Effects

As with all drugs, many of phencyclidine's severe adverse effects occur at large doses. At these doses, phencyclidine can produce cataleptic-like effects on movements. The effect is associated with antagonism of nicotinic cholinergic receptors at neuromuscular junctions.

As first described in the history of dissociative anesthetics, a schizophrenia-like state is another adverse effect. This episode of schizophrenia persists for days and even weeks. In the study conducted by Morgan and colleagues (2004) described previously, the phencyclidine-like drug ketamine produced effects that measured as schizophrenia-like symptoms on a psychiatric scale. The production of schizophrenia-like states led to the *glutamate hypothesis of schizophrenia*. The glutamate hypothesis basically states that schizophrenia symptoms manifest from diminished glutamate neurotransmission. Chapter 15 provides more information about this hypothesis for schizophrenia.

Tolerance, Dependence, and the Use of Dissociative Anesthetics

Generally, phencyclidine or ketamine users administer these drugs once a week or less. The separation of drug administrations by days or weeks prevents the development of tolerance. However, for those who take phencyclidine or ketamine on a regular basis, greater doses become necessary to achieve similar pharmacological effects, a clear indication of tolerance.

For the same dosing reasons already described, dependence on phencyclidine, ketamine, or other dissociative anesthetics seldom occurs. When it does, it manifests as psychological withdrawal symptoms. These symptoms include craving the drug or feeling lethargic and depressed. These drugs rarely produce physical dependence (Lerner & Burns, 1978).

Stop & Check

1. At which doses do the anesthetic effects of a dissociative anesthetic drug occur?

2. Which effects of dissociative anesthetic drugs relate to interference of long-term potentiation?

3. How do the reinforcing effects of dissociative anesthetics compare to the hallucinogen LSD?

1. Numbness occurs at low doses and become more pronounced at moderate doses. **2.** Memory disruptive effects **3.** Unlike LSD, animals learn to self-administer dissociative anesthetics. In addition, humans report enjoying the dissociative anesthetic drug ketamine. Overall, dissociative anesthetics appear to exhibit greater reinforcing effects than LSD.

Other Psychedelic Drugs

As is apparent from the drugs covered so far in this chapter, the class of psychedelic drugs is an ever-growing list, including newly synthesized drugs, discovered constituents in plants, and reassessed effects of already known substances. To this end, a coverage of all psychedelic drugs is beyond the scope of this text. However, three other types of psychedelic drugs need mentioning.

dextromethorphan
Opioid cough suppressant found in many over-the-counter cold medications.

The first is **dextromethorphan**, an opioid receptor cough suppressant found in many over-the-counter cold medications. Because of its presence in Robitussin cough syrups, recreational dextromethorphan users, who mainly consist of adolescents, refer to consuming large amounts of cough syrup to achieve psychedelic effects as *Robo-tripping.* At cough suppressant doses, dextromethorphan functions primarily as an opioid receptor agonist, just like the prescription opioid cough suppressant codeine. At higher doses, dextromethorphan functions as a glutamate NMDA receptor antagonist, an action similar to phencyclidine. Together, these actions produce pharmacological effects similar to both opioid receptor agonists, like morphine, and NMDA receptor antagonists, like phencyclidine.

Users can achieve enjoyable and stimulating drug effects after ingesting 100 mg of dextromethorphan, roughly equivalent to 25ml of over-the-counter cough syrup. Psychedelic effects, similar to those produced by dissociative anesthetics, occurs at doses near 475 mg, equivalent to about 120 ml, or one full 4-ounce bottle of cough syrup. Psychedelic effects consist of visual perceptual changes, feelings of transcendence, and mystical experiences (Reissig et al., 2012).

salvinorin A
Psychoactive constituent of the psychedelic plant *Salvia divinorum.*

The second drug is **Salvinorin A**, the psychoactive constituent in *Salvia divinorum. Salvia divinorum* is referred to as *magic mint* and *diviner's sage,* and is currently not a controlled substance in the United States or in most countries (Drug Enforcement Administration, 2012c). Recreational users administer Salvinorin A by chewing or smoking *Salvia* leaves. Unlike LSD, Salvinorin A exhibits no activity at 5-HT$_{2A}$ receptors (Roth et al., 2002). It differs from LSD by also functioning as an agonist for kappa opioid receptors. The discovery of this pharmacological action suggests that kappa opioid receptors play a role in sensory perception (Chavkin et al., 2004; Roth et al., 2002). Salvinorin A also produces modest increases in dopamine levels in the nucleus accumbens in rats (Braida et al., 2008). Salvinorin A users report experiencing visions and perceptions, such as becoming objects, revisiting places from the past, depersonalization, uncontrollable laughter, and perceptions of being several places at once from amounts as low as 0.2–1.0 mg (Siebert, 1994).

Animal research findings suggest that Salvinorin A also produces reinforcing effects. Salvinorin A administration produces a conditioned place preference in zebrafish and rats (Braida et al., 2008; Braida et al., 2007). Third, rats self-administer lower doses of intravenously administered Salvinorin A (Braida et al., 2008).

scopolamine Muscarinic receptor antagonist that produces true visual hallucinations, delusional thinking, and disorientation about time and place.

atropine Muscarinic receptor antagonist that produces true visual hallucinations, delusional thinking, and disorientation about time and place.

Muscarinic receptor antagonists such as scopolamine and atropine represent another type of psychedelic drug. Both scopolamine and atropine occur naturally in plants such as *Atropa belladonna*, which is known as deadly night shade, and *Datura stramonium*, which is also known as Jamestown weed. These substances have ancient histories of human use, including medicinal and religious practices (Schultes, 1969). **Scopolamine** and **atropine** produce true visual hallucinations, delusional thinking, and disorientation about time and place by acting as antagonists for muscarinic cholinergic receptors in the central and peripheral nervous systems (Goudie et al., 2001; Watanabe et al., 1978). Scopolamine or atropine use also causes dry mouth, hypertension, and urinary retention, owing to blockade of choliner-gic receptors in the parasympathetic nervous system (Shervette, Schydlower, Fearnow, & Lampe, 1979).

Stop & Check

1. What is the psychedelic compound found in over-the-counter cough syrups such as Robitussin DM?

2. Although Salvinorin A elicits hallucinogenic effects through activating 5-HT$_{2A}$ receptors, what other pharmacological action might contribute to the compound's psychedelic effects?

3. Why are scopolamine and atropine unattractive recreational psychedelic substances?

1. Dextromethorphan **2.** Salvinorin A also functions as an agonist for kappa opioid receptors. **3.** Scopolamine, atropine, and other muscarinic receptor antagonists exhibit confusion and delusional thinking. In particular, these drugs exhibit profound inhibition of memory.

FROM ACTIONS TO EFFECTS
Synesthesia

Some psychedelic drug users experience a phenomenon called *synesthesia*. During synesthesia, the correct perception of a sensory stimulus accompanies an incorrect perception of a sensory stimulus. For example, a person experiencing synesthesia may correctly see the colors of an object, but also perceive sounds radiating from those colors.

Although occurring during some hallucinogenic experiences, synesthesia commonly arises without an apparent cause. In fact, about 1 in 23 individuals (referred to as *synesthetes*) routinely experience synesthesia in normal everyday situations. Synesthetes report these experiences as normal and generally pleasant (Hubbard, 2007). Further, studies indicate no reliable association between psychiatric conditions and synesthesia.

Several neurobiological models exist to explain synesthesia. One model implicates potential abnormalities in portions of the brain where multiple sensory modalities meet. For example, the temporo-parietal-occipital junction, the meeting point for the parietal, occipital, and temporal lobes, may lack proper inhibitory feedback functioning during synesthesia. Improper feedback may, in turn, lead to additional sensory perceptions to a single sensory stimulus. Other models suggest that synesthesia reflects an abnormality in processes that integrate sensory information into a single multisensory scene (Hubbard, 2007).

REVIEW! Visual processing first takes place in the occipital lobe. The parietal lobe assesses touch information and contributes to visual processing. The temporal lobe processes auditory information as well as visual processing. Chapter 2 (pg. 44).

Although the neurobiology of innately occurring synesthesia remains uncertain, drug-induced synesthesia presents a clearer picture. Perception researchers Brang and Ramachandran (2008) described several lines of evidence linking 5-HT$_{2A}$ receptor activation to hallucinogen-induced synesthesia. The first line of evidence is that 5-HT$_{2A}$ receptor agonists such as LSD produce synesthesia. Second, antidepressant drugs acting as serotonin reuptake inhibitors inhibit synesthesia. The elevated serotonin levels caused by serotonin reuptake inhibitors lead to the activation of 5-HT$_{1A}$ receptors that, in turn, *reduce* 5-HT$_{2A}$ activation, a mechanism that counteracts synesthesia. Chapter 14 provides more information about the interactions between 5-HT$_{1A}$ and 5-HT$_{2A}$ receptors.

Third, antidepressant drugs acting as norepinephrine reuptake inhibitors also inhibit synesthesia. Similar to the second mechanism described already, elevated norepinephrine levels lead to greater activation of α_2 adrenoceptors, which also reduce 5-HT$_{2A}$ receptor activation. Fourth, melatonin causes synesthesia in some individuals. Melatonin inhibits serotonin levels, reducing the inhibitory influence 5-HT$_{1A}$ receptors have on 5-HT$_{2A}$ receptors. By removing the inhibitor, 5-HT$_{2A}$ receptor-induced synesthesia becomes more likely to occur. Based on these four reasons, Brang and Ramachandran (2008) suggest that 5-HT$_{2A}$ receptors, are in fact, *synesthesia receptors*.

Stop & Check

1. Is synesthesia a mental disorder?
2. Which receptor likely accounts for hallucinogen-induced synesthesia?

1. Synesthesia is not considered a mental disorder: It correlates poorly with psychiatric disorders, and individuals do not find synesthetic experiences disturbing or disruptive. 2. The 5-HT$_{2A}$ receptor

▶CHAPTER SUMMARY

Psychedelic drugs include a long list of substances that vary in effects, ranging from hallucinations, sensory distortion, delusions, and dissociation. The three primary psychedelic drug classes include hallucinogens, mixed stimulant–psychedelics, and dissociative anesthetics. The representative drug for hallucinogens, LSD, closely resembles the chemical structure of neurotransmitter serotonin and subsequently functions as an agonist for many serotonin receptors. Activation of 5-HT$_{2A}$ receptors in particular leads to visual hallucinations as well as synesthesia. In addition to hallucinations, LSD produces a suggestible state that can lead to altered perceptions of reality.

Mixed stimulant–psychedelic drugs exhibit effects similar to both psychostimulant drugs such as amphetamine and hallucinogenic drugs such as LSD. MDMA, the representative drug for mixed stimulant–psychedelic drugs, elevates sensory perceptions at lower doses by enhancing serotonin neurotransmission and produces additional psychostimulant effects at higher doses by enhancing dopamine neurotransmission.

Dissociative anesthetics such as phencyclidine and ketamine produce both depressant and psychostimulant effects along with anesthesia, feelings of disconnectedness from the body, and memory-impairing effects. These effects arise from enhancing serotonin and dopamine neurotransmission as well as from blocking glutamate NMDA receptors, which are important for memory function.

Many other psychedelic drugs exist. Dextromethorphan found in Robitussin cough syrup elicits morphine-like euphoria and dissociative anesthetic-like psychedelic effects. Salvinorin A, found in the plant *Salvia divinorum*, produces hallucinogenic effects by serving as a opioid kappa receptor agonist. Muscarinic receptor antagonists, such as scopolamine, produce hallucinations, delirium, confusion, delusions, and poor judgment.

KEY TERMS

Psychedelic drugs

Hallucinogens

Lysergic acid diethylamide (LSD)

Modal object completion

True hallucination

Pseudo-hallucinations

Trip

Synesthesia

Flashback

Hallucinogen persisting perception disorder

Mixed stimulant–psychedelic drugs

MDMA ("Ecstasy")

Entactogen

Empathogen

Rave

Dissociative anesthetics

Phencyclidine (PCP)

Long-term potentiation

Dextromethorphan

Salvinorin A

Scopolamine

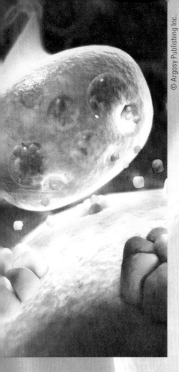
© Argosy Publishing Inc.

Treatments for Depression and Bipolar Disorder

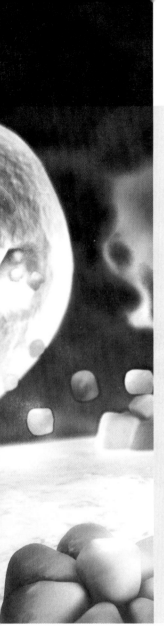

Did Reserpine Revolutionize the Study of Antidepressant Medications?

In 1952, reserpine was first isolated from the *Rauwolfia serpentina*, a plant known for its tranquilizing properties. In healthy volunteers, researchers not only verified reserpine's tranquilizing effects but also noticed that it produced a depressed mood. Attempts to understand this drug's actions divided opinion into two camps. On the one hand, Bernard Brodie and others argued that serotonin depletion accounted for reserpine's effects; on the other hand, Arvid Carlsson and others argued that dopamine and norepinephrine accounted for its effects. This debate sparked important discoveries about the production, release, and reuptake of monoamine neurotransmitters. When a drug was serendipitously found reducing depression in humans, researchers saw that these first antidepressant drugs reversed reserpine-induced depression in animals. Moreover, the wealth of research centered on reserpine convinced researchers that monoamine neurotransmitters were central to the actions of antidepressant drugs.

Despite the important discoveries resulting from studies on reserpine, it appears to be a part of forgotten history. As psychopharmacologist Silvio Garattini (2006) notes, "the new pharmacology texts no longer even mention this drug that was so instrumental in the generation of new knowledge about the chemical mediators in the brain that gave rise to the field of psychopharmacology."

The preceding chapters of this text concerned changes in brain function and behavior caused by psychoactive substances. Thus, normal behavior became abnormal after a drug was administered. For mental illness, we have the opposite. Behavior may appear abnormal before treatment, but with successful drug treatment it may then become normal. The subsequent chapters of this text will shift from drugs of abuse to those used for treating mental disorders, which we refer to as *therapeutic drugs* or *pharmacotherapeutic drugs*.

Mental Disorders

. . . .

mental disorder
Impairment in normal behavioral, cognitive, or emotional functioning.

Just as we have referred to the *Diagnostic and Statistical Manual* (DSM) for defining substance dependencies, we can also refer to this manual for defining different types of mental disorders. We generally define a **mental disorder** as an impairment in normal behavioral, cognitive, or emotional functioning. For clinically diagnosing a mental disorder, the DSM requires that an individual experience significant stress from the disorder and that the disorder does not arise from a medical condition with a clear physiological cause. For example, the DSM does not qualify Alzheimer's disease as a *mental disorder* because, as described in Chapter 3, Alzheimer's disease derives from clear deterioration of brain tissue. This distinction makes sense less today than years past, when neuroscience technology had not advanced sufficiently to glean physiological causes for mental disorders. We will learn much about the neurobiology of DSM mental disorders in these remaining chapters and focus on how therapeutic drugs alter biological processes to improve mental functioning. The subsequent chapters will cover the following major mental disorders: depression, bipolar disorder, anxiety, and schizophrenia.

Mental disorders are highly prevalent throughout the world and occur across all demographics. According to the World Health Organization (WHO), an estimated 450 million people qualify for a mental disorder diagnosis, whereas many others have various symptoms associated with mental disorders. Based on 2002 estimates, WHO reported that 154 million individuals have depression, and 877,000 commit suicide annually. WHO also found that despite the tremendous impact that poor mental health has on a society, only 1 percent of health costs are devoted to mental health in low- to middle-income countries.

Depression

. . . .

major depressive disorder Disorder characterized by at least five depressive symptoms that last 2 weeks or longer.

According to the DSM-IV, **major depressive disorder** is characterized by at least five symptoms occurring within the same 2 week period. These symptoms can include a depressed mood, lack of interest or pleasure in most activities, change in body weight, change in sleep patterns, fatigue, feelings of worthlessness, difficulties in thinking or in concentrating, and recurrent thoughts of death. Moreover, these symptoms significantly interfere with normal everyday activities such as going to work, doing daily chores, and socializing with family and friends.

dysthymic disorder
Disorder consisting of a depressed mood that occurs nearly every day for at least 2 years.

Clinical depression also may occur in a milder form called **dysthymic disorder**. The primary symptoms for dysthymic disorder include a depressed mood that occurs nearly every day for at least 2 years. In addition, individuals diagnosed with dysthymic disorder must have at least two symptoms for depression.

Nonspecific descriptions may be used for some symptoms of depression. For example, "changes in body weight" doesn't specify whether this consists of weight loss or weight gain. However, in depression, we could find that either of these changes occurs. A severely depressed individual may eat excessively, possibly because eating provides temporary improvements in mood, or may eat too little, possibly because the individual lacks an appetite. The same may be true for sleeping; an individual may sleep most of the day or suffer long bouts of insomnia.

Although we generally relate psychotic symptoms, such as hallucinations or delusional thinking, to schizophrenia, they can occur in other mental disorders as well, including depression. The DSM-IV describes this particular form of depression as **major depression with psychotic features.** In this form of depression, hallucinations and delusions relate to depressed mood and negative thoughts. For example, an individual may have delusions that she has cancer all throughout her body or that no one wants her to live. An individual may hear voices stating the same types of things.

major depression with psychotic features
Form of depression characterized by the presence of depression, hallucinations, and delusions related to depressed mood and negative thoughts.

Stop & Check

1. What is the major distinction between a neurological disorder and a mental disorder?

2. How is major depressive disorder different from dysthymic disorder?

1. If the condition causing abnormal behavior has a clear organic cause, then it is a neurological disorder. Otherwise, it is a mental disorder that can be diagnosed by the DSM. **2.** Major depressive disorder requires more diagnosis symptoms than dysthymic disorder, and the symptoms for major depressive disorder need only last 2 weeks, whereas a depressed mood for dysthymic disorder must consistently occur for 2 years.

The Prevalence of Clinical Depression

Depression is the fourth leading cause of disability worldwide because of its prevalence and its dramatic effects on life (Murray & Lopez, 1997). According to a U.S. national survey conducted by Kessler and colleagues (2005), the prevalence of major depressive disorder during a lifetime is 16 percent (**figure 13.1**). Approximately, one out of six individuals with major depression commit suicide, and the Centers for Disease Control and Prevention (CDC) estimates that as many as 12 to 25 suicide attempts are made for every suicide death. Women are twice as likely to be diagnosed with major depressive disorder as men, whereas men are nearly twice as likely to commit suicide as women.

Across age groups, the prevalence of depression appears to be relatively balanced, as shown in figure 13.1. Suicide is the third highest cause of death in teenagers, but it is 4–6 times more likely to occur in male adolescents and young adults than in female adolescents and young adults. Elderly adults are also at high risk for depression. Twenty percent of suicide deaths in the United States occur in adults who are 65 and older. In addition, these adults are more likely to have successful suicide attempts than other age groups. Despite this prevalence, only 8 percent of older Americans see a mental health professional in a given year.

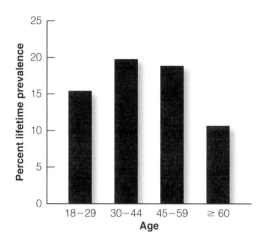

figure 13.1 The lifetime likelihood of experiencing depression is approximately 16 percent, and this is approximately the same in most age groups. (Data from Kessler et al., 2005.)

A potential reason for depression in the elderly may be poor blood flow to the brain. In advanced age, the vasculature throughout the body, including the brain, tends to harden and become less permeable to blood flow, which is critical for maintaining brain activity. In such a state, reduced brain activity may contribute to a depressed mood. The term for depressed symptoms associated with poor blood flow in the brain is called **vascular depression** (Alexopoulos et al., 1997).

vascular depression
Depressed symptoms associated with poor blood flow in the brain.

Just as we find a high prevalence of depression, we also find a high prevalence of antidepressant prescriptions. In fact, the CDC states that antidepressants are the third most prescribed drugs among those 12 and older in United States and the most prescribed drug among those between 18 and 44 years of age. Women are more than twice as likely to take antidepressants drugs than men, and more than 1 in 5 women ages 40 to 59 take antidepressant medications. In addition to the high frequency of being prescribed antidepressant drugs, most patients take these medications for at least 2 years (Pratt, Brody, & Gu, 2011).

Stop & Check

1. Women are more likely to be diagnosed with major depressive disorder, but men are more likely to commit _____.
2. Despite a high prevalence of depression and a greater likelihood to successfully commit suicide, _____ individuals seldom see a mental health professional.
3. _____ depression refers to depressed symptoms associated with poor blood flow in the brain.

1. suicide **2.** elderly **3.** Vascular

Neuroimaging Techniques and Functioning Differences in Depression

The development of advanced neuroimaging equipment has significantly aided our understanding of depression. The structural abnormalities in depression involve many structures, including the amygdala, prefrontal cortex, hippocampus, and nucleus accumbens. The *amygdala*, a brain structure important for fear and aggression, appears overactive in depression. Using positron emission tomography (PET), Drevets and colleagues showed that individuals with depression exhibit increased cerebral blood flow in the left amygdala (Drevets et al., 1992). This same research group later found increased glucose uptake, a further indication that neuronal activity also occurs in the amygdala during depression (Drevets et al., 2002).

Magnetic resonance imaging (MRI) studies also reveal volume reductions in the hippocampus in depression. In a extensive review of imaging studies among depressed patients, Campbell and colleagues (2004) found that the majority of studies found such reductions compared to nondepressed individuals. As presented later in this chapter, researchers have an interest in the hippocampus because of the ability of antidepressant drugs to promote neuron growth in this structure.

Although the amygdala appears overactive in depression, studies indicate underactivity in the left dorsal prefrontal cortex during depression (Savitz & Drevets, 2009). For example, in a study conducted by Drevets, Bogers, and Raichle (2002), PET assessments using F-18-fluorodeoxyglucose in unmedicated patients with unipolar depression consistently revealed decreased metabolism in the dorsal prefrontal cortex. The volume of gray and white matter also appears reduced in the left and right dorsal prefrontal cortex in depression and seems to be related to the severity of depression (Chen et al., 2007).

Volume reductions also suggest irregularities in the basal ganglia. The basal ganglia includes the nucleus accumbens, an important structure for reward- and goal-directed behavior, and the other basal ganglia structures that facilitate movement. Although movement disorders are not a feature of depression, approximately half of all Parkinson's disease patients report a major depressive episode before the first occurrence of Parkinson's symptoms (Santamaria, Tolosa, & Valles, 1986).

Experimental deep brain stimulation treatments for depression also suggest that the nucleus accumbens is underactive in depression. In one such procedure, Schlaepfer and colleagues (2008) implanted brain electrodes into the nucleus accumbens of three patients. After surgery, activating the electrode led to improvements in depression. In addition to these improvements, the patients spontaneously remarked about interests in doing something novel or something they had not done in many years. One patient, for example, said that she wanted to take up bowling again, and another patient wished to visit the Cologne Cathedral because it was nearby and he had never done so before.

Stop & Check

1. The _____, a structure important for anxiety, is overactive in depression.

2. In depression, the left _____ appears to be underactive and to have reduced gray and white matter volume.

3. The volume reduction in the _____ is of particular interest because antidepressant drugs increase proliferation in this structure.

1. amygdala **2.** dorsolateral prefrontal cortex **3.** hippocampus

Antidepressant Drugs and Depression

The first antidepressant drugs emerged during the 1950s when pharmacological treatments for mental illness were virtually unknown. The first antidepressant drug, iproniazid (Marsilid), was developed for the treatment of tuberculosis in 1953 (Fox & Gibas, 1953). Experimental animal findings showed that iproniazid reversed sedation and miosis produced by a drug called *reserpine*. (See **box 13.1** for information on the use of animal behavior models.) During later clinical testing for tuberculosis in 1960, Alfred Pletscher and colleagues observed mood elevations among their patients (Pletscher, 2006). Saunders and colleagues (1959) reported the first clinical data showing reduced depressive symptoms after iproniazid treatment. Since then, the pharmaceutical industry has developed dozens of different antidepressant medications, which vary in their pharmacological actions, clinical efficacy, and adverse effects. We classify antidepressant drugs according to their pharmacological actions and chemical structures, which has led to the following categories: monoamine oxidase (MAO) inhibitors, tricyclic antidepressant drugs, selective serotonin reuptake inhibitors, serotonin–norepinephrine reuptake inhibitors, and atypical antidepressant drugs (**table 13.1**). Largely because of early

table 13.1

Selected Antidepressant Drugs				
Monoamine oxidase inhibitors	**Tricyclic antidepressant drugs**	**Selective serotonin reuptake inhibitors**	**Serotonin–norepinephrine reuptake inhibitors**	**Atypical antidepressant drugs**
Phenelzine (Nardil)	Imipramine (Tofranil)	Citalopram (Celexa)	Duloxetine (Cymbalta)	Bupropion (Wellbutrin)
Tranylcypromine (Parnate)	Amiriptyline (Elavil)	Dapoxetine (Priligy)	Venlafaxine (Effexor)	Mirtazapine (Remeron)
Iproniazid (Marsilid)	Desipramine (Pertofrane)	Escitalopram (Lexapro)		Reboxetine (Edronax)
Selegiline (Emsam)	Clomipramine (Anafranil)	Fluoxetine (Prozac)		
Moclobemide (Aurorix)		Fluvoxamine (Luvox)		
		Indalpine (Upstene)		
		Paroxetine (Paxil)		
		Sertraline (Zoloft)		

box **13.1** Animal Behavioral Models for Identifying Antidepressant Drugs

An important challenge during drug development is an ability to behaviorally identify effective medications. Researchers have developed animal behavioral procedures that, although not resembling depression, accurately predict antidepressant efficacy. The primary models used include the forced swim test, tail suspension test, and differential reinforcement of a low-rate, 72-second task.

The **forced swim test** is an animal behavioral model of depression that measures the length of time an animal, usually a rat or mouse, will swim in a cylinder of water. When a rat determines escape is impossible, it assumes a floating posture and only commits movements necessary to keeps its head above water. Researchers coin this floating posture as *behavioral despair*, although the behavioral analytic term *extinction* also applies. The test arose from data by Porsolt and colleagues (1977) showing the successful screening of clinically proven antidepressant drugs from nonantidepressant drugs.

The **tail-suspension test** is an animal behavioral model of depression that measures the length of time an animal, usually a mouse, will struggle to escape while being suspended by its tail. The amount of time the animal gives up struggling, or despairs, reduces

after antidepressant treatment (Cryan, Mombereau, & Vassout, 2005). Researchers occasionally call the tail suspension test a *dry land* version of the forced swimming test.

A **differential reinforcement of low-rate reinforcement schedule** (DRL-72 sec) requires an animal to withhold lever presses for food until after 72 seconds have elapsed. If a rat presses the lever too soon, the 72-second counter resets. Only responses occurring after the full 72 seconds have passed result in food pellets. In this procedure, antidepressant drugs cause an increase in the reinforcement rate, defined as the number of food pellets earned over time, meaning that animals tend to wait longer before responding. In addition, response rates, defined as the number of responses that occur over a period of time, either increase or remain unchanged after acute administration of an antidepressant drug. Nonantidepressant drugs produce different behavioral effects in the DRL-72 second task. For example, benzodiazepine anxiolytic drugs generally decrease both reinforcement and response rates. Figure 2 shows the effects of several tricyclic antidepressant effects on reinforcement and response rates in this task (O'Donnell, Marek, & Seiden, 2005).

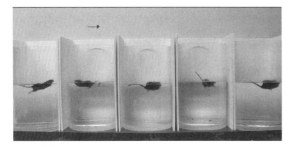 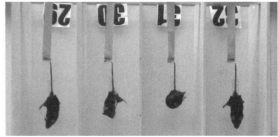

box **13.1**, figure **1**

Periods of immobility during a forced swim test (left) or tail suspension task (right) are used as indexes of antidepressant response. (Photo courtesy of Adem Can, PhD, and Todd D. Gould, MD, Department of Psychiatry, University of Maryland School of Medicine, Baltimore MD)

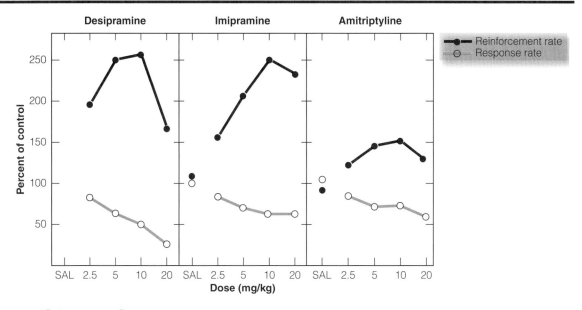

box **13.1**, figure **2**
Antidepressant drugs improve the efficiency of responding in rats trained on a differential reinforcement of low-rate 72-second operant schedule. Specifically, antidepressant drugs increase the reinforcement rate (shown by the solid symbols) and reduce the response rates (open symbols) compared to a control test (i.e., saline test). The data are graphed as percentages of control in order to easily show how each value can be compared to the control tests. (O'Donnell et al., 2005. By permission.)

Unlike animal models for depression, we do not have specific animals models to identify treatments for bipolar disorder. In particular, most successful medications for bipolar disorder derive from treatments for other disorders—that is, antidepressant medications used for bipolar disorder were identified in animal models for depression. Likewise, antipsychotic drugs used for bipolar disorder were identified in animal

models for schizophrenia. Thus, determining the usefulness of a drug to treat bipolar disorder usually occurs exclusively at the clinical level after screening it for efficacy in other disorders such as depression and schizophrenia.

tail-suspension test Animal behavioral model of depression that measures the length of time an animal, usually a mouse, will struggle to escape while being suspended by its tail.

forced swim test Animal behavioral model of depression that measures the length of time an animal, usually a rat or mouse, will swim in a cylinder of water.

differential reinforcement of low-rate reinforcement schedule Behavioral test that requires an animal to withhold lever presses for food until after 72 seconds elapse.

monoamine hypothesis
Hypothesis stating that a monoamine neurotransmitter deficiency causes depressive mood.

MAO inhibitors
Antidepressant drugs that prevent MAO from breaking down monoamine neurotransmitters, including serotonin, dopamine, norepinephrine, and other monoamine compounds such as tyramine.

irreversible MAO inhibitors Antidepressant drugs that irreversibly inhibit MAO.

reversible MAO inhibitors Antidepressant drug that either temporarily binds to MAO or allows other compounds to displace the drug from MAO.

cheese reaction
Overactivated sympathetic nervous system functioning that leads to increased heart rate, hypertension, sweating, and inhibited digestion.

selective MAO$_B$ inhibitors Antidepressant drugs that primarily inhibit MAO$_B$ enzymes and exhibit weaker inhibition of MAO$_A$ enzymes.

reversible inhibitor of MAO$_A$ (RIMA)
Antidepressant drug that selectively inhibits MAO$_A$ but allows for displacement from MAO$_A$ by other compounds such as tyramine.

MAO inhibitors, researchers developed the monoamine hypothesis of depression. The **monoamine hypothesis** states that a monoamine deficiency causes depressive mood. Although decades of research have passed since these first drugs came out, we still develop antidepressant drugs based on this hypothesis (Skolnick & Basile, 2006).

Monoamine Oxidase Inhibitors

Researchers have discovered and named two types of MAO: MAO$_A$ and MAO$_B$. We find MAO$_A$ in the brain, peripheral nervous system, and the intestinal tract, whereas MAO$_B$ is found mainly in the brain and, to a lesser extent, in the peripheral nervous system. In the brain, MAO$_A$ resides in dopamine and norepinephrine neurons, and MAO$_B$ resides in serotonin and norepinephrine neurons (Mills, 1997).

Iproniazid became known as the first clinically used antidepressant drug among the **MAO inhibitors**. They act by binding to MAO and preventing it from breaking down monoamine neurotransmitters, including serotonin, dopamine, and norepinephrine, as well as other monoamine compounds such as tyramine. Depending on the particular drug, an MAO inhibitor may bind irreversibly or reversibly to MAO. For **irreversible MAO inhibitors**, the drug never releases from MAO. To make up for the loss of MAO functions, neurons synthesize more MAO. For **reversible MAO inhibitors**, the drug either temporarily binds to MAO or other compounds such as tyramine to displace the drug from MAO.

An adverse effect termed the *cheese reaction* led to a significant clinical limitation for the first MAO inhibitors. Clinicians characterize the **cheese reaction** as activated sympathetic nervous system function leading to increased heart rate, hypertension, sweating, and inhibited digestion. This reaction occurs when MAO inhibition increases the levels of norepinephrine and tyramine, both of which activate sympathetic nervous system functions. Doctors advise patients to reduce their consumption of foods containing high amounts of tryamine such as dairy products, meat, and grain products when taking MAO inhibitors.

Modern MAO inhibitors reduce, although to do not eliminate, the risk of a cheese reaction. The first type of modern MAO inhibitor, **selective MAO$_B$ inhibitors** such as selegiline (Emsam) primarily inhibit MAO$_B$ enzymes and exhibit weaker binding to MAO$_A$ enzymes. This configuration decreases a cheese reaction risk while enhancing levels of dopamine, norepinephrine, and serotonin. Selegiline also can be administered through a skin patch, allowing the drug to bypass the intestinal tract, where it would otherwise cause tyramine buildup and a cheese reaction.

The second type of modern MAO inhibitors, a **reversible inhibitor of MAO$_A$ (RIMA)**, selectively inhibit MAO$_A$ but allow for displacement from MAO$_A$ by tyramine. By allowing MAO$_A$ to break down tyramine, patients have a lower risk of a cheese reaction. Moclobemide (Aurorix, Manerix) is a RIMA clinically available for depression in Canada and Europe, but the weak efficacy of the drug failed to gain approval by the Food and Drug Administration for depression treatment in the United States (Youdim, 2006).

Stop & Check

1. What was the first antidepressant drug, iproniazid, actually developed for?

2. A deficiency of dopamine, norepinephrine, or serotonin is the basis for the _____ hypothesis of depression.

3. MAO_A is found in the intestinal tract, peripheral nervous system, and the brain, whereas MAO_B is primarily found in the _____.

4. Why might a reversible MAO_A inhibitor be preferable to a irreversible MAO inhibitor to treat depression?

1. tuberculosis **2.** monoamine **3.** brain **4.** A reversible MAO_A inhibitor enhances levels of the monoamines dopamine, norepinephrine, and serotonin, but has a low cheese reaction risk because it can be displaced by tyramine. An irreversible MAO inhibitor causes a buildup of tyramine, which contributes to sympathetic nervous system activation and the subsequent cheese reaction.

Tricyclic Antidepressant Drugs

tricyclic antidepressant drugs Antidepressant drugs that lock the reuptake of norepinephrine and serotonin and function as antagonists for various receptors.

Tricyclic antidepressant drugs block the reuptake of norepinephrine and serotonin and function as antagonists for various receptors, often including muscarinic acetylcholine receptors (Lenox & Frazer, 2002). The name of the category refers to these drugs' shared chemical structures of three connected benzene rings. Chemists developed the first drug in this category, imipramine, in an attempt to produce drugs similar to the first antipsychotic drug chlorpromazine (Thorazine) for the purpose of treating schizophrenia (Davis, 2006). Although failing to effectively treat schizophrenia, clinicians noticed improvements in mood, prompting clinical testing for depression instead (Kuhn, 1958).

As the definition of tricyclic antidepressant drugs provides, imipramine and other tricyclic antidepressant drugs produce certain pharmacological actions similar to MAO inhibitors. Tricylic antidepressants achieve an elevation of serotonin and norepinephrine levels at synapses just like MAO inhibitors. However, tricyclic antidepressants do not inhibit MAO, but instead prevent the reuptake of serotonin and norepinephrine into the neurons that released them. This provides elevated levels of serotonin and norepinephrine without causing the cheese reaction produced by MAO inhibitors.

However, the tricyclic antidepressants have unique adverse effects of their own. First, their pharmacological actions are less selective than MAO inhibitors. Tricyclic antidepressants not only block the reuptake of serotonin and norepinephrine but also bind to many receptors throughout the body, including antagonist actions at muscarinic receptors. Through this property, tricyclic antidepressant drugs prevent parasympathetic acetylcholine from binding to these receptors at target sites in the body, resulting in adverse effects such as dry mouth, dry eyes, constipation, urinary retention (from a lack of bladder relaxation), and various other effects related to these nervous systems. As a result of dry eyes, blurred vision also may occur. By blocking muscarinic receptors in the brain, these drugs also carry a risk of cognitive and memory difficulties (Lenox & Frazer, 2002).

Many tricyclic antidepressants also block α_1 adrenoceptors, causing potentially dangerous cardiovascular effects. Many of these drugs act as histamine H_1 receptor antagonists, which cause sedative effects just as antihistamine cold medicines do. In addition, tricyclic antidepressants are known to cause weight gain, which can lead to a variety of health concerns, including type II diabetes (Brown, Majumdar, & Johnson, 2008; Lenox & Frazer, 2002).

REVIEW! Adrenoceptors are the receptors for the neurotransmitter norepinephrine. Chapter 3 (pg. 87).

Stop & Check	**1.** Tricyclic antidepressants reduce depressive symptoms by preventing the reuptake of _____.
	2. What effect might the adverse effects of tricyclic antidepressant drugs have on patient compliance?

1. serotonin and norepinephrine **2.** These adverse effects decrease the likelihood of patients reliably taking these medications. Parasympathetic nervous system inhibition can cause a number of bothersome effects, including dry mouth, blurred vision, constipation, cognitive disruption, and urinary retention. In particular, weight gain often deters patient compliance.

Selective Serotonin Reuptake Inhibitors (SSRIs)

The pharmacological actions of tricyclic antidepressant drugs established a directed effort to develop drugs that selectively inhibited the reuptake of serotonin or norepinephrine. Based on these pharmacological actions and other experimental support for the specific influence of serotonin on mood, Arvid Carlsson* worked with Astra Pharmaceuticals to develop zimelidine (Zelmid) for the treatment of depression (Shorter, 1997). Thus, zimelidine was the first selective serotonin reuptake inhibitor. A **selective serotonin reuptake inhibitor (SSRI)** blocks serotonin transporters, resulting in greater serotonin levels within synapses. Beginning in 1981, zimelidine was marketed in Europe for a limited time, but was abruptly withdrawn from the market because it damaged myelin sheathing around central and peripheral nervous system axons.

selective serotonin reuptake inhibitor (SSRI) Antidepressant drug that blocks serotonin transporters resulting in greater serotonin levels within synapses.

Researchers at Eli Lilly Company discovered a far safer SSRI—fluoxetine—which is best known by its trade name Prozac. Fluoxetine met FDA approval for the treatment of depression in 1987. Finding it was generally safer compared to MAO inhibitors and tricyclic antidepressant drugs, fluoxetine became one of the most prescribed drugs in history (Shorter, 1997).

Due to the perceived safety, SSRIs have readily been prescribed for depression in teens and children. However, in 2005 the FDA issued a boxed warning

---

*Arvid Carlsson won the Nobel Prize in Physiology or Medicine in 2000 for his discovery of dopamine's functional role in the brain.

label for SSRIs that was meant to alert prescribers and patients of increased suicide risk in teens and children (Food and Drug Administration, 2005). This warning was based on a review of published clinical studies in teens that together indicated a higher suicide rate (4 percent) compared to placebo-treated patients (2 percent). This warning does not ban the use of these medications in children and teens, but rather, indicates that physicians must carefully monitor suicidal tendencies after prescribing these medications.

serotonin syndrome
Antidepressant drug-induced life-threatening condition characterized by agitation, restlessness, disturbances in cognitive functioning, and possibly hallucinations.

Other significant concerns remain for SSRIs. They may cause a **serotonin syndrome**, a life-threatening condition characterized by agitation, restlessness, disturbances in cognitive functioning, and possibly hallucinations. This syndrome is usually avoided by taking low or moderate doses of an SSRI, although a drug reaction with another serotonin compound, such as a different antidepressant drug or lithium, a common treatment for bipolar disorder, can increase serotonin syndrome risk (Sternbach, 1991).

serotonin discontinuation syndrome Syndrome caused by abrupt withdrawal of an antidepressant drug, resulting in sensory disturbances, sleeping disturbances, disequilibrium, flulike symptoms, and gastrointestinal effects.

Just as taking SSRIs might lead to a serotonin syndrome, abrupt withdrawal from SSRI treatment may cause a serotonin *discontinuation* syndrome. The **serotonin discontinuation syndrome** is characterized by sensory disturbances, sleeping disturbances, disequilibrium, flulike symptoms, and gastrointestinal effects. As with most drugs used long term, a careful and progressive reduction in dose is necessary to successfully reduce taking an SSRI (Sternbach, 1991).

sexual side effects
Sexual dysfunction, including erectile dysfunction, inability to achieve orgasm, and loss of sexual drive caused by antidepressant drugs.

Elevations in serotonin levels are likely to cause **sexual side effects**, including erectile dysfunction, inability to achieve orgasm, and loss of sexual drive. This negatively affects one's quality of life and is an important contributor to poor patient compliance with these medications. Many drug developers have sought new antidepressant drugs that have the safety of a SSRI, but avoid this particular adverse effect (Skolnick & Basile, 2006).

Stop & Check

1. SSRIs enhance serotonin levels by blocking _____.
2. High doses of an SSRI may cause a _____, which is characterized by agitation, restlessness, cognitive disruption, and hallucinations.
3. Abrupt withdrawal from SSRI treatment causes a _____.

1. serotonin transporters **2.** serotonin syndrome **3.** serotonin discontinuation syndrome

serotonin norepinephrine reuptake inhibitors (SNRIs)
Antidepressant drugs that enhance levels of serotonin and norepinephrine by blocking serotonin and norepinephrine transporters.

Serotonin–Norepinephrine Reuptake Inhibitors (SNRIs)

Serotonin–norepinephrine reuptake inhibitors (SNRIs), which are also called *dual serotonin and norepinephrine reuptake inhibitors*, enhance levels of serotonin and norepinephrine by blocking serotonin and norepinephrine transporters. The push for a new class of antidepressant drugs resulted from the adverse effects of SSRIs, particularly its sexual side effects, and a significant population of patients who failed to respond adequately to SSRIs or other

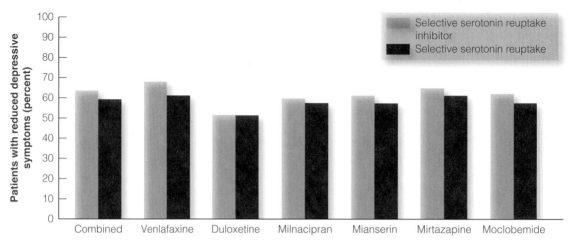

According to a review of antidepressant clinical trials, SNRIs consistently reveal greater improvements in depressive symptoms than SSRIs. However, these differences were seldom robust. (Papakostas et al., 2007. By permission.)

antidepressant drugs (Skolnick & Basile, 2006). This climate led to the development of venlafaxine (Effexor), the first of the class of SNRIs. Venlafaxine (Effexor) received FDA approval for the treatment of depression in 1993. Venlafaxine and other SNRIs are at least as effective as SSRIs for the treatment of depression, and some studies conclude that SNRIs are more effective.

Papakostas and colleagues (2007) conducted a meta-analysis on clinical depression studies that used either an SSRI or an SNRI to determine which class was the most effective. The literature review was extensive, including more than 90 trials and more than 17,000 patients. In each comparison, an SNRI always produced a slightly greater improvement compared to an SSRI. The effects were modest, but consistent (**figure 13.2**).

Atypical Antidepressant Drugs

atypical antidepressant drugs Antidepressant drugs that reduce depression through mechanisms that differ from those of other antidepressant classifications.

Atypical antidepressant drugs reduce depression through mechanisms that differ from those of other antidepressant classifications. They are neither MAO inhibitors nor tricyclic antidepressants. Nor do atypical antidepressant drugs selectively block either serotonin reuptake, norepinephrine reuptake, or both. Thus, this category is a bit of a catchall for antidepressant drugs that do not fit into other antidepressant drug categories.

One of the most prescribed atypical antidepressant drugs is bupropion (Wellbutrin). Bupropion is a reuptake inhibitor for norepinephrine and dopamine and therefore is unique among the antidepressants for its lack of serotonin elevation. Given the lack of serotonin effects, bupropion does not carry a risk for serotonin syndrome, and it does not have a risk of sexual side effects (Ascher et al., 1995).

Stop & Check

1. How does the efficacy and safety of SNRIs compare to SSRIs?
2. What is atypical about atypical antidepressant drugs?

1. SNRIs are at least as effective for depression as SSRIs, and many clinical studies indicate a modestly greater efficacy by SNRIs. Both SNRIs and SSRIs have similar adverse effects. 2. The mechanisms of action for atypical antidepressant drugs differ from those of other antidepressant drug classes.

Limitations in Antidepressant Drug Effectiveness and Development

Although antidepressant drug classes differ pharmacologically, they share many of the same limitations for treating depression. We consider three issues in this section: length of response time, treatment resistance, and strong placebo effects in clinical trials. The "From Actions to Effects" section later in this chapter also considers pharmacogenetic factors in antidepressant response.

Length of Response Time

All antidepressant drugs have a lengthy response time. For those who eventually respond to antidepressant drugs, clinically significant effects occur after 2 weeks of treatment and generally show full effects after 4 weeks. If patients fail to respond sufficiently after 4 weeks, then the likelihood of successful treatment with the drug diminishes. The long response time is particularly troublesome for patients with a high risk of suicide (Nierenberg et al., 2000).

Treatment Resistance

treatment-resistant depression Diagnosis made after successive failed attempts to significantly reduce depressive symptoms.

Many patients may fail to respond adequately to antidepressant treatment. We identify an individual as having **treatment-resistant depression** after successive failed attempts to significantly reduce depressive symptoms, including a treatment course with an SSRI. Fava and Davidson (1996) estimated that between 29 and 46 percent of patients fail to fully recover with antidepressant drug treatment. In these cases, clinicians may increase the dose of the SSRI, add another medication, or switch altogether to a different antidepressant drug. Finding antidepressant drugs with a shorter response time is an important goal for antidepressant researchers (Trivedi et al., 2006).

Placebo Effects in Clinical Studies

Placebo effects present an important issue for drug developers during clinical trials for antidepressant drugs. To gain FDA approval, novel antidepressant drugs must be tested in clinical trials that compare the novel drug to placebo or another antidepressant drug. When conducting clinical trials with antidepressant drugs, a clinically significant improvement often occurs in placebo-treated patients. This requires a novel antidepressant drug to produce clinical effects that significantly exceed those found with placebo. Given these strong placebo effects combined with the cautious nature of clinical drug testing, researchers may fail to find clinically significant antidepressant drugs effects.

REVIEW! During clinical trials for new drugs, researchers start by testing low doses because of the potential risk of adverse effects. Chapter 1 (pg. 26).

Stop & Check

1. How many weeks does it take for antidepressant drugs to become effective?
2. Treatment-resistant depression is often identified after failed treatment with a(n) _____.
3. A particular problem in antidepressant clinical trials is that patients often improve when taking a(n) _____.

1. at least two weeks **2.** SSRI **3.** placebo

Antidepressant Drugs and Monoamine Neurotransmitter Systems

Although imaging procedures conducted in depressed patients help us to identify brain regions involved in depression, these techniques tell us nothing about the neurochemical abnormalities found in depression. Thus, we are largely left to study the actions of antidepressant drugs as a means to interfere potential neurochemical abnormalities in depression. We refer to this approach as a **pharmacologic dissection of mental disorders**. While this approach is not ideal, it has led to the development of many therapeutic psychoactive drugs on the market today.

pharmacologic dissection of mental disorders Approach that infers neuronal abnormalities in a mental disorder from the pharmacological actions of successful treatments.

Most Antidepressant Drugs Elevate Brain Serotonin Levels

One of the main hypotheses for antidepressant actions concerns increases in serotonin release. We derive this hypothesis by finding that nearly all antidepressants drugs, including the SSRIs, increase serotonin release. Yet, bupropion, which increases dopamine and norepinephrine release, provides an important exception to this hypothesis.

Several lines of evidence suggest that dopamine is critical for antidepressant effects and that changes in dopamine neurotransmission may account for delayed treatment response. We begin by noting that acute administration of most antidepressant drugs fail to increase dopamine release or cause other changes in dopamine neurotransmission within the limbic system (Pozzi, Invernizzi, Garavaglia, & Samanin, 1999). Yet during the course of chronic administration with antidepressant drugs, including the tricyclic antidepressant drugs tianeptine, imipramine, and the SSRI fluoxetine, dopamine levels increase in the nucleus accumbens (D'Aquila, Collu, Gessa, & Serra, 2000). These actions in the nucleus accumbens may treat lack of joy in depression.

Chronic administration with fluoxetine also increases the availability of dopamine D_2 receptors in the limbic system. In a study by Maj and colleagues (1996), a greater density of limbic system D_2 receptors was found in rats chronically treated with fluoxetine compared to rats treated with the vehicle. In another study, chronic administration with fluoxetine, the tricyclic antidepressant drug desipramine, or the MAO inhibitor tranylcypromine, produced increases in nucleus accumbens levels of mRNA that encode for synthesizing D_2 receptors (Ainsworth, Smith, & Sharp, 1998). Given that dopamine neurotransmission changes generally occur after chronic, rather than acute, administration, many researchers suspect that these changes account for the lengthy response time for antidepressant drugs (Skolnick & Basile, 2006).

Stop & Check

1. All current antidepressant drugs increase the levels of one or more _____ neurotransmitters.

2. Chronic administration with an antidepressant drug may increase the number of _____ receptors in the limbic system, possibly accounting for a lengthy response time for antidepressant response.

1. monoamine (alternatively, dopamine, norepinephrine, or serotonin) **2.** D_2 receptors

Antidepressant Drugs Increase Dopamine Concentrations in the Prefrontal Cortex

While we find that acute administration of most antidepressant drugs fails to increase dopamine concentrations in the limbic system, acute antidepressant drug administration tends to increase dopamine concentrations in the prefrontal cortex. Using microdialysis procedures in rats, acute administration (i.e., a single administration) of an SSRI or tricyclic antidepressant have been shown to significantly increase dopamine levels in the rat prefrontal cortex. Chronic administration with the tricyclic antidepressants desipramine and clomiramine have been shown to raise the normal, baseline level of dopamine in the prefrontal cortex. However, this is not a universal finding, as chronic administration with fluoxetine fails to produce this effect.

A potential link between prefrontal cortical dopamine levels and antidepressant effects may account for recent observations of antidepressant efficacy from the dissociative anesthetic drug ketamine. Ketamine's possible antidepressant effects were first reported by Berman and colleagues (2000), who assessed intravenous infusion of a low ketamine dose to seven volunteers with

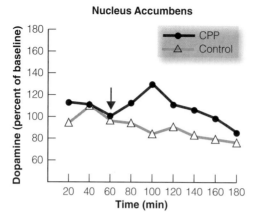

In rats, direct administration of the NMDA receptor antagonist CPP into the prefrontal cortex (injection time shown by the downward arrow) caused a significant elevation of dopamine levels in the nucleus accumbens. Dopamine was sampled from the nucleus accumbens using a microdialysis probe. The drug was administered in the prefrontal cortex through a cannula. (With kind permission from Springer Science+Business Media: Del Arco, A. (2008). Blockade of NMDA receptors in the prefrontal cortex increases dopamine and acetylcholine release in the nucleus accumbens and motor activity. Psychopharmacology (Berl), 201(3), 325–38, fig. 2. doi: 10.1007/s00213-008-1288-3.)

figure 13.3

major depressive disorder. Patients exhibited an immediate symptom reduction that lasted as long as 3 days after treatment. A subsequent study found that ketamine's antidepressant effects lasted as long as 1 week (Zarate et al., 2006).

REVIEW! Ketamine is an NMDA noncompetitive receptor antagonist and dissociative anesthetic that causes visual hallucinations, out-of-body experiences, cognitive impairment, and psychosis. Chapter 12 (pg. 341).

These antidepressant effects appear to result from ketamine's effects in the prefrontal cortex. In laboratory rats and mice, ketamine administration increases both dopamine and glutamate concentrations in the prefrontal cortex. Moreover, Li and colleagues (2010) revealed rapid prefrontal cortical synaptic changes after acute administration. In turn, direct administration of CPP* into the prefrontal cortex leads to increased dopamine concentrations in the nucleus accumbens (Del Arco, Segovia, & Mora, 2008) (**figure 13.3**).

Neuronal Growth Occurs During Antidepressant Treatment

Chronic administration with antidepressant drugs causes neuronal proliferation in the hippocampus (Dranovsky & Hen, 2006; Duman, Malberg, & Thome, 1999; Sahay & Hen, 2007). Because an increase in neuron density occurs over weeks during chronic administration, researchers suspect a link between these changes and the response delay for antidepressant effects. Thus, learning how antidepressant drugs increase proliferation in the hippocampus may aid in developing ways to shorten the response time to these drugs.

*3-[(R)-2-carboxypiperazin-4-yl]-propyl-1- phophonic acid

The SSRI fluoxetine (Prozac) has been shown to increase the activation of TrkB receptors, which are activated by BDNF. In turn, activation of TrkB receptors has been shown to increase the production of neurons in the hippocampus (Li et al., 2008). Together, these findings suggest that SSRIs may produce new cells in the hippocampus via the BDNF system.

REVIEW! Brain-derived neurotrophic factor (BDNF) is a neurotrophin, which facilitates neurogrowth and neuroconnectivity. Chapter 3 (pg. 93).

Stop & Check

1. Many antidepressant drugs increase _____ levels in the prefrontal cortex.
2. A single injection of _____ may produce immediate and long-lasting improvement in depression.
3. In addition to dopamine receptivity described previously, a lengthy response time for antidepressant drugs also may depend on neuron proliferation in the _____.
4. An SSRI such as fluoxetine may increase proliferation by activating _____ receptors for BDNF.

1. dopamine **2.** ketamine **3.** hippocampus **4.** TrkB

Bipolar Disorder

bipolar disorder Mental disorder characterized by abnormal changes between depressive and manic mood states.

Bipolar disorder is a mental disorder that is characterized by abnormal changes between depressive and manic mood states, representing both "poles" of mood. Depression in bipolar disorder exhibits the same features of depression characterized earlier in this chapter. In many ways, mania exhibits opposite features of depression. Mania consists of an abnormal elevated or irritated mood, arousal or energy levels. Manic behavior may occur as fast speaking, rapidly changing ideas and impulsive decision making. During a manic episode, individuals may engage in excessive spending, reckless behaviors, drastic decision making, drug abuse and hypersexuality. **Table 13.2** provides a listing of these and other behaviors found in mania.

The DSM-IV defines two types of bipolar disorder that differ primarily by the severity of mania. **Type I bipolar disorder** consists of exhibiting depression and episodes of severe mania. When presented with a severe manic episode, a mental health professional need not require evidence of depression to make a type I diagnosis. **Type II bipolar disorder** consists of exhibiting depression along with episodes of less-severe mania. We also use the term *hypomania* to refer to this form of mania.

type I bipolar disorder Type of bipolar disorder that exhibits depression and episodes of severe mania.

type II bipolar disorder Type of bipolar disorder that exhibits depression along with episodes of less-severe mania.

Some researchers propose a type III bipolar disorder. This suggestion comes from evidence that antidepressant drugs cause some patients to shift into a manic state. Because this occurs in only a subpopulation of patients,

table **13.2**

Behaviors Associated with Mania in Bipolar Disorder	
Mood changes	A long period of feeling high or an overly happy or outgoing mood Extremely irritable mood, agitation, feeling jumpy or wired
Behavioral changes	Talking very fast, jumping from one idea to another, having racing thoughts Being easily distracted Increasing goal-directed activities, such as taking on new projects Being restless Sleeping little Having an unrealistic belief in one's abilities Behaving impulsively and taking part in a lot of pleasurable high-risk behaviors such as spending sprees, impulsive sex, and impulsive business investments

(Taken from www.nimh.nih.gov/health/publications/bipolar-disorder/complete-index.shtml#pub3.)

this may represent a distinct type of bipolar disorder. Currently, the DSM does not recognize a third type of this disorder (Akiskal & Pinto, 1999).

Many patients with bipolar disorder receive an incorrect diagnosis when first presenting to a clinician. Reasons for misdiagnosis occur from gathering limited or incorrect clinical histories from patients in order to determine a history of both manic and depressive episodes. The most common incorrect diagnosis is *depression*, which tends to occur most frequently in bipolar disorder. Further, individuals in manic states seldom see a reason to seek help, feeling that nothing is wrong with them. Thus, an individual may more likely seek help while feeling depressed (Bowden, 2001).

Bipolar disorder is far less prevalent than unipolar depression. According to a national survey conducted by the National Institute of Mental Health in 2006, the lifetime prevalence of any type of bipolar disorder in the United States is 4.4 percent. The average age for the first diagnosis of a bipolar disorder is 20.8 years old (Merikangas et al., 2007).

Neurobiology of Bipolar Disorder

Neuroimaging studies have revealed that areas of reduced activity in the frontal and temporal lobes of the right hemisphere have a tendency to produce manic episodes, whereas those occurring in the left hemisphere have a tendency to produce depressive episodes. Several studies have shown that the volume of the basal ganglia and thalamus tends to be larger in patients with bipolar disorder.

Functional MRI in bipolar disorder reveals areas of excessive activity in cortical white matter areas from unknown causes. Subsequently, these areas of activity are called *unidentified bright objects* (UBOs). The occurrence of UBOs in bipolar disorder reportedly ranges between 5 percent and 50 percent. The presence of UBOs in white matter areas might interfere with interconnectivity between the frontal and temporal cortex, which may relate to reduced activity in these regions as previously noted (Berns & Nemeroff, 2003).

Stop & Check

1. How do type I and type II bipolar disorders differ?
2. What effects might antidepressant drugs have on bipolar disorder?
3. In bipolar disorder, mania is associated with reduced activity in the frontal and temporal lobes, whereas depressive symptoms are associated with reduced activity in the _____.
4. _____ may interfere with frontal and temporal lobe interconnectivity, possibly mediating mania in bipolar dipolar disorder.

1. Severe mania is observed in type I bipolar disorder, whereas hypomania occurs in type II bipolar disorder. 2. Although the depressive symptoms of bipolar disorder can improve, antidepressant drugs can cause some patients to switch from a depressed state to a manic state. For this reason, some researchers propose a third type of bipolar disorder for this subpopulation. 3. left hemisphere 4. UBOs

Bipolar Disorder, Mood Stabilizers, and Other Drugs

Many of the treatments for bipolar disorder were first developed and approved for the treatment of other mental disorders. Thus, we have few drugs that are considered purely *mood stabilizers*—that is, drugs that reduce both depressive and manic symptoms. Beyond mood stabilizers, other treatments include anticonvulsant drugs and antipsychotic drugs. Although clinicians may also prescribe antidepressant drugs to bipolar disorder patients, they seldom administered antidepressant drugs alone, instead preferring to combine them with another bipolar treatment.

Lithium Is One of the Oldest and Most Effective Treatments for Bipolar Disorder

Lithium was the first mood stabilizer found effective for bipolar disorder. Its effectiveness for bipolar disorder was first realized by John Cade in 1949. Cade served as a physician and superintendent of a hospital in Australia, a position he assumed after spending three years in a Japanese prisoner-of-war camp. After noticing that lithium chloride appeared to calm down guinea pigs, he administered the compound to several manic patients, finding striking reductions in mania. After other investigators confirmed these findings in Europe and the United States, lithium became a primary treatment for bipolar disorder (Cade, 1949; Shorter, 1997).

Since this discovery, hundreds of studies have reported on the mood-stabilizing effects of lithium in bipolar disorder. We can determine the general consensus of lithium's efficacy by reviewing randomized double-blind, placebo-controlled trials conducted in patients with bipolar disorder. Geddes and colleagues (2004) conducted an assessment of five studies with this design. They found that lithium overall proved consistently more effective than placebo for preventing manic symptoms. However, they failed to see substantial reductions in depressive symptoms. Thus, we find that lithium provides greater efficacy for mania than for depression.

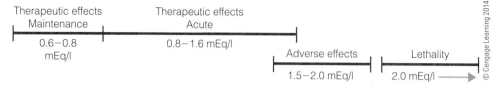

Lithium Concentrations and Their Effects

figure **13.4**

The dose window for the therapeutic effects of lithium stray near those that produce serious adverse effects. Largely because of this, lithium dosing is adjusted based on levels in blood as expressed as concentration in millequivalents of blood per liter (mEq/l). After the desired effects are achieved, lower concentrations of lithium will maintain these effects.

Lithium treatment poses a risk of serious adverse effects. The risk for these adverse effects accompany a narrow therapeutic index and narrow therapeutic dose range. Blood monitoring is used to carefully adjust lithium dosing (**figure 13.4**). When first beginning lithium therapy, therapeutically effective concentrations fall within a range of 0.8 to 1.2 milliequivalents per liter (mEq/l) of blood. After lithium has accumulated in the body over the course of approximately 2 weeks, the concentration must be reduced to 0.6 to 0.8 mEq/l to avoid adverse effects. At this stage, these lower concentrations sufficiently maintain therapeutic effects (Ferrier et al., 1995).

REVIEW! A therapeutic index represents the difference between lethal and therapeutic drug doses. Chapter 1 (pg. 9).

At lithium blood concentrations of 1.5 to 2.0 mEq/l, gastrointestinal effects become prominent, including nausea, vomiting, and diarrhea. Adverse effects may occur at therapeutic blood concentrations as well, including thirst and increased urination, largely because of lithium-induced inhibition of kidney function. Lithium may also produce tremor at therapeutic doses. Higher lithium concentrations, beginning at approximately 2.0 to 2.5 mEq/l, may produce renal failure and muscle rigidity. Moreover, these concentrations pose a serious risk of coma and death. Taken together, even an accidental second ingestion of lithium might increase lithium blood concentrations to near fatal levels.

Lithium's Mechanisms of Action Lithium (Li^+) is element number 3 on the periodic table and is part of the same grouping as sodium (Na^+, atomic number = 11) and potassium (K^+, atomic number = 19). As you may recall from Chapter 3, Na^+ and K^+ play important roles in generating action potentials. Lithium enters neurons through Na^+ channels. Once inside a neuron, lithium takes part in a large variety of intracellular actions, including second-messenger actions and gene expression. This presents an important challenge to researchers endeavoring to study the pharmacological actions important for lithium's mood-stabilizing properties. We find general consensus that lithium's efficacy for bipolar disorder derives from neuroprotective effects against neurodegeneration, which, as noted, may lead to cortical abnormalities (Chiu & Chuang, 2010).

We find these neuroprotective effects in preclinical studies. In particular, lithium promotes the survival of neurons during excitotoxicity. Lithium also protects neuron development during detrimental conditions, including the

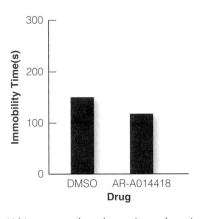 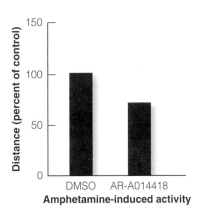

Lithium may reduce depressive and manic symptoms, at least in part, through inhibition of GSK-3, an enzyme that promotes apoptosis and regulates inflammation. A selective inhibitor of GSK-3 activity called *AR-A014418* has been shown to decrease immobility time in rats in a forced swim task, suggesting an antidepressant effect (left figure). In this figure, dimethyl sulfoxide (DMSO) was the vehicle for AR-A014418 and was tested alone to provide a control group. AR-A014418 also reduced hyperactivity induced by amphetamine as well as overall spontaneous activity (right figure). (Gould, T. D., Einat, H., Bhat, R., & Manji, H. K. (2004). AR-A014418, a selective GSK-3 inhibitor, produces antidepressant-like effects in the forced swim test. *The International Journal of Neuropsychopharmacology*, 7(04), 387–390. doi: doi:10.1017/S146114, p. 4. Reproduced with permission.)

figure 13.5

absence of growth factor, heat shock, and high doses of anticonvulsant drugs. A key action for lithium's neuroprotective effects may involve inhibition of the enzyme glycogen synthase kinase 3 (Chiu & Chuang, 2010).

REVIEW! Excitotoxicity consists of neuronal death caused by overstimulation by glutamate. Chapter 3 (pg. 98).

glycogen synthase kinase 3 (GSK-3) Protein kinase that promotes apoptosis and regulates inflammation.

Although it is involved in many processes, **glycogen synthase kinase 3 (GSK-3)** promotes apoptosis and regulates inflammation. In mice, overexpression of the GSK-3 gene causes an increase in behavioral activity, whereas inhibition of GSK-3 enzyme activity decreases behavioral activity (O'Brien et al., 2004). These results suggest that GSK-3 inhibition may lead to decreases in hyperactivity, which is somewhat analogous to mania in humans. In another study, an inhibitor of GSK-3 enzymes led to decreased immobility time in a forced swim test, an indication of antidepressant effects (**figure 13.5**) (Gould, Einat, Bhat, & Manji, 2004).

Stop & Check

1. Although effective for bipolar disorder, lithium's adverse effects are coupled with a narrow _____ index, requiring careful monitoring of blood concentrations.

2. How does lithium enter neurons?

3. Although lithium has many neurobiological effects, perhaps the most implicated action for treating bipolar disorder is inhibition of the _____ enzyme.

1. therapeutic **2.** Lithium enters neurons through sodium channels. **3.** GSK3

Anticonvulsant Drugs

Clinicians also used anticonvulsant drugs to treat bipolar disorder, including carbamazepine (Tegretol), valproic acid (or valproate; trade name is Depakote), oxcarbazepine (Trileptal), and lamotrigine (Lamictal). Most anticonvulsant drugs serve as positive modulators for $GABA_A$ receptors, although we find that other $GABA_A$ positive modulators such as barbiturates appear ineffective for treatment of bipolar disorder. Instead, other actions produced by anticonvulsant drugs may account for reduced symptoms in bipolar disorder.

Beyond facilitating GABA neurotransmission, anticonvulsant drugs produce a variety of other effects on neurons. First, many of the anticonvulsant drugs for bipolar disorder inhibit Na^+ channel functioning. At therapeutic doses, Na^+ channel inhibition largely affects high-frequency action potentials. This action not only likely plays a role in their antiseizure effects, but also may reduce manic symptoms in bipolar disorder. Second, many of these anticonvulsant drugs inhibit GSK-3 activity, a mechanism of action comparable to the effects of lithium (Chiu & Chuang, 2010; Keck, McElroy, & Nemeroff, 1992).

Atypical Antipsychotic Drugs

Although clinicians use antipsychotic drugs for the treatment of schizophrenia, antipsychotic drugs are also used for the treatment of bipolar disorder. In particular, the *atypical* antipsychotic drugs have become safer first-line treatments compared to lithium. These drugs include quetiapine (Seroquel), aripiprazole (Abilify), olazapine (Zeprexa), and risperidone (Risperdal), among others. The compounds serve to reduce and prevent mania from occurring in this disorder.

One of the most common treatment approaches involves a combination of both an atypical antidepressant drugs and an antidepressant drug. Eli Lilly pharmaceutical sponsored one of the first demonstrations of this combined approach for treating bipolar disorder. During the course of 8 weeks, Tohen and colleagues (2003) administered placebo, olanzapine alone, or a treatment combination of olanzapine and fluoxetine in patients with type I bipolar disorder. They found significantly reduced depression scores after treatment with the drug combination compared to either placebo or olanzapine given alone. Manic symptoms occurred too infrequently in the placebo-treated patients to allow for studying treatment effects on mania in this study.

Treatment time course serves as the most clinically important finding in this study. After 3 weeks of treatment, 50 percent of participants were responsive to the olanzapine and fluoxetine combination compared to only 30 percent of olanzapine-treated patients. Thus, the addition of fluoxetine decreased the amount of time it took for a reduction in depressive symptoms to occur.

This study provided an important shift in treatment strategies for bipolar disorder. In an extensive review of clinical studies evaluating antipsychotic drugs and other traditional medications for depressive symptoms in bipolar disorder, the fluoxetine–olanzapine combination provided the greatest effects. The atypical antipsychotic drug quetiapine was shown to be the second most effective for depressive symptoms, whereas other antipsychotic drugs and the more traditional treatments for bipolar disorder were inconsistently effective for depressive symptoms (Vieta et al., 2010).

The ability of quetiapine alone to be effective for depressive symptoms is a bit of mystery because, after all, the receptor binding profile for quetiapine is very similar to other atypical antipsychotic drugs, including olanzapine. The unique efficacy quetiapine has for depression may not actually be a result of the quetiapine molecule but of *N-desalkylquetiapine*, one of the metabolites for quetiapine. N-desalkylquetiapine chemically resembles a tricyclic antidepressant drug, and pharmacological studies reveal that N-desalkylquetiapine inhibits reuptake of serotonin and norepinephrine (Jensen et al., 2008). In this way, quetiapine treatment may functionally serve like a combination of an atypical antipsychotic drug and an antidepressant drug.

Stop & Check

1. Like lithium, anticonvulsant drugs effective for bipolar disorder inhibit the _____ enzyme.
2. Another common bipolar treatment is a combination of an atypical antipsychotic drug and a(n) _____ drug.
3. How might the effects of quetiapine be similar to those produced by a combination of olanzapine and fluoxetine?

1. GSK3 **2.** antidepressant drug **3.** Quetiapine is an atypical antipsychotic drug, but the active metabolite for quetiapine, N-desalkylquetiapine, may have antidepressant effects.

FROM ACTIONS TO EFFECTS
Pharmacogenetic Factors and Treatment Response in Depression

Early in this this chapter, we presented important limitations in the efficacy of antidepressant mediations. Another limitation involves genetic differences. Pharmacogenetics may inhibit a patient's response to antidepressant drugs. For example, genetic differences may alter the ability of an antidepressant drug to cross the blood–brain barrier. In a study conducted by Uhr and colleagues (2008), variations in the $ABCB_1$ gene were examined because this gene encodes for P-glycoprotein, a transporter important for the ability of certain antidepressants drugs to cross the blood–brain barrier. In patients who had a polymorphism in the $ABCB_1$ gene, full recovery from depression was less likely if they were treated with a drug transported by P-glycoprotein, such as the tricyclic antidepressant drug amitriptyline (Elavil), the SSRIs paroxetine (Paxil) and citalopram (Celexa), or the SNRI venlafaxine (Effexor). However, they found no such correlation with the antidepressant drug mirtazapine (Remeron), which does not rely on P-glycoprotein to cross the blood–brain barrier.

Pharmacogenetic factors may also alter serotonin transporter function, an important site of action for many antidepressant drugs. The gene for the serotonin transporter is *SLC6A4*, and it includes a region important for serotonin transporter function called the *serotonin-transporter-gene–linked polymorphic region*. Clinicians find a poorer treatment response and shorter time until depressive symptoms return in patients who have a short variation of this region (Horstmann & Binder, 2009; Serretti, Kato, De Ronchi, & Kinoshita, 2007).

Finally, genetic expression of neurotrophins may affect antidepressant treatment response. These investigations stem from findings that chronic antidepressant drug administration promotes neural proliferation in the hippocampus. In particular, several studies have focused on the polymorphism called *Val66Met* existing on the gene for BDNF. This polymorphism reduces BDNF levels and may subsequently lead to reduced density of TrkB receptors (Bath et al., 2008; Egan et al., 2003). As noted previously, antidepressant drugs may promote proliferation by indirectly activating TrkB receptors. Patients with this polymorphism tend to have poorer treatment response to antidepressant drugs (Horstmann & Binder, 2009; Shimizu, Hashimoto, & Iyo, 2004).

Stop & Check

1. How might a short variation of the serotonin-transporter-gene–linked polymorphic region impact the effectiveness of antidepressant drugs?

2. Two pharmacokinetic factors important for antidepressant drugs that are affected by pharmacogenetic factors are _____.

3. Gene polymorphisms for neurotrophins may diminish the effects on antidepressant drugs on _____.

1. An individual with this polymorphism may have fewer functional serotonin reuptake transporters. Fewer serotonin reuptake transporters are fewer targets for SSRIs or other antidepressant drugs that block serotonin reuptake. **2.** the ability to cross the blood–brain barrier (P-glycoprotein activity) and drug metabolism (CYP2D6 polymorphisms). **3.** proliferation in the hippocampus

---

▶ CHAPTER SUMMARY

A major depressive disorder is characterized by at least five depressive symptoms, such as feelings of worthlessness or thoughts of death, that persist for two weeks. Dysthymic disorder consists of fewer symptoms, but these symptoms persist for at least two years. Depression is highly prevalent across age groups and carries a significant risk of suicide.

Neurobiologically, depression appears to be associated with overactivity in the amygdala, reduced activity in the left dorsal prefrontal cortex, and reduced volume of the hippocampus. The classes of antidepressant drugs include MAO inhibitors, tricyclic antidepressant drugs,

SSRIs, SNRIs, and atypical antidepressant drugs. Important challenges to using antidepressant drugs to treat depression include a lengthy response time, treatment resistance, large placebo effects in clinical trials, and pharmacogenetic differences.

Bipolar disorder is a mental disorder that is characterized by abnormal changes between depressive and manic mood states. Mania is most severe in type I bipolar disorder and less severe in type II disorder. Bipolar disorder is associated with a larger basal ganglia and thalamus, as well as instances of unusually high cortical activity called *unidentified bright objects* (UBOs). Cortical metabolic activity has been shown to change significantly between high activity during manic episodes and low activity during depressive episodes.

A long-used and still common treatment for bipolar disorder is lithium, which is effective for reducing manic symptoms and, to a lesser extent, depressive symptoms. However, lithium's severe adverse effects coupled with a small therapeutic index makes lithium less desirable if other effective treatments are available. Subsequently, bipolar disorder may be treated with anticonvulsant drugs or antipsychotic drugs. In particular, combined treatment with an antipsychotic drug and an antidepressant drug may be effective for improving depression in bipolar disorder.

KEY TERMS

Mental disorder

Major depressive disorder

Dysthymic disorder

Major depression with psychotic features

Vascular depression

Monoamine hypothesis

MAO inhibitors

Irreversible MAO inhibitors

Reversible MAO inhibitors

Cheese reaction

Selective MAO_B inhibitors

Reversible inhibitor of MAO_A (RIMA)

Tricyclic antidepressant drugs

Selective serotonin reuptake inhibitor (SSRI)

Serotonin syndrome

Serotonin discontinuation syndrome

Sexual side effects

Serotonin norepinephrine reuptake inhibitors (SNRIs)

Atypical antidepressant drugs

Treatment-resistant depression

Pharmacologic dissection of mental disorders

Bipolar disorder

Type I bipolar disorder

Type II bipolar disorder

Forced swim test

Glycogen synthase kinase 3 (GSK-3)

Tail-suspension test

Differential reinforcement of low-rate reinforcement schedule

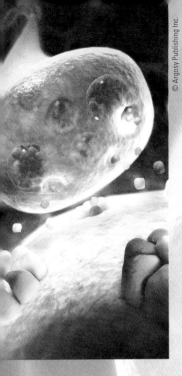

© Argosy Publishing Inc.

CHAPTER **14**

Treatments for Anxiety Disorders

- ▶ DSM Definitions of Anxiety Disorders
- ▶ The Amygdala's Role in Anxiety
- ▶ Anxious Feelings, the Amygdala, and the Sympathetic Nervous System
- ▶ Stress and the HPA Axis
- ▶ Anxiolytic and Antidepressant Drugs and the Treatment of Anxiety
- ▶ From Actions to Effects: How Do Antidepressant Drugs Reduce Anxiety?
- ▶ Chapter Summary

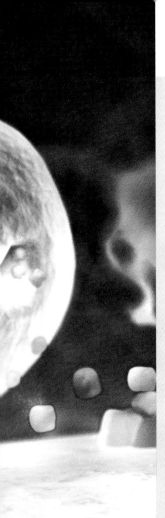

Was Miltown Too Good to Be True?

In the first half of the 20th century, barbiturate drugs served as prescription medications for relieving anxiety. Yet by the 1950s, the dangers of barbiturates gained widespread attention. This decade saw a dramatic increase in both accidental and suicidal deaths from barbiturate use. In 1951, the addictive properties of barbiturates led *The New York Times* to declare them more dangerous than heroin or cocaine (Lopez-Munoz, Ucha-Udabe, & Alamo, 2005).

The world was ready for safer barbiturate-like drugs when meprobamate (Miltown) hit the market. Wallace Laboratories sold meprobamate as a tranquilizer to rid anxiousness, but the company falsely claimed there was no risk of addiction. Tone (2005) describes meprobamate use as an "overnight sensation," accounting for 57 million prescriptions to Americans in 1957 alone. Convinced of its safety, physicians freely prescribed meprobamate to relieve everyday tensions. When pharmacies ran out of meprobamate, they posted signs to alert their customers. Television comic Milton Berle once told viewers that they were only addicted to Miltown if they took more than their doctors. The popularity of meprobamate soon faded; by the mid-1960s, most patients had switched to a safer alternative: the benzodiazepines (Tone, 2005).

DSM Definitions of Anxiety Disorders

The fourth edition of the *Diagnostic and Statistical Manual of Mental Disorders* (DSM-IV) classifies anxiety disorders as (1) panic disorders, (2) specific phobias (e.g., fear of heights and fear of spiders), (3) social phobias (social anxiety disorder), (4) obsessive–compulsive disorders, (5) post-traumatic stress disorders, and (6) generalized anxiety disorders. Many individuals with anxiety disorders also have **agoraphobia**, a profound fear of being in a situation from which escape is difficult or embarrassing, particularly if a panic attack occurs.

Panic attacks may appear in any anxiety disorder and occur as the primary feature of panic disorder. The DSM-IV TR defines a **panic attack** as

> a discrete period in which there is the sudden onset of intense apprehension, fearfulness, or terror, often associated with feelings of impending doom. During these attacks, symptoms such as shortness of breath, palpitations, chest

agoraphobia Anxiety about being in situations from which escape is difficult or embarrassing.

panic attack Strong physiological fear response associated with intense apprehension, fearfulness, or terror.

pain or discomfort, choking or smothering sensations, and fear of "going crazy" or losing control are present (American Psychiatric Association, 2000, p. 429).

Individuals who experience their first panic attack often mistake it for a heart attack.

specific phobias
Significant anxiety provoked by exposure to specific feared objects or situations.

Specific phobias consist of "significant anxiety provoked by exposure to a specific feared object or situation" (APA, 2000). These include a number of common fears such as a fear of heights (acrophobia) or of spiders (arachnophobia) and less common fears such as a fear of clowns (coulrophobia). New specific phobias, particularly unique ones, arise from case studies that apply the general characteristics of a phobia described in the DSM. A phobia occurs as something far more severe than a general dislike for something. In other words, someone who dislikes heights may still decide to climb a ladder or look down from an upper-story window. Instead, a phobia manifests as a strong repulsion to such situations—that is, an acrophobic person may go to great lengths to avoid heights. Depending on the type, a phobia may cause significant disruptions in normal daily living activities.

social phobia Fear of being in or performing in social or public situations.

Social phobia, also referred to as *social anxiety disorder*, is a fear of being in or performing in social or public situations. These situations provoke an immediate anxiety response, one that may be severe enough to elicit a panic attack. With a 12-percent prominence rate, we find social phobia second only to specific phobia as the most common type of anxiety disorder (Kessler et al., 2005).

obsessive–compulsive disorder Anxiety arising over obsession; accompanied by compulsive behavior that endeavors to reduce this anxiety.

Obsessive–compulsive disorder (OCD) consists of anxiety arising over obsession and compulsive behavior that endeavors to reduce this anxiety. The DSM defines obsession as "persistent ideas, thoughts, impulses, or images that are experienced as intrusive and inappropriate and that cause marked anxiety or distress" (APA, 2000). Common obsessions include thoughts about germs or other contaminations, unresolved doubts (such as whether doors have been left open or home appliances have been left on), and not having objects in a precise order. Because of these anxiety-causing obsessions, individuals with OCD engage in compulsive behaviors that reduce this anxiety. Thus, common compulsions include excessive hand washing, checking doors or appliances, and organizing objects, respectively.

post-traumatic stress disorder (PTSD)
Persistent state of physiological arousal or exaggerated response to certain stimuli, particularly those associated with a traumatic event.

Post-traumatic stress disorder (PTSD) is characterized by a persistent state of physiological arousal or exaggerated response to certain stimuli, particularly those associated with a traumatic event. According to the DSM-IV, a person's response to the traumatic event "must involve intense fear, helplessness, or horror." Individuals with PTSD often have moments of recall of the traumatic event, possibly occurring in dreams. Some individuals may experience flashbacks in which reality temporarily gives way to a reliving of the traumatic event (APA, 2000).

generalized anxiety disorder Excessive worry about events, individuals, or activities.

Finally, **generalized anxiety disorder** is characterized by excessive worry about events, individuals, or activities. Individuals with generalized anxiety disorder may constantly feel worried and subsequently exhausted. This worry often generalizes to various perceived physical ailments, often leading to unnecessary medical care.

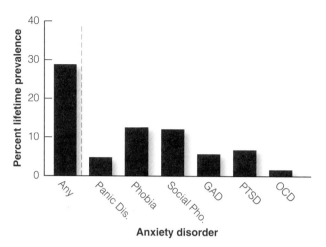

figure **14.1**   Anxiety disorders are among the most prevalent mental disorders. (Data from Kessler et al., 2005.)

Anxiety disorders are highly prevalent and may develop as a result of both environmental and genetic factors. Kessler and colleagues (2005) estimate that 28.8 percent of U.S. individuals have had an anxiety disorder in their lifetime (**figure 14.1**). The majority of these individuals experienced either some type of specific phobia or social phobia. A fourth of those experiencing an anxiety disorder reported having PTSD. Childhood physical and sexual abuse correlates highly with having an anxiety disorder in adulthood (Cougle, Timpano, Sachs-Ericsson, Keough, & Riccardi, 2010). Overall, genetic risk accounts for 30 percent to 40 percent of anxiety disorder diagnoses (Norrholm & Ressler, 2009). In particular, genetics accounts for 47 percent of the likelihood of developing PTSD after experiencing a traumatic event (Sartor et al., 2012).

Given their prevalence, anxiety disorders have a significant economic burden on society. For example, Greenberg and colleagues (1999) reported that the annual cost of treating anxiety disorders in 1990 was approximately $42.3 billion. The economic cost models for anxiety disorders not only assess direct psychiatric care but also prescription costs, unnecessary medical care, and various other factors. This study also estimated that anxiety disorders account for approximately $4.1 billion per year in lost workplace productivity.

Stop & Check

1. Anxiety disorders may be accompanied by _____, an anxiety about being in situations where escape is difficult or embarrassing.
2. A profound fear of something such as heights, spiders, or confined spaces is defined as a(n) _____, according to the DSM.
3. Which anxiety disorder has the clearest genetic predisposition?

1. agoraphobia **2.** specific phobia **3.** Post-traumatic stress disorder

The Amygdala's Role in Anxiety

As presented in Chapter 4, research identifies the amygdala as a critical structure for fear and anxiety. Increased activity in the structure is associated with fear, anxiety, and aggression in numerous animal and human studies. In humans, increased activity in the amygdala causes states of fear and anxiety, and amygdala dysfunction occurs in every type of anxiety disorder, with the possible exception of OCD (Davis & Whalen, 2001; Shin & Liberzon, 2010). Rather, researchers associate OCD with abnormal functioning in the thalamus, cingulate cortex, prefrontal cortex, orbitofrontal cortex, basal ganglia, and nucleus accumbens (Graybiel & Rauch, 2000; Laplane et al., 1989).

The amygdala appears responsible for relating stimuli or events to fear and for mediating the physiological and psychological reactions to fear. Studies in both animals and humans consistently reveal increased activity in the amygdala during fear conditioning, a process in which a stimulus is associated with an aversive event such as a shock. Moreover, increases in amygdala activity occur when receiving oral warnings, watching videos of humans being fear conditioned, and seeing pictures of faces with frightened expressions. Researchers find associations between deficient amygdala functioning in humans, which may result from infections, injury, or parasites, with placid reactions to aversive stimuli and self-inflicted injury (Shin & Liberzon, 2010).

The amygdala receives information from many parts of the brain (**figure 14.2**). The nervous system sends sensory information, including visual, auditory, touch, and pain, from the thalamus to the amygdala via two pathways. First, the thalamo-amygdala pathway sends crude and unprocessed sensory information directly from the thalamus to the amygdala. We refer to this as the *short route* for sensory information from the thalamus. As largely unprocessed information, this pathway provides the amygdala only basic features of a stimulus, such as a loud noise, but does not indicate what the stimulus actually is (Davis & Whalen, 2001).

Second, the thalamo-cortical-amygdala pathway sends sensory information to the amygdala after processing in the cerebral cortex. We refer to this as the *long route* for sensory information from the thalamus, and this requires a slightly longer amount of time to reach the amygdala. Because the sensory information is processed in the cortex, the information contains information about what the stimulus is. For example, instead of a "loud noise" as the short pathway may communicate, a person may afterward discern a "dog's bark" as the long pathway may communicate (Davis & Whalen, 2001).

The hippocampus sends information on the context surrounding the stimulus to the amygdala. Thus, if the context of the environment is important for the amygdala's response to the stimulus, then information sent from the hippocampus will modify this response. Thus, a person may have a weak fear response when seeing a large dog—the stimulus in this example—behind

INPUTS TO AMYGDALA

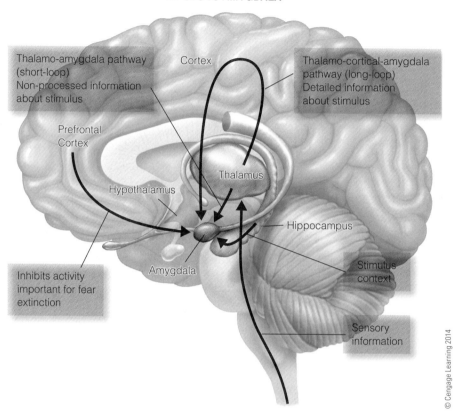

Thalamo-amygdala pathway (short-loop)
Non-processed information about stimulus

Cortex

Thalamo-cortical-amygdala pathway (long-loop)
Detailed information about stimulus

Prefrontal Cortex

Thalamus

Hypothalamus

Hippocampus

Inhibits activity important for fear extinction

Amygdala

Stimulus context

Sensory information

© Cengage Learning 2014

figure 14.2 The amygdala receives sensory inputs from the body and sends information to the prefrontal cortex, hypothalamus, and other areas important for anxiety responses.

a large fence—the stimulus context. Inputs to the amygdala from the prefrontal cortex act to reduce amygdala activity, resulting in an inhibited reaction to fearful stimuli. We also find the prefrontal cortex important for extinction of fear conditioning or, in other words, unlearning that particular stimuli are fearful (Davis & Whalen, 2001). We cover the role the amygdala and other structures play in how we experience fear or anxiety in the next section.

Stop & Check

1. A key structure mediating fear and anxiety is the _____.
2. Of the two loops for routing sensory information from the thalamus to the amygdala, which is most likely to facilitate a fear caused by a sudden, bright flash of light?

1. amygdala 2. The short loop, which routes crude, unprocessed information from the thalamus directly to the amygdala.

Anxious Feelings, the Amygdala, and the Sympathetic Nervous System

Just as the amygdala receives fear-related stimuli, the amygdala also sends information for fear-related responses (**figure 14.3**). After receiving fear-related stimuli, the amygdala sends output signals to the prefrontal cortex, hypothalamus, and locus coeruleus, among other structures. The prefrontal cortex plays a role in determining how we behave in a fearful situation—that is, whether we should approach or avoid a fearful stimulus. The hypothalamus and locus coeruleus facilitate physiological reactions to fear.

The feelings of fear largely manifest from an activated sympathetic nervous system. Signals from the amygdala and the hypothalamus travel to the locus coeruleus, and the locus coeruleus ultimately causes the release of

OUTPUTS FROM AMYGDALA

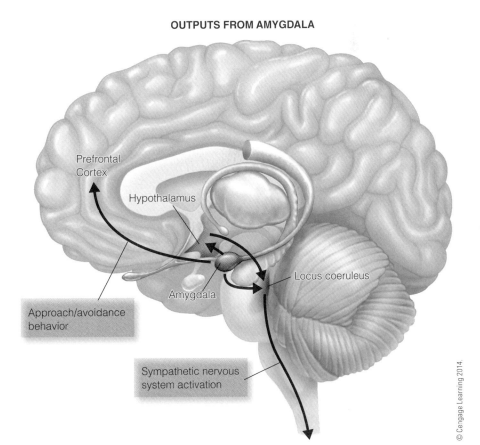

Prefrontal Cortex

Hypothalamus

Locus coeruleus

Amygdala

Approach/avoidance behavior

Sympathetic nervous system activation

© Cengage Learning 2014.

figure 14.3 Outputs from the amygdala go to the prefrontal cortex, hypothalamus, and locus coeruleus. Although the prefrontal cortex is important for approach and avoidance behaviors, the hypothalamus and locus coeruleus are important for sympathetic nervous system activation.

acetylcholine from preganglionic nerves in the sympathetic nervous system. This in turn causes the release of epinephrine (adrenaline) and norepinephrine (noradrenaline) from the adrenal gland. If the sympathetic nervous system is active enough, then respiration, heartbeat, blood pressure, and sweating increase (Davis & Whalen, 2001).

Many anxiety sufferers report having a fear of panic attacks, which consist of strong physiological responses noted by trembling, rapid forceful beating of the heart, restricted breathing, sweating, and dampening of visual or auditory sensations. Objective assessments confirm the physiological effects associated with panic attacks. For example, in a study conducted by Hoehn-Saric and colleagues (2004), individuals with panic disorder or generalized anxiety disorder self-reported anxiety levels at regular intervals throughout the course of several days. These individuals also wore portable physiological recording equipment in an effort to link objective physiological measures with subjective reports of anxiety as they went about their normal daily lives. This study found that physiological measures of increased heart rate and perspiration confirmed self-reports of these events.

These real-life assessments validate experimentally induced methods of producing panic, including hyperventilation-induced panic and CO_2-induced panic. Both methods produce increases in a participant's reported level of panic and physiological responses to panic. Anxiety studies have also reported that individuals with panic disorder appear more sensitive to CO_2-induced panic than individuals with other anxiety disorders (Papp et al., 1993; Welkowitz, Papp, Martinez, Browne, & Gorman, 1999). Anxiety medication use or prior cognitive behavioral therapy reduces CO_2-induced panic severity (Gorman, Martinez, Coplan, Kent, & Kleber, 2004).

general adaptation syndrome Stress syndrome occurring in three progressive phases: alarm stage, resistance, and exhaustion.

Stress and the HPA Axis

We can consider our reactions to short- and long-term stress according to the **general adaptation syndrome** proposed by Selye (1950) (**table 14.1**). This syndrome has three stages. The first stage is called *alarm* and is characterized

table **14.1**

General Adaptation Syndrome		
Stage	**Characteristics**	**Physiology**
1: Alarm	Increased physiological arousal in preparation for an emergency situation	Hypothalamus activates sympathetic nervous system
2: Resistance	Sustained level of physiological arousal	Hypothalamus elicits the release of ACTH from pituitary gland; adrenal gland releases cortisol
3: Exhaustion	Fatigue, susceptibility to disease	Immune system and metabolic activity of organs throughout the body are underactive

by increased physiological arousal in preparation for an emergency situation. The alarm stage consists of the acute reactions to fearful stimuli, including activation of the sympathetic nervous system.

The second stage of the general adaptation syndrome is called *resistance* and is characterized by a sustained level of physiological arousal in response to prolonged stress. During this stage, the hypothalamus releases corticotrophin releasing factor, which in turn elicits the release of adrenocorticotropic hormone (ACTH) from the pituitary gland. ACTH causes the adrenal gland to release cortisol, a stress-related hormone that causes several other effects in the body, including increases in metabolic activity, immune system activity, and glucose and other nutrients. Given their combined distinct role in stress responses, these structures are referred to as the **hypothalamic–pituitary–adrenal (HPA) axis** (**figure 14.4**).

hypothalamic–pituitary–adrenal axis A system involved in physiological responses to stress.

The third and final stage of the general adaptation syndrome is *exhaustion*. In this stage, the body can no longer maintain the high, sustained levels of physiological arousal that occurred during the second stage. This leads to impaired immune system function and reduced metabolic activity of organs throughout

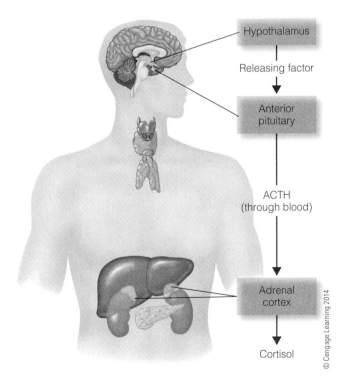

© Cengage Learning 2014

figure 14.4 The HPA axis includes the hypothalamus, pituitary gland, and adrenal gland. In response to sustained stress, the hypothalamus elicits the anterior pituitary gland to release ACTH, which in turn causes the adrenal cortex to release cortisol.

the body. An individual who is in the exhaustion phase is susceptible to disease and feels fatigued.

Prolonged increases in cortisol levels are associated with damage to the hippocampus, an important structure for cognition and a site of action for serotonin reuptake inhibitors, which are used for the treatment of anxiety and depression. In this structure, high levels of cortisol are associated with damaged and destroyed neurons, decreased hippocampal size, and memory impairments (Sapolsky, 1992). Further, chronic stress conditions are related to reduced dendrite sizes on neurons and cause memory impairments in rats (Kleen, Sitomer, Killeen, & Conrad, 2006).

For these reasons, researchers consider cortisol a *stress hormone* and have heavily studied its potential role in disorders associated with prolonged stress such as PTSD. Yet changes in cortisol levels in PTSD are inconsistent, revealing both increases and decreases in cortisol levels compared to healthy controls. When referring to changes in hormone or neurochemical levels, researchers often categorize these changes in two phases. A *tonic phase* is generally a baseline state; for PTSD, this might be altered cortisol levels before a traumatic event or altered cortisol levels during a normal day after being diagnosed with PTSD. A *phasic phase* occurs during a stressful event, which for PTSD might have been the actual traumatic event that led to PTSD or the presence of stimuli that might trigger reminders about the traumatic event.

Several studies found consistently lower tonic cortisol levels in individuals with PTSD (Mason, Giller, Kosten, Ostroff, & Podd, 1986; Yehuda et al., 1990). Other studies, however, have shown increased tonic cortisol levels in individuals with PTSD (De Bellis et al., 1999; Pitman & Orr, 1990). Phasic levels of cortisol in PTSD are more consistent across studies. Researchers find high phasic cortisol levels immediately after traumatic events, including military battles and rape (Howard, Olney, Frawley, Peterson, & Guerra, 1955; Resnick, Yehuda, Pitman, & Foy, 1995). Moreover, phasic cortisol levels increase when an individual is exposed to reminders about the traumatic event (Elzinga, Schmahl, Vermetten, van Dyck, & Bremner, 2003).

Stop & Check

1. Panic attacks can be experimentally induced through hyperventilation or exposure to _____.

2. During a fear-provoking situation, the approach–avoidance behavior is mediated by the _____.

3. Feelings of fear, such as increased heart rate and faster breathing, result from activation of the _____.

4. The _____ plays an important role in the body's reaction to stress.

1. CO_2 gas 2. prefrontal cortex 3. sympathetic nervous system 4. HPA axis

Anxiolytic and Antidepressant Drugs and the Treatment of Anxiety

Barbiturates

Drugs prescribed to treat anxiety are called **anxiolytic drugs**. The first **anxiolytic drugs** consisted of sedative barbiturates introduced in the early 1900s after German chemists Emil Fischer and Josef von Mering developed barbital (Fischer & von Mering, 1903; Shorter, 1997). Barbital served as the first known sedative barbiturate synthesized as a derivative of an earlier compound, barbituric acid, discovered years earlier by Adolf von Baeyer, who may have named it after his girlfriend, Barbara. Von Baeyer also became the founder of Bayer Pharmaceuticals, which developed many of the 50 known therapeutic barbiturate compounds (Lopez-Munoz et al., 2005). Soon after their discovery, barbiturates were commonly used in psychiatric hospitals and prescribed by general family physicians for sleep, nervousness, and other purposes (Shorter, 1997).

We subclassify barbiturates by time course. Long-acting barbiturates generally take at least 1 hour to take effect, but produce these effects for 10 to 12 hours. The barbiturates have poor lipid solubility and slow metabolism. Ultrashort-acting barbiturates produce effects within 10 to 20 seconds and maintain drug effects for approximately 30 minutes. These barbiturates are highly soluble in lipids, quickly store in fats, and rapidly metabolize. We classify barbiturates falling between these time courses as short- or intermediate-acting barbiturates (**table 14.2**).

Other uses for barbiturates include anesthesia and reduced seizures. Phenobarbital and other barbiturates at the time also were used to aid a general anesthetic such as ether to induce full anesthesia. In the early 1930s, a new barbiturate called *hexobarbital* (Evipal from Bayer Pharmaceuticals) became the first barbiturate capable of producing general anesthesia (Lopez-Munoz et al., 2005; Weese & Scharpff, 1932). Barbiturates were also the first drugs capable of reducing the frequency and severity of epileptic seizures.

table **14.2**

Barbiturates Classified by Duration for Onset and Duration of Drug Action				
Class of barbiturate	**Selected barbiturates**	**Lipid solubility**	**Duration for onset**	**Duration of action**
Ultrashort	Thiopental (Pentothal) Methohexital (Brevital)	High	A few minutes	~30 min
Short- or intermediate-acting	Secobarbital (Seconal) Pentobarbital (Nembutal)	Medium	~30 min	~8 hr
Long	Phenobarbital (Luminol) Mephobarbitaol (Mebaral)	Low	~1hr	~12 hr

Stop & Check

1. A drug prescribed specifically for the treatment of anxiety is a called a(n) _____.

2. Why are some barbiturates, like phenobarbital, longer acting than other barbiturates?

1. anxiolytic drug. **2.** Longer acting barbiturates tend to have lower lipid solubility and a longer metabolism process than shorter acting barbiturates.

Barbiturates Serve as Drugs of Abuse

During the decades that preceded the introduction of benzodiazepines in the 1960s, short-acting barbiturates were commonly abused. Users referred to barbiturates as *downers*, among other names. Along with reduced anxiety, barbiturates produced feelings of well-being and lowered inhibitions.

Barbiturates also appear to have positive reinforcing effects. Nonhuman primates readily self-administer barbiturates. Further, barbiturates increase the breaking points on progressive ratio schedules (Griffiths, Findley, Brady, Dolan-Gutcher, & Robinson, 1975; Morgan, 1990). In human laboratory studies, participants prefer barbiturates just as well as morphine (McClane & Martin, 1976) and short-acting barbiturates more than longer-lasting barbiturates (Morgan, 1990).

REVIEW! A break point refers to the number of responses an organism will emit to earn a drug injection. Chapter 5 (pg. 141).

Griffiths and colleagues (1980) asked human participates to rate how much they "liked" the effects produced by the barbiturate pentobarbital compared to the benzodiazepine diazepam. Consistent with other studies, they reported pentobarbital as well liked, particularly when compared to diazepam. On the other hand, they reported diazepam as somewhat liked, but this liking did not increase as the doses of diazepam increased. Thus, the effects of barbiturates appear more rewarding than the effects of benzodiazepines.

Chronic Barbiturate Administration Increases the Risk of Respiratory Depression

Most deaths occurring from barbiturate overdose result from respiratory depression. Many accidental overdoses likely occurred because of a barbiturate's memory-impairing effects, resulting in a an individual taking a barbiturate after forgetting that one had been taken earlier (Lopez-Munoz et al., 2005).

The risk of accidental overdose increases during long-term usage because of a shrinking therapeutic index. Initially, we find a barbiturate's therapeutic dose range far lower than its lethal dose range. However, chronic use causes tolerance to therapeutic effects but not to respiratory depressant effects. As a result, the therapeutic doses shift dangerously close to lethal doses. At this point, even an accidental second administration of a barbiturate might lead to severe respiratory depression.

barbiturate abstinence syndrome Anxiety, muscle weakness, and abdominal pain caused by abrupt cessation of barbiturate use.

Abrupt Withdrawal Causes a Barbiturate Abstinence Syndrome

Abrupt cessation from chronic barbiturate administration can lead to a **barbiturate abstinence syndrome** that is characterized by anxiety, muscle weakness, and abdominal pain. Moreover, in severe cases, seizures may develop, particularly for individuals taking higher doses of barbiturates. Thus, abrupt cessation from barbiturate treatment is dangerous, so users must gradually reduce the amount of a barbiturate administered or switch to a medication that will offset the effects of this abstinence syndrome (Westgate & Stiebler, 1964).

Barbiturates Produce Pharmacological Effects Through Facilitating GABA Neurotransmission

GABA,* the most common inhibitory neurotransmitter in the nervous system, is key for therapeutic and aversive effects of barbiturates. Barbiturates selectively bind to a site, referred to as the *barbiturate site*, on $GABA_A$ receptors. (see **figure 14.5**). Through this site, barbiturates function as a positive modulator, which enhances the inhibitory effects of GABA.

We find $GABA_A$ receptors throughout the brain, but structures of interest here include the amygdala, thalamus, cerebral cortex, and medulla as illustrated in **figure 14.6**. The anxiolytic effects of barbiturates derive from inhibition of amygdala activity. Inhibition of thalamic and cortical activity accounts for the effects of barbiturates on seizures, memory, attention, and other cognitive functions. The sedative effects of barbiturates occur by suppressing cortical functioning and structures important for cortical arousal.

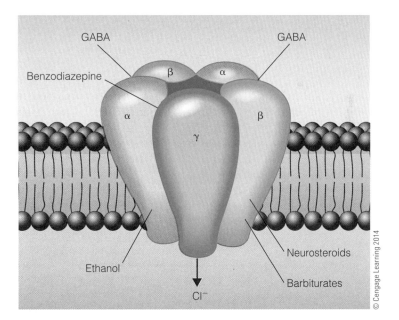

© Cengage Learning 2014

figure **14.5** The $GABA_A$ receptor contains a binding site for barbiturates. Binding to this site facilitates the binding of GABA to the GABA receptor.

*Gamma-aminobutyric acid

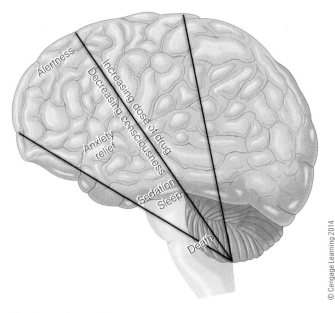

The doses of a CNS depressant such as a barbiturate decrease consciousness as the dose is increased. Alertness is affected first and is linked to suppression of cortical functioning, particularly the prefrontal cortex. A higher dose will provide anxiety relief, resulting from an inhibition of functioning in the amygdala. Even higher doses will affect brain-stem areas, resulting in sedation and sleep. If doses are high enough, the medulla will no longer elicit breathing.

figure **14.6**

The effects of barbiturates on respiratory function result from inhibition of the medulla (Ito, Suzuki, Wellman, & Ho, 1996; Meldrum, 1982).

Stop & Check

1. In humans, the rewarding effects of barbiturates appear equivalent to those of the opioid _____.
2. The major cause of overdose death with barbiturates is _____.
3. The primary mechanism of action for barbiturates is the facilitation of _____ receptor activation by GABA.

1. morphine **2.** respiratory depression **3.** GABA$_A$

Benzodiazepines

Benzodiazepines became available in the 1960s amid the growing illicit barbiturate use and increased occurrence of barbiturate overdose. The potential for such medications was realized after nonbarbituate tranquilizers such as Miltown became popular in the 1950s; however, these medications also provided abuse potential and other adverse effects. In 1960, chlordiazepoxide, better known by its trade name *Librium*, became the first benzodiazepine drug to reach the market (Tone, 2005).

During this decade, Librium became the most commonly prescribed drug in the United States, only to be surpassed soon after by diazepam (Valium). We attribute the discoveries of Librium and Valium to Leo Sternbach, a chemist working for Roche Pharmaceuticals. These and the dozens of benzodiazepines to follow produced less sedation than barbiturates, making them far more appealing for outpatient treatment. In 1981, the Upjohn Company produced alprazolam (Xanax), which still remains a commonly prescribed benzodiazepine today. Roche Pharmaceuticals discovered clonazepam (Klonopin), which also remains a frequently prescribed drug (Shorter, 1997).

Physicians may prescribe a benzodiazepine as a chronic treatment or for use on an "as needed" basis. Depending on these uses, certain benzodiazepines serve better than others. Short-acting benzodiazepines such as alprazolam and clonazepam take 1 to 2 hours for full effect and have a 12- to 24-hour elimination half-life. Physicians may prescribe these drugs to take as needed for anxiety. Thus, a patient may take these medications when experiencing anxiety or when expecting anxiety. Physicians may also prescribe short-lasting benzodiazepines for insomnia, although newer nonbenzodiazepine medications such as Ambien serve as first-line treatments for insomnia today. We find intermediate- and long-lasting benzodiazepines used chronically to relieve or prevent generalized anxiety disorder, seizures, and other conditions where long-lasting minor sedative–hypnotic effects are desired.

Metabolism accounts for the differences in length of drug action among benzodiazepines (**figure 14.7**). Unlike short-acting benzodiazepines,

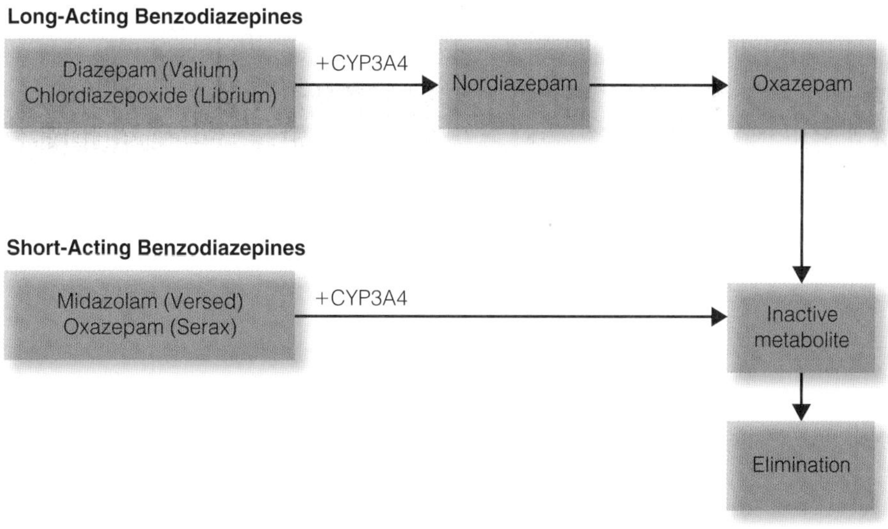

figure **14.7** The duration of action for benzodiazepines depends on the process of metabolism. The two long-lasting benzodiazepines shown here are metabolized by the CYP3A4 enzyme in nordiazepam. Nordiazepam also has benzodiazepine effects, as does its metabolite oxazepam. Oxazepam is also a short-lasting benzodiazepine and does not have an active metabolite. (Data from Marin et al., 1964.)

intermediate- and long-lasting benzodiazepines produce active metabolites with benzodiazepine actions. In particular, the benzodiazepine drug nordiazepam serves as an active metabolite for many benzodiazepines. Thus, nordiazepam and other active benzodiazepine metabolites produce further benzodiazepine effects. Moreover, enzymes convert nordiazepam to oxazepam (Serax), a short-acting benzodiazepine with no active metabolites (Marin, Coles, Merrell, & McMillin, 2008; Tobin, Lorenz, Brousseau, & Conner, 1964).

Pharmacogenetic factors also play a role in benzodiazepine metabolism. Benzodiazepines are broken down (i.e., oxidized) primarily by the cytochrome P450 (CYP) enzyme subfamilies CYP-2C19 and CYP-3A4. However, a polymorphism of the CYP-2C19 gene, specifically a CYP2C19*2 polymorphism, causes poor metabolism of benzodiazepines. As a result, patients with this polymorphism exhibit a stronger and longer-lasting treatment response likely because of greater levels of nonmetabolized benzodiazepines in the body. Polymorphisms of the CYP-3A4 gene have not revealed differences in the ability to metabolize benzodiazepines.

The CYP3A5 enzyme is uniquely involved in metabolism of the benzodiazepines alprazolam and midazolam. Researchers associate a CYP3A5*3 polymorphism with poor metabolism of alprazolam and subsequently higher levels of alprazolam in blood plasma. This particular polymorphism occurs in approximately 85–98 percent of Europeans, but in only 55–64 percent of African Americans (Tiwari, Souza, & Muller, 2009).

Benzodiazepines Have Weaker Abuse Potential Than Barbiturates

Like barbiturate drugs, benzodiazepines are generally considered by physicians to be substances of abuse. This determination results partly from the development of a benzodiazepine withdrawal syndrome, a physiological form of dependence characterized by anxiety, mania, suicidality, and convulsions that occurs after abrupt withdrawal of a chronically used benzodiazepine. The physiological withdrawal symptoms of benzodiazepines may last for several months. A lower probability of this withdrawal syndrome occurs after gradually reducing the dose of a benzodiazepine over time. The appearance of physical dependence along with inferences that benzodiazepine act similarly to barbiturates supports a notion that benzodiazepine has abuse potential.

The abuse liability of benzodiazepines has been debated. Woods and Winger (1995) have argued that benzodiazepines have low abuse potential. First, even though a physical dependency on benzodiazepines can develop, psychological dependence, which is characterized by craving a drug, seldom develops. Second, patients generally do not develop a tolerance to benzodiazepines. Third, reviews of clinical reports indicate that most patients appropriately use benzodiazepines. Fourth, patients normally use benzodiazepines for brief periods of time rather than for long-term frequent usage, an unlikely characteristic for an abused drug.

However, a drug abuse history significantly increases the risk of abusing benzodiazepines. Routine users of gamma-hydroxybutyric acid (GHB) have indicated that the benzodiazepine flunitrazepam produced rewarding subjective effects (Abanades et al., 2007). Further, moderate alcohol drinkers prefer the

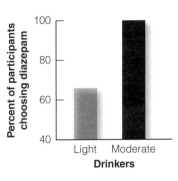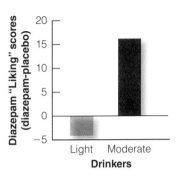

figure **14.8**   Compared to light drinkers, moderate drinkers preferred the benzodiazepine diazepam (Valium) over placebo when (left) given the ability to choose diazepam and (right) when indicating how well they liked diazepam on a "liking" scale. (Data from deWit et al., 1989.)

effects of benzodiazepine pills compared to placebo (deWit, Pierri, & Johanson, 1989) (**figure 14.8**). Although the precise factors that account for a greater likelihood of abusing benzodiazepines are not yet known, it is interesting to note that GHB, alcohol, and benzodiazepines all facilitate the effects of GABA.

Stop & Check

1. Like barbiturates, _____ also are characterized by their time of onset and duration of their drug effects.

2. Polymorphism of the CYP-2C19 gene affects the _____ of benzodiazepines, accounting partly for individual differences in sensitivity to benzodiazepine drug effects.

3. Although benzodiazepines are perceived to have abuse potential, several lines of evidence suggest otherwise, including a lack of escalation of drug _____ in patients.

1. benzodiazepines **2.** metabolism **3.** dose

Benzodiazepines Facilitate GABA Neurotransmission Through Specific Types of GABA$_A$ Receptors

Like barbiturates, benzodiazepines affect the GABA$_A$ receptor. However, this class of drugs binds to different sites on the receptor. To briefly review parts of the GABA$_A$ receptor from Chapter 3, the **GABA$_A$ receptor** is an ionotropic receptor comprised of five subunits (figure 14.5). Of the five subunits, two are of the α type and two are of the β type. The fifth is a bit of a wildcard: It can be a γ, ρ, δ, or ε subunit. Although there are several types of GABA$_A$ receptor subunits, each subunit has multiple subtypes. There are six subtypes of the α subunit, four subtypes of the β subunit, and six subunits of the γ subunit currently known.

The GABA$_A$ receptor provides two binding sites for the neurotransmitter GABA. These sites exist in regions formed where an α subunit joins a β subunit. GABA must occupy both sites to open the GABA$_A$ receptor. Benzodiazepines

GABA$_A$ receptor
Ionotropic receptor comprised of five subunits and activated to the neurotransmitter GABA.

serve as GABA$_A$ positive modulators by binding to a site, referred to as a *benzodiazepine site*, on specific α subunits (Amin & Weiss, 1993; Sigel & Buhr, 1997).

Benzodiazepines have a high affinity for a benzodiazepine site contained within an α$_1$ subunit (Sigel & Buhr, 1997). However, benzodiazepines have a lower affinity for the benzodiazepine sites contained within α$_2$, α$_3$, or α$_5$ subunits (Klepner, Lippa, Benson, Sano, & Beer, 1979; Pritchett, Luddens, & Seeburg, 1989). Benzodiazepines bind poorly to α$_4$ and α$_6$ subunits (Derry, Dunn, & Davies, 2004; Pritchett et al., 1989). Putting this altogether, we essentially have two different types of benzodiazepine sites. We refer to the high affinity site, contained on the α$_1$ subunit, as the **BZ I site**; we refer to the low affinity site, contained in α$_2$, α$_3$, or α$_5$ subunits, as the **BZ II site**.

As shown in **figure 14.9**, the locations of these receptors in the brain help explain the behavioral effects of benzodiazepines. We find BZ I sites highly expressed in the cerebellum, substantia nigra, and thalamus (Wisden, Laurie, Monyer, & Seeburg, 1992). Although they are not structures implicated in anxiety, they explain why benzodiazepines disrupt balance and coordination (cerebellum), reduce seizure activity, and produce sedative and hypnotic effects by inhibiting cortical arousal (substantia nigra and thalamus) (Veliskova,

BZ I site Allosteric site on the GABA$_A$ receptor that can be bound to by benzodiazepines.

BZ II site Allosteric site on the GABA$_A$ receptor that can be bound to by benzodiazepines, but with weaker affinity compared to the BZ I site.

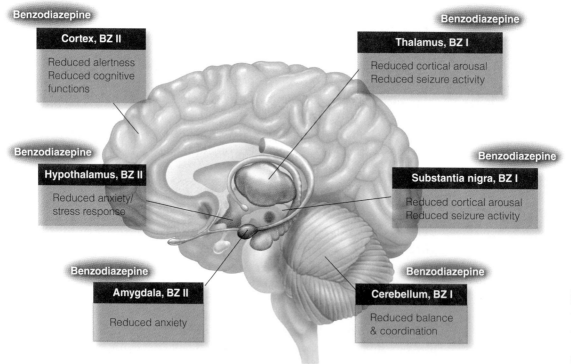

figure **14.9** The behavioral effects of benzodiazepines depend on the location of BZ I or BZ II sites in structures throughout the brain.

Velisek, Nunes, & Moshe, 1996; Veliskova, Velsek, & Moshe, 1996). On the other hand, we find BZ II sites highly expressed in the amygdala and hypothalamus, two areas traditionally important for anxiety and stress, and various parts of the cerebral cortex (Wisden et al., 1992). During benzodiazepine treatment for anxiety, benzodiazepines produce behavioral effects by acting at both types of BZ sites. These actions lead to their anxiolytic effects and undesirable effects such as sedation and physical dependence.

Given the different locations of BZ I and BZ II sites, drugs can be developed that may selectively bind to one site but not the other. This, in fact, is a basis for a new class of sleep aids that includes zolpidem (Ambien) and eszopiclone (Lunesta) and acts selectively through the BZ I but not BZ II site (Sanger, 2004; Wieland & Luddens, 1994). Thus, Ambien and Lunesta have no efficacy for anxiety, although they do have uses for other disorders such as insomnia and epilepsy.

Are There Endogenous Benzodiazepines?

endozepines Endogenous or naturally occurring benzodiazepines.

The involvement of benzodiazepine receptors for the facilitation of GABA binding has led to a search for endogenous benzodiazepines referred to as **endozepines**. Currently, benzodiazepine receptors remain orphan receptors, meaning that an endogenous substance has not been confirmed. Of the many candidates for an endozepine, researchers found that an endogenous substance termed **diazepam-binding-inhibitor** reduced the binding of benzodiazepine to BZ sites (Wildmann, Niemann, & Matthaei, 1986).

diazepam-binding-inhibitor Endogenous substance that reduces the binding of benzodiazepine to BZ sites.

Anticonvulsant Drugs for Treating Anxiety

Anticonvulsant drugs, which are used for the treatment of seizures, facilitate the neurotransmission of GABA. As barbiturates and benzodiazepines also facilitate GABAergic neurotransmission, anticonvulsants also appear to exhibit anti-anxiety effects. A variety of anticonvulsants have been found effective for treating anxiety, including valproic acid, carbamazepine, gabapentin, lamortrigine, vigabatrin, and pregabalin. In general, anticonvulsant drugs have shown promising results in case studies and clinical trials for the treatment of anxiety, but we need further studies to determine their safety and efficacy compared to benzodiazepines and antidepressant compounds (Gorman, Kent, & Coplan, 2002).

Stop & Check

1. Although a benzodiazepine binding site exists in the alpha subunit of $GABA_A$ receptors, benzodiazepines have a greater affinity for the BZI site, which is found on α_1 subunits, and have a lower affinity for the _____ site, which is contained in α_2, α_3, or α_5 subunits.

2. Benzodiazepines reduce seizure activity by binding to BZI sites on $GABA_A$ receptors in the substantia nigra and _____.

3. Why might anticonvulsant drugs be effective for anxiety?

1. BZII **2.** thalamus **3.** Anticonvulsant drugs such as benzodiazepines and barbiturates facilitate the activation of GABA.

Antidepressant Drugs and the Treatment of Anxiety Disorders

Although this chapter has so far focused on the anxiolytic drugs, barbiturates and benzodiazepines, the first-line treatments for anxiety disorders have shifted from these medications to antidepressant drugs. Among the antidepressant drugs, we find the selective serotonin reuptake inhibitors (SSRIs) and the serotonin–norepinephrine reuptake inhibitors (SNRIs) most used for treating anxiety.

SSRIs and SNRIs Reduce and Prevent Anxiety

SSRIs and SNRIs have become the first-line treatments for anxiety disorders. As described in Chapter 13, SSRIs and SNRIs both prevent the reuptake of serotonin through a serotonin transporter, although SNRIs also prevent the reuptake of norepinephrine through a norepinephrine transporter. As for the treatment of depression, we attribute the anti-anxiety effects of SSRIs and SNRIs to enhanced elevations of serotonin in the brain. Furthermore, like treating depression, SSRI and SNRIs require at least 2 weeks to improve the symptoms of anxiety.

The SSRIs paroxetine (Paxil) and fluoxetine (Prozac) have both demonstrated an efficacy in clinical trials for panic disorder, social phobia, generalized anxiety disorder, and post-traumatic disorder (Gorman et al., 2002). Moreover, researchers have found paroxetine effective versus placebo for the treatment of specific phobias (Benjamin, Ben-Zion, Karbofsky, & Dannon, 2000). Paroxetine, fluoxetine, and sertraline (Zoloft) have met FDA approval for the treatment of certain types of anxiety disorders.

Clinical studies also find SNRI effective for anxiety disorders. Duloxetine (Cymbalta) met approval by the Food and Drug Administration (FDA) in 2008 for the treatment of general anxiety, based on a series of positive clinical studies (Carter & McCormack, 2009). Venlafaxine (Effexor) also has proven effective, and has been approved by the FDA for generalized anxiety disorder and social phobia.

Clinical studies generally find SSRIs and SNRIs effective for the treatment of OCD, although the response time appears longer than for other anxiety disorders, often ranging up to 10–12 weeks. The SSRI fluvoxamine (Luvox) has long been considered the first-line treatment of OCD and disorders possibly similar to OCD such as impulse control disorders, eating disorders, and Tourette's syndrome (Goodman, Ward, Kablinger, & Murphy, 1997). Antipsychotic drugs may augment the effects of SSRIs on OCD. Diniz and colleagues (2010) found that the atypical antipsychotic drug quetiapine (Seroquel) improved the response to an SSRI in OCD patients who failed to respond SSRI treatment alone.

Although SSRIs and SNRIs have become the first-line treatments for anxiety, approximately one-third of patients do not respond adequately. This failure rate is found in depression as well, and Chapter 13 offers some suggestions for why this might occur. **Table 14.3** shows some of the pro and cons of antidepressant drugs versus benzodiazepines for the treatment of anxiety.

Buspirone (BuSpar) Reduces Anxiety by Acting on 5-HT$_{1A}$ Receptors

Buspirone (BuSpar) is a partial agonist for the serotonin (5-HT)$_{1A}$ receptor that produces anxiolytic effects. Although generally not considered effective

table **14.3**

SSRIs/SNRIs Versus Benzodiazepines for the Treatment of Anxiety		
	SSRI/SNRI	**Benzodiazepine**
Abuse potential	Unlikely	Possible, especially in former or current illicit drug users
Physical dependence	Serotonin discontinuation syndrome when withdrawal is abrupt	Physiological withdrawal symptoms with abrupt discontinuation
Efficacy	Effective for all types of anxiety; approximately 1/3 of patients are unresponsive	Not effective for OCD; most patients responsive
Response time	2–4 weeks (8–10 weeks for OCD)	Immediate

© Cengage Learning 2014.

for panic disorder or social phobia, buspirone appears as effective as benzodiazepines for the treatment of generalized anxiety disorder. Unlike benzodiazepines, buspirone neither exhibits abuse potential nor potentiates the effects of depressant drugs (DeMartinis, Rynn, Rickels, & Mandos, 2000; van Vliet, den Boer, Westenberg, & Pian, 1997).

Similar to SSRI and SNRIs, buspirone takes several weeks to become effective. Absorption issues limit its utility. Buspirone rapidly breaks in the stomach by CYP-3A4 enzymes, reducing the amount of buspirone for absorption by 90 percent. To address this limitation, researchers have developed a nasal form of buspirone that so far has produced greater bioavailability in rats (Khan, Patil, Yeole, & Gaikwad, 2009), but it has yet to be evaluated clinically in humans.

Stop & Check

1. Antidepressant drugs such as SSRI and SNRIs have become first-line treatments for _____.

2. Unlike the response time for other anxiety disorders, the response time for _____ often ranges from 10 to 12 weeks.

3. Although effective for anxiety in animal models, poor _____ in humans severely limits its clinical uses.

1. anxiety disorders **2.** OCD **3.** absorption

FROM ACTIONS TO EFFECTS
How Do Antidepressant Drugs Reduce Anxiety?

As presented in Chapter 13, a key pharmacological action of most antidepressant drugs consists of increased concentrations of serotonin. Moreover, chronic administration of antidepressant drugs leads to greater serotonin concentrations resulting from desensitization of serotonin transporters and, depending on the antidepressant drugs,

box **14.1** Animal Models for Screening Anxiety Treatments

As with other classes of drugs, *anxiolytics*—drugs that reduce anxiety—are identified in animal behavioral models before they are tested in humans. Many of these models are developed for face validity and thus use tasks that can produce behaviors indicative of stress, fear, or anxiety.

The activity of rodents in an open field provides a simple assessment of anxiety. After being placed in the field, rodents spend much of their time running along the walls or edge of the space rather than the open center. We refer to this as *thigmotaxia*, and it is indicative of fear or anxiety. Drugs effective for anxiety increase the time spent in the center area of the field (Hall, 1934).

The **elevated plus maze** is perhaps the most commonly used model because of its ease, speed, simplicity of equipment, and screening quality (box 14.1, figure 1).

The maze has four arms connected in the shape of a plus symbol, and as the name further implies, the maze is elevated above the ground by about 3 feet. Two of the four arms have tall walls, whereas the other two arms are open. After placing an animal, usually a rat or mouse, in the center of the maze, researchers measure anxiety according to how long the animal spends in the arms with walls compared to the arms without walls. A drug's anxiolytic effects are demonstrated when treated animals spend more time in the arms without walls (Pellow & File, 1986). Although benzodiazepines generally increase the time spent within open arms, SSRIs do not always show this effect (Takeuchi, Owa, Nishino, & Kamei, 2010).

In the **Vogel conflict test**, an animal, usually a rat or mouse, learns to press lever for a lick of water. At times

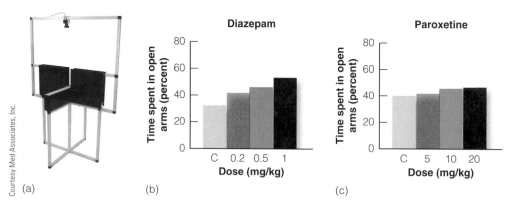

Courtesy Med Associates, Inc.

(a) (b) (c)

box **14.1**, figure **1**

An elevated plus maze is a common model for screening anti-anxiety compounds. (A) An elevated plus maze has two closed arms and two open arms. Anxiety is shown as an avoidance of the open arms. (B) In a study by Takeuchi et al. (2010) using mice, the benzodiazepine diazepam (Valium) was shown to increase time spent in the open arms. (C) In contrast, the SSRI paroxetine (Paxil) was not shown to increase time spent in the open arms. (Takeuchi, T., Owa, T., Nishino, T., & Kamei, C. (2010). Assessing anxiolytic- like effects of selective serotonin reuptake inhibitors and serotonin-noradrenaline reuptake inhibitors using the elevated plus maze in mice. *Methods Find Exp Clin Pharmacol* 2010, 32 (2). 113–121. Copyright © 2010 Prous Science, S.A.U. or its licensors. All rights reserved.)

α_2 heteroceptors. **Figure 14.10** presents these pharmacological actions as well as others discussed in this section.

In addition to the actions already reviewed, evidence suggests that 5-HT_{1A} receptors serve a critical function for serotonin's effects on anxiety. For example, 5-HT_{1A} receptor knock-out mice exhibit greater levels of anxiety compared to normal

during this task, a lick will result in a brief, mild electric shock. This presents a conflict: A drink to relieve thirst also causes an aversive shock. The stress or anxiety caused in this task is relieved by anxiolytic drugs—that is, the drugs result in animals taking more licks (Vogel, Beer, & Clody, 1971).

Fear conditioning is a process in which animals learn to associate stimuli with an aversive shock. In a human version of this task, researchers deliver a mild electric shock to a participant's skin while the participant observes a stimulus. During subsequent sessions, the participant demonstrates fear conditioning by startling whenever researchers present the stimulus. Despite the known role of the amygdala in fear conditioning, benzodiazepines seldom inhibit fear responses in this task (Baas et al., 2009; Grillon, 2008).

In the schedule-induced polydipsia paradigm referred to in this chapter (figure 14.11), experiments are conducted in animals seeking food pellets in an operant chamber that contains a water bottle. In a typical setup, the food pellets are delivered every 60 seconds; a sipper tube for the water bottle is always available. Rats are hungry before these sessions but not thirsty. During the intervals between food pellet deliveries, rats tend to drink water from the water bottle. Over time, water consumption in this task develops into excessive drinking, or *polydipsia*. Rats may consume more water during a 30-minute test session than they do throughout an entire day. Schedule-induced polydipsia may be mediated by anxiety, and chronic administration of antidepressant drugs reduces polydipsia.

elevated plus maze Most commonly used model in assessing anxiety in mice and rats.

Vogel conflict test Test that establishes a conflict between reward and punishment in response to a presented stimulus; used especially to test anxiolytic drugs.

Fear conditioning Process in which animals learn to associate stimuli with an aversive shock.

Stop & Check

Q. A common thread among animal anxiety models is that they all require an animal to produce responses in anxiety-provoking situations. Thus, any drug that reduces these responses can be inferred to reduce anxiety. However, is there a problem with this inference?

A. One criticism of these models is that a lack of responding suggests an anti-anxiety effect. Many other drug effects, however, could also reduce activity in these tasks—for example, a paralyzing agent, a cataleptic drug, or a sedating drug. Thus, *reduced activity* in a behavioral model is a nonspecific drug effect. To avoid this problem, researchers evaluate experimental drugs in more than one behavioral model, including those that assess other possible reasons for reduced behavioral activity. Moreover, these data are interpreted in conjunction with a drug's known biological effects. Together, these findings reveal a picture about a drug's potential for treating anxiety.

---

mice (Gross, Santarelli, Brunner, Zhuang, & Hen, 2000; Olivier et al., 2001). In rats, direct injection of the 5-HT$_{1A}$ receptor partial agonist 8-OH-DPAT into the amygdala decreases anxiety in an *elevated plus maze* (Zangrossi, Viana, & Graeff, 1999). **Box 14.1** describes the elevated plus maze procedure and other models used for screening treatments for anxiety.

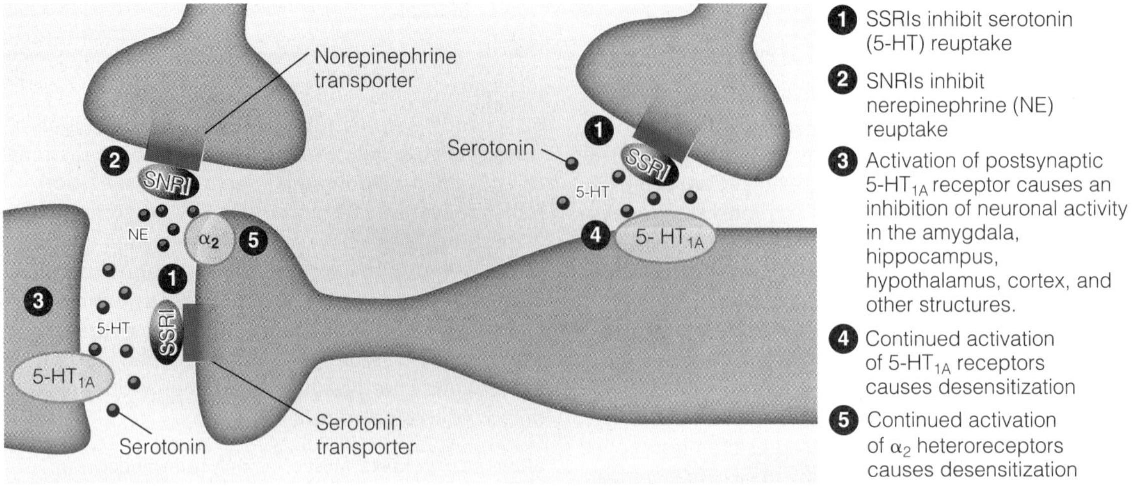

figure 14.10

SSRIs and SNRIs produce desensitization at presynaptic receptors on 5-HT neurons. Desensitization, in turn, enhances the release of 5-HT, possibly accounting for the effects of SSRIs and SNRIs on anxiety.

REVIEW! Genetic alterations cause missing proteins such as receptors in knock-out mice. Chapter 2 (pg. 56).

As shown in figure 14.10, we find 5-HT_{1A} receptors located presynaptically on serotonin neurons. In this role, 5-HT_{1A} receptors function as autoreceptors, serving to inhibit serotonin release from the neuron. Rather than finding these receptors at the axon terminal, we instead find them on the somas and dendrites of serotonin neurons. Thus, these we refer to these types of receptors as *somato-dendritic autoreceptors*. During acute administration, increased serotonin concentrations activate these receptors, causing inhibition of serotonin neurons.

If the desired goal is an enhancement of serotonin levels to treat anxiety, then 5-HT_{1A} receptors first appear to provide a puzzling scenario; that is, when an SSRI or SNRI enhances serotonin levels, this serotonin binds to 5-HT_{1A} autoreceptors and inhibits further serotonin release. Although this likely occurs when first taking an SSRI or SNRI, researchers find that receptor changes occur during the course of chronic treatment.

As we find for serotonin transporters, chronic administration of an antidepressant drug, particularly an SSRI or an SNRI, desensitizes 5-HT_{1A} autoreceptors. This occurs as either a reduced number of 5-HT_{1A} autoreceptors or a decreased sensitivity for serotonin. As a result, 5-HT_{1A} autoreceptors provide less inhibition of serotonin neurons, thereby increasing serotonin release (Blier & Abbott, 2001).

Pharmacologically enhancing serotonin levels may shorten the response time for antidepressant drugs. We can demonstrate these effects experimentally in animals. For example, Hogg and Dalvi (2004) used a schedule-induced polydipsia paradigm to evaluate the effects of repeated administration with the SSRI

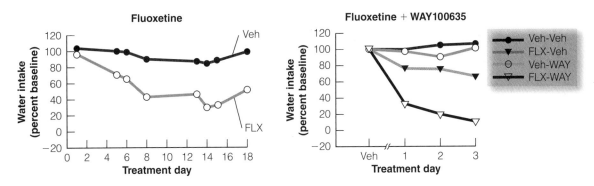

figure 14.11 Fluoxetine (FLX, left) reduces water intake after 6 days of administration in rats using a schedule-induced polydipsia paradigm. The administration of the 5-HT$_{1A}$ receptor antagonist WAY100635 (WAY) with fluoxetine significantly reduced the number of days it took for water intake to be reduced. In fact, this reduction was shown on the first day of drug treatment. Veh = vehicle. (Hogg & Dalvi, 2004. By permission.)

fluoxetine with or without a combination with the 5-HT$_{1A}$ receptor antagonist WAY100635 (**figure 14.11**; see box 14.1 for a description of this procedure). Fluoxetine reduced water intake over 4 days of treatment, suggesting that fluoxetine reduced anxiety. However, in a group of rats treated with the 5-HT$_{1A}$ receptor antagonist WAY100635 in combination with fluoxetine, the reduction in water intake occurred much sooner. Administration of a 5-HT$_{1A}$ receptor antagonist prevented activation of 5-HT$_{1A}$ autoreceptors, which reduced their inhibition of serotonin neurons. We find this to be functionally similar to the desensitization of 5-HT$_{1A}$ autoreceptors that occurs during chronic antidepressant treatment.

In addition to their importance, we also find that postsynaptic 5-HT$_{1A}$ autoreceptors play a role in reducing anxiety. Postsynaptic 5-HT$_{1A}$ receptors exist in the cortex, hippocampus, hypothalamus, and amygdala (Aznar, Qian, Shah, Rahbek, & Knudsen, 2003). Prolonged activation of postsynaptic 5-HT$_{1A}$ receptors causes sensitization rather than desensitization of these receptors. Sensitized postsynaptic 5-HT$_{1A}$ receptors may enhance serotonin's inhibitory effects on those neurons and ultimately reduce activity in those structures. Activation of inhibitory postsynaptic 5-HT$_{2A}$ receptors in these structures may serve a similar role.

Finally, postsynaptic receptors for norepinephrine may also contribute to reductions in anxiety. Norepinephrine neurons from the locus coeruleus elicit sympathetic nervous activity that, as described earlier, may account for the physiological effects of fear, anxiety, and acute stress. Norepinephrine neurons from the locus coeruleus also project to the amygdala, and the activation of postsynaptic norepinephrine β_1 adrenoceptors in the amygdala enhances anxiety. Again, the ability of SNRIs, which increase norepinephrine levels, to treat anxiety seems counterintuitive. But, just as desensitization of 5-HT$_{1A}$ autoreceptors ultimately facilitates reductions in anxiety, so do does desensitization of β_1 adrenoceptors. Eventually, fewer active β_1 adrenoceptors result in a weaker activation of the amygdala, and subsequently, a reduction in anxiety (Duncan et al., 1989; Ordway et al., 1991).

Stop & Check

1. Long-term administration with an SSRI or SNRI can desensitize 5-HT_{1A} receptors, resulting in a(n) _____ in serotonin levels.

2. Long-term administration of an SNRI can desensitize α_2 heteroceptors on serotonin neurons, resulting in a(n) _____ in serotonin levels.

3. Long-term administration of a SNRI can desensitize β_1 adrenoceptors in the amygdala, resulting in a(n) _____ in anxiety.

1. increase 2. increase 3. decrease

▶ CHAPTER SUMMARY

The DSM includes five major types of anxiety disorders: panic disorder, specific phobia, social phobia, generalized anxiety disorder, and obsessive compulsive disorder (OCD). The amygdala plays an important role for anxiety disorders. Other limbic system structures, including the hippocampus and cingulate cortex, might also play a role in anxiety disorders as demonstrated in studies using fear conditioning. The hypothalamic-pituitary-adrenal (HPA) axis mediates the feelings associated with panic attacks and mediates the body's response to long-term stress. Sustained stress leads to activation of the HPA axis and increased levels of cortisol, the body's stress hormone. Drugs effective for anxiety include anxiolytic drugs, antidepressant drugs, and 5-HT_{1A} receptor agonists. Barbiturates, the first anxiolytic drugs, caused CNS depressant effects, carried a risk for respiratory failure, and had a high abuse liability. Barbiturates facilitated the effects of the inhibitory neurotransmitter GABA by binding to barbiturate sites on $GABA_A$ receptors. Benzodiazepines replaced barbiturates for the treatment of anxiety and are still used today. Benzodiazepines also are CNS depressants, but carry less risk of respiratory suppression and have a lower risk of abuse. Benzodiazepines facilitate the effects of GABA through binding to either BZ I or BZ II sites on $GABA_A$ receptors.

Antidepressant drugs have become the first-line treatments for anxiety disorders largely because of their efficacy and low abuse liability. The 5-HT_{1A} receptor agonist buspirone has shown promise in many animal studies; clinically, however, pharmacokinetic issues severely limit absorption and subsequently its therapeutic effects. The 5-HT_{1A} receptors play an important role in anxiety and may be important for the efficacy of SSRIs and SNRIs for the treatment of anxiety.

KEY TERMS

Agoraphobia

Panic attack

Specific phobias

Social phobia

Obsessive–compulsive disorder

Post-traumatic stress disorder (PTSD)

Generalized anxiety disorder

General adaptation syndrome

Hypothalamic–pituitary–adrenal axis

Anxiolytic drugs

Barbiturate abstinence syndrome

$GABA_A$ receptor

BZ I site

BZ II site

Endozepines

Diazepam-binding-inhibitor

Elevated plus maze

Vogel conflict test

Fear conditioning

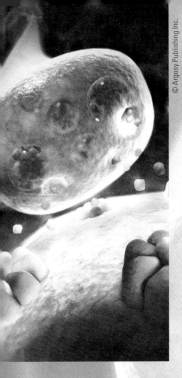

© Argosy Publishing Inc.

CHAPTER **15**

Antipsychotic Drugs

▶ Schizophrenia

▶ Schizophrenia's Complex Neurobiological Profile

▶ A Brief History of Schizophrenia and Its Treatment

▶ Antipsychotic Drugs and the Treatment of Schizophrenia

▶ Typical and Atypical Antipsychotic Drugs

▶ From Actions to Effects: Antipsychotic Drug Actions and Dopamine Neurotransmission in Schizophrenia

▶ Chapter Summary

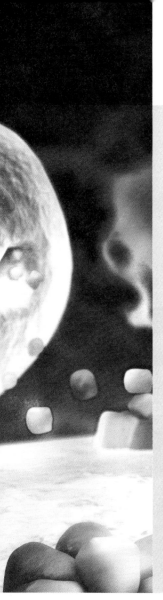

Kraepelin's Influence in Distinguishing Neurological from Mental Disorders

As the chair of psychiatry at the University of Munich from 1903 to 1922, Emil Kraepelin worked with his colleagues in researching mental deterioration. From studying patients in the hospital ward, Kraepelin determined that major distinctions existed for dementia occurring in the young compared to the elderly. One of Kraepelin's colleagues, Alois Alzheimer, revealed that dementia in many elderly patients corresponded to degeneration of the cerebral cortex, hippocampus, and other parts of the brain. On the other hand, dementia occurring in young adults, which Kraepelin described as *dementia praecox*—and which was later named *schizophrenia*—appeared to reveal no neuroanatomical signs of decline. In his textbooks on psychiatric disorders, Kraepelin categorized all mental disorders stemming from a clear biological cause (e.g., the later-named Alzheimer's disease) as *neurological disorders* while categorizing those without clear biological causes as *psychiatric disorders* (e.g., dementia praecox). This distinction, among other important works on the classification of mental disorders, played a foundational role in the creation of the American Psychiatric Association's *Diagnostic and Statistical Manual of Mental Disorders* (DSM) as well as the International Classification of Diseases, the two primary classification systems for mental disorders used today.

From Shorter (1997) and Hippius and Müller (2008).

Schizophrenia

schizophrenia Severe, life-long mental illness consisting of disturbed thought processes and poor emotional responsiveness.

Schizophrenia is a severe, life-long mental illness consisting of disturbed thought processes and poor emotional responsiveness. The symptoms of schizophrenia consist of either **positive symptoms** or **negative symptoms.** The terms *positive* and *negative* refer to the presence of abnormal behaviors or the reduction in normal behaviors, respectively. Examples of positive symptoms include hallucinations, delusions, and thoughts of persecution, whereas negative symptoms include reduced emotional responsiveness, social withdrawal, reduced movement, and lack of motivation.

positive symptoms
Addition of abnormal behaviors such as hallucinations, delusions, and thoughts of persecution to diagnosis of schizophrenia.

negative symptoms
Within diagnosis of schizophrenia, reduction of normal behaviors such as reduced emotional responsiveness, social withdrawal, reduced movement, and lack of motivation.

treatment resistant
Patients with schizophrenia who exhibit minimal or no improvements after two trials with either typical or atypical antipsychotic drugs.

The DSM-IV describes five types of schizophrenia: (1) a *paranoid* type characterized by prominent positive symptoms; (2) a *catatonic* type characterized by predominantly negative symptoms, including immobility; (3) a *disorganized* type characterized by disorganized behaviors and silly or immature emotional expression; (4) an *undifferentiated* type that does not appropriately fit these other categories; and (5) a *residual* type for patients who now exhibit less prominent symptoms of schizophrenia, but did so in the past.

Longitudinal studies find that 50–70 percent of individuals diagnosed with schizophrenia exhibit chronic symptoms; the remaining 30–50 percent of patients tend to exhibit residual features of schizophrenia (Bota, Munro, Nguyen, & Preda, 2011). Moreover, we find that approximately one-third of those with schizophrenia qualify as treatment-resistant patients. Those defined as **treatment resistant** exhibit no or minimal improvements after two trials with either a typical or an atypical antipsychotic drug.

Although clinicians diagnose schizophrenia based on the presence of positive and negative symptoms, researchers find striking and consistent impairments in cognitive functioning (Silver, Feldman, Bilker, & Gur, 2003). Nearly all individuals with schizophrenia have moderate to severe deficits in cognitive functioning, including working memory, reference memory, attention, and executive functioning compared to the general population (Green, Kern, & Heaton, 2004; Keefe & Fenton, 2007; Wilk et al., 2004) (see **figure 15.1**). Cognitive impairment may be present before the first episode of schizophrenia (Keefe & Fenton, 2007).

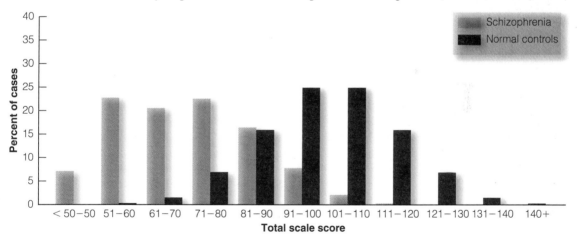

Individuals with schizophrenia tend to score lower on tests for cognitive performance compared to healthy individuals. In this figure, patients with schizophrenia were compared to healthy controls on the Repeatable Battery for the Assessment of Neuropsychological Status, which measures memory, attention, and other aspects of cognitive functioning. Scores on the scale are plotted in increments of 10 on the *x*-axis. The percentage of participants scoring within each range is plotted from the *y*-axis. The average score for healthy participants was 100, and the average score for individuals with schizophrenia was 70, a score that only 2 percent of the healthy participants had. (Keefe, R. S., & Fenton, W. S. (2007). How should DSM-V criteria for schizophrenia include cognitive impairment? *Schizophr Bull*, 33(4), 912–920. doi: sbm046 [pii] 10.1093/schbul/sbm046, p.8. by permission of Oxford University Press.)

figure **15.1**

box **15.1** Prepulse Inhibition

The prepulse inhibition procedure consists of determining one's ability to demonstrate a weaker reflexive response to a sudden stimulus after exposure to a weaker form of the stimulus immediately before. In humans, researchers normally use auditory stimuli and assess eyeblink as the response, as measured in intensity using measures of muscle movement around the eye.

For example, Braff and colleagues (1999) assessed the effects of a brief 112-decibel blast of white noise on intensity of eyeblink startle response. Then during selected trials, a quieter pulse of white noise occurred 40 milliseconds before the 112-decibel white noise. For those without schizophrenia, the preceded noise significantly diminished their subsequent startle to the louder noise that immediately followed. Yet individuals with schizophrenia had a significantly poorer reduction in startle response under these same circumstances. We infer from these findings that those with schizophrenia have a weaker ability to filter out these auditory stimuli.

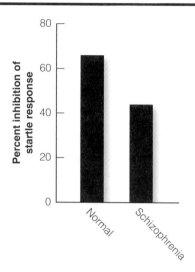

box **15.1**, figure **1**

Individuals with schizophrenia demonstrated a diminished ability to inhibit a startle response compared to normal controls in a prepulse inhibition test. (Data from Braff, et al., 1999.)

sensory-gating deficit A schizophrenic's diminished capacity to filter out unimportant stimuli in his or her environment.

Moreover, many patients with schizophrenia demonstrate a **sensory-gating deficit** that is characterized by a diminished capacity to filter out unimportant stimuli in their environment. Attendance to these unimportant stimuli may lead to misperceptions of their environment, possibly facilitating delusional behavior (Adler et al., 1998). Researchers assess sensory-gating deficits in schizophrenia by using a prepulse inhibition procedure as described in **box 15.1**.

Researchers find that cognitive impairment contributes to poor functional outcomes. Functional outcomes consist of a patient's inclusion into a community, behaving normally in social situations, and successfully employing psychosocial skills. Examples of functional outcomes in schizophrenia include employability, ability to conduct daily living activities, and the ability to form friendships (Green, 1996; Green, Kern, Braff, & Mintz, 2000). To address cognitive impairment in schizophrenia, the National Institute on Mental Health (NIMH) sponsored a research initiative called Measurement and Treatment Research to Improve Cognition in Schizophrenia (MATRICS). The MATRICS program seeks to identify cognitive features of schizophrenia and determine the best treatment strategies for reducing these impairments. In particular, the MATRICS recommendations play an important role in NIMH's funding priorities for studying novel pharmacological mechanisms for treating schizophrenia (Marder & Fenton, 2004).

A first diagnosis for schizophrenia is usually found in one's late teens or early 20s. We seldom find schizophrenia occurring before puberty or after age 40 (Lewis & Lieberman, 2000). Schizophrenia is relatively prominent among psychiatric disorders, affecting 1 percent of the world's population, equating to approximately 3 million individuals in the United States (Regier et al., 1993). The prevalence of schizophrenia occurs equally in males and females, although males may develop this disorder 2–4 years earlier than females and exhibit more severe symptoms. A modestly increased prevalence of schizophrenia occurs in northern geographic regions and for individuals born during winter months, the latter possibly related to winter diseases such as influenza (Davies, Welham, Chant, Torrey, & McGrath, 2003). Schizophrenia provides a significant societal impact, with no more than 73 percent of individuals able to find any employment and only 14.5 percent of individuals finding competitive employment (Rosenheck et al., 2006). Depression rates among individuals with schizophrenia are high, with as much as 10 percent committing suicide each year (Caldwell & Gottesman, 1990; Miles, 1977; Pompili et al., 2007). In general, researchers find a 16–18 year shorter life span among those with schizophrenia compared to the general population (Laursen, 2011).

Schizophrenia clearly has a genetic basis, although this is not the only determining factor. In the general population, as already noted, we find a 1-percent rate of prevalence. This risk factor increases slightly to about 2–4 percent when there is a cousin, uncle or aunt, or nephew or niece with schizophrenia. However, having one parent with schizophrenia increases the risk to 13 percent, and having both parents with schizophrenia increases the risk to about 50 percent. Having an identical twin with schizophrenia also provides a 50-percent chance of developing schizophrenia (**figure 15.2**). The remaining risks for developing

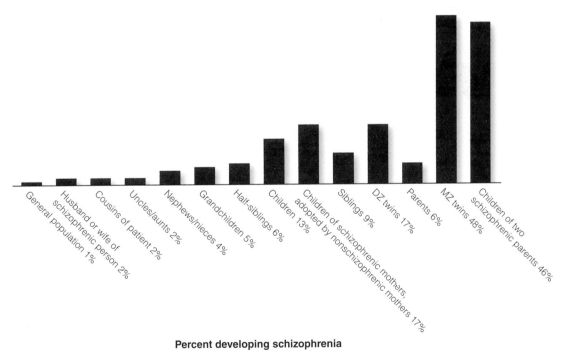

Percent developing schizophrenia

figure **15.2**   The risk of developing schizophrenia increases with genetic closeness to a relative who has schizophrenia. (Based on data from Gottesman, 1991.)

schizophrenia come from the environment, which may consist of responses to stress, life events, or other factors (Tsuang, 2000; van Os, Kenis, & Rutten, 2010).

In the years before a first diagnosis of schizophrenia, patients usually exhibit early but subtle signs of schizophrenia. These preschizophrenia signs are collectively referred to as the **prodromal phase of schizophrenia**, which is characterized by schizophrenia-like symptoms that occur less frequently and with less severity than the symptoms found in schizophrenia. These include, in particular, deficits in working memory, attention, sensory gating, and sociability. Of these, attention impairments appear most predictive of the prodrome phase. In addition to these behavioral and cognitive features, those identified with prodromal phase characteristics also exhibit reduced volume of cortical gray matter (Stone et al., 2009).

prodromal phase of schizophrenia
Schizophrenia-like symptoms that occur less frequently and with less severity than the symptoms found in schizophrenia.

Stop & Check

1. Reduced emotional expression and social isolation are both examples of _____ symptoms of schizophrenia.

2. Although not considered part of the diagnosis criteria, impairments in _____ functioning are commonly found in patients with schizophrenia.

1. negative 2. cognitive

Schizophrenia's Complex Neurobiological Profile

Schizophrenia derives from a complexity of neurobiological traits, including genetic abnormalities, reduced volume of brain structures, and abnormal connectivity among brain structures (Lewis & Lieberman, 2000; Ross, Margolis, Reading, Pletnikov, & Coyle, 2006). Yet most of these characteristics remain under investigation largely because of the clinical differences between the subtypes of schizophrenia and lack of a clear neuropathology of schizophrenia, particularly when compared to disorders with clear neurobiology abnormalities such as Parkinson's disease and Alzheimer's disease (Ross et al., 2006). To this extent, important questions exist about how the brain manifests the symptoms of schizophrenia.

Among the genes studied for risk of schizophrenia, we find perhaps the most evidence implicating the *disrupted in schizophrenia 1* (DISC1) gene (Hodgkinson et al., 2004; Roberts, 2007). Associations occur between abnormal DISC1 genes and occurrence of schizophrenia in Scottish and Finnish individuals (Ekelund et al., 2001; Millar et al., 2000). The DISC1 gene encodes for the DISC1 protein, which plays an important role in a cascade of signaling events that take place within neurons, as well as the development of neurons (Mao et al., 2009). In particular, DISC1 genes may affect cell migration, which can lead to architectural abnormalities in cellular networks (Wong & Van Tol, 2003).

Structural differences in schizophrenia may vary across patients as shown through inconsistent findings across neuroimaging studies. The most consistent observations suggest reduced volume sizes of structures in the left hemisphere, including the lateral and third ventricles, and temporal lobe. Less consistently, studies find reduced volume of the frontal lobe, including the prefrontal cortex, and the thalamus in the left hemisphere (Byne, Hazlett, Buchsbaum, & Kemether, 2009; Ross et al., 2006). Furthermore, imaging and postmortem studies tend to reveal a modest volume reduction of the hippocampus in both hemispheres (Lewis & Lieberman, 2000). Functional imaging studies on the hippocampus also reveal abnormal levels of activity during auditory hallucinations, memory tasks, and rest (Heckers, 2001).

Volume reductions may arise from altered circuitry within these structures. Postmortem studies find possible disorganization of axons in cortical white matter (Akbarian et al., 1996; Arnold, Talbot, & Hahn, 2005). Individuals with schizophrenia also appear to have fewer projections from the thalamus going to the prefrontal cortex (Lewis & Lieberman, 2000). The result of these or other possible altered circuitry may cause differences in neurotransmission, which we consider in the context of antipsychotic drug actions later in this chapter.

Taken together, researchers see the many different abnormalities described above as support for the neurodevelopmental hypothesis for schizophrenia. The **neurodevelopment hypothesis** for schizophrenia states that abnormal nervous system development leads to irregular neuronal signaling in the brain, resulting in the characteristics of schizophrenia (Weinberger, 1996). As Lewis and Lieberman (2000) describe, genetics causes alterations in neuronal growth and development, which likely impacts synaptogenesis and myelination, before and after birth. These abnormalities might eventually cause the prodromal phase of schizophrenia, as described earlier, during adolescence. The transition from a prodromal phase to the full onset of schizophrenia may later arise in reaction to environmental factors, such as those described earlier (**figure 15.3**).

neurodevelopment hypothesis Hypothesis for schizophrenia stating that abnormal nervous system development leads to irregular neuronal signaling in the brain, resulting in the characteristics of schizophrenia.

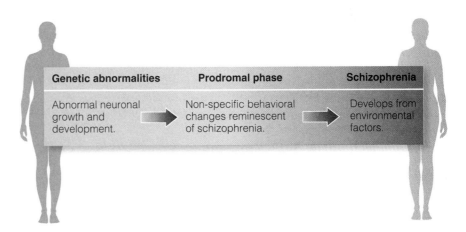

Schizophrenia may develop from a combination of genetic and environmental factors. Genetic factors may alter the normal development, growth, and connectivity among neurons, which may predispose an individual to develop prodromal features of schizophrenia. A response to environmental events may cause someone to shift from the prodromal phase to full onset of schizophrenia. (Adapted from Lewis and Lieberman, 2000.)

figure **15.3**

A Brief History of Schizophrenia and Its Treatment

Stories of madness have been documented throughout human history, but the first clinical diagnosis for schizophrenia was only made in 1871 by Ewald Hecker in Görlitz, Germany. Hecker gave several psychotic young patients a diagnosis of *hebephrenia*, a term coined by his clinical director, Karl Kahlbaum. In 1893, Kraepelin first named this disorder *dementia praecox*, noting the striking cognitive decline by relatively young individuals, particularly compared to dementias he studied in the elderly. Some years later, in 1911, Dr. Eugen Bleuler coined the term *schizophrenia* because of what he saw as a "splitting of psychic functions" in this disorder and a consistent lack of increasing cognitive decline like that seen in Alzheimer's disease (Shorter, 1997).

Early attempts to treat schizophrenia appear barbaric by today's standards. During the early 20th century, psychiatric staff often employed confinement methods as early purported treatments, which often included the use of an isolation cell or straight jacket. Staff members also restrained patients in ice baths for hours or days at a time. Some psychiatrists induced fevers in their patients, which resulted in a temporary abatement of symptoms afterward. By the 1930s, convulsive shock therapies, using either insulin or electricity, sometimes offered real gains in symptom remission, although only temporarily and with significant risk to the patient.

Also during this time, the first of a series of techniques, collectively referred to as *frontal lobotomies*, began to be offered as a long-lasting treatment for schizophrenia, although they provided no symptom improvements and were made at great cost to the patient's health, assuming the patient even survived the procedure (Freeman & Watts, 1945; Shorter, 1997). There were several different ways developed to produce frontal lobotomies, but all of these methods involved penetrating the frontal lobe with an instrument, often simply a rod, and then moving the instrument around to destroy brain tissue. The result was often described as a state of drowsiness and disorientation. There also was significant risk of death from these procedures from hemorrhaging in the brain. Dr. Walter Freeman is most noted for promoting frontal lobotomy techniques for treating schizophrenia, and he is particularly known for the *transorbital leucotomy*. The first procedures involved the use of ordinary ice picks, thus leading to so-called ice-pick lobotomies. During this procedure, Freeman punched the instrument up into the frontal lobe through the inner corner of the eye socket. He then moved it around within the frontal lobe to destroy brain tissue (Kucharski, 1984; Shorter, 1997).

Some years later, in 1952, Dr. Henri Laborit occasioned administering a preanesthetic agent called *chlorpromazine* to manic patients at St. Anne's Hospital in Paris. He found a calmness occurring in these patients, including those with psychosis. The efficacy of chlorpromazine for schizophrenia was formally studied by Dr. Jean Delay and Dr. Pierre Deniker, who published their findings that same year (Delay, Deniker, & Harl, 1952). Chlorpromazine and therapeutically similar drugs that followed revolutionized the treatment of schizophrenia. Of the procedures predating the antipsychotic drugs, only electroconvulsive shock therapy remains, although it is a substantially improved version compared to the 1930s and 1940s and is used as a last resort for those patients who fail to improve with antipsychotic drug treatment (Chanpattana & Sackeim, 2010).

Antipsychotic Drugs and the Treatment of Schizophrenia

dopamine hypothesis Hypothesis for schizophrenia stating that positive symptoms arise from excessive dopamine release in the limbic system.

Most theories concerning the neuropathology of schizophrenia consider abnormalities in dopamine and glutamate neurotransmission. Much of what we know about these irregularities comes from studying the actions of antipsychotic drugs and experimentally inducing temporary psychotic states in healthy human volunteers with dopaminergic and glutamatergic drugs.

The first and most basic account for schizophrenia is the original **dopamine hypothesis** for schizophrenia, which states that positive symptoms arise from excessive dopamine release in the limbic system (Meltzer & Stahl, 1976) (**figure 15.4**). The hypothesis derives from the discovery that antipsychotic drugs act as antagonists for D_2 receptors and that amphetamine, through

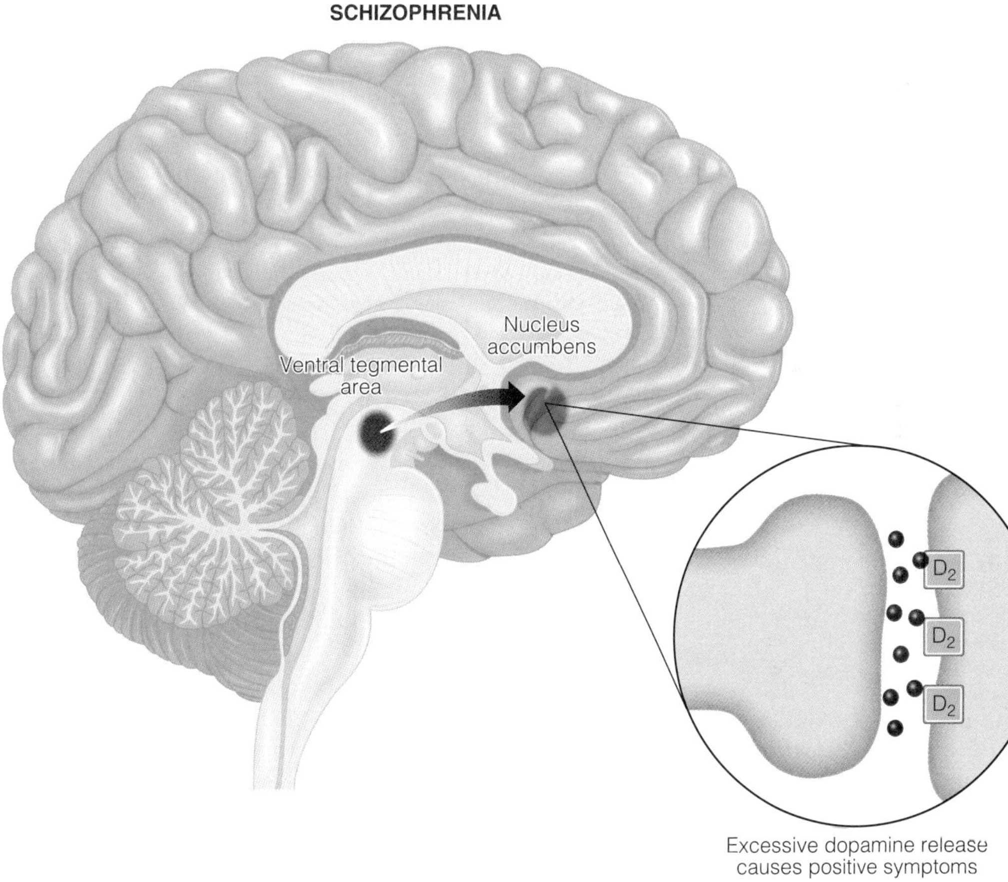

SCHIZOPHRENIA

Nucleus accumbens

Ventral tegmental area

D_2

D_2

D_2

Excessive dopamine release causes positive symptoms

© Cengage Learning 2014

figure 15.4 According to the dopamine hypothesis for schizophrenia, increased dopamine release from mesolimbic dopamine neurons causes the positive symptoms of schizophrenia. Mesolimbic dopamine neurons terminate in structures of the limbic system such as the nucleus accumbens shown here.

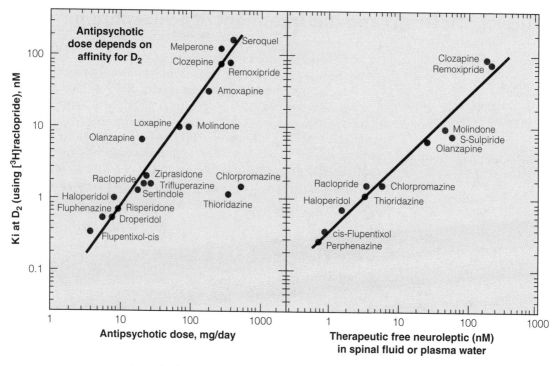

Dopamine D$_2$ Receptors and Therapeutic Efficacy. There is a strong association between strength of binding for the D$_2$ receptor (*y*-axis) and the dose of an antipsychotic drug necessary to produce antipsychotic effects (*x*-axis). (Adapted by permission from Macmillan Publishers Ltd: Antipsychotic drug doses and neuroleptic/dopamine receptors," by P. Seeman, T. Lee, M. Chau-Wong, and K. Wong, *Nature*, 261, 1976, pp. 717–719. Copyright © 1976 Macmillan Magazines Limited.)

figure **15.5**

glutamate hypothesis Hypothesis for schizophrenia stating that diminished levels of glutamate release throughout the cerebral cortex and limbic system may lead to the symptoms of schizophrenia.

increasing dopamine release, causes psychotic symptoms (Seeman & Lee, 1975; Wallis, Mc, & Scott, 1949). As shown in **figure 15.5**, antipsychotic drug doses effective for schizophrenia correlated highly to their strength of binding to D$_2$ receptors (Seeman, 2005; Seeman & Lee, 1975).

Although we still find the dopamine hypothesis useful for understanding antipsychotic drug actions, we also find glutamate dysregulated in schizophrenia. According to the **glutamate hypothesis** for schizophrenia, diminished levels of glutamate release throughout the cerebral cortex and limbic system may lead to the symptoms of schizophrenia (Paz, Tardito, Atzori, & Tseng, 2008; Sesack, Carr, Omelchenko, & Pinto, 2003). Support for this hypothesis comes from human drug overdose cases and experimental studies with the dissociative anesthetics phencyclidine and ketamine (Jacob, Carlen, Marshman, & Sellers, 1981; Krystal et al., 1994). An appealing feature of this hypothesis is that ketamine and phencyclidine cause users to exhibit behaviors similar to positive and negative symptoms in schizophrenia as well as cognitive impairment.

By evaluating dopamine and glutamate interactions in the brain, we find complimentary features in both hypotheses in schizophrenia. Figure 15.7 in the "From Actions to Effects" section provides a schematic of how both dopamine and glutamate systems may interact in schizophrenia. As shown in this figure, diminished levels of glutamate may account for both reduced dopamine levels in the prefrontal cortex and excessive dopamine levels in the limbic system (Sesack et al., 2003).

REVIEW! The dissociative anesthetic drugs ketamine and phencyclidine function as antagonists for glutamate NMDA receptors. Chapter 12 (pg. 341).

Stop & Check

1. The first antipsychotic drug was _____, which Laborit first provided to manic patients.
2. The hypothesis for positive symptoms in schizophrenia states elevated concentrations of _____ are found in the limbic system.

1. chlorpromazine 2. dopamine

Typical and Atypical Antipsychotic Drugs

We divide the wide variety of antipsychotic drugs into two broad categories: typical antipsychotic drugs and atypical antipsychotic drugs (**table 15.1**). However, many different names are used to describe these categories. Researchers and clinicians may instead refer to typical antipsychotic drugs as *first-generation* or *classical* antipsychotic drugs. We also find the term *neuroleptic* synonymous with a typical antipsychotic drug, although many people misapply this term to describe all types of antipsychotic drugs. Atypical antipsychotic drugs may be called *second-generation* or *novel* antipsychotic drugs. Finally, some researchers describe a third class of antipsychotic drugs,

t a b l e **15.1**

Antipsychotic Drugs	
Typical antipsychotic drugs	**Atypical antipsychotic drugs**
Chlorpromazine (Thorazine)	Clozapine (Clozaril)
Haloperidol (Haldol)	Olanzapine (Zeprexa)
Perphenazine (Trilafon)	Risperidone (Risperdal)
Thioridazine (Mellaril)	Quetiapine (Seroquel)
	Ziprasidone (Geodon)
	Paliperidone (Invega)
	Amisulpride (Solian)
	Aripiprazole (Abilify)
	Asenapine (Saphris)
	Iloperidone (Fanapt)

© Cengage Learning 2014

generally referred to as *third-generation* antipsychotic drugs, to describe newer agents that may differ pharmacologically from drugs in these other categories (Meltzer, 2002). This chapter will first describe the development and pharmacology of typical antipsychotic drugs and then those of atypical antipsychotic drugs. Finally, it follows with a discussion about possible third-generation antipsychotic drugs.

Typical Antipsychotic Drugs: The First Effective Medications for Schizophrenia

As noted previously, the first of the typical antipsychotic drugs was chlorpromazine. A number of chlorpromazine-like drugs followed, including the typical antipsychotic haloperidol, a butyrophenone compound synthesized in 1958. As a class, **typical antipsychotic drugs** reduce the positive symptoms of schizophrenia, have weak efficacy for negative symptoms and cognitive impairment, and produce extrapyramidal side effects at therapeutic doses (**table 15.2**). The pharmacological actions of antipsychotic drugs derive from antagonism of dopamine D_2 receptors. Typical antipsychotic drugs may require as long as 6–8 weeks to produce full efficacy (Agid, Kapur, Arenovich, & Zipursky, 2003; Emsley, Rabinowitz, & Medori, 2006).

Figure 15.6 shows these actions using the dopamine hypothesis of schizophrenia. As previously noted, this hypothesis consists of elevated levels of dopamine and its subsequent activation of dopamine D_2 receptors. Typical antipsychotic drugs reduce positive symptoms by counteracting elevated dopamine release through antagonism of D_2 receptors. These actions also account for extrapyramidal side effects (Meltzer & Stahl, 1976).

typical antipsychotic drugs Class of antipsychotic drugs that reduce the positive symptoms of schizophrenia, have weak efficacy for negative symptoms and cognitive impairment, and produce extrapyramidal side effects at therapeutic doses.

table **15.2**

Typical Versus Atypical Antipsychotic Drug Effects and Mechanisms		
	Typical antipsychotic	**Atypical antipsychotic**
Positive symptoms	Effective	Effective
Negative symptoms	Generally ineffective	Modestly effective
Cognitive impairment	Generally ineffective	Modestly effective
Extrapyramidal side effects	Occur at therapeutically effective doses. Generally requires treatment with an anticholinergic drug.	Unlikely to occur at minimally therapeutically effective doses
Tardive dyskinesia	Likely to develop after long-term use	Very unlikely
Mechanism of action	Mainly through blockade of dopamine D_2 receptors	Through blockade of D_2 receptors and serotonin $(5\text{-}HT)_{2A}$ receptors. However, many other receptors implicated in these effects.

© Cengage Learning 2014

SCHIZOPHRENIA + ANTIPSYCHOTIC

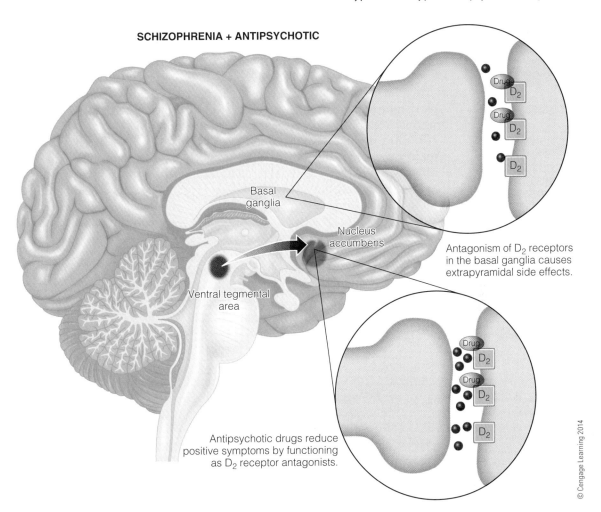

Basal ganglia

Nucleus accumbens

Ventral tegmental area

Antagonism of D_2 receptors in the basal ganglia causes extrapyramidal side effects.

Antipsychotic drugs reduce positive symptoms by functioning as D_2 receptor antagonists.

© Cengage Learning 2014

figure **15.6**

Antipsychotic drugs reduce the positive symptoms of schizophrenia (top) by acting as an antagonists for D_2 receptors, which counteract the activity of mesolimbic dopamine neurons. Yet antagonism of D_2 receptors in the basal ganglia impairs normal dopamine neurotransmission, leading to extrapyramidal side effects.

Extrapyramidal side effects (EPS) Adverse effects consisting of tremor, muscle rigidity, and involuntary movements associated with antipsychotic drugs.

Extrapyramidal side effects (EPS) consist of tremor, muscle rigidity, and involuntary movements (Owens, 1999). As we see in figure 15.6, the nigrostriatal dopamine pathway, which terminates in the basal ganglia, likely functions normally in schizophrenia. D_2 receptor antagonism reduces dopamine neurotransmission in this pathway, causing diminished control of movement. In many ways, EPS resembles the features of Parkinson's disease, which also derive from disrupted dopamine neurotransmission in this pathway.

Today, physicians seldom prescribe typical antipsychotic drugs for schizophrenia, but the low costs of these medications make them more readily available in economically impoverished parts of the world. In patients who are treated with a typical antipsychotic drug, physicians usually also prescribe a muscarinic receptor antagonist such as benztropine to reduce EPS severity (e.g., Brune et al., 1962). Unfortunately, muscarinic receptor antagonists further impair cognitive functioning in schizophrenia (Spohn & Strauss, 1989). Long-term usage with a typical antipsychotic drug, even when also prescribed with an anticholinergic drug, may result in an EPS-related condition called *tardive dyskinesia*.

tardive dyskinesia
Motor disorder primarily affecting muscles of the face that may occur after long-term antipsychotic drug use.

Tardive dyskinesia is a motor disorder that affects muscles primarily around the mouth and other parts of the face. Characteristic features of tardive dyskinesia include facial tics and rhythmic, involuntary movements of the jaw such as chewing or teeth grinding, involuntary use of the tongue such as in lip licking, or excessive lip smacking and pursing. These adverse effects may not occur until after a patient stops taking the medication. In fact, tardive dyskinesia can persist for months and even years after cessation from typical antipsychotic treatment (Owens, 1999).

neuroleptic malignant syndrome (NMS) Flulike symptoms such as sweating, fever, and other symptoms such as blood pressure changes and autonomic nervous system irregularities induced by antipsychotic drugs.

Typical antipsychotic drugs also may produce **neuroleptic malignant syndrome (NMS)**. Some of the symptoms of NMS resemble those of influenza, including sweating and fever, whereas other symptoms include blood pressure changes, autonomic nervous system irregularities such as changes in heart and breathing rate, and muscle rigidity (Caroff, 1980). These symptoms are severe and life threatening; any appearance tends to occur during the first few weeks of treatment.

hyperprolactinemia
Disorder characterized by abnormally high blood levels of prolactin over prolonged periods of time, resulting in reduced lactation, loss of libido, disruptions in menstrual cycles, erectile dysfunction, and hypogonadism.

Typical antipsychotic drugs also are noted for **hyperprolactinemia**, which occurs from abnormally high blood levels of prolactin over prolonged periods of time. The symptoms of hyperprolactinemia include reduced lactation, loss of libido, disruptions in menstrual cycles, erectile dysfunction, and hypogonadism. Dopamine D_2 receptors regulate the release of prolactin from the anterior hypothalamus (Meltzer, Koenig, Nash, & Gudelsky, 1989).

Atypical Antipsychotic Drugs: First-Line Treatments for Schizophrenia

Clozapine (Clozaril) was the first atypical antipsychotic drug. It was synthesized in 1959 only a few years after the discovery of chlorpromazine. Yet researchers disregarded clozapine as an antipsychotic drug because of a lack of EPS in animal models. In other words, because all known antipsychotic drugs at the time produced EPS in humans, researchers identified potential antipsychotic drugs by their ability to produce EPS in animals. Thus, we do not find clozapine used clinically for schizophrenia until the 1970s and 1980s (Hippius, 1989; Matz, Rick, Thompson, & Gershon, 1974). The remarkable efficacy of clozapine led to the development of many other atypical antipsychotic drugs, including olanzapine (Zeprexa) and risperidone (Risperdal) (table 15.1).

atypical antipsychotic drugs Antipsychotic drugs that reduce positive and negative symptoms and carry a low risk of EPS at therapeutic doses.

As a class, **atypical antipsychotic drugs** reduce positive and negative symptoms and carry a low risk of EPS at therapeutic doses. Because of reduced EPS risk, the World Health Organization (WHO) recommends atypical antipsychotic drugs as first-line treatments for schizophrenia. Similar to typical antipsychotic drugs, atypical antipsychotic drugs may also require as long as 6–8 weeks to produce full efficacy (Agid et al., 2003; Emsley et al., 2006).

From clinical studies, we find that atypical antipsychotic drugs produce modest to moderate gains in negative symptoms. Moreover, clinical studies also find consistent, albeit modest, gains in cognitive functioning (Meltzer & McGurk, 1999; Woodward, Purdon, Meltzer, & Zald, 2005). Thus, we find some improvement in functional outcomes after atypical antipsychotic drug treatment, although these are less than desired (Green et al., 2000; Kaneda, Jayathilak, & Meltzer, 2010). Atypical antipsychotic drugs may also reduce depression in schizophrenia, and clinical studies find that clozapine, olanzapine, and risperidone reduce suicide risk among individuals with schizophrenia (Barak, Mirecki, Knobler, Natan, & Aizenberg, 2004; Meltzer, 2001). We also find improvements from some atypical antipsychotic drugs for *treatment-resistant* schizophrenia. Clozapine, for example, provides significant clinical improvement in 70 percent of treatment resistant patients (Kane, Honigfeld, Singer, & Meltzer, 1988).

Atypical antipsychotic drugs carry the risk of serious adverse effects. As already noted, atypical antipsychotic drugs are capable of treating schizophrenia at doses that do not produce EPS. However, most atypical antipsychotic drugs will produce EPS at a sufficiently high dose. Atypical antipsychotic drugs also carry a risk of neuroleptic malignant syndrome (Trollor, Chen, & Sachdev, 2009). Although having lower risk than typical antipsychotic drugs, atypical antipsychotic drugs may also produce hyperprolactinemia. Thus, when compared to typical antipsychotic drugs, atypical antipsychotic drugs have a lower risk, but not a complete absence of these adverse effects.

Clinicians also carefully monitor for three other types of adverse effects. First, many atypical antipsychotic drugs produce significant increases in body weight (Kroeze et al., 2003; Wirshing et al., 1999). Increases in body weight accompany a substantial risk of type II diabetes (Tschoner et al., 2009). Second, many atypical antipsychotic drugs produce a cardiovascular effect called **QT interval prolongation**. The QT interval refers to readings found on an electrocardiogram, which is used to monitor the components of heartbeat. Although prolonging the QT intervals appears safe in itself, this condition can degenerate into a more serious condition called *torsades de pointes*, which may lead to cardiac arrest (Stollberger, Huber, & Finsterer, 2005).

QT interval prolongation Prolonged heartbeat as revealed on from the QT interval of an electrocardiogram.

Third, some atypical antipsychotic drugs pose a slight risk of producing **agranulocytosis**, a disorder characterized by reduced white blood cell counts in the immune system. Clozapine is most noted for this adverse effects. As a result, patients prescribed clozapine must have weekly or monthly blood draws to monitor white blood cell counts (Amsler, Teerenhovi, Barth, Harjula, & Vuopio, 1977).

agranulocytosis Disorder characterized by reduced white blood cell counts in the immune system.

There Are Two Primary Hypotheses for the Actions of Atypical Antipsychotic Drugs

As noted earlier, the principal mechanism of action for typical antipsychotic drugs consists of dopamine D_2 receptor blockade. We find more complex mechanisms of actions in atypical antipsychotic drugs. These mechanisms fall largely into two hypotheses for atypical antipsychotic drugs.

table **15.3**

Receptor Binding Affinities for Haloperidol and Clozapine		
Receptor	Haloperidol	Clozapine
D_2	1.4	150
Serotonin (5-HT)$_{2A}$	25	3.3
5-HT$_{2C}$	>5,000	13
Muscarinic cholinergic receptors (M_1–M_5)	4,670	34
Alpha$_1$ adrenoceptors	19	23
Alpha$_2$ adrenoceptors	>5,000	160

The numbers in the table represent the binding affinity (K_i values in nM) of haloperidol and clozapine for certain receptors in the brain. The lower the number on the table, the greater the binding affinity (i.e., the greater strength of binding) the drug has for the receptor. For example, haloperidol has a greater affinity for the D_2 receptor than it does for the 5-HT$_{2A}$ receptor, whereas the opposite is true for clozapine. Clozapine has a greater affinity for muscarinic receptors and for alpha$_2$ adrenoceptors than haloperidol does, and both drugs have a similar affinity for the alpha$_1$ adrenoceptor.

Data from Schotte et al., 1996.

The first hypothesis states that atypical antipsychotic drug effects derive from preferential antagonism of serotonin (5-HT$_{2A}$) receptors compared to dopamine D_2 receptors. As shown in **table 15.3**, receptor binding studies support this hypothesis by finding that the vast majority of atypical antipsychotic drugs fit this profile (Meltzer, Matsubara, & Lee, 1989; Schotte et al., 1996). Note that for the atypical antipsychotic drugs shown, greater affinities, expressed as K_i's, occur for the 5-HT$_{2A}$ receptor compared to the D_2 receptor.

The second, or *fast D_2-off*, hypothesis, states that atypical antipsychotic effects derive from a rapid dissociation from the D_2 receptor, which distinguishes them from typical antipsychotic drugs that slowly dissociate from the D_2 receptor (Kapur & Seeman, 2000). In other words, atypical antipsychotic drugs do not block D_2 receptors for as long as typical antipsychotic drugs do. To date, however, we find no clinically available atypical antipsychotic drugs developed from the fast D_2-off hypothesis. Instead, pharmaceutical companies find that following the 5-HT$_{2A}$-D_2 receptor hypothesis results in the greatest likelihood of successfully producing atypical antipsychotic drugs.

Pharmacological Effects Generated from Other Receptor Actions

As shown in table 15.3, antipsychotic drugs bind to more than dopamine and serotonin receptors. Although the primary hypotheses for antipsychotic drugs concern the role of dopamine and serotonin receptors, other receptors may contribute to either antipsychotic effects or side effects. The α_2 adrenoceptor for norepinephrine, for example, provides an important example of other receptor actions contributing to antipsychotic efficacy. In a preclinical study by Hertel and colleagues (1999), combined administration of an

α_2 adrenoceptor antagonist with a dopamine D_2 receptor antagonist led to atypical antipsychotic druglike effects on conditioned avoidance responding, catalepsy assessments (see **box 15.2**), and prefrontal cortical dopamine release, which may account for improvements in cognitive functioning and negative symptoms, as discussed later in this chapter. For certain atypical antipsychotic drugs such as clozapine, α_2 adrenoceptor antagonism may contribute to antipsychotic effects.

For some atypical antipsychotic drugs, muscarinic receptor antagonism causes dry eyes and dry mouth. Clozapine's antagonism of histamine H_1 receptors causes sedation, similar to how an antihistamine causes sedation, during the first several days of treatment (Ahnaou, Megens, & Drinkenburg, 2003). Receptor binding studies also implicate H_1 receptors, as well as $5\text{-}HT_{2C}$ receptors, in antipsychotic drug-induced weight gain and subsequent risk of type II diabetes (Kroeze et al., 2003; Reynolds, Hill, & Kirk, 2006).

Third-Generation Antipsychotic Drugs

Third-generation antipsychotic drugs consist of any medication that does not conform to the other categories of antipsychotic drugs. In particular, potential third-generation antipsychotic drugs have deviated from the pharmacological actions found among typical and atypical antipsychotic drugs, rather than having unique therapeutic effects. Currently, the only clinically available compound that might qualify as a third-generation antipsychotic drug is aripiprazole (Abilify). Unlike typical and atypical antipsychotic drugs, aripiprazole functions as a weak partial agonist for dopamine D_2 receptors at therapeutic doses. Yet aripiprazole also shares antagonist effects at $5\text{-}HT_{2A}$ receptors, making this drug some what similar to atypical antipsychotic drugs (Burris et al., 2002). Clinically, aripiprazole appears slightly less effective than the atypical antipsychotic drug olanzapine, but might be safer for type II diabetes risk (Fleischhacker et al., 2009).

Administration Forms for Antipsychotic Drugs

Pharmaceutical companies provide all typical and atypical antipsychotic drugs in pill form, allowing for oral administration. However, patient compliance considerations lead companies to develop other administration routes as well. In a hospital, patients, out of possible mistrust of health care staff, may refuse to take a medication or attempt to hide medication under their tongues. During in-patient care, patients may receive intramuscular injections of antipsychotic drugs instead. Drug developers have also sought to provide antipsychotic drugs in dissolvable pill or nasal spray form (Miller, Ashford, Archer, Rudy, & Wermeling, 2008; Potkin, Cohen, & Panagides, 2007).

Many antipsychotic drugs produce active metabolites. For example, the active metabolite of risperidone, called *paliperidone* (Invega), was recently developed as an atypical antipsychotic drug (Dlugosz & Nasrallah, 2007).

box 15.2 Conditioned Avoidance and Catalepsy Measures Distinguish Atypical from Typical Antipsychotic Drugs

As noted previously, researchers find an important challenge in identifying treatments in animals for uniquely human disorders. For finding treatments for schizophrenia, researchers tend to avoid modeling the entire disorder, but rather model some distinct feature of the disorder. Another strategy involves characterizing the distinct changes in animal behavior, whatever they may be, after administration of clinically proven antipsychotic drugs. After identifying these behaviors, we then screen experimental compounds by determining if they elicit similar behaviors. From these perspectives on antipsychotic drug development, we find two procedures highly effective for screening atypical antipsychotic drugs: conditioned avoidance responding and catalepsy.

Conditioned avoidance responding consists of a learning model that requires animals, usually rats or mice, to associate a warning stimulus with an impending aversive stimulus such as mild electric shock. An animal then learns to avoid the aversive stimulus by emitting some type of response, such as pressing a lever or crossing into a different compartment. All known clinically effective typical and atypical antipsychotic drugs decrease accuracy in this procedure. Thus, antipsychotic effects manifest as poor avoidance of aversive stimulation.

Because the conditioned avoidance procedure fails to separate typical from atypical antipsychotic drugs, we add an assessment of *catalepsy* in these experiments. Catalepsy assessments consist of recording how long an animal remains in a certain posture. As presented in this chapter, typical—but not atypical—antipsychotic drugs produce EPS at therapeutically effective doses. By using catalepsy as an index of EPS in animals, researchers can determine if EPS occurs at doses effective in reducing accuracy in the conditioned avoidance response task.

For example, Holly and colleagues (2011) evaluated the atypical antipsychotic drug clozapine and the typical antipsychotic drug haloperidol using these two procedures. As shown in figure 1 of this box, both clozapine and haloperidol led to significant decreases in avoidance of the aversive stimulation. Haloperidol, however, produced these decreases in avoidance at doses that significantly increased catalepsy, whereas clozapine produced no effects on catalepsy. By putting these findings together, clozapine produces antipsychotic effects without producing EPS, a key feature of atypical antipsychotic effects.

Although this is the first active metabolite approved clinically as an atypical antipsychotic drug, the active metabolite of clozapine, N-desmethylclozapine (Pimavanserin), has also shown promising antipsychotic effects in animal models (Lameh et al., 2007; Philibin et al., 2009).

Stop & Check

1. In addition to primarily treating positive symptoms of schizophrenia, typical antipsychotic drugs also produce _____ at therapeutic doses.

2. An important pharmacological distinction between atypical and typical antipsychotic drugs is that atypical antipsychotic drugs act as an antagonist for both D_2 receptors and _____ receptors.

1. extrapyramidal side effects 2. 5-HT$_{2A}$

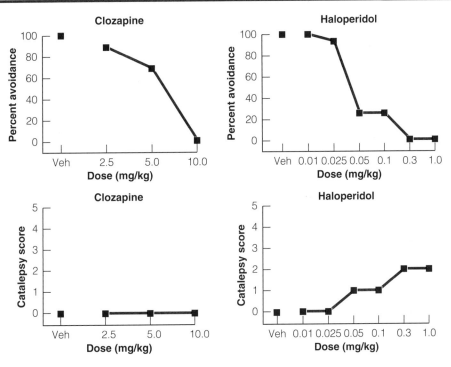

box 15.2, figure 1
Both the atypical antipsychotic drug clozapine (left) and the typical antipsychotic drug haloperidol (right) decrease the percentage of trials a laboratory rat avoided aversive stimulation (top panels). Haloperidol, but not clozapine, increased scores divided in time increments during a catalepsy assessment. The x-axis for all graphs shows the dose of each drug expressed in mg/kg.　(Holly, Ebrecht, & Prus, 2011. By permission.)

FROM ACTIONS TO EFFECTS
Antipsychotic Drug Actions and Dopamine Neurotransmission in Schizophrenia

Beyond differences in receptor actions between typical and atypical antipsychotic drugs, microdialysis studies reveal important differences in dopamine neurotransmission between these drug classes. Moreover, these neurotransmission differences correspond to the role of dopamine in the glutamate hypothesis of schizophrenia. As shown in **figure 15.7**, the glutamate hypothesis, together with other evidence, reveals diminished cortical levels of dopamine and enhanced limbic system levels of dopamine in schizophrenia. Figure 15.7 focuses on the prefrontal cortex and nucleus accumbens for these regions, respectively. Researchers relate diminished dopamine levels in the

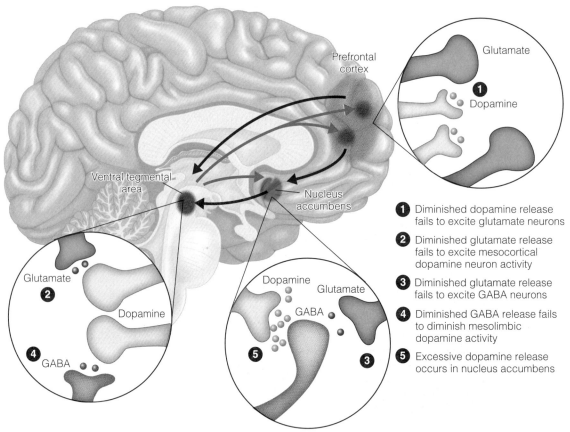

figure 15.7

In schizophrenia, disruption in neurotransmission occurs for glutamate and dopamine. In this image we find underactive mesocortical dopamine neurons that originate in the ventral tegmental area and terminate in prefrontal cortex and other parts of the cortex. Thus, dopamine levels in the prefrontal cortex may be too low. Diminished dopamine activity in the prefrontal cortex cause less activation of glutamate neurons that innervate the ventral tegmental area and facilitate a positive feedback loop. Through another glutamate pathway, lower glutamate activity also lowers the activation GABA neurons that terminate in the ventral tegmental area. Diminished GABA neuron activity may disinhibit mesolimbic dopamine neurons, leading to increased dopamine release in the nucleus accumbens and perhaps other parts of the limbic system.

prefrontal cortex to cognitive impairment and negative symptoms. The different effects that atypical and typical antipsychotic drugs have on dopamine levels in the prefrontal cortex relates to their general clinical effects for cognitive impairment and negative symptoms.

Microdialysis studies find that atypical, but not typical antipsychotic drugs, increase dopamine concentrations in the prefrontal cortex. For example, in a study by Kuroki and colleagues (1999), the atypical antipsychotic drugs clozapine and risperidone significantly increased dopamine concentrations in the rat medial prefrontal cortex. However,

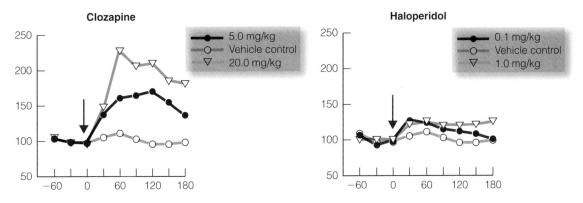

figure 15.8
Antipsychotic Drugs and Prefrontal Cortex Dopamine Levels. Microdialysis procedures reveal that atypical antipsychotic drugs such as clozapine (left) produce increased dopamine concentrations in the prefrontal cortex, although typical antipsychotic drugs such as haloperidol tend to have minimal effects on dopamine concentrations in the prefrontal cortex (right). The arrow indicates when the injection of clozapine or haloperidol was given. The y-axis shows the percentage of dopamine level change compared to baseline plotted at the 100-percent level. The x-axis shows the time before (with minus signs) and after drug injection. (Kuroki, T., Meltzer, H. Y., & Ichikawa, J. (1999). Effects of antipsychotic drugs on extracellular dopamine levels in rat medial prefrontal cortex and nucleus accumbens. *J Pharmacol Exp Ther*, 288(2), 774–781. By permission.)

the typical antipsychotic drug haloperidol failed to increase dopamine concentrations in the prefrontal cortex (**figure 15.8**).

To determine why atypical, but not typical antipsychotic drugs, elevated prefrontal cortical dopamine levels, Liegeois, Ichikawa, and Meltzer (2002) assessed the effects of drugs selective for 5-HT$_{2A}$ receptors and D$_2$ receptors on prefrontal cortical dopamine concentrations. They found that neither the 5-HT$_{2A}$ receptor antagonist M100907 nor haloperidol, a D$_2$ receptor antagonist, significantly increased dopamine concentrations in the prefrontal cortex. After combining the two drugs, however, these researchers found significant increases in dopamine concentrations in the prefrontal cortex. Based on these findings, the actions of atypical antipsychotic drugs on 5-HT$_{2A}$ and D$_2$ receptors may account for their effects on cortical dopamine neurotransmission and possibly their ability to improve cognitive impairment and negative symptoms in schizophrenia.

Stop & Check

1. How do dopamine levels in the prefrontal cortex relate to cognitive impairment in schizophrenia?

2. How might atypical antipsychotic drugs—but not typical antipsychotic drugs—increase prefrontal cortical dopamine levels?

1. Diminished prefrontal cortical dopamine levels may lead to cognitive impairment in schizophrenia. 2. Combined actions of 5-HT$_{2A}$ and D$_2$ receptor antagonism appear to increase prefrontal cortical dopamine concentrations.

▶CHAPTER SUMMARY

Schizophrenia is a severe thought disorder diagnosed by the presence of positive symptoms and negative symptoms. In addition, many patients exhibit deficits in cognitive functioning, which is an important predictor of functional outcomes. Schizophrenia occurs from genetic and environmental factors. The main treatments for schizophrenia consist of typical and atypical antipsychotic drugs. Typical antipsychotic drugs reduce positive symptoms of schizophrenia and produce extrapyramidal side effects at therapeutically effective doses. They produce antipsychotic effects by serving as antagonists for D_2 receptors. Atypical antipsychotic drugs are effective for positive symptoms and, to some degree, negative symptoms and cognitive impairment. They are also capable of producing these therapeutic effects at doses that do not produce EPS. The therapeutic effects of atypical antipsychotic drugs are produced through preferential antagonism of $5\text{-}HT_{2A}$ receptors compared to D_2 receptors. Many antipsychotic drugs produce significant weight gain and subsequently carry the risk of type II diabetes.

KEY TERMS

Schizophrenia

Positive symptoms

Negative symptoms

Treatment resistant

Sensory-gating deficit

Prodromal phase of schizophrenia

Neurodevelopmental hypothesis

Dopamine hypothesis

Glutamate hypothesis

Typical antipsychotic drugs

Extrapyramidal side effects (EPS)

Tardive dyskinesia

Neuroleptic malignant syndrome (NMS)

Hyperprolactinemia

Atypical antipsychotic drugs

QT interval prolongation

Agranulocytosis

REFERENCES

AAALAC. (2012). What is AAALAC? Retrieved from www.aaalac.org/about/index.cfm

Abanades, S., Farré, M., Segura, M., Pichini, S., Barral, D., Pacifici, R., . . . De La Torre, R. (2006). Gamma-hydroxybutyrate (GHB) in humans: Pharmacodynamics and pharmacokinetics. *Annals of the New York Academy of Sciences, 1074*, 559–576. doi: 1074/1/559 [pii]

Abanades, S., Farré, M., Barral, D., Torrens, M., Closas, N., Langohr, K., . . . de la Torre, R. (2007). Relative abuse liability of γ-hydroxybutyric acid, flunitrazepam, and ethanol in club drug users. *Journal of Clinical Psychopharmacology, 27*(6), 625–638 10.1097/jcp.1090b1013e31815a32542

Abood, M. E., & Martin, B. R. (1992). Neurobiology of marijuana abuse. *TiPS, 13*, 201–206.

Abraham, H. D., McCann, U. D., & Ricaurte, G. A. (2002). Psychedelic drugs *Neuropsychopharmacology: The fifth generation of progress.* Brentwood, NJ: American College of Neuropsychopharmacology.

Adinoff, B., Bone, G. H., & Linnoila, M. (1988). Acute ethanol poisoning and the ethanol withdrawal syndrome. *Medical Toxicology and Adverse Drug Experience, 3*(3), 172–196.

Adler, L. E., Olincy, A., Waldo, M., Harris, J. G., Griffith, J., Stevens, K., . . . Freedman, R. (1998). Schizophrenia, sensory gating, and nicotinic receptors. *Schizophrenia Bulletin, 24*(2), 189–202.

Agar, M. (1974). Talking about doing: Lexicon and event. *Language in Society, 3*, 83–89.

Aggarwal, S. K., Carter, G. T., Sullivan, M. D., ZumBrunnen, C., Morrill, R., & Mayer, J. D. (2009). Medicinal use of cannabis in the United States: Historical perspectives, current trends, and future directions. *Journal of Opioid Management, 5*, 153–168.

Agid, O., Kapur, S., Arenovich, T., & Zipursky, R. B. (2003). Delayed-onset hypothesis of antipsychotic action: A hypothesis tested and rejected. *Archives of General Psychiatry, 60*(12), 1228–1235. doi: 10.1001/archpsyc.60.12.1228

Agurell, S., Holmstedt, B., Lindgren, J. E., & Schultes, R. E. (1969). Alkaloids in certain species of Virol and other South American plants of the ethnopharmacologic interest. *Acta Chemica Scandinavica, 23*, 903–916.

Ahmed, B., Jacob, P., III, Allen, F., & Benowitz, N. (2011). Attitudes and practices of hookah smokers in the San Francisco Bay Area. *Journal of Psychoactive Drugs, 43*(2), 146–152.

Ahnaou, A., Megens, A. A., & Drinkenburg, W. H. (2003). The atypical antipsychotics risperidone, clozapine and olanzapine differ regarding their sedative potency in rats. *Neuropsychobiology, 48*(1), 47–54. doi: 10.1159/000071829

Akbarian, S., Kim, J. J., Potkin, S. G., Hetrick, W. P., Bunney, W. E., & Jones, E. G. (1996). Maldistribution of interstitial neurons in prefrontal white matter of the brains of schizophrenic patients. *Archives of General Psychiatry, 53*, 425–436.

Alcoholics Anonymous. (2012). AA fact file. Retrieved from www.aa.org/pdf/products/m-24_aafactfile

Al-Hebshi, N. N., & Skaug, N. (2005). Khat (Catha edulis)-an updated review. *Addiction Biology, 10*(4), 299–307. doi: 10.1080/13556210500353020

Ainsworth, K., Smith, S. E., & Sharp, T. (1998). Repeated administration of fluoxetine, desipramine and tranylcypromine increases dopamine D2-like but not D1-like receptor function in the rat. *Journal of Psychopharmacology, 12*(3), 252–257.

Akiskal, H. S., & Pinto, O. (1999). The evolving bipolar spectrum: prototypes I, II, III, and IV. *Psychiatric Clinics of North America, 22*, 517–534.

Alexopoulos, G. S., Meyers, B. S., Young, R. C., Campbell, S., Silbersweig, D., & Charlson, M. (1997). "Vascular depression" hypothesis. *Archives of General Psychiatry, 54*(10), 915–922. doi: 10.1001/archpsyc.1997.01830220033006

Alper, A. T., Akyol, A., Hasdemir, H., Nurkalem, Z., Guler, O., Guvenc, T. S., . . . Gurkan, K. (2008). Glue (toluene) abuse: Increased QT dispersion and relation with unexplained syncope. *Inhalation Toxicology, 20*(1), 37–41. doi: 10.1080/08958370701758304

American Dental Association. (2005). For the dental patient: Methamphetamine use and oral health. *Journal of the American Dental Association, 136*, 1491.

American Psychiatric Association. (2000). *Diagnostic and statistical manual of mental disorders* (4th ed.). Arlington, VA: Author.

American Psychiatric Association. (2012). Inhalant use disorder. Retrieved from www.dsm5.org/proposedrevision/pages/proposedrevision.aspx?rid=457

American Psychiatric Association. (2012). R10 cannabis withdrawal. Retrieved from www.dsm5.org/

ProposedRevision/Pages/propose-drevision.aspx?rid=430

Amin, J., & Weiss, D. S. (1993). GABAA receptor needs two homologous domains of the beta-subunit for activation by GABA but not by pentobarbital. *Nature*, 366(6455), 565–569. doi: 10.1038/366565a0

Amsler, H. A., Teerenhovi, L., Barth, E., Harjula, K., & Vuopio, P. (1977). Agranulocytosis in patients treated with clozapine. *Acta Psychiatrica Scandinavoca Supplement*, 56(4), 241–248. doi: 10.1111/j.1600-0447.1977.tb00224.x

Anderson, A. L., Reid, M. S., Li, S. H., Holmes, T., Shemanski, L., Slee, A., . . . Elkashef, A. M. (2009). Modafinil for the treatment of cocaine dependence. *Drug and Alcohol Dependence*, 104(1–2), 133-139. doi: 10.1016/j.drugalcdep.2009.04.015

Anderson, B. L., Dang, E. P., Floyd, R. L., Sokol, R., Mahoney, J., & Schulkin, J. (2010). Knowledge, opinions, and practice patterns of obstetrician-gynecologists regarding their patients' use of alcohol. *Journal of Addiction Medicine*, 4(2), 114–121 10.1002/dta.254

Andresen, H., Aydin, B. E., Mueller, A., & Iwersen-Bergmann, S. (2011). An overview of gamma-hydroxybutyric acid: Pharmacodynamics, pharmacokinetics, toxic effects, addiction, analytical methods, and interpretation of results. *Drug Testing and Analysis*. doi: 10.1002/dta.254

Angrist, B., Gershon, S., Sathananthan, G., Walker, R. W., Lopez-Ramos, B., Mandel, L. R., & Vandenheuvel, W. J. (1976). Dimethyltryptamine levels in blood of schizophrenic patients and control subjects. *Psychopharmacology (Berl)*, 47, 29–32.

Anonymous. (1966). Concentration camp for dogs. *Life*, 60(5), 7.

Anonymous. (2009). Marching for science. Nature Neuroscience, 12, 523 10.1038/nn0509-523

Arinaminpathy, Y., Sansom, M. S. P., & Biggin, P. C. (2002). Molecular dynamics simulations of the ligand-binding domain of the ionotropic glutamate receptor GluR2. *Biophysical Journal*, 82(2), 676–683. doi: 10.1016/s0006-3495(02)75430-1

Ariyoshi, N., Miyamoto, M., Umetsu, Y., Kunitoh, H., Dosaka-Akita, H., Sawamura, Y.-i., . . . Kamataki, T. (2002). Genetic polymorphism of CYP2A6 gene and tobacco-induced lung cancer risk in male smokers. *Cancer Epidemiology, Biomarkers, and Prevention*, 11(9), 890–894.

Armitage, A. K., & Turner, D. M. (1970). Absorption of nicotine in cigarette and cigar smoke through the oral mucosa. *Nature*, 226(5252), 1231–1232.

Armstrong, N., & Gouaux, E. (2000). Mechanisms for activation and antagonism of an AMPA-sensitive glutamate receptor: Crystal structures of the GluR2 ligand binding core. *Neuron*, 28(1), 165–181. doi: 10.1016/s0896-6273(00)00094-5

Arnér, S., & Meyerson, B. A. (1988). Lack of analgesic effect of opioids on neuropathic and idiopathic forms of pain. *Pain*, 33(1), 11–23. doi: 10.1016/0304-3959(88)90198-4

Arnold, S. E., Talbot, K., & Hahn, C. G. (2005). Neurodevelopment, neuroplasticity, and new genes for schizophrenia. *Progress in Brain Research*, 147, 319–345.

Arria, A. M., & O'Brien, M. C. (2011). The "high" risk of energy drinks. *Journal of the American Medical Association*, 305(6), 600–601. doi: jama.2011.109 [pii]

Ascher, J. A., Cole, J. O., Jean-Noel, C., Feighner, J. P., Ferris, R. M., Fibiger, H. C., . . . Richelson, E. (1995). Bupropion: A review of its mechanism of antidepressant activity. *Journal of Clinical Psychiatry*, 56, 395–401.

Ashton, C. H. (2001). Pharmacology and effects of cannabis: A brief review. *British Journal of Psychiatry*, 178(2), 101–106. doi: 10.1192/bjp.178.2.101

Aura, J., & Riekkinen, P., Jr. (1999). Blockade of NMDA receptors located at the dorsomedial prefrontal cortex impairs spatial working memory in rats. *Neuroreport*, 10(2), 243–248.

Austin, G. A. (1985). *Alcohol in Western society from antiquity to 1800: A chronological history*. Santa Barbara: ABC-Clio Information Services.

Axelrod, J. (1961). Enzymatic formation of psychotomimetic metabolites from normally occurring compounds. *Science*, 134, 343.

Aznar, S., Qian, Z., Shah, R., Rahbek, B., & Knudsen, G. M. (2003). The 5-HT1A serotonin receptor is located on calbindin- and parvalbumin-containing neurons in the rat brain. *Brain Research*, 959(1), 58–67.

Baas, J. M., Mol, N., Kenemans, J. L., Prinssen, E. P., Niklson, I., Xia-Chen, C., . . . van Gerven, J. (2009). Validating a human model for anxiety using startle potentiated by cue and context: the effects of alprazolam, pregabalin, and diphenhydramine. *Psychopharmacology (Berl)*, 205(1), 73–84. doi: 10.1007/s00213-009-1516-5

Baker, F., Ainsworth, S. R., Dye, J. T., Crammer, C., Thun, M. J., Hoffmann, D., . . . Shopland, D. R. (2000). Health risks associated with cigar smoking. *Journal of the American Medical Association*, 284(6), 735–740. doi: 10.1001/jama.284.6.735

Baker, J. R., Jatlow, P., & McCance-Katz, E. F. (2007). Disulfiram effects on responses to intravenous cocaine administration. *Drug and Alcohol Dependence*, 87(2–3), 202–209. doi: 10.1016/j.drugalcdep.2006.08.016

Baker, L. E., Searcy, G. D., Pynnonen, D. M., & Poling, A. (2008). Differentiating the discriminative stimulus effects of gamma-hydroxybutyrate and ethanol in a three-choice drug discrimination procedure in rats. *Pharmacology Biochemistry and Behavior*, 89(4), 598–607. doi: 10.1016/j.pbb.2008.02.016

Bale, A. S., Tu, Y., Carpenter-Hyland, E. P., Chandler, L. J., & Woodward, J. J. (2005). Alterations in glutamatergic and gabaergic ion channel activity in hippocampal neurons following exposure to the abused inhalant toluene. *Neuroscience*, 130(1), 197–206. doi: 10.1016/j.neuroscience.2004.08.040

Ballenger, J. C., & Post, R. M. (1978). Kindling as a model for alcohol withdrawal syndromes. *British Journal of Psychiatry*, 133, 1–14.

Balster, R. L., Johanson, C. E., Harris, R. T., & Schuster, C. R. (1973). Phencyclidine self-administration in the rhesus monkey. *Pharmacology Biochemistry and Behavior, 1*(2), 167–172. doi: 10.1016/0091-3057(73)90094-4

Balster, R. L. (1998). Neural basis of inhalant abuse. *Drug and Alcohol Dependence, 51*(1–2), 207–214.

Barak, Y., Mirecki, I., Knobler, H. Y., Natan, Z., & Aizenberg, D. (2004). Suicidality and second generation antipsychotics in schizophrenia patients: A case-controlled retrospective study during a 5-year period. *Psychopharmacology (Berl), 175*(2), 215–219. doi: 10.1007/s00213-004-1801-2

Barnes, M. P. (2006). Sativex: Clinical efficacy and tolerability in the treatment of symptoms of multiple sclerosis and neuropathic pain. *Expert Opinion on Pharmacotherapy, 7*(5), 607–615. doi: 10.1517/14656566.7.5.607

Barrett, R. J., White, D. K., & Caul, W. F. (1992). Tolerance, withdrawal, and supersensitivity to dopamine mediated cues in a drug-drug discrimination. *Psychopharmacology (Berl), 109*(1–2), 63–67.

Bass, M. (1970). Sudden sniffing death. *Journal of the American Medical Association, 212*(12), 2075-2079.

Bath, K. G., Mandairon, N., Jing, D., Rajagopal, R., Kapoor, R., Chen, Z.-Y., . . . Lee, F. S. (2008). Variant brain-derived neurotrophic factor (Val66Met) alters adult olfactory bulb neurogenesis and spontaneous olfactory discrimination. *Journal of Neuroscience, 28*(10), 2383–2393. doi: 10.1523/jneurosci.4387-07.2008

Battista, N., Di Tommaso, M., Bari, M., & Maccarrone, M. (2012). The endocannabinoid system: An overview. *Frontiers in Behavioral Neuroscience, 6*, 1–7.

Baumann, M. H., Ayestas, M. A., Jr., Partilla, J. S., Sink, J. R., Shulgin, A. T., Daley, P. F., . . . Cozzi, N. V. (2012). The designer methcathinone analogs, mephedrone and methylone, are substrates for monoamine transporters in brain tissue.

Neuropsychopharmacology, 37(5), 1192–1203. doi: 10.1038/npp.2011.304

Beckstead, M. J., Weiner, J. L., Eger, E. I., Gong, D. H., & Mihic, S. J. (2000). Glycine and gamma-aminobutryic acid(A) recepor function is enhanced by inhaled drugs of abuse. *Molecular Pharmacology, 57*, 1199–1205.

Begas, E., Kouvaras, E., Tsakalof, A., Papakosta, S., & Asprodini, E. K. (2007). In vivo evaluation of CYP1A2, CYP2A6, NAT-2 and xanthine oxidase activities in a Greek population sample by the RP-HPLC monitoring of caffeine metabolic ratios. *Biomedical Chromatography, 21*(2), 190–200. doi: 10.1002/bmc.736

Beltramo, M., Stella, N., Calignano, A., Lin, S. Y., Makriyannis, A., & Piomelli, D. (1997). Functional role of high-affinity anandamide transport, as revealed by selective inhibition. *Science, 277*(5329), 1094–1097. doi: 10.1126/science.277.5329.1094

Benjamin, J., Ben-Zion, I. Z., Karbofsky, E., & Dannon, P. (2000). Double-blind placebo-controlled pilot study of paroxetine for specific phobia. *Psychopharmacology (Berl), 149*(2), 194–196.

Berman, R. M., Cappiello, A., Anand, A., Oren, D. A., Heninger, G. R., Charney, D. S., & Krystal, J. H. (2000). Antidepressant effects of ketamine in depressed patients. *Biological Psychiatry, 47*(4), 351–354. doi: 10.1016/s0006-3223(99)00230-9

Berns, G. S., & Nemeroff, C. B. (2003). The neurobiology of bipolar disorder. *Seminars in Medical Genetics, 123C*, 76–84.

Bernstein, G. A., Carroll, M. E., Thuras, P. D., Cosgrove, K. P., & Roth, M. E. (2002). Caffeine dependence in teenagers. *Drug and Alcohol Dependence, 66*(1), 1–6.

Beseler, C. L., & Hasin, D. S. (2010). Cannabis dimensionality: Dependence, abuse, and consumption. *Addictive Behaviors, 35*, 961–969.

Bjork, J. M., Hommer, D. W., Grant, S. J., & Danube, C. (2004). Impulsivity in abstinent alcohol-dependent patients: relation to

control subjects and type 1-/type 2-like traits. *Alcohol, 34*(2–3), 133–150.

Blake, C. A., Barker, K. L., & Sobel, B. E. (2006). The role of modern biology and medicine in drug development in academia and industry. *Experimental biology and medicine, 231*(11), 1680–1681.

Blanchard, J., & Sawers, S. J. (1983). The absolute bioavailability of caffeine in man. *European Journal of Clinical Pharmacology, 24*(1), 93–98.

Blankman, J. L., Simon, G. M., & Cravatt, B. F. (2007). A comprehensive profile of brain enzymes that hydrolyze the endocannabinoid 2-arachidonoylglycerol. *Chemistry and Biology, 14*(12), 1347–1356. doi: S1074-5521(07)00399-7 [pii]

Blier, P., & Abbott, F. V. (2001). Putative mechanisms of action of antidepressant drugs in affective and anxiety disorders and pain. *Journal of Psychiatry and Neuroscience, 26*, 37–43.

Bolser, D. C. (2006). Cough suppressant and pharmacologic protussive therapy. *Chest, 129*(1 suppl), 238S–249S. doi: 10.1378/chest.129.1_suppl.238S

Booth, M. (1998). *Opium: A history.* New York: St. Martin's Press.

Booth, M. (2005). *Cannabis : A history.* New York: Picador.

Borio, G. (2011). The tobacco timeline. Retrieved from archive.tobacco.org/History/Tobacco_History.html

Bossong, M., Brunt, T., Van Dijk, J., Rigter, S., Hoek, J., Goldschmidt, H., & Niesink, R. (2010). mCPP: an undesired addition to the ecstasy market. *Journal of Psychopharmacology, 24*(9), 1395–1401. doi: 10.1177/0269881109102541

Bota, R. G., Munro, S., Nguyen, C., & Preda, A. (2011). Course of schizophrenia: What has been learned from longitudinal studies? In M. Ritsner (Ed.), *Handbook of schizophrenia spectrum disorders* (Vol. II., pp. 281–300). Netherlands: Springer.

Boules, M., Oliveros, A., Liang, Y., Williams, K., Shaw, A., Robinson, J., . . . Richelson, E.

(2011). A neurotensin analog, NT69L, attenuates intravenous nicotine self-administration in rats. *Neuropeptides, 45*(1), 9–16. doi: 10.1016/j.npep.2010.09.003

Bowden, C. L. (2001). Strategies to reduce misdiagnosis of bipolar depression. *Psychiatric Services, 52*(1).

Bradberry, C. W., Nobiletti, J. B., Elsworth, J. D., Murphy, B., Jatlow, P., & Roth, R. H. (1993). Cocaine and cocaethylene: Microdialysis comparison of brain drug levels and effects on dopamine and serotonin. *Journal of Neurochemistry, 60*(4), 1429–1435.

Bradley, C. (1937) Behavior of children receiving benzedrine. *American Journal of Psychiatry, 94*, 577–585.

Brady, K. T., Lydiard, R. B., Malcolm, R., & Ballenger, J. C. (1991). Cocaine-induced psychosis. *Journal of Clinical Psychiatry, 52*(12), 509–512.

Braff, D. L., Swerdlow, N. R., & Geyer, M. A. (1999). Symptom correlates of prepulse inhibition deficits in male schizophrenic patients. *American Journal of Psychiatry, 156*(4), 596–602.

Braida, D., Limonta, V., Capurro, V., Fadda, P., Rubino, T., Mascia, P., . . . Sala, M. (2008). Involvement of κ-opioid and endocannabinoid system on Salvinorin A-induced reward. *Biological Psychiatry, 63*(3), 286–292. doi: 10.1016/j.biopsych.2007.07.020

Braida, D., Limonta, V., Pegorini, S., Zani, A., Guerini-Rocco, C., Gori, E., & Sala, M. (2007). Hallucinatory and rewarding effect of salvinorin A in zebrafish: κ-opioid and CB1-cannabinoid receptor involvement. *Psychopharmacology, 190*(4), 441–448. doi: 10.1007/s00213-006-0639-1

Brang, D., & Ramachandran, V. S. (2008). Psychopharmacology of synesthesia: The role of serotonin S2a receptor activation. *Medical Hypotheses, 70*(4), 903–904. doi: S0306-9877(07)00580-4 [pii]

Brauer, L. H., Hatsukami, D., Hanson, K., & Shiffman, S. (1996). Smoking topography in tobacco chippers and dependent smokers. *Addictive Behaviors,*

21(2), 233–238. doi: 0306-4603 (95)00054-2 [pii]

Brecher, E. M. (1972). *Licit and illicit drugs*. Mount Vernon, NY: Consumers Union of the United States.

Brill, H., & Hirose, T. (1969). The rise and fall of the methamphetamine epidemic in Japan, 1945–1955. *Seminars in Psychiatry, 19731*, 179–194.

Brink, C.B., Harvey, B.H., Bodenstein, J., Venter, D.P., & Oliver, D.W. (2004) Recent advances in drug action and therapeutics: Relevance of novel concepts in G-protein-coupled receptor and signal transduction pharmacology. *British Journal of Clinical Pharmacology, 57*, 373–387. DOI 10.1007/s00213-012-2680-6

Brown, A. J. (2007). Novel cannabinoid receptors. *British Journal of Pharmacology, 152*(5), 567–575. doi: 10.1038/sj.bjp.0707481

Brown, J., McKone, E., & Ward, J. (2010). Deficits of long-term memory in ecstasy users are related to cognitive complexity of the task. *Psychopharmacology, 209*(1), 51–67. doi: 10.1007/s00213-009-1766-2

Brown, L. C., Majumdar, S. R., & Johnson, J. A. (2008). Type of antidepressant therapy and risk of type 2 diabetes in people with depression. *Diabetes Research and Clinical Practice, 79*(1), 61–67. doi: 10.1016/j.diabres.2007.07.009

Bruci, Z., Papoutsis, I., Athanaselis, S., Nikolaou, P., Pazari, E., Spiliopoulou, C., & Vyshka, G. (2012). First systematic evaluation of the potency of *Cannabis sativa* plants grown in Albania. *Forensic Science International.* doi: 10.1016/j.forsciint.2012.04.032

Brune, G. G., Morpurgo, C., Bielkus, A., Kobayashi, T., Tourlentes, T. T., & Himwich, H. E. (1962). Relevance of drug-induced extrapyramidal reactions to behavioral changes during neuroleptic treatment. I. Treatment with trifluoperazine singly and in combination with trihexyphenidyl. *Comprehensive Psychiatry, 3*, 227–234.

Burris, K. D., Molski, T. F., Xu, C., Ryan, E., Tottori, K., Kikuchi, T., . . . Molinoff, P. B. (2002). Aripiprazole, a

novel antipsychotic, is a high-affinity partial agonist at human dopamine D2 receptors. *Journal of Pharmacology and Experimental Therapeutics, 302*(1), 381–389.

Busch, A. K., & Johnson, W. C. (1950). L.S.D. 25 as an aid in psychotherapy: Preliminary report of a new drug. *Diseases of the Nervous System, 11*(8), 241–243.

Buysse, D., Bate, G., & Kirkpatrick, P. (2005). Fresh from the pipeline: Ramelteon. *Nature Reviews Drug Discovery, 4*(11), 881–882. doi: 10.1038/nrd1881

Byck, R. (Ed.). (1974). *Cocaine papers by Sigmund Freud*. New York: New American Library.

Byne, W., Hazlett, E., Buchsbaum, M., & Kemether, E. (2009). The thalamus and schizophrenia: current status of research. *Acta Neuropathologica, 117*(4), 347–368. doi: 10.1007/s00401-008-0404-0

Cade, J. F. J. (1949). Lithium salts in the treatment of psychotic excitement. *Medical Journal of Australia, 2*(10), 349–351.

Cadet, J. L., & Krasnova, I. N. (2007). Interactions of HIV and methamphetamine: Cellular and molecular mechanisms of toxicity potentiation. *Neurotoxicity Research, 12*(3), 181–204.

Caine, S. B., Thomsen, M., Gabriel, K. I., Berkowitz, J. S., Gold, L. H., Koob, G. F., . . . Xu, M. (2007). Lack of self-administration of cocaine in dopamine D1 receptor knock-out mice. *Journal of Neuroscience, 27*(48), 13140–13150. doi: 10.1523/jneurosci.2284-07.2007

Cairney, S., Maruff, P., Burns, C., & Currie, B. (2002). The neurobehavioural consequences of petrol (gasoline) sniffing. *Neuroscience and Biobehavioral Reviews, 26*(1), 81–89. doi: 10.1016/s0149-7634(01)00040-9

Caldwell, C. B., & Gottesman, II. (1990). Schizophrenics kill themselves too: A review of risk factors for suicide. *Schizophrenia Bulletin, 16*(4), 571–589.

Campbell, A. D., & McBride, W. J. (1995). Serotonin-3 receptor and ethanol-stimulated dopamine release in the nucleus accumbens. *Pharmacology Biochemistry and Behavior, 51*(4), 835–842.

Campbell, S., Marriott, M., Nahmias, C., & MacQueen, G. M. (2004). Lower hippocampal volume in patients suffering from depression: A meta-analysis. *American Journal of Psychiatry, 161,* 598–607.

Carbone, L. (2000). Justification for the use of animals. In J. Silverman, M. A. Suckow, & S. Murthy (Eds.), *The IACUC handbook* (2nd ed.). Boca Raton, FL: Taylor & Francis Group.

Carboni, E., Imperato, A., Perezzani, L., & Di Chiara, G. (1989). Amphetamine, cocaine, phencyclidine, and nomifensine increase extracellular dopamine concentrations preferentially in the nucleus accumbens of freely moving rats. *Neuroscience, 28*(3), 653–661.

Carlsson, A., Lindqvist, M., Magnusson, T., & Waldeck, B. (1958). On the presence of 3-hydroxytyramine in brain. *Science, 127*(3296), 471.

Carmona, R. H. (2005). A 2005 message to women from the U.S. Surgeon General: Advisory on alcohol use in pregnancy. Retrieved from www.surgeongeneral.gov/news/2005/02/sg02222005.html

Caroff, S. N. (1980). The neuroleptic malignant syndrome. *Journal of Clinical Psychiatry, 41*(3), 79–83.

Carson-Dewitt, R. (Ed.). (2003). *Drugs, alcohol, and tobacco: Learning about addictive behavior,* Vol. 1. New York: Macmillan.

Carter, L., Griffiths, R., & Mintzer, M. (2009). Cognitive, psychomotor, and subjective effects of sodium oxybate and triazolam in healthy volunteers. *Psychopharmacology (Berl), 206*(1), 141–154. doi: 10.1007/s00213-009-1589-1

Carter, N. J., & McCormack, P. L. (2009). Duloxetine: A review of its use in the treatment of generalized anxiety disorder. *CNS Drugs, 23*(6), 523–541. 10.2165/00023210-200923060-00006.

Casale, J. F., & Klein, R. F. X. (1993). Illicit production of cocaine. *Forensic Science Review, 5,* 95–107.

CDC (Centers for Disease Control and Prevention). (2008). *National ambulatory medical care survey.* Retrieved from www.cdc.gov/nchs/data/ahcd/namcs_summary/namcssum2008.pdf

CDC. (2008). Smoking-attributable mortality, years of potential life lost, and productivity losses—United States 2000–2004. *Morbidity and Mortality Weekly Report, 57,* 1226–1228.

CDC. (2010). Traumatic brain injury in the United States: Emergency department visits, hospitalizations, and deaths 2002–2006. Retrieved from www.cdc.gov/TraumaticBrainInjury/

CDC. (2011). *Emergency department visits after use of a drug sold as "Bath Salts"—Michigan, November 13, 2010–March 31, 2011.* Washington, DC: U.S. Government Printing Office.

CDC. (2011). Summary health statistics for U.S. adults: National health interview survey, 2010. *Vital and Health Statistics, 10*(252).

Center for Disease Control (2011) Effects of blood alcohol concentration. Retrieved November 25, 2012 from http://www.cdc.gov/Motorvehiclesafety/Impaired_Driving/bac.html

Chandler, A. L., & Hartman, M. A. (1960). Lysergic acid diethylamide (LSD-25) as a facilitating agent in psychotherapy. *Archives of General Psychiatry, 2,* 286.

Chanpattana, W., & Sackeim, H. A. (2010). Electroconvulsive therapy in treatment-resistant schizophrenia: Prediction of response and the nature of symptomatic improvement. *The Journal of ECT, 26*(4), 289–298.

Chapman, L. F. (1970). Experimental induction of hangover. *Quarterly Journal of Studies on Alcohol, 5,* 67–86.

Chavkin, C., James, I., & Goldstein, A. (1982). Dynorphin is a specific endogenous ligand of the kappa opioid receptor. *Science, 215*(4531), 413–415. doi: 10.1126/science.6120570

Chavkin, C., Sud, S., Jin, W., Stewart, J., Zjawiony, J. K., Siebert, D. J., . . . Roth, B. L. (2004). Salvinorin A, an active component of the hallucinogenic sage *Salvia divinorum* is a highly efficacious κ-opioid receptor agonist:

Structural and functional considerations. *Journal of Pharmacology and Experimental Therapeutics, 308*(3), 1197–1203. doi: 10.1124/jpet.103.059394

Chen, C.-H., Ridler, K., Suckling, J., Williams, S., Fu, C. H. Y., Merlo-Pich, E., & Bullmore, E. (2007). Brain imaging correlates of depressive symptom severity and predictors of symptom improvement after antidepressant treatment. *Biological Psychiatry, 62*(5), 407–414. doi: 10.1016/j.biopsych.2006.09.018

Chen, J. G., Sachpatzidis, A., & Rudnick, G. (1997). The third transmembrane domain of the serotonin transporter contains residues associated with substrate and cocaine binding. *Journal of Biological Chemistry, 272*(45), 28321–28327.

Chen, Y., & Sommer, C. (2006). Nociceptin and its receptor in rat dorsal root ganglion neurons in neuropathic and inflammatory pain models: Implications on pain processing. *Journal of the Peripheral Nervous System, 11*(3), 232–240. doi: 10.1111/j.1529-8027.2006.0093.x

Chesher, G. B., Bird, K. D., Jackson, D. M., Perrignon, A., & Starmer, G. A. (1990). The effects of orally administered Δ9-tetrahydrocannabinol in man on mood and performance measures: A dose-response study. *Pharmacology Biochemistry and Behavior, 35*(4), 861–864. doi: 10.1016/0091-3057(90)90371-n

Childress, A. C., Sallee, F. R., & Berry, S. A. (2011). Single-dose pharmacokinetics of NWP06, an extended-release methylphenidate suspension, in children and adolescents with ADHD. *Postgraduate Medicine, 123*(5), 80–88. doi: 10.3810/pgm.2011.09.2462

Chin, R. L., Sporer, K. A., Cullison, B., Dyer, J. E., & Wu, T. D. (1998). Clinical course of gamma-hydroxybutyrate overdose. *Annals of Emergency Medicine, 31*(6), 716–722.

Chinnawirotpisan, P., Theeragool, G., Limtong, S., Toyama, H., Adachi, O. O., & Matsushita, K. (2003). Quinoprotein alcohol dehydrogenase is involved in catabolic acetate production, while NAD-dependent alcohol dehydrogenase in ethanol assimilation in *Acetobacter pasteurianus* SKU1108. *Journal of Bioscience and Bioengineering, 96*(6), 564–571. doi: S1389-1723(04)70150-4 [pii]

Chiu, C.-T., & Chuang, D.-M. (2010). Molecular actions and therapeutic potential of lithium in preclinical and clinical studies of CNS disorders. *Pharmacology and Therapeutics, 128*(2): 281–304. doi: 10.1016/j.pharmthera.2010.07.006

Christrup, L. L. (1997). Morphine metabolites. *Acta Anaesthesiologica Scandinavica, 41*(1), 116–122. doi: 10.1111/j.1399-6576.1997.tb04625.x

Clark, P. A., Capuzzi, K., & Fick, C. (2011). Medical marijuana: Medical necessity versus political agenda. *Medical Science Monitor, 17,* 249–261.

Cloninger, C. R. (1987). Neurogenetic adaptive mechanisms in alcoholism. *Science, 236*(4800), 410–416.

Coe, J. W., Brooks, P. R., Vetelino, M. G., Wirtz, M. C., Arnold, E. P., Huang, J., . . . O'Neill, B. T. (2005). Varenicline: An alpha4beta2 nicotinic receptor partial agonist for smoking cessation. *Journal of Medicinal Chemistry, 48*(10), 3474–3477. doi: 10.1021/jm050069n

Coffey, C., Carlin, J. B., Degenhardt, L., Lynskey, M., Sanci, L., & Patton, G. C. (2002). Cannabis dependence in young adults: An Australian population study. *Addiction, 97*(2), 187–194.

Cohen, C., Perrault, G., Voltz, C., Steinberg, R., & Soubrie, P. (2002). SR141716, a central cannabinoid (CB(1)) receptor antagonist, blocks the motivational and dopamine-releasing effects of nicotine in rats. *Behavioural Pharmacology, 13*(5–6), 451–463.

Cohen, S. (1977). Inhalant abuse: An overview of the problem. *NIDA Research Monograph, 15,* 2–11.

Cole, J. C., Bailey, M., Sumnall, H. R., Wagstaff, G. F., & King, L. A. (2002). The content of ecstasy tablets: Implications for the study of their long-term effects. *Addiction,*

97(12), 1531–1536. doi: 10.1046/j.1360-0443.2002.00222.x

Comb, M., Seeburg, P. H., Adelman, J., Eiden, L., & Herbert, E. (1982). Primary structure of the human Met- and Leu-enkephalin precursor and its mRNA. *Nature, 295*(5851), 663–666.

Comer, S. D., Collins, E. D., & Fischman, M. W. (2001). Buprenorphine sublingual tablets: Effects on IV heroin self-administration by humans. *Psychopharmacology, 154*(1), 28–37. doi: 10.1007/s002130000623

Cone, E. J., & Johnson, R. E. (1986). Contact highs and urinary cannabinoid excretion after passive exposure to marijuana smoke. *Clinical Pharmacology and Therapy, 40,* 247–256.

Conger, J. J. (1956). Reinforcement theory and the dynamics of alcoholism. *Quarterly Journal of Studies on Alcohol, 17,* 296–305.

Connolly, G. N., Richter, P., Aleguas, A., Jr, Pechacek, T. F., Stanfill, S. B., & Alpert, H. R. (2010). Unintentional child poisonings through ingestion of conventional and novel tobacco products. *Pediatrics, 125*(5), 896–899. doi: 10.1542/peds.2009-2835

Cook, C., Biddlestone, L., Coop, A., & Beardsley, P. (2006). Effects of combining ethanol (EtOH) with gamma-hydroxybutyrate (GHB) on the discriminative stimulus, locomotor, and motor-impairing functions of GHB in mice. *Psychopharmacology (Berl), 185*(1), 112–122. doi: 10.1007/s00213-005-0276-0

Cook, C. E., Perez-Reyes, M., Jeffcoat, A. R., & Brine, D. R. (1983). Phencyclidine disposition in humans after small doses of radiolabeled drug. *Federation proceedings, 42*(9), 2566–2569.

Cottler, L. B., Womack, S. B., Compton, W. M., & Ben-Abdallah, A. (2001). Ecstasy abuse and dependence among adolescents and young adults: applicability and reliability of DSM-IV criteria. *Human Psychopharmacology: Clinical and Experimental, 16*(8), 599–606. doi: 10.1002/hup.343

Cougle, J. R., Timpano, K. R., Sachs-Ericsson, N., Keough, M. E., & Riccardi, C. J. (2010). Examining

the unique relationships between anxiety disorders and childhood physical and sexual abuse in the National Comorbidity Survey-Replication. *Psychiatry Research, 177*(1–2), 150–155. doi: S0165-1781(09)00108-5 [pii]

Cravatt, B. F., Giang, D. K., Mayfield, S. P., Boger, D. L., Lerner, R. A., & Gilula, N. B. (1996). Molecular characterization of an enzyme that degrades neuromodulatory fatty-acid amides. *Nature, 384*(6604), 83–87. doi: 10.1038/384083a0

Cruz, S. L., & Dominguez, M. (2011). Misusing volatile substances for their hallucinatory effects: A qualitative pilot study with Mexican teenagers and a pharmacological discussion of their hallucinations. *Substance Use and Misuse, 46*(suppl. 1), 84–94. doi: 10.3109/10826084.2011.580222

Cruz, S. L., Mirshahi, T., Thomas, B., Balster, R. L., & Woodward, J. J. (1998). Effects of the abused solvent toluene on recombinant N-methyl-d-aspartate and non-N-methyl-d-aspartate receptors expressed in *Xenopus* oocytes. *Journal of Pharmacology and Experimental Therapeutics, 286*(1), 334–340.

Cryan, J. F., Mombereau, C., & Vassout, A. (2005). The tail suspension test as a model for assessing antidepressant activity: Review of pharmacological and genetic studies in mice. *Neuroscience & Biobehavioral Reviews, 29*(4–5), 571–625. doi: 10.1016/j.neubiorev.2005.03.009

Cui, D., & Morris, M. E. (2009). The drug of abuse γ-hydroxybutyrate is a substrate for sodium-coupled monocarboxylate transporter (SMCT) 1 (SLC5A8): Characterization of SMCT-mediated uptake and inhibition. *Drug Metabolism and Disposition, 37*(7), 1404–1410. doi: 10.1124/dmd.109.027169

Curran, V., Brignell, C., Fletcher, S., Middleton, P., & Henry, J. (2002). Cognitive and subjective dose-response effects of acute oral Δ⁹-tetrahydrocannabinol (THC) in infrequent cannabis users. *Psychopharmacology, 164*(1), 61–70. doi: 10.1007/s00213-002-1169-0

Dackis, C. A., Kampman, K. M., Lynch, K. G., Pettinati, H. M., &

O'Brien, C. P. (2004). A double-blind, placebo-controlled trial of modafinil for cocaine dependence. *Neuropsychopharmacology, 30*(1), 205–211.

Dahan, A., Yassen, A., Romberg, R., Sarton, E., Teppema, L., Olofsen, E., & Danhof, M. (2006). Buprenorphine induces ceiling in respiratory depression but not in analgesia. *British Journal of Anaesthesiology, 96*(5), 627–632. doi: 10.1093/bja/ael051

D'Aquila, P. S., Collu, M., Gessa, G. L., & Serra, G. (2000). The role of dopamine in the mechanism of action of antidepressant drugs. *European Journal of Pharmacology, 405*(1–3), 365–373. doi: S0014299900005665 [pii]

Davies, G., Welham, J., Chant, D., Torrey, E. F., & McGrath, J. (2003). A systematic review and meta-analysis of Northern Hemisphere season of birth studies in schizophrenia. *Schizophrenia Bulletin, 29*(3), 587–593.

Davis, C., Curtis, C., Levitan, R. D., Carter, J. C., Kaplan, A. S., & Kennedy, J. L. (2011). Evidence that "food addiction" is a valid phenotype of obesity. *Appetite, 57*(3), 711–717. doi: 10.1016/j.appet.2011.08.017

Davis, J. M. (2006). Tri-cyclic antidepressants, neurotransmitters, and neuropsychopharmacology. In T. A. Ban & R. U. Udabe (Eds.), *The neurotransmitter era in neuropsychopharmacology.* Buenos Aires: Editorial Polemos.

Davis, M., & Whalen, P. J. (2001). The amygdala: Vigilance and emotion. *Molecular Psychiatry, 6*(1), 13–34.

De Bellis, M. D., Baum, A. S., Birmaher, B., Keshavan, M. S., Eccard, C. H., Boring, A. M., . . . Ryan, N. D. (1999). A.E. Bennett Research Award. Developmental traumatology. Part I: Biological stress systems. *Biological Psychiatry, 45*(10), 1259–1270. doi: S000632239900044X [pii]

de Boer, J. Z., Hale, J. R., & Chanton, J. (2001). New evidence for the geological origins of the ancient Delphic oracle (Greece). *Geology, 29*, 707–710.

Del Arco, A., Segovia, G., & Mora, F. (2008). Blockade of NMDA receptors in the prefrontal cortex increases dopamine and acetylcholine release in the nucleus accumbens and motor activity. *Psychopharmacology, 201*(3), 325–338. doi: 10.1007/s00213-008-1288-3

de la Garza, R., & Johanson, C. E. (1985). Discriminative stimulus properties of cocaine in pigeons. *Psychopharmacology (Berl), 85*(1), 23–30.

De La Torre, R., Farré, M., Ortuño, J., Mas, M., Brenneisen, R., Roset, P. N., . . . Camí, J. (2000). Non-linear pharmacokinetics of MDMA ('ecstasy') in humans. *British Journal of Clinical Pharmacology, 49*(2), 104–109. doi: 10.1046/j.1365-2125.2000.00121.x

De La Torre, R., Farré, M., Roset, P. N., López, C. H., Mas, M., Ortuño, J., . . . Camí, J. (2000). Pharmacology of MDMA in humans. *Annals of the New York Academy of Sciences, 914*(1), 225–237. doi: 10.1111/j.1749-6632.2000.tb05199.x

Delay, J., Deniker, P., & Harl, J. M. (1952). [Therapeutic use in psychiatry of phenothiazine of central elective action (4560 RP)]. *Annals of Medicine and Psychology (Paris), 110*(2 1), 112-117.

De Leonibus, E., Verheij, M. M. M., Mele, A., & Cools, A. (2006). Distinct kinds of novelty processing differentially increase extracellular dopamine in different brain regions. *European Journal of Neuroscience, 23*(5), 1332–1340. doi: 10.1111/j.1460-9568.2006.04658.x

DeMartinis, N., Rynn, M., Rickels, K., & Mandos, L. (2000). Prior benzodiazepine use and buspirone response in the treatment of generalized anxiety disorder. *Journal of Clinical Psychiatry, 61*(2), 91–94.

Deng, J., Shen, C., Wang, Y. J., Zhang, M., Li, J., Xu, Z. Q., . . . Zhou, H. D. (2010). Nicotine exacerbates tau phosphorylation and cognitive impairment induced by amyloid-beta 25–35 in rats. *European Journal of Pharmacology, 637*(1–3), 83–88. doi: S0014-2999(10)00226-8 [pii]

De Petrocellis, L., Melck, D., Bisogno, T., Milone, A., & Di Marzo, V. (1999). Finding of the endocannabinoid signalling system in Hydra, a very primitive organism: Possible role in the feeding response. *Neuroscience, 92*(1), 377–387. doi: 10.1016/s0306-4522(98)00749-0

Derry, J. M. C., Dunn, S. M. J., & Davies, M. (2004). Identification of a residue in the gamma-aminobutyric acid type A receptor alpha subunit that differentially affects diazepam-sensitive and -insensitive benzodiazepine site binding. *Journal of Neurochemistry, 88*(6), 1431–1438.

De Schepper, H. U., Cremonini, F., Park, M. I., & Camilleri, M. (2004). Opioids and the gut: Pharmacology and current clinical experience. *Neurogastroenterology and Motility, 16*(4), 383–394. doi: 10.1111/j.1365-2982.2004.00513.x

deWit, H., Pierri, J., & Johanson, C. E. (1989). Reinforcing and subjective effects of diazepam in nondrug-abusing volunteers. *Pharmacology Biochemistry and Behavior, 33*(1), 205–213.

de Wit, S., & Dickinson, A. (2009). Associative theories of goal-directed behaviour: A case for animal-human translational models. *Psychological Research, 73*(4), 463–476. doi: 10.1007/s00426-009-0230-6

Diana, M., Mereu, G., Mura, A., Fadda, F., Passino, N., & Gessa, G. (1991). Low doses of gamma-hydroxybutyric acid stimulate the firing rate of dopaminergic neurons in unanesthetized rats. *Brain Research, 566*(1–2), 208–211.

Ding, Z.-M., Oster, S., Hall, S., Engleman, E., Hauser, S., McBride, W., & Rodd, Z. (2011). The stimulating effects of ethanol on ventral tegmental area dopamine neurons projecting to the ventral pallidum and medial prefrontal cortex in female Wistar rats: Regional difference and involvement of serotonin-3 receptors. *Psychopharmacologia, 216*(2), 245–255. doi: 10.1007/s00213-011-2208-5

Ding, Z. M., Toalston, J. E., Oster, S. M., McBride, W. J., & Rodd, Z. A. (2009). Involvement of local serotonin-2A but not serotonin-1B receptors in the reinforcing effects of ethanol within the posterior ventral tegmental area of female Wistar rats. *Psychopharmacology, 204*(3), 381–390. doi: 10.1007/s00213-009-1468-9

Dingemanse, J., & Appel-Dingemanse, S. (2007). Integrated pharmacokinetics and pharmacodynamics in drug development. *Clinical pharmacokinetics, 46*(9), 713–737.

Diniz, J. B., Shavitt, R. G., Pereira, C. A., Hounie, A. G., Pimentel, I., Koran, L. M., . . . Miguel, E. C. (2010). Quetiapine versus clomipramine in the augmentation of selective serotonin reuptake inhibitors for the treatment of obsessive-compulsive disorder: A randomized, open-label trial. *Journal of Psychopharmacology, 24*(3), 297–307. doi: 0269881108099423 [pii]

Djordjevic, M. V., Hoffman, D., Glynn, T., & Connolly, G. N. (1995). U.S. commercial brands of moist snuff, 1994: I. Assessment of nicotine, moisture, and pH. *Tobacco Control, 4*, 62–66.

Dlugosz, H., & Nasrallah, H. A. (2007). Paliperidone: a new extended-release oral atypical antipsychotic. *Expert Opinion on Pharmacotherapy, 8*(14), 2307–2313.

Doherty, J. D., Stout, R. W., & Roth, R. H. (1975). Metabolism of (1-14C)gamma-hydroxybutyric acid by rat brain after intraventricular injection. *Biochemical Pharmacology, 24*(4), 469–474.

Domino, E. F., & Luby, E. D. (2012). Phencyclidine/schizophrenia: One view toward the past, the other to the future. *Schizophrenia Bulletin, 38*: 914–919.

Donjacour, C. E. H. M., Aziz, N. A., Roelfsema, F., Frölich, M., Overeem, S., Lammers, G. J., & Pijl, H. (2011). Effect of sodium oxybate on growth hormone secretion in narcolepsy patients and healthy controls. *American Journal of Physiology—Endocrinology and Metabolism, 300*(6), E1069–E1075. doi: 10.1152/ajpendo.00623.2010

dos Reis, A., Jr. (2009). Sigmund Freud (1856–1939) and

Karl Koller (1857–1944) and the discovery of local anesthesia. *Revista Brasileira Anestesiologia, 59*(2), 244–257.

Doyon, S. (2001). The many faces of ecstasy. *Current Opinion in Pediatrics, 13*(2), 170–176.

Dranovsky, A., & Hen, R. (2006). Hippocampal neurogenesis: regulation by stress and antidepressants. *Biological Psychiatry, 59*(12), 1136–1143. doi: S0006-3223(06)00581-6 [pii]

Drdla, R., Gassner, M., Gingl, E., & Sandkuhler, J. (2009). Induction of synaptic long-term potentiation after opioid withdrawal. *Science, 325*(5937), 207–210. doi: 10.1126/science.1171759

Drevets, W., Videen, T., Price, J., Preskorn, S., Carmichael, S., & Raichle, M. (1992). A functional anatomical study of unipolar depression. *Journal of Neuroscience, 12*(9), 3628–3641.

Drevets, W. C., Bogers, W., & Raichle, M. E. (2002). Functional anatomical correlates of antidepressant drug treatment assessed using PET measures of regional glucose metabolism. *European Neuropsychopharmacology, 12*(6), 527–544. doi: 10.1016/s0924-977x(02)00102-5

Drevets, W. C., Price, J. L., Bardgett, M. E., Reich, T., Todd, R. D., & Raichle, M. E. (2002). Glucose metabolism in the amygdala in depression: Relationship to diagnostic subtype and plasma cortisol levels. *Pharmacology Biochemistry and Behavior, 71*(3), 431–447. doi: 10.1016/s0091-3057(01)00687-6

Drug Enforcement Administration. (2010). Exempt chemical mixtures containing gamma-butyrolactone. Retrieved from www.deadiversion.usdoj.gov/fed_regs/rules/2010/fr06293.htm

Drug Enforcement Administration. (2011). *3-4-methylenedioxypyrovalerone (MDPV)*. Washington, DC: United States Department of Justice.

Drug Enforcement Administration. (2012a). Gamma hydrobutyric acid. Retrieved from www.deadiversion.usdoj.gov/drugs_concern/ghb/ghb.htm

Drug Enforcement Administration. (2012b). Scheduling actions. Retrieved from www.deadiversion.usdoj.gov/schedules/orangebook/a_sched_alpha.pdf

Drug Enforcement Administration. (2012c). *Salvia divinorum*. Retrieved from www.justice.gov/dea/concern/salvia_divinorum.html

Duarte, D. F. (2005). Una breve história do ópio e dos opióides. *Revista Brasileira de Anestesiologia, 55*, 135–146.

Dubowski, K. M. (1985). Absorption, distribution and elimination of alcohol: highway safety aspects. *Journal of Studies on Alcohol, Supplement 10*, 98–108.

Dufour, M. C. (1999). What is moderate drinking? Defining "drinks" and drinking levels. *Alcohol Research and Health, 23*, 5–14.

Duman, R. S., Malberg, J., & Thome, J. (1999). Neural plasticity to stress and antidepressant treatment. *Biological Psychiatry, 46*(9), 1181–1191. doi: S0006-3223(99)00177-8 [pii]

Duncan, G. E., Paul, I. A., Powell, K. R., Fassberg, J. B., Stumpf, W. E., & Breese, G. R. (1989). Neuroanatomically selective down-regulation of beta adrenergic receptors by chronic imipramine treatment: Relationships to the topography of [3H]imipramine and [3H]desipramine binding sites. *Journal of Pharmacology and Experimental Therapeutics, 248*(1), 470–477.

Duvauchelle, C. L., Ikegami, A., Asami, S., Robens, J., Kressin, K., & Castaneda, E. (2000). Effects of cocaine context on NAcc dopamine and behavioral activity after repeated intravenous cocaine administration. *Brain Research, 862*(1–2), 49–58.

Duvauchelle, C. L., Ikegami, A., & Castaneda, E. (2000). Conditioned increases in behavioral activity and accumbens dopamine levels produced by intravenous cocaine. *Behavioral Neuroscience, 114*(6), 1156–1166.

Egan, M. F., Kojima, M., Callicott, J. H., Goldberg, T. E., Kolachana, B. S., Bertolino, A., . . . Weinberger, D. R. (2003). The BDNF val66met polymorphism affects activity-dependent secretion of BDNF and human memory and hippocampal function. *Cell, 112*(2), 257–269. doi: 10.1016/s0092-8674(03)00035-7

Ekelund, J., Hovatta, I., Parker, A., Paunio, T., Varilo, T., Martin, R., . . . Peltonen, L. (2001). Chromosome 1 loci in Finnish schizophrenia families. *Human Molecular Genetics, 10*, 1611–1617.

Ellinwood, E. H., King, G., & Lee, T. H. (2000). Chronic amphetamine use and abuse. In F. E. Bloom & D. J. Kupfer (Eds.), *Psychopharmacology: The fourth generation of progress.* Brentwood, TN: American College of Neuropsychopharmacology.

Elliott, S., & Burgess, V. (2005). The presence of gamma-hydroxybutyric acid (GHB) and gamma-butyrolactone (GBL) in alcoholic and non-alcoholic beverages. *Forensic Science International, 151*(2–3), 289–292. doi: 10.1016/j.forsciint.2005.02.014

Ellis, R. J., Toperoff, W., Vaida, F., van den Brande, G., Gonzales, J., Gouaux, B., . . . Atkinson, J. H. (2009). Smoked medicinal cannabis for neuropathic pain in HIV: a randomized, crossover clinical trial. *Neuropsychopharmacology, 34*(3), 672–680. doi: 10.1038/npp.2008.120

El-Mallakh, R. S., & Walker, K. L. (2010). Hallucinations, pseudohallucinations, and parahallucinations. *Psychiatry: Interpersonal and Biological Processes, 73*, 34–42.

Elmes, D. G., Kantowitz, B. H., & Roediger, H. L. (2006). *Research methods in psychology* (8th ed.). New York: Cengage Learning.

ElSohly, M. A., & Salamone, S. J. (1999). Prevalence of drugs used in cases of alleged sexual assault. *Journal of Analytical Toxicology, 23*(3), 141–146. doi: 10.1093/jat/23.3.141

Elzinga, B. M., Schmahl, C. G., Vermetten, E., van Dyck, R., & Bremner, J. D. (2003). Higher cortisol levels following exposure to traumatic reminders in abuse-related PTSD. *Neuropsychopharmacology, 28*(9), 1656–1665.

Emboden, W. A. (1972). Ritual use of *Cannabis sativa L.*: A historical-ethnographic survey. In P. T. Furst

(Ed.), *Flesh of the gods: The ritual use of hallucinogens.* New York: Praeger.

Emerson, T. S., & Cisek, J. E. (1993). Methcathinone: A Russian designer amphetamine infiltrates the rural Midwest. *Annals of Emergency Medicine, 22*(12), 1897–1903.

Emsley, R., Rabinowitz, J., & Medori, R. (2006). Time course for antipsychotic treatment response in first-episode schizophrenia. *American Journal of Psychiatry, 163*(4), 743–745. doi: 10.1176/appi.ajp.163.4.743

Ernst, M., Matochik, J. A., Heishman, S. J., Van Horn, J. D., Jons, P. H., Henningfield, J. E., & London, E. D. (2001). Effect of nicotine on brain activation during performance of a working memory task. *Proceedings of the National Academy of Sciences of the United States of America, 98*(8), 4728–4733. doi: 10.1073/pnas.061369098

Erritzoe, D., Frokjaer, V. G., Holst, K. K., Christoffersen, M., Johansen, S. S., Svarer, C., . . . Knudsen, G. M. (2011). In vivo imaging of cerebral serotonin transporter and serotonin2A receptor binding in 3,4-Me thylenedioxymethamphetamine (MDMA or "Ecstasy") and hallucinogen users. *Archives of General Psychiatry, 68*(6), 562–576. doi: 68/6/562 [pii]

Ervin, G. N., & Nemeroff, C. B. (1988). Interactions of neurotensin with dopamine-containing neurons in the central nervous system. *Progress in Neuropsychopharmacology and Biological Psychiatry, 12 Suppl*, S53–69.

Etches, R. C., Sandler, A. N., & Daley, M. D. (1989). Respiratory depression and spinal opioids. *Canadian Journal of Anaesthesiology, 36*(2), 165–185. doi: 10.1007/BF03011441

European Monitoring Centre for Drugs and Drug Addiction. (2009). *Annual report 2009: The state of the drugs problem in Europe.* Luxembourg: Publications Office of the European Union.

Eveloff, H. H. (1968). The LSD syndrome. A review. *California Medicine, 109*(5), 368–373.

Everett, G. M. (1972). Effects of amyl nitrite ("poppers") on sexual experience. *Medical Aspects of Human Sexuality, 6*, 146–151.

Fantegrossi, W. E., Ullrich, T., Rice, K. C., Woods, J. H., & Winger, G. (2002). 3,4-Me thylenedioxymethamphetamine (MDMA, "Ecstasy") and its stereoisomers as reinforcers in rhesus monkeys: serotonergic involvement. *Psychopharmacology (Berl), 161*(4), 356–364. doi: 10.1007/s00213-002-1021-6

Farré, M., & Camí, J. (1991). Pharmacokinetic considerations in abuse liability evaluation. *British Journal of Addiction, 86*(12), 1601–1606. doi: 10.1111/j.1360-0443.1991.tb01754.x

Fava, M., & Davidson, K. G. (1996). Definition and epidemiology of treatment-resistant depression. *Psychiatric Clinics of North America, 19*(2), 179–200.

FDA-approved labeling for Xyrem oral solution. (2005). Palo Alto, CA: Jazz Pharmaceuticals. Retrieved from www.fda.gov/downloads/Drugs/DrugSafety/ucm089830.pdf

Felder, C. C., Briley, E. M., Axelrod, J., Simpson, J. T., Mackie, K., & Devane, W. A. (1993). Anandamide, an endogenous cannabimimetic eicosanoid, binds to the cloned human cannabinoid receptor and stimulates receptor-mediated signal transduction. *Proceedings of the National Academy of Sciences, 90*, 7656–7660.

Ferrier, I.N., Tyrer, S.P., & Bell, A.J. (1995) Lithium therapy. *Advances in Psychiatric Treatment, 1*, 102-108. 10.1192/apt.1.4.102

Fillmore, M. T., Marczinski, C. A., & Bowman, A. M. (2005). Acute tolerance to alcohol effects on inhibitory and activational mechanisms of behavioral control. *Journal of Studies on Alcohol and Drugs, 66*(5), 663–672.

Fischer, E., & von Mering, J. (1903). Uber eine neue Klasse von Schlafmitteln. *Therapie der Gegenwart, 44*, 97–101.

Fish, E., DeBold, J., & Miczek, K. (2002). Repeated alcohol: Behavioral sensitization and alcohol-heightened aggression in mice. *Psychopharmacology, 160*(1),

39–48. doi: 10.1007/s00213-001-0934-9

Fisone, G., Borgkvist, A., & Usiello, A. (2004). Caffeine as a psychomotor stimulant: Mechanism of action. *Cellular and Molecular Life Sciences, 61*(7), 857–872. doi: 10.1007/s00018-003-3269-3

Fleischhacker, W. W., McQuade, R. D., Marcus, R. N., Archibald, D., Swanink, R., & Carson, W. H. (2009). A double-blind, randomized comparative study of aripiprazole and olanzapine in patients with schizophrenia. *Biological Psychiatry, 65*(6), 510–517. doi: 10.1016/j.biopsych.2008.07.033

Foltin, R. W., Fischman, M. W., Brady, J. V., Bernstein, D. J., Capriotti, R. M., Nellis, M. J., & Kelly, T. H. (1990). Motivational effects of smoked marijuana: Behavioral contingencies and low-probability activities. *Journal of Experimental Analysis of Behavior, 53*(1), 5–19. doi: 10.1901/jeab.1990.53-5

Food and Drug Administration (FDA). (2002). New drug and biological drug products: Evidence needed to demonstrate effectiveness of new drugs when human efficacy studies are not ethical or feasible. *Federal Register, 67*(105).

Food and Drug Administration. (2005). Public health advisory: Suicidality in adults being treated with antidepressant medications. Retrieved from www.fda.gov/Drugs/DrugSafety/

Food and Drug Administration. (2007). Adderall labeling information. Application number NDA 011522. Washington, DC: Author.

Fowler, J. S., Volkow, N. D., Wang, G. J., Pappas, N., Logan, J., MacGregor, R., . . . Cilento, R. (1996). Inhibition of monoamine oxidase B in the brains of smokers. *Nature, 379*(6567), 733–736. doi: 10.1038/379733a0

Fox, H. H., & Gibas, J. T. (1953). Synthetic tuberculostats. VII Monoalkyl derivatives of isonicotinylhydrazine. *Journal of Organic Chemistry, 18*, 994–1002.

Frary, C. D., Johnson, R. K., & Wang, M. Q. (2005). Food sources and intakes of caffeine in the diets of persons in the United States. *Journal of the American Dietetic Association, 105*, 110–113.

Frederiksen, L. W., Martin, J. E., & Webster, J. S. (1979). Assessment of smoking behavior. *Journal of Applied Behavioral Analysis, 12*(4), 653–664. doi: 10.1901/jaba.1979.12-653

Fredholm, B. B. (2011). Notes on the history of caffeine use. *Methylxanthines.* Vol. 200, pp. 1–9). Berlin: Springer.

Fredholm, B. B., & Arnaud, M. J. (2011). Pharmacokinetics and metabolism of natural methylxanthines in animal and man. *Methylxanthines.* (Vol. 200, pp. 33–91). Berlin: Springer.

Freeman, W., & Watts, J. W. (1945). Prefrontal lobotomy the problem of schizophrenia. *American Journal of Psychiatry, 101,* 739–748.

Freud, S. (1974). *The cocaine papers.* New York: Stonehill Publishing and Robert Byck.

Fryer, J. D., & Lukas, R. J. (1999). Noncompetitive functional inhibition at diverse, human nicotinic acetylcholine receptor subtypes by bupropion, phencyclidine, and ibogaine. *Journal of Pharmacology and Experimental Therapeutics, 288*(1), 88–92.

Fudala, P. J., & Woody, G. E. (2002). Current and experimental therapeutics for the treatment of opioid addiction. In K. L. Davis, D. Charney, J. T. Coyle & C. Nemeroff (Eds.), *Neuropsychopharmacology: The fifth generation of progress.* Philadelphia: Lippincott, Williams, & Wilkins.

Galloway, G. P., Newmeyer, J., Knapp, T., Stalcup, S. A., & Smith, D. (1996). A controlled trial of imipramine for the treatment of methamphetamine dependence. *Journal of Substance Abuse Treatment, 13*(6), 493–497. doi: 10.1016/s0740-5472(96)00154-7

Ganesan, K., Raza, S. K., & Vijayaraghavan, R. (2010). Chemical warfare agents. *Journal of Pharmacy & Bioallied Sciences, 2*(3), 166–178. doi: 10.4103/0975-7406.68498

Garattini, S. (2006) Reserpine and the opening of the neurotransmitter era in neuropsychopharmacology. In T. A. Ban & R. U. Udabe (Eds.), *The neurotransmitter era in neuropsychopharmacology* (pp. 127–138). Buenos Aires: Editorial Polemos.

Garcia, J., Kimeldorf, D. J., & Koellino, R. A. (1955). Conditioned aversion to saccharin resulting from exposure to gamma radiation. *Science, 122*(3160), 157–158.

Garrett, M. D., Walton, M. I., McDonald, E., Judson, I., & Workman, P. (2003). The contemporary drug development process: Advances and challenges in preclinical and clinical development. *Progress in Cell Cycle Research, 5,* 145–158.

Gebissa, E. (2010). Khat in the Horn of Africa: Historical perspectives and current trends. *Journal of Ethnopharmacology, 132*(3), 607–614. doi: 10.1016/j.jep.2010.01.063

Geddes, J. R., Burgess, S., Hawton, K., Jamison, K., & Goodwin, G. M. (2004). Long-term lithium therapy for bipolar disorder: Systematic review and meta-analysis of randomized controlled trials. *American Journal of Psychiatry, 161*(2), 217–222. doi: 10.1176/appi.ajp.161.2.217

Gems, D. (1999). Alexander Shulgin and Ann Shulgin, PIHKAL, a chemical love story. Alexander Shulgin and Ann Shulgin, TIHKAL, the continuation. *Theoretical Medicine and Bioethics, 20,* 477–479.

Georgotas, A., & Zeidenberg, P. (1979). Observations on the effects of four weeks of heavy marihuana smoking on group interaction and individual behavior. *Comprehensive Psychiatry, 20*(5), 427–432. doi: 0010-440X(79)90027-0 [pii]

Gerasimov, M. R. (2004). Brain uptake and biodistribution of [11C] toluene in nonhuman primates and mice. In P. M. Conn (Ed.), *Methods in Enzymology* (Vol. 385, pp. 334–349). San Diego: Academic Press.

Gerasimov, M. R., Schiffer, W. K., Marstellar, D., Ferrieri, R., Alexoff, D., & Dewey, S. L. (2002). Toluene inhalation produces regionally specific changes in extracellular dopamine. *Drug and Alcohol Dependence, 65*(3), 243–251. doi: 10.1016/s0376-8716(01)00166-1

Gerber, G. J., & Stretch, R. (1975). Drug-induced reinstatement of extinguished self-administration behavior in monkeys. *Pharmacology Biochemistry and Behavior, 3*(6), 1055–1061.

Gertsch, J., Pertwee, R. G., & Di Marzo, V. (2010). Phytocannabinoids beyond the *Cannabis* plant: Do they exist? *British Journal of Pharmacology, 160*(3), 523–529. doi: BPH745 [pii]

Ginsburg, B. C., Pinkston, J. W., & Lamb, R. J. (2011). Reinforcement magnitude modulation of rate dependent effects in pigeons and rats. *Experimental and Clinical Psychopharmacology, 19*(4), 285–294. doi: 10.1037/a0024311

Glaser, H. H., & Massengale, O. N. (1962). Glue-sniffing in children. *Journal of the American Medical Association, 181*, 301.

Glennon, R. A. (2011). Cathinone. Retrieved from www.pharmacy.vcu.edu/medchem/articles/cat/cat.html

Goldman, D. A. (2001). Thalidomide use: Past history and current implications for practice. *Oncology Nursing Forum, 28*(3), 471–477, 478–479.

Gomes, T., Juurlink, D. N., Dhalla, I. A., Mailis-Gagnon, A., Paterson, J. M., & Mamdani, M. M. (2011). Trends in opioid use and dosing among socio-economically disadvantaged patients. *Open Medicine, 5*, e12–e22.

Gonzales, D., Rennard, S. I., Nides, M., Oncken, C., Azoulay, S., Billing, C. B., . . . Reeves, K. R. (2006). Varenicline, an alpha-4beta2 nicotinic acetylcholine receptor partial agonist, vs sustained-release bupropion and placebo for smoking cessation: A randomized controlled trial. *Journal of the American Medical Assocaition, 296*(1), 47–55. doi: 10.1001/jama.296.1.47

Gonzales, R. A., & Weiss, F. (1998). Suppression of ethanol-reinforced behavior by naltrexone is associated with attenuation of the ethanol-induced increase in dialysate dopamine levels in the nucleus accumbens. *Journal of Neuroscience, 18*(24), 10663–10671.

Goodman, W. K., Ward, H., Kablinger, A., & Murphy, T. (1997). Fluvoxamine in the treatment of obsessive-compulsive disorder and related conditions.

Journal of Clinical Psychiatry, 58(suppl. 5), 32–49.

Goodwin, D. W., Powell, B., & Stern, J. (1971). Behavioral tolerance to alcohol in moderate drinkers. *American Journal of Psychiatry, 127*(12), 1651–1653. doi: 10.1176/appi.ajp.127.12.1651

Gorman, J. M., Kent, J. M., & Coplan, J. D. (2002). Current and emerging therapeutics of anxiety and stress disorders. In K. L. Davis, D. Charney, J. T. Coyle & C. Nemeroff (Eds.), *Neuropsychopharmacology: The fifth generation of progess*, pp. 967–980. Brentwood, TN: American College of Neuropsychopharmacology.

Gorman, J. M., Martinez, J., Coplan, J. D., Kent, J., & Kleber, M. (2004). The effect of successful treatment on the emotional and physiological response to carbon dioxide inhalation in patients with panic disorder. *Biological Psychiatry, 56*(11), 862–867.

Gossop, M., Bradley, B., & Phillips, G. T. (1987). An investigation of withdrawal symptoms shown by opiate addicts during and subsequent to a 21-day in-patient methadone detoxification procedure. *Addictive Behaviors, 12*(1), 1–6. doi: 10.1016/0306-4603(87)90002-5

Goto, Y., & Grace, A. A. (2005). Dopaminergic modulation of limbic and cortical drive of nucleus accumbens in goal-directed behavior. *Nature Neuroscience, 8*(6), 805–812. doi: 10.1038/nn1471

Goudie, A. J., Baker, L. E., Smith, J. A., Prus, A. J., Svensson, K. A., Cortes-Burgos, L. A., . . . Haadsma-Svensson, S. (2001). Common discriminative stimulus properties in rats of muscarinic antagonists, clozapine and the D 3 preferring antagonist PNU-99194A: an analysis of possible mechanisms. *Behavioural Pharmacology, 12*(5), 303–315.

Gould, T. D., Einat, H., Bhat, R., & Manji, H. K. (2004). AR-A014418, a selective GSK-3 inhibitor, produces antidepressant-like effects in the forced swim test. *International Journal of Neuropsychopharmacology, 7*(04), 387–390. doi: 10.1017/S1461145704004535

Grant, B. F., & Harford, T. C. (1990). Concurrent and simultaneous use of alcohol with cocaine: results of national survey. *Drug and Alcohol Dependence, 25*(1), 97–104.

Grant, K. A., Valverius, P., Hudspith, M., & Tabakoff, B. (1990). Ethanol withdrawal seizures and the NMDA receptor complex. *European Journal of Pharmacology, 176*(3), 289–296.

Grattan-Miscio, K., & Vogel-Sprott, M. (2005). Effects of alcohol and performance incentives on immediate working memory. *Psychopharmacology, 181*(1), 188–196. doi: 10.1007/s00213-005-2226-2

Graybiel, A. M., & Rauch, S. L. (2000). Toward a neurobiology of obsessive-compulsive disorder. *Neuron, 28*(2), 343–347. doi: S0896-6273(00)00113-6 [pii]

Green, M. F. (1996). What are the functional consequences of neurocognitive deficits in schizophrenia? *American Journal of Psychiatry, 153*(3), 321–330.

Green, M. F., Kern, R. S., Braff, D. L., & Mintz, J. (2000). Neurocognitive deficits and functional outcome in schizophrenia: Are we measuring the "right stuff"? *Schizophrenia Bulletin, 26*(1), 119–136.

Green, M. F., Kern, R. S., & Heaton, R. K. (2004). Longitudinal studies of cognition and functional outcome in schizophrenia: implications for MATRICS. *Schizophrenia Research, 72*(1), 41–51. doi: S0920-9964(04)00344-5 [pii]

Greenberg, P. E., Sisitsky, T., Kessler, R. C., Finkelstein, S. N., Berndt, E. R., Davidson, J. R., . . . Fyer, A. J. (1999). The economic burden of anxiety disorders in the 1990s. *Journal of Clinical Psychiatry, 60*(7), 427–435.

Grella, C. E., Hser, Y. I., & Hsieh, S. C. (2003). Predictors of drug treatment re-entry following relapse to cocaine use in DATOS. *Journal of Substance Abuse Treatment, 25*(3), 145–154.

Griffiths, R. R., Bigelow, G. E., Liebson, I., & Kaliszak, J. E. (1980). Drug preference in humans: double-blind choice comparison of pentobarbital, diazepam and placebo. *Journal of Pharmacology and Experimental Therapeutics, 215*(3), 649–661.

Griffiths, R. R., & Chausmer, A. L. (2000). Caffeine as a model drug of dependence: Recent developments in understanding caffeine withdrawal, the caffeine dependence syndrome, and caffeine negative reinforcement. *Nihon Shinkei Seishin Yakurigaku Zasshi, 20*(5), 223–231.

Griffiths, R. R., Findley, J. D., Brady, J. V., Dolan-Gutcher, K., & Robinson, W. W. (1975). Comparison of progressive-ratio performance maintained by cocaine, methylphenidate and secobarbital. *Psychopharmacologia, 43*(1), 81–83.

Grillon, C. (2008). Models and mechanisms of anxiety: Evidence from startle studies. *Psychopharmacology (Berl), 199*(3), 421–437. doi: 10.1007/s00213-007-1019-1

Gross, C., Santarelli, L., Brunner, D., Zhuang, X., & Hen, R. (2000). Altered fear circuits in 5-HT(1A) receptor KO mice. *Biological Psychiatry, 48*(12), 1157–1163. doi: S0006322300010416 [pii]

Guillem, K., Vouillac, C., Azar, M. R., Parsons, L. H., Koob, G. F., Cador, M., & Stinus, L. (2005). Monoamine oxidase inhibition dramatically increases the motivation to self-administer nicotine in rats. *Journal of Neuroscience, 25*(38), 8593–8600. doi: 10.1523/jneurosci.2139-05.2005

Guillon, J. M. (2010). Place and role of safety pharmacology in drug development. *Annales pharmaceutiques françaises, 68*(5), 291–300.

Gulya, K., Grant, K. A., Valverius, P., Hoffman, P. L., & Tabakoff, B. (1991). Brain regional specificity and time-course of changes in the NMDA receptor-ionophore complex during ethanol withdrawal. *Brain Research, 547*(1), 129–134. doi: 0006-8993(91)90583-H [pii]

Gundersen, H., Specht, K., Grüner, R., Ersland, L., & Hugdahl, K. (2008). Separating the effects of alcohol and expectancy on brain activation: An fMRI working memory study. *NeuroImage, 42*(4), 1587–1596. doi: 10.1016/j.neuroimage.2008.05.037

Guttman, M., Leger, G., Reches, A., Evans, A., Kuwabara, H., Cedarbaum, J. M., & Gjedde, A. (1993). Administration of the new COMT inhibitor OR-611 increases striatal uptake of fluorodopa. *Movement Disorders, 8*(3), 298–304. doi: 10.1002/mds.870080308

Haile, C. N., Kosten, T. R., & Kosten, T. A. (2009). Pharmacogenetic treatments for drug addiction: Cocaine, amphetamine, and methamphetamine. *American Journal of Drug and Alcohol Abuse, 35*(3), 161–177. doi: 911581221 [pii] 10.1080/00952990902825447

Hajnal, A., Smith, G. P., & Norgren, R. (2004). Oral sucrose stimulation increases accumbens dopamine in the rat. *American Journal of Physiology—Regulatory, Integrative and Comparative Physiology, 286*(1), R31–R37. doi: 10.1152/ajpregu.00282.2003

Hall, C. S. (1934). Emotional behavior in the rat. I. Defecation and urination as measures of individual differences in emotionality. *Journal of Comparative Psychology, 18*(3).

Hall, W. (2010). What are the policy lessons of national alcohol prohibition in the United States, 1920–1933? *Addiction, 105*(7), 1164–1173. doi: 10.1111/j.1360-0443.2010.02926.x

Hall, W., & Zador, D. (1997). The alcohol withdrawal syndrome. *The Lancet, 349*(9069), 1897–1900. doi: 10.1016/s0140-6736(97)04572-8

Hameedi, F. A., Rosen, M. I., McCance-Katz, E. F., McMahon, T. J., Price, L. H., Jatlow, P. I., . . . Kosten, T. R. (1995). Behavioral, physiological, and pharmacological interaction of cocaine and disulfiram in humans. *Biological Psychiatry, 37*(8), 560–563. doi: 10.1016/0006-3223(94)00361-6

Haney, M., Gunderson, E. W., Rabkin, J., Hart, C. L., Vosburg, S. K., Comer, S. D., & Foltin, R. W. (2007). Dronabinol and marijuana in HIV-positive marijuana smokers. Caloric intake, mood, and sleep. *Journal of Acquired Immune Deficiency Syndrome, 45*(5), 545–554. doi: 10.1097/QAI.0b013e31811ed205

Harburg, E. (1981). Negative affect, alcohol consumption and hangover symptoms among normal drinkers in a small community. *Journal of Studies on Alcohol and Drugs, 42*, 998–1012.

Hart, C. L., Ward, A. S., Haney, M., Comer, S. D., Foltin, R. W., & Fischman, M. W. (2002). Comparison of smoked marijuana and oral Δ⁹-tetrahydrocannabinol in humans. *Psychopharmacology (Berl), 164*(4), 407–415. doi: 10.1007/s00213-002-1231-y

Hashibe, M., Straif, K., Tashkin, D. P., Morgenstern, H., Greenland, S., & Zhang, Z.-F. (2005). Epidemiologic review of marijuana use and cancer risk. *Alcohol, 35*(3), 265–275. doi: 10.1016/j.alcohol.2005.04.008

Hasin, D. S., Stinson, F. S., Ogburn, E., & Grant, B. F. (2007). Prevalence, correlates, disability, and comorbidity of DSM-IV alcohol abuse and dependence in the United States: Results from the National Epidemiologic Survey on Alcohol and Related Conditions. *Archives of General Psychiatry, 64*(7), 830–842. doi: 10.1001/archpsyc.64.7.830

Hasler, F., Bourquin, D., Brenneisen, R., Bar, T., & Vollenweider, F. X. (1997). Determination of psilocin and 4-hydroxyindole-3-acetic acid in plasma by HPLC-ECD and pharmacokinetic profiles of oral and intravenous psilocybin in man. *Pharmaceutica Acta Helvetiae, 72*(3), 175–184.

Hatsukami, D. K., & Fischman, M. W. (1996). Crack cocaine and cocaine hydrochloride. *Journal of the American Medical Association, 276*(19), 1580–1588. doi: 10.1001/jama.1996.03540190052029

Hatzidimitriou, G., McCann, U. D., & Ricaurte, G. A. (1999). Altered serotonin innervation patterns in the forebrain of monkeys treated with (±)3,4-methylenedioxymethamphetamine seven years previously: Factors influencing abnormal recovery. *Journal of Neuroscience, 19*(12), 5096–5107.

Heather, N. (1989). Disulfiram treatment for alcoholism. *British Medical Journal, 299*(6697), 471–472. doi: 10.1136/bmj.299.6697.471

Heckers, S. (2001). Neuroimaging studies of the hippocampus in schizophrenia. *Hippocampus,*

11(5), 520–528. doi: 10.1002/hipo.1068

Hebert, L. E., Scherr, P. A., Bienias, J. L., Bennett, D. A., & Evans, D. A. (2003). Alzheimer disease in the U.S. population: Prevalence estimates using the 2000 census. *Archives of Neurology, 60*(8), 1119–1122.

Henningfield, J. E., Fant, R. V., Radzius, A., & Frost, S. (1999). Nicotine concentration, smoke pH, and whole tobacco aqueous pH of some cigar brands and types popular in the United States. *Nicotine and Tobacco Research, 1*(2), 163–168. doi: 10.1080/14622299050011271

Henningfield, J. E., & Keenan, R. M. (1993). Nicotine delivery kinetics and abuse liability. *Journal of Consulting and Clinical Psychology, 61*(5), 743–750.

Henningfield, J. E., Radzius, A., & Cone, E. J. (1995). Estimation of available nicotine content of six smokeless tobacco products. *Tobacco Control, 4*, 57–61.

Hepler, R. S., & Frank, I. R. (1971) Marihuana smoking and intraocular pressure. *Journal of the American Medical Association, 217*, 1392.

Herculano-Houzel, S. (2009). The human brain in numbers: A linearly scaled-up primate brain. *Frontiers in Human Neuroscience, 3.* doi: 10.3389/neuro.09.031.2009

Herkenham, M., Lynn, A. B., Little, M. D., Johnson, M. R., Melvin, L. S., de Costa, B. R., & Rice, K. C. (1990). Cannabinoid receptor localization in brain. *Proceedings of the National Academy of Sciences of the USA, 87*(5), 1932–1936.

Hertel, P., Fagerquist, M. V., & Svensson, T. H. (1999). Enhanced cortical dopamine output and antipsychotic-like effects of raclopride by alpha2 adrenoceptor blockade. *Science, 286*(5437), 105–107.

Hillbom, M., Pieninkeroinen, I., & Leone, M. (2003). Seizures in alcohol-dependent patients: Epidemiology, pathophysiology, and management. *CNS Drugs, 17*(14), 1013–1030.

Hillig, K. W., & Mahlberg, P. G. (2004). A chemotaxonomic analysis of cannabinoid variation in *Cannabis* (Cannabaceae).

American Journal of Botany, 91(6), 966–975. doi: 10.3732/ajb.91.6.966

Hilts, P. J. (1994, August 2). Is nicotine addictive? It depends on whose criteria you use. *The New York Times*, p. 1.

Hines, L. M., Stampfer, M. J., Ma, J., Gaziano, J. M., Ridker, P. M., Hankinson, S. E., . . . Hunter, D. J. (2001). Genetic variation in alcohol dehydrogenase and the beneficial effect of moderate alcohol consumption on myocardial infarction. *New England Journal of Medicine, 344*(8), 549–555. doi: 10.1056/NEJM200102223440802

Hippius, H. (1989). The history of clozapine. *Psychopharmacology, 99*, S3–S5.

Hippius, H., & Müller, N. (2008). The work of Emil Kraepelin and his research group in München. *European Archives of Psychiatry and Clinical Neuroscience, 258* (suppl. 2): 3–11.

Hodgkinson, C. A., Goldman, D., Jaeger, J., Persaud, S., Kane, J. M., Lipsky, R. H., & Malhotra, A. K. (2004). Disrupted in schizophrenia 1 (DISC1): Association with schizophrenia, schizoaffective disorder, and bipolar disorder. *American Journal of Human Genetics, 75*(5), 862–872.

Hoehn-Saric, R., McLeod, D. R., Funderburk, F., & Kowalski, P. (2004). Somatic symptoms and physiologic responses in generalized anxiety disorder and panic disorder: An ambulatory monitor study. *Archives in General Psychiatry, 61*, 913–921.

Hogg, S., & Dalvi, A. (2004). Acceleration of onset of action in schedule-induced polydipsia: combinations of SSRI and 5-HT1A and 5-HT1B receptor antagonists. *Pharmacology Biochemistry and Behavior, 77*(1), 69–75. doi: S0091305703002971 [pii]

Holly, E. N., Ebrecht, B., & Prus, A. J. (2011). The neurotensin-1 receptor agonist PD149163 inhibits conditioned avoidance responding without producing catalepsy in rats. *European Neuropsychopharmacology, 21*(7), 526–531. doi: S0924-977X(10)00280-4 [pii]

Holmes, A., Li, Q., Murphy, D. L., Gold, E., & Crawley, J. N. (2003).

Abnormal anxiety-related behavior in serotonin transporter null mutant mice: The influence of genetic background. *Genes, Brain, and Behavior, 2*(6), 365–380. doi: 10.1046/j.1601-1848.2003.00050.x

Homberg, J., De Boer, S., Raasø, H., Olivier, J., Verheul, M., Ronken, E., . . . Cuppen, E. (2008). Adaptations in pre- and post-synaptic 5-HT1$_A$ receptor function and cocaine supersensitivity in serotonin transporter knockout rats. *Psychopharmacology, 200*(3), 367–380. doi: 10.1007/s00213-008-1212-x

Hooft, P. J., & van de Voorde, H. P. (1994). Reckless behaviour related to the use of 3,4-methylenedioxymethamphetamine (Ecstasy): Apropos of a fatal accident during car-surfing. *International Journal of Legal Medicine, 106*(6), 328–329. doi: 10.1007/bf01224781

Horlocker, T. T., Burton, A. W., Connis, R. T., Hughes, S. C., Nickinovich, D. G., Palmer, C. M., . . . Wu, C. L. (2009). Practice guidelines for the prevention, detection, and management of respiratory depression associated with neuraxial opioid administration. *Anesthesiology, 110*(2), 218–230. doi: 10.1097/ALN.0b013e31818ec946

Hormes, J. T., Filley, C. M., & Rosenberg, N. L. (1986). Neurologic sequelae of chronic solvent vapor abuse. *Neurology, 36*(5), 698–702.

Horstmann, S., & Binder, E. B. (2009). Pharmacogenomics of antidepressant drugs. *Pharmacology and Therapeutics, 124*(1), 57–73. doi: S0163-7258(09)00132-6 [pii]

Hosztafi, S. (2001). The history of heroin. *Acta Pharmaceutica Hungarica, 71*(2), 233–242.

Howard, J. M., Olney, J. M., Frawley, J. P., Peterson, R. E., & Guerra, S. (1955). Adrenal function in the combat casualty. *AMA Archives of Surgery, 71*(1), 47–58.

Howard, O., & Perron, B. E. (2009). Nitrous oxide inhalation among adolescents: Prevalence, correlates, and co-occurrence with volatile solvent inhalation. *Journal of Psychoactive Drugs, 41*, 337–347.

Howland, J., Rohsenow, D. J., Bliss, C. A., Almeida, A. B., Calise,

T. V., Heeren, T., & Winter, M. (2010). Hangover predicts residual alcohol effects on psychomotor vigilance the morning after intoxication. *Journal of Addiction Research and Therapy, 1*(101). doi: 1000101 [pii]

Hser, Y. I., Hoffman, V., Grella, C. E., & Anglin, M. D. (2001). A 33-year follow-up of narcotics addicts. *Archives of General Psychiatry, 58*(5), 503–508.

Hu, X., Primack, B. A., Barnett, T. E., & Cook, R. L. (2011). College students and use of K2: an emerging drug of abuse in young persons. *Substance Abuse Treatment, Prevention, and Policy, 6*(16).

Hubbard, E. M. (2007). Neurophysiology of synesthesia. *Current Psychiatry Reports, 9*(3), 193–199.

Hubert, G. W., Jones, D. C., Moffett, M. C., Rogge, G., & Kuhar, M. J. (2008). CART peptides as modulators of dopamine and psychostimulants and interactions with the mesolimbic dopaminergic system. *Biochemical Pharmacology, 75*(1), 57–62. doi: 10.1016/j.bcp.2007.07.028

Hubbard, R. L., Craddock, S. G., & Anderson, J. (2003). Overview of 5-year followup outcomes in the drug abuse treatment outcome studies (DATOS). *Journal of Substance Abuse Treatment, 25*(3), 125–134.

Hughes, J., Kosterlitz, H. W., & Leslie, F. M. (1975). Effect of morphine on adrenergic transmission in the mouse vas deferens: Assessment of agonist and antagonist potencies of narcotic analgesics. *British Journal of Pharmacology, 53*, 371–381.

Hughes, J., Smith, T., Morgan, B., & Fothergill, L. (1975). Purification and properties of enkephalin: The possible endogenous ligand for the morphine receptor. *Life Sciences, 16*(12), 1753–1758.

Hughes, J. R., Oliveto, A. H., Liguori, A., Carpenter, J., & Howard, T. (1998). Endorsement of DSM-IV dependence criteria among caffeine users. *Drug and Alcohol Dependence, 52*(2), 99–107.

Hungund, B. L., Szakall, I., Adam, A., Basavarajappa, B. S., & Vadasz, C. (2003). Cannabinoid CB1 receptor knockout mice exhibit markedly reduced voluntary alcohol consumption and lack alcohol-induced dopamine release in the nucleus accumbens. *Journal of Neurochemistry, 84*(4), 698–704. doi: 10.1046/j.1471-4159.2003.01576.x

Hustveit, O., Maurset, A., & Oye, I. (1995). Interaction of the chiral forms of ketamine with opioid, phencyclidine, sigma, and muscarinic receptors. *Pharmacology and Toxicology, 77*(6), 355–359.

Ifland, J. R., Preuss, H. G., Marcus, M. T., Rourke, K. M., Taylor, W. C., Burau, K., . . . Manso, G. (2009). Refined food addiction: A classic substance use disorder. *Medical Hypotheses, 72*(5), 518–526. doi: 10.1016/j.mehy.2008.11.035

Ikeda, H., Stark, J., Fischer, H., Wagner, M., Drdla, R., Jager, T., & Sandkuhler, J. (2006). Synaptic amplifier of inflammatory pain in the spinal dorsal horn. *Science, 312*(5780), 1659–1662. doi: 10.1126/science.1127233

International Conference on Harmonization. (1996). *Guideline for industry: Structure and content of clinical study reports* (Vol. 61FR37320). Federal Register: International Conference on Harmonisation of Technical Requirements for Registration of Pharmaceuticals for Human Use.

Ishida, K., Murata, M., Katagiri, N., Ishikawa, M., Abe, K., Kato, M., . . . Taguchi, K. (2005). Effects of Î²-phenylethylamine on dopaminergic neurons of the ventral tegmental area in the rat: A combined electrophysiological and microdialysis study. *Journal of Pharmacology and Experimental Therapeutics, 314*(2), 916–922. doi: 10.1124/jpet.105.084764

Israel, Y., Khanna, J. M., Orrego, H., Rachamin, G., Wahid, S., Britton, R., . . . Kalant, H. (1979). Studies on metabolic tolerance to alcohol, hepatomegaly, and alcoholic liver disease. *Drug and Alcohol Dependence, 4*(1–2), 109–118.

Ito, T., Suzuki, T., Wellman, S. E., & Ho, I. K. (1996). Pharmacology of barbiturate tolerance/dependence: $GABA_A$ receptors and molecular aspects. *Life Sciences, 59*(3), 169–195.

Jacob, M. S., Carlen, P. L., Marshman, J. A., & Sellers, E. M. (1981). Phencyclidine ingestion: Drug abuse and psychosis. *International Journal of Addiction, 16*(4), 749–758.

Jacob, P., III, Abu Raddaha, A. H., Dempsey, D., Havel, C., Peng, M., Yu, L., & Benowitz, N. L. (2011). Nicotine, carbon monoxide, and carcinogen exposure after a single use of a water pipe. *Cancer Epidemiology, Biomarkers, and Prevention, 20*(11), 2345–2353. doi: 10.1158/1055-9965.EPI-11-0545

Jacobson, S. W., Jacobson, J. L., & Sokol, R. J. (1994). Effects of fetal alcohol exposure on infant reaction time. *Alcoholism: Clinical and Experimental Research, 18*(5), 1125–1132. doi: 10.1111/j.1530-0277.1994.tb00092.x

James, D., Adams, R. D., Spears, R., Cooper, G., Lupton, D. J., Thompson, J. P., & Thomas, S. H. (2011). Clinical characteristics of mephedrone toxicity reported to the U.K. National Poisons Information Service. *Emergency Medicine Journal, 28*(8), 686–689. doi: 10.1136/emj.2010.096636

James, J., & Rogers, P. (2005). Effects of caffeine on performance and mood: Withdrawal reversal is the most plausible explanation. *Psychopharmacology, 182*(1), 1–8. doi: 10.1007/s00213-005-0084-6

Jenkins, J., & Hubbard, S. (1991). History of clinical trials. *Seminars in oncology nursing, 7*(4), 228–234.

Jensen, N. H., Rodriguiz, R. M., Caron, M. G., Wetsel, W. C., Rothman, R. B., & Roth, B. L. (2008). N-desalkylquetiapine, a potent norepinephrine reuptake inhibitor and partial 5-HT1A agonist, as a putative mediator of quetiapine's antidepressant activity. *Neuropsychopharmacology, 33*(10), 2303–2312. doi: 1301646 [pii]

Jentsch, J. D., & Roth, R. H. (1999). The neuropsychopharmacology of phencyclidine: From NMDA receptor hypofunction to the dopamine hypothesis of schizophrenia. *Neuropsychopharmacology, 20*(3), 201–225. doi: 10.1016/S0893-133X(98)00060-8

Joeres, R., Klinker, H., Heusler, H., Epping, J., Zilly, W., & Richter, E. (1988). Influence of smoking on caffeine elimination in healthy volunteers and in patients with alcoholic liver cirrhosis. *Hepatology, 8*(3), 575–579.

Joerger, M., Wilkins, J., Fagagnini, S., Baldinger, R., Brenneisen, R., Schneider, U., . . . Weber, M. (2012). Single-dose pharmacokinetics and tolerability of oral delta-9-tetrahydrocannabinol in patients with amyotrophic lateral sclerosis. *Drug Metabolism Letters, 6*(2), 102–108. doi: 10.2174/1872312811206020102

Johanson, C. E., Lundahl, L. H., Lockhart, N., & Schubiner, H. (2006). Intravenous cocaine discrimination in humans. *Experimental and Clinical Psychopharmacology, 14*(2), 99–108. doi: 2006-07129-001 [pii]

Johnson, C. L., & Sansone, R. A. (1993). Integrating the twelve-step approach with traditional psychotherapy for the treatment of eating disorders. *International Journal of Eating Disorders, 14*(2), 121–134.

Johnston, I. R. (1982). The role of alcohol in road crashes. *Ergonomics, 25*(10), 941–946.

Johnston, L. D., O'Malley, P. M., Bachman, J. G., & Schulenberg, J. E. (2011). Monitoring the future national results on adolescent drug use: Overview of key findings. *General Hospital Psychiatry, 33*, 3–4.

Johnston, L. D., O'Malley, P. M., & Bachman, J. G. (2003). *Monitoring the future national survey results on drug use, 1975–2002. Vol. I: Secondary school students.* Bethesday, MD: National Institute on Drug Abuse.

Jones, E. (1953). *The life and work of Sigmond Freud* (Vol. 1). New York: Basic Books.

Jones, S. R., Garris, P. A., & Wightman, R. M. (1995). Different effects of cocaine and nomifensine on dopamine uptake in the caudate-putamen and nucleus accumbens. *Journal of Pharmacology and Experimental Therapeutics, 274*(1), 396–403.

Juliano, L. M., Evatt, D. P., Richards, B. D., & Griffiths, R. R. (2012). Characterization of individuals seeking treatment for caffeine dependence. *Psychology of Addictive Behaviors.* doi: 10.1037/a0027246

Juliano, L. M., Fucito, L. M., & Harrell, P. T. (2011). The influence of nicotine dose and nicotine dose expectancy on the cognitive and subjective effects of cigarette smoking. *Experimental and Clinical Psychopharmacology, 19*(2), 105–115. doi: 10.1037/a0022937

Kalant, H. (2001). Medicinal use of cannabis: History and current status. *Medicinal Use of Cannabis, 6*, 80–91.

Kalat, J. W. (2009). *Biological psychology* (10th ed.). Belmont, CA: Wadsworth.

Kalayasiri, R., Sughondhabirom, A., Gueorguieva, R., Coric, V., Lynch, W. J., Lappalainen, J., . . . Malison, R. T. (2007). Dopamine β-hydroxylase gene (DβH) -1021C→T influences self-reported paranoia during cocaine self-administration. *Biological Psychiatry, 61*(11), 1310–1313. doi: 10.1016/j.biopsych.2006.08.012

Kalivas, P. W. (2002). Neurocircuitry of addiction. In K. L. Davis, D. Charney, J. T. Coyle & C. Nemeroff (Eds.), *Neuropsychopharmacology: The fifth generation of progress.* Brentwood, NJ: American College of Neuropsychopharmacology.

Kalivas, P. W. (2009). The glutamate homeostasis hypothesis of addiction. *Nature Reveus Neuroscience, 10*(8), 561-572. doi: 10.1038/nrn2515

Kalivas, P. W., Churchill, L., & Klitenick, M. A. (1993). GABA and enkephalin projection from the nucleus accumbens and ventral pallidum to the ventral tegmental area. *Neuroscience, 57*(4), 1047–1060.

Kalix, P. (1981). Cathinone, an alkaloid from khat leaves with an amphetamine-like releasing effect. *Psychopharmacology (Berl), 74*(3), 269–270.

Kampman, K. M. (2010). What's new in the treatment of cocaine addiction? *Current Psychiatry Reports, 12*(5), 441–447. doi: 10.1007/s11920-010-0143-5

Kampman, K. M., Pettinati, H., Lynch, K. G., Dackis, C., Sparkman, T., Weigley, C., & O'Brien, C. P. (2004). A pilot trial of topiramate for the treatment of cocaine dependence. *Drug and Alcohol Dependence,* 75(3), 233–240. doi: 10.1016/j.drugalcdep.2004.03.008

Kane, J., Honigfeld, G., Singer, J., & Meltzer, H. (1988). Clozapine for the treatment-resistant schizophrenic: A double-blind comparison with chlorpromazine. *Archives of General Psychiatry, 45*(9), 789–796.

Kaneda, Y., Jayathilak, K., & Meltzer, H. (2010). Determinants of work outcome in neuroleptic-resistant schizophrenia and schizoaffective disorder: Cognitive impairment and clozapine treatment. *Psychiatry Research, 178*, 57–62.

Kapur, S., & Seeman, P. (2000). Antipsychotic agents differ in how fast they come off the dopamine D2 receptors: Implications for atypical antipsychotic action. *Journal of Psychiatry and Neuroscience, 25*(2), 161–166.

Kapur, S., & Seeman, P. (2002). NMDA receptor antagonists ketamine and PCP have direct effects on the dopamine D(2) and serotonin 5-HT(2) receptors-implications for models of schizophrenia. *Molecular Psychiatry, 7*(8), 837–844. doi: 10.1038/sj.mp.4001093

Kaye, S., Darke, S., & Duflou, J. (2009). Methylenedioxymethamphetamine (MDMA)-related fatalities in Australia: Demographics, circumstances, toxicology and major organ pathology. *Drug and Alcohol Dependence, 104*(3), 254–261. doi: 10.1016/j.drugalcdep.2009.05.016

Keck, P. E., McElroy, S. L., & Nemeroff, C. B. (1992). Anticonvulsants in the treatment of bipolar disorder. *Journal of Neuropsychiatry and Clinical Neurosciences, 4*, 395–405.

Keefe, R. S., & Fenton, W. S. (2007). How should DSM-V criteria for schizophrenia include cognitive impairment? *Schizophrenia Bulletin, 33*(4), 912–920. doi: sbm046 [pii]

Ker, K., Edwards, P. J., Felix, L. M., Blackhall, K., & Roberts, I. (2010). Caffeine for the prevention of injuries and errors in shift workers. *Cochrane Database Systems Review* (5), CD008508. doi: 10.1002/14651858.CD008508

Kerner, K. (1988). Current topics in inhalant abuse. In R. A. Crider & B. A. Rouse (Eds.), *Epidemiology of inhalant abuse*. Rockville, MD: National Institute on Drug Abuse.

Kessler, R. C., Berglund, P., Demler, O., Jin, R., Merikangas, K. R., & Walters, E. E. (2005). Lifetime prevalence and age-of-onset distributions of DSM-IV disorders in the National Comorbidity Survey Replication. *Archives of General Psychiatry, 62*(6), 593–602. doi: 62/6/593 [pii]

Khalil, A. A., Steyn, S., & Castagnoli, N. (1999). Isolation and characterization of a monoamine oxidase inhibitor from tobacco leaves. *Chemical Research in Toxicology, 13*(1), 31–35. doi: 10.1021/tx990146f

Khan, S., Patil, K., Yeole, P., & Gaikwad, R. (2009). Brain targeting studies on buspirone hydrochloride after intranasal administration of mucoadhesive formulation in rats. *Journal of Pharmacy and Pharmacology, 61*(5), 669–675. doi: 10.1211/jpp/61.05.0017

Klasser, G. D., & Epstein, J. (2005). Methamphetamine and its impact on dental care. *Journal of the Canadian Dental Association, 71*(10), 759–762.

Kleen, J. K., Sitomer, M. T., Killeen, P. R., & Conrad, C. D. (2006). Chronic stress impairs spatial memory and motivation for reward without disrupting motor ability and motivation to explore. *Behavioral Neuroscience, 120*, 842–851.

Klepner, C. A., Lippa, A. S., Benson, D. I., Sano, M. C., & Beer, B. (1979). Resolution of two biochemically and pharmacologically distinct benzodiazepine receptors. *Pharmacology Biochemistry and Behavior, 11*(4), 457–462.

Kleykamp, B. A., Griffiths, R. R., & Mintzer, M. Z. (2010). Dose effects of triazolam and alcohol on cognitive performance in healthy volunteers. *Experimental and Clinical Psychopharmacology, 18*(1), 1–16. doi: 2010-02775-001 [pii]

Kolbrich, E. A., Goodwin, R. S., Gorelick, D. A., Hayes, R. J., Stein, E. A., & Huestis, M. A. (2008). Physiological and subjective responses to controlled oral 3,4-methylenedioxymethamphetamine administration. *Journal of Clinical Psychopharmacology, 28*(4), 432–440. doi: 10.1097/JCP.0b013e31817ef470

Kometer, M., Cahn, B. R., Andel, D., Carter, O. L., & Vollenweider, F. X. (2011). The 5-HT2A/1A agonist psilocybin disrupts modal object completion associated with visual hallucinations. *Biological Psychiatry, 69*(5), 399–406. doi: 10.1016/j.biopsych.2010.10.002

Koob, G. F., & Volkow, N. D. (2009). Neurocircuitry of addiction. *Neuropsychopharmacology, 35*(1), 217–238.

Kopelman, M. D., Thomson, A. D., Guerrini, I., & Marshall, E. J. (2009). The Korsakoff syndrome: Clinical aspects, psychology, and treatment. *Alcohol and Alcoholism, 44*(2), 148–154. doi: 10.1093/alcalc/agn118

Krabbendam, L., Visser, P. J., Derix, M. M. A., Verhey, F., Hofman, P., Verhoeven, W., Tuinier, S., & Jolles, J. (2000) Normal cognitive performance in patients with chronic alcoholism in contrast to patients with Korsakoff's syndrome. *Journal of Neuropsychiatry and Clinical Neuroscience, 12*, 44–50.

Kroeze, W. K., Hufeisen, S. J., Popadak, B. A., Renock, S. M., Steinberg, S., Ernsberger, P., . . . Roth, B. L. (2003). H1-histamine receptor affinity predicts short-term weight gain for typical and atypical antipsychotic drugs. *Neuropsychopharmacology, 28*(3), 519–526.

Krystal, J. H., Cramer, J. A., Krol, W. F., Kirk, G. F., & Rosenheck, R. A. (2001). Naltrexone in the treatment of alcohol dependence. *New England Journal of Medicine, 345*(24), 1734–1739. doi: 10.1056/NEJMoa011127

Krystal, J. H., Karper, L. P., Seibyl, J. P., Freeman, G. K., Delaney, R., Bremner, J. D., . . . Charney, D. S. (1994). Subanesthetic effects of the noncompetitive NMDA antagonist, ketamine, in humans. Psychotomimetic, perceptual, cognitive, and neuroendocrine responses. *Archives of General Psychiatry, 51*(3), 199–214.

Krystal, J. H., Petrakis, I. L., Mason, G., Trevisan, L., & D'Souza, D. C. (2003). N-methyl-D-aspartate glutamate receptors and alcoholism: Reward, dependence, treatment, and vulnerability. *Pharmacology and Therapeutics, 99*(1), 79–94.

Kucharski, A. (1984). History of frontal lobotomy in the United States, 1935–1955. *Neurosurgery, 14*(6), 765–772.

Kuhn, R. (1958). The treatment of depressive states with G-22355 (imipramine hydrochloride). *American Journal of Psychiatry, 115*, 459-464.

Kuroki, T., Meltzer, H. Y., & Ichikawa, J. (1999). Effects of antipsychotic drugs on extracellular dopamine levels in rat medial prefrontal cortex and nucleus accumbens. *Journal of Pharmacology and Experimental Therapeutics, 288*(2), 774–781.

Kurtzman, T. L., Otsuka, K. N., & Wahl, R. A. (2001). Inhalant abuse by adolescents. *Journal of Adolescent Health, 28*(3), 170–180. doi: 10.1016/s1054-139x(00)00159-2

LaLumiere, R. T., & Kalivas, P. W. (2008). Glutamate release in the nucleus accumbens core is necessary for heroin seeking. *Journal of Neuroscience, 28*(12), 3170–3177. doi: 10.1523/jneurosci.5129-07.2008

Lameh, J., Burstein, E. S., Taylor, E., Weiner, D. M., Vanover, K. E., & Bonhaus, D. W. (2007). Pharmacology of N-desmethylclozapine. *Pharmacology and Therapeutics, 115*(2), 223-231.

Laplane, D., Levasseur, M., Pillon, B., Dubois, B., Baulac, M., Mazoyer, B., . . . Baron, J. C. (1989). Obsessive-compulsive and other behavioural changes with bilateral basal ganglia lesions: A neuropsychological, magnetic resonance imaging, and positron tomography study. *Brain, 112* (Part 3), 699–725.

Laursen, T. M. (2011). Life expectancy among persons with schizophrenia or bipolar disorder. *Schizophrenia Research, 131*, 101–104.

LeBeau, M., Andollo, W., Hearn, W. L., Baselt, R., Cone, E., Finkle, B., . . . Saady, J. (1999). Recommendations for toxicological investigations of drug-facilitated sexual assaults. *Journal of Forensic Science, 44*(1), 227–230.

Leicht, M. E., Gamma, A., & Vollenweider, F. X. (2001). Gender differences in the subjective effects of MDMA. *Psychopharmacology, 154*, 161–168.

Lenox, R. H., & Frazer, A. (2002). Mechanisms of action of antidepressants and mood stabilizers. In K. L. Davis, D. Charney, J. T. Coyle & C. Nemeroff (Eds.), *Neuropsychopharmacology: The fifth generation of progress.* Brentwood, TN: American College of Neuropsychopharmacology.

Leonhart, M. M. (2011). Denial of petition to initiate proceedings to reschedule marijuana. (DEA-352N). *Federal Register.*

Lerner, A. G., Gelkopf, M., Skladman, I., Oyffe, I., Finkel, B., Sigal, M., & Weizman, A. (2002). Flashback and hallucinogen persisting perception disorder: Clinical aspects and pharmacological treatment approach. *Israel Journal of Psychiatry and Related Sciences, 39*, 92–99.

Lerner, S. E., & Burns, S. R. (1978). Phencyclidine use among youth: History, epidemiology, and acute and chronic intoxication. *NIDA Research Monographs, 21*, 66–118.

Lewin, L. (1924). *Phantastica, narcotic and stimulating drugs: Their use and abuse.* London: Routledge & Kegan Paul.

Lewis, D. A., & Lieberman, J. A. (2000). Catching up on schizophrenia: natural history and neurobiology. *Neuron, 28*, 325–334.

Lewis, J. E. (2005). *Testimony at United States Senate Committee on Environment and Public Works.* Retrieved from www.fbi.gov/news/testimony/investigating-and-preventing-animal-rights-extremism

Li, N., Lee, B., Liu, R. J., Banasr, M., Dwyer, J. M., Iwata, M., . . . Duman, R. S. (2010). mTOR-dependent synapse formation underlies the rapid antidepressant effects of NMDA antagonists. *Science, 329*(5994), 959–964. doi: 329/5994/959 [pii]

Li, Y., Luikart, B. W., Birnbaum, S., Chen, J., Kwon, C.-H., Kernie, S. G., . . . Parada, L. F. (2008). TrkB regulates hippocampal neurogenesis and governs sensitivity to antidepressive treatment. *Neuron, 59*(3), 399–412.

Li, Y.-F., LaCroix, C., & Freeling, J. (2009). Specific subtypes of nicotinic cholinergic receptors involved in sympathetic and parasympathetic cardiovascular responses. *Neuroscience Letters, 462*(1), 20–23. doi: 10.1016/j.neulet.2009.06.081

Lieber, C. S. (1997). Ethanol metabolism, cirrhosis, and alcoholism. *Clinica Chimica Acta, 257*(1), 59–84.

Liecht, M. E., Gamma, A., & Vollenweider, F. X. (2001) Gender differences in the subjective effects of MDMA. *Psychopharmacology, 154*, 161–168.

Liegeois, J. F., Ichikawa, J., & Meltzer, H. Y. (2002). 5-HT(2A) receptor antagonism potentiates haloperidol-induced dopamine release in rat medial prefrontal cortex and inhibits that in the nucleus accumbens in a dose-dependent manner. *Brain Research, 947*(2), 157–165.

Liguori, A., D'Agostino, R. B., Dworkin, S. I., Edwards, D., & Robinson, J. H. (1999). Alcohol effects on mood, equilibrium, and simulated driving. *Alcoholism: Clinical and Experimental Research, 23*(5), 815–821. doi: 10.1111/j.1530-0277.1999.tb04188.x

Lile, J. A., Kelly, T. H., Pinsky, D. J., & Hays, L. R. (2009). Substitution profile of delta9-tetrahydrocannabinol, triazolam, hydromorphone, and methylphenidate in humans discriminating delta9-tetrahydrocannabinol. *Psychopharmacology (Berl), 203*(2), 241–250. doi: 10.1007/s00213-008-1393-3

Lineberry, T. W., & Bostwick, J. M. (2006). Methamphetamine abuse: A perfect storm of complications. *Mayo Clinic Proceedings, 81*(1), 77–84. doi: 10.4065/81.1.77

Littleton, J. (1995). Acamprosate in alcohol dependence: How does it work? *Addiction, 90*, 1179–1188.

Loimer, N., Schmid, R. W., Presslich, O., & Lenz, K. (1989). Continuous naloxone administration suppresses opiate withdrawal symptoms in human opiate addicts during detoxification treatment. *Journal of Psychiatric Research,* 23(1), 81–86. doi: 10.1016/0022-3956(89)90020-4

Longabaugh, R., & Morgenstern, J. (1999). Cognitive–behavioral coping-skills therapy for alcohol dependence: Current status and future directions. *Alcohol Research and Health, 23*(2), 78–85.

Lopez-Muñoz, F., Ucha-Udabe, R., & Alamo, C. (2005). The history of barbiturates a century after their clinical introduction. *Neuropsychiatric Disease Treatment, 1*(4), 329–343.

Lopreato, G. F., Phelan, R., Borghese, C. M., Beckstead, M. J., & Mihic, S. J. (2003). Inhaled drugs of abuse enhance serotonin-3 receptor function. *Drug and Alcohol Dependence, 70*, 11–15.

Lotfipour, S., Arnold, M. M., Hogenkamp, D. J., Gee, K. W., Belluzzi, J. D., & Leslie, F. M. (2011). The monoamine oxidase (MAO) inhibitor tranylcypromine enhances nicotine self-administration in rats through a mechanism independent of MAO inhibition. *Neuropharmacology, 61*, 95–104. doi: 10.1016/j.neuropharm.2011.03.007

Loyola Marymount University (2006) Blood Alcohol Content. Retrieved November 25, 2012 from http://www.lmu.edu/Page25066.aspx

Lubman, D. I., Hides, L., & Yucel, M. (2006). Inhalant misuse in youth: The need for a coordinated response. *Medical Journal of Australia, 185*, 327–330.

Lubman, D. I., Yucel, M., & Lawrence, A. J. (2008). Inhalant abuse among adolescents: Neurobiological considerations. *British Journal of Pharmacology, 154*(2), 316–326. doi: 10.1038/bjp.2008.76

Lufty, K., & Cowan, A. (2004). Buprenorphine: A unique drug with complex pharmacology. *Current Neuropharmacology, 2*, 395–402.

Machu, T. K., & Harris, R. A. (1994). Alcohols and anesthetics enhance the function of 5-hydroxytryptamine3 receptors expressed in Xenopus laevis oocytes. *Journal of Pharmacology and Experimental Therapeutics, 271*(2), 898–905.

MacMillan, M. (2008). Phineas Gage: Unraveling the myth. *The Psychologist, 21*, 836–839.

MacPhail, R. C., & Gollub, L. R. (1975). Separating the effects of response rate and reinforcement frequency in the rate-dependent effects of amphetamine and scopolamine on the schedule-controlled performance of rats and pigeons. *Journal of Pharmacology and Experimental Therapeutics, 194*(2), 332–342.

Madden, J. A., Konkol, R. J., Keller, P. A., & Alvarez, T. A. (1995). Cocaine and benzoylecgonine constrict cerebral arteries by different mechanisms. *Life Sciences, 56*(9), 679–686.

Maitre, M. (1997). The γ-hydroxybutyrate signalling system in brain: Organization and functional implications. *Progress in Neurobiology, 51*(3), 337–361. doi: 10.1016/s0301-0082(96)00064-0

Maj, J., Dziedzicka-Wasylewska, M., Rogoz, R., Rogoz, Z., & Skuza, G. (1996). Antidepressant drugs given repeatedly change the binding of the dopamine D2 receptor agonist, [3H]N-0437, to dopamine D2 receptors in the rat brain. *European Journal of Pharmacology, 304*(1–3), 49–54.

Malinauskas, B. M., Aeby, V. G., Overton, R. F., Carpenter-Aeby, T., & Barber-Heidal, K. (2007). A survey of energy drink consumption patterns among college students. *Nutrition Journal, 6*, 35. doi: 10.1186/1475-2891-6-35

Malit, L. A., Johnstone, R. E., Bourke, D. I., Kulp, R. A., Klein, V., & Smith, T. C. (1975). Intravenous delta9-tetrahydrocannabinol: Effects on ventilatory control and cardiovascular dynamics. *Anesthesiology, 42*, 666–673.

Mamelak, M. (1989). Gamma-hydroxybutyrate: An endogenous regulator of energy metabolisms. *Neuroscience and Biobehavioral Reviews, 13*, 187–198.

Mao, Z. M., Arnsten, A. F., & Li, B. M. (1999). Local infusion of an alpha-1 adrenergic agonist into the prefrontal cortex impairs spatial working memory performance in monkeys. *Biological Psychiatry, 46*(9), 1259–1265.

Mao, Y., Ge, X., Frank, C. L., Madison, J. M., Koehler, A. N., Doud, M. K., . . . Tsai, L. H. (2009). Disrupted in schizophrenia 1 regulates neuronal progenitor proliferation via modulation of GSK3beta/beta-catenin signaling. *Cell, 136*(6), 1017–1031. doi: S0092-8674 (09)00021-X [pii]

Marching for science. (2009). *Nature Neuroscience, 12*, 523.

Marczynski, T. J., Yamaguchi, N., Ling, G. M., & Grodzinska, L. (1964). Sleep induced by the administration of melatonin (5-methoxyn-acetyltryptamine) to the hypothalamus in unrestrained cats. *Experientia, 20*(8), 435–437.

Marder, S. R., & Fenton, W. (2004). Measurement and treatment research to improve cognition in schizophrenia: NIMH MATRICS initiative to support the development of agents for improving cognition in schizophrenia. *Schizophrenia Research, 72*(1), 5–9. doi: 10.1016/j.schres.2004.09.010

Maric, T., Sedki, F., Ronfard, B., Chafetz, D., & Shalev, U. (2012). A limited role for ghrelin in heroin self-administration and food deprivation-induced reinstatement of heroin seeking in rats. *Addiction Biology, 17*(3), 613–622. doi: 10.1111/j.1369-1600.2011.00396.x

Marin, S. J., Coles, R., Merrell, M., & McMillin, G. A. (2008). Quantitation of benzodiazepines in urine, serum, plasma, and meconium by LC-MS-MS. *Journal of Analytical Toxicology, 32*(7), 491–498.

Marmor, J. B. (1998). Medical marijuana. *Western Journal of Medicine, 168*, 540–543.

Martell, B. A., Orson, F. M., Poling, J., Mitchell, E., Rossen, R. D., Gardner, T., & Kosten, T. R. (2009). Cocaine vaccine for the treatment of cocaine dependence in methadone-maintained patients: A randomized, double-blind, placebo-controlled efficacy trial. *Archives of General Psychiatry, 66*(10), 1116–1123. doi: 10.1001/archgenpsychiatry.2009.128

Mason, B. J. (2001). Treatment of alcohol-dependent outpatients with acamprosate: A clinical review. *Journal of Clinical Psychiatry, 62*(suppl), 42–48.

Mason, J. W., Giller, E. L., Kosten, T. R., Ostroff, R. B., & Podd, L. (1986). Urinary free-cortisol levels in posttraumatic stress disorder patients. *Journal of Nervous and Mental Disease, 174*(3), 145–149.

Mason, P. E., & Kerns, W. P., II. (2002). Gamma hydroxybutyric acid (GHB) intoxication. *Academic Emergency Medicine, 9*(7), 730–739.

Mathew, R. J., Wilson, W. H., Turkington, T. G., & Coleman, R. E. (1998). Cerebellar activity and disturbed time sense after THC. *Brain Research, 797*(2), 183–189. doi: 10.1016/s0006-8993(98)00375-8

Matsumoto, Y., Ohmori, K., & Fujiwara, M. (1992). Microglial and astroglial reactions to inflammatory lesions of experimental autoimmune encephalomyelitis in the rat central nervous system. *Journal of Neuroimmunology, 37*(1–2), 23–33.

Matz, R., Rick, W., Thompson, H., & Gershon, S. (1974). Clozapine—a potential antipsychotic agent without extrapyramidal manifestations. *Current Therapeutic Research, Clinical and Experimental, 16*(7), 687–695.

Maxwell, C. R., Spangenberg, R. J., Hoek, J. B., Silberstein, S. D., & Oshinsky, M. L. (2010). Acetate causes alcohol hangover headache in rats. *PLoS One, 5*(12), e15963. doi: 10.1371/journal.pone.0015963

Mayes, R., Bagwell, C., & Erkulwater, J. (2008). ADHD and the rise in stimulant use among children. *Harvard Review of Psychiatry, 16*(3), 151–166. doi: 10.1080/10673220802167782

Mayo Foundation. (2011). Caffeine content for coffee, tea, soda, and more. Retrieved from www.webcitation.org/67XR8IBJQ

McBride, W. J., Murphy, J. M., & Ikemoto, S. (1999). Localization of brain reinforcement mechanisms: Intracranial self-administration and intracranial place-conditioning studies. *Behavioural Brain Research, 101*(2), 129–152. doi: 10.1016/s0166-4328(99)00022-4

McCance, E. F., Price, L. H., Kosten, T. R., & Jatlow, P. I. (1995). Cocaethylene: Pharmacology, physiology, and behavioral effects in humans. *Journal of Pharmacology and Experimental Therapeutics, 274*(1), 215–223.

McCann, U. D., Ridenour, A., Shaham, Y., & Ricaurte, G. A. (1994). Serotonin neurotoxicity after (+/–)3,4-methylenedioxymethamphetamine (MDMA; "Ecstasy"): A controlled study in humans. *Neuropsychopharmacology, 10*(2), 129–138.

McClane, T. K., & Martin, W. R. (1976). Subjective and physiologic effects of morphine, pentobarbital, and meprobamate. *Clinical Pharmacology and Therapy, 20*(2), 192–198. doi: 0009-9236(76)90049-7 [pii]

McDowell, D. M., & Kleber, H. D. (1994). MDMA: Its history and pharmacology. *Psychiatric Annals, 24*, 127–130.

McGlothlin, W. H., & West, L. J. (1968). The marihuana problem: An overview. *American Journal of Psychiatry, 125*(3), 126–134.

McShane, R., Areosa Sastre, A., & Minakaran, N. (2006). Memantine for dementia. *Cochrane Database of Systematic Reviews* (Online)(2), CD003154.

Medical-memorandum. (1960). Amphetamine overdosage in an athlete. *British Medical Journal, 2*, 589.

Mehra, R., Moore, B. A., Crothers, K., Tetrault, J., & Fiellin, D. A. (2006). The association between marijuana smoking and lung cancer: A systematic review. *Archives of Internal Medicine, 166*(13), 1359–1367. doi: 10.1001/archinte.166.13.1359

Meier, K. E., & Mendoza, S. A. (1976). Effect of ethanol on the water permeability and short-circuit current of the urinary bladder of the toad and the response to vasopressin, adenosine-3′,5′-monophosphate and theophylline. [In Vitro Research Support, U.S. Gov't, P.H.S.]. *Journal of Pharmacology and Experimental Therapeutics, 196*(1), 231–237.

Melamede, R. (2005). Cannabis and tobacco are not equally carcinogenic. *Harm Reduction Journal, 2*(21).

Meldrum, B. (1982). Pharmacology of GABA. *Clinical Neuropharmacology, 5*(3), 293–316.

Meltzer, H. Y. (2001). Treatment of suicidality in schizophrenia. *Annals of the New York Academy of Sciences, 932*, 44–58, 58–60.

Meltzer, H. Y. (2002). Mechanism of action of atypical antipsychotic drugs. In K. L. Davis & American College of Neuropsychopharmacology. (Eds.), *Neuropsychopharmacology : The fifth generation of progress*, pp. xxi, 2010 . Philadelphia: Lippincott Williams & Wilkins.

Meltzer, H. Y., Arvanitis, L., Bauer, D., & Rein, W. (2004). Placebo-controlled evaluation of four novel compounds for the treatment of schizophrenia and schizoaffective disorder. *American Journal of Psychiatry, 161*(6), 975–984.

Meltzer, H. Y., Koenig, J. I., Nash, J. F., & Gudelsky, G. A. (1989). Melperone and clozapine: Neuroendocrine effects of atypical neuroleptic drugs. *Acta Psychiatrica Scandinavica Supplement, 352*, 24–29.

Meltzer, H. Y., Matsubara, S., & Lee, J. C. (1989). Classification of typical and atypical antipsychotic drugs on the basis of dopamine D-1, D-2 and serotonin2 pKi values. *Journal of Pharmacology and Experimental Therapeutics, 251*(1), 238–246.

Meltzer, H. Y., & McGurk, S. R. (1999). The effects of clozapine, risperidone, and olanzapine on cognitive function in schizophrenia. *Schizophrenia Bulletin, 25*(2), 233–255.

Meltzer, H. Y., & Prus, A. J. (2006). NK3 receptor antagonists for the treatment of schizophrenia. *Drug Discovery Today: Therapeutic Strategies, 3*, 555–560.

Meltzer, H. Y., & Stahl, S. M. (1976). The dopamine hypothesis of schizophrenia: A review. *Schizophrenia Bulletin, 2*(1), 19–76.

Merikangas, K. R., Akiskal, H. S., Angst, J., Greenberg, P. E., Hirschfeld, R. M. A., Petukhova, M., & Kessler, R. C. (2007). Lifetime and 12-month prevalence of bipolar spectrum disorder in the National Comorbidity Survey replication. *Archives of General Psychiatry, 64*(5), 543–552. doi: 10.1001/archpsyc.64.5.543

Merritt, J. C., Crawford, W. J., Alexander, P. C., Anduze, A. L., & Gelbart, S. S. (1980). Effect of marijuana on intraocular and blood pressure in glaucoma. *Ophthalmology, 87*, 222–228.

Meunier, J.-C. (1997). Nociceptin/orphanin FQ and the opioid receptor-like ORL1 receptor. *European Journal of Pharmacology, 340*(1), 1–15. doi: 10.1016/s0014-2999(97)01411-8

Mihic, S. J., Ye, Q., Wick, M. J., Koltchine, V. V., Krasowski, M. D., Finn, S. E., . . . Harrison, N. L. (1997). Sites of alcohol and volatile anaesthetic action on GABA(A) and glycine receptors. *Nature, 389*(6649), 385–389. doi: 10.1038/38738

Miles, C. P. (1977). Conditions predisposing to suicide: A review. *Journal of Nervous and Mental Disease, 164*(4), 231–246.

Millar, J. K., Wilson-Annan, J. C., Anderson, S., Christie, S., Taylor, M. S., Semple, C. A., . . . Porteous, D. J. (2000). Disruption of two novel genes by a translocation co-segregating with schizophrenia. *Human Molecular Genetics, 9*, 1415–1523.

Miller, J. L., Ashford, J. W., Archer, S. M., Rudy, A. C., & Wermeling, D. P. (2008). Comparison of intranasal administration of haloperidol with intravenous and intramuscular administration: A pilot pharmacokinetic study. *Pharmacotherapy, 28*(7), 875–882. doi: 10.1592/phco.28.7.875

Miller, K. E. (2008). Wired: Energy drinks, jock identity, masculine norms, and risk taking. *Journal of American College Health, 56*(5), 481–489. doi: 10.3200/JACH.56.5.481-490

Miller, N. S., & Schwartz, R. H. (1997). MDMA (Ecstasy) and the rave: A review. *Pediatrics, 100*+.

Miller, W. R., Walters, S. T., & Bennett, M. E. (2001). How effective is alcoholism treatment in the United States? *Journal of Studies on Alcohol and Drugs, 62*, 221–220.

Mills, K. C. (1997). Serotonin syndrome: A clinical update. *Critical Care Clinics, 13*(4), 763–783. doi: 10.1016/s0749-0704(05)70368-7

Minematsu, N., Nakamura, H., Furuuchi, M., Nakajima, T., Takahashi, S., Tateno, H., & Ishizaka, A. (2006). Limitation of cigarette consumption by CYP2A6*4, *7 and *9 polymorphisms. *European Respiratory Journal, 27*(2), 289–292. doi: 10.1183/09031936.06.00056305

Miotto, K., Darakjian, J., Basch, J., Murray, S., Zogg, J., & Rawson, R. (2001). Gamma-hydroxybutyric acid: Patterns of use, effects, and withdrawal. *American Journal on Addictions, 10*(3), 232–241.

Mithoefer, M. C., Wagner, M. T., Mithoefer, A. T., Jerome, L., & Doblin, R. (2011). The safety and efficacy of ±3,4-methylenedioxymethamphetamine-assisted psychotherapy in subjects with chronic, treatment-resistant posttraumatic stress disorder: The first randomized controlled pilot study. *Journal of Psychopharmacology, 25*(4), 439–452. doi: 10.1177/0269881110378371

Miyamoto, M., Nishikawa, H., Doken, Y., Hirai, K., Uchikawa, O., & Ohkawa, S. (2004). The sleep-promoting action of ramelteon (TAK-375) in freely moving cats. [Comparative Study]. *Sleep, 27*(7), 1319–1325.

Mohamed, W. M., Ben Hamida, S., Cassel, J. C., de Vasconcelos, A. P., & Jones, B. C. (2011). MDMA: interactions with other psychoactive drugs. *Pharmacology Biochemistry and Behavior, 99*(4), 759–774. doi: 10.1016/j.pbb.2011.06.032

Mohamed, W. M. Y., Hamida, S. B., Pereira de Vasconcelos, A., Cassel, J. C., & Jones, B. C. (2009). Interactions between 3,4-Methylenedioxymethamphetamine and Ethanol in Humans and Rodents. *Neuropsychobiology, 60*(3–4), 188–194.

Montagu, K. A. (1957). Catechol compounds in rat tissues and in brains of different animals. *Nature, 180*(4579), 244–245.

Montpied, P., Morrow, A. L., Karanian, J. W., Ginns, E. I., Martin, B. M., & Paul, S. M. (1991). Prolonged ethanol inhalation decreases gamma-aminobutyric acidA receptor alpha subunit mRNAs in the rat cerebral cortex. *Molecular Pharmacology, 39*(2), 157–163.

Moreno, A. Y., Mayorov, A. V., & Janda, K. D. (2011). Impact of distinct chemical structures for the development of a methamphetamine vaccine. *Journal of the American Chemical Society, 133*(17), 6587–6595. doi: 10.1021/ja108807j

Morgan, C. A., Mofeez, A., Brandner, B., Bromley, L., & Curran, H. V. (2004). Ketamine impairs response inhibition and is positively reinforcing in healthy volunteers: A dose–response study. *Psychopharmacology, 172*(3), 298–308. doi: 10.1007/s00213-003-1656-y

Morgan, W. W. (1990). Abuse liability of barbiturates and other sedative-hypnotics. *Advances in Alcohol and Substance Abuse, 9*(1–2), 67–82.

Morgenstern, J., Kahler, C. W., Frey, R. M., & Labouvie, E. (1996). Modeling therapeutic response to 12-step treatment: Optimal responders, nonresponders, and partial responders. *Journal of Substance Abuse, 8*(1), 45–59.

Moriyama, Y., Mimura, M., Kato, M., & Kashima, H. (2006). Primary alcoholic dementia and alcohol-related dementia. *Psychogeriatrics, 6*(3), 114–118. doi: 10.1111/j.1479-8301.2006.00168.x

Morley, K. C., & McGregor, I. S. (2000). (±)-3,4-Methylenedioxymethamphetamine (MDMA, ["Ecstasy"] increases social interaction in rats. *European Journal of Pharmacology, 408*(1), 41–49. doi: 10.1016/s0014-2999(00)00749-4

Morrison, P. D., Zois, V., McKeown, D. A., Lee, T. D., Holt, D. W., Powell, J. F., . . . Murray, R. M. (2009). The acute effects of synthetic intravenous delta9-tetrahydrocannabinol on psychosis, mood and cognitive functioning. *Psychological Medicine, 39*(10), 1607–1616. doi: S0033291709005522 [pii]

Mucha, R. F., van der Kooy, D., O'Shaughnessy, M., & Bucenieks, P. (1982). Drug reinforcement studied by the use of place conditioning in rat. *Brain Research, 243*(1), 91–105. doi: 0006-8993(82)91123-4 [pii]

Muller, C., Viry, S., Miehe, M., Andriamampandry, C., Aunis, D., & Maitre, M. (2002). Evidence for a γ-hydroxybutyrate (GHB) uptake by rat brain synaptic vesicles. *Journal of neurochemistry, 80*(5), 899–904. doi: 10.1046/j.0022-3042.2002.00780.x

Munro, S., Thomas, K. L., & Abu-Shaar, M. (1993). Molecular characterization of a peripheral receptor for cannabinoids. *Nature, 365*(6441), 61–65. doi: 10.1038/365061a0

Murray, C. J. L., & Lopez, A. D. (1997). Global mortality, disability, and the contribution of risk factors: Global Burden of Disease study. *The Lancet, 349*(9063), 1436–1442. doi: 10.1016/s0140-6736(96)07495-8

Mutzell, S. (1998). A 20-year longitudinal prospective study of 284 heroin addicts in Stockholm County, Sweden. *Archives of Public Health, 56*, 307–316.

Myers, C. S., Taylor, R. C., Moolchan, E. T., & Heishman, S. J. (2007). Dose-related enhancement of mood and cognition in smokers administered nicotine nasal spray. *Neuropsychopharmacology, 33*(3), 588–598.

Natale, M., Kowitt, M., Dahlberg, C. C., & Jaffe, J. (1978). Effect of psychotomimetic (LSD and dextroamphetamine) on the use of figurative language during psychoanalysis. *Journal of Consulting and Clinical Psychology, 46*, 157–158.

National Drug Intelligence Center. (2004, September). Intelligence report: GHB trafficking and abuse. (2004-L0424-015). Retrieved from www.justice.gov/archive/ndic/pubs10/10331/10331t.htm

National Institutes of Health. (2012). Retrieved February 14, 2012, from Clinicaltrials.gov

National Institute on Alcohol Abuse and Alcoholism (NIAAA). (1995). Diagnostic criteria for alcohol abuse and dependence. *Alcohol Alert, 30* (PH 359). Retrieved from http://pubs.niaaa.nih.gov/publications/aa30.htm

National Institute on Alcohol Abuse and Alcoholism. (2012). What is a standard drink? Retrieved from http://pubs.niaaa.nih.gov/publications/Practitioner/PocketGuide/pocket_guide2.htm

National Research Council. (2011). *Guide for the care and use of laboratory animals* (8th ed.). Washington, DC: National Academies Press.

Nichols, D. E., & Oberlender, R. (1990). Structure-activity relationship of MDMA and related compounds: A new class of psychoactive drugs? *Annals of the New York Academy of Sciences, 600*, 613–625.

Nierenberg, A. A., Farabaugh, A. H., Alpert, J. E., Gordon, B. A., Worthington, J. J., Rosenbaum, J. F., & Fava, M. (2000). Timing of onset of antidepressant response with fluoxetine treatment. *American Journal of Psychiatry, 157*, 1423–1428.

Nisell, M., Nomikos, G. G., & Svensson, T. H. (1994). Infusion of nicotine in the ventral tegmental area or the nucleus accumbens of the rat differentially affects accumbal dopamine release. *Pharmacology and Toxicology, 75*(6), 348–352.

Nonnemaker, J. M., Crankshaw, E. C., Shive, D. R., Hussin, A. H., & Farrelly, M. C. (2011). Inhalant use initiation among U.S. adolescents: Evidence from the National Survey of Parents and Youth using discrete-time survival analysis. *Addictive Behaviors, 36*(8), 878–881. doi: 10.1016/j.addbeh.2011.03.009

Norrholm, S. D., & Ressler, K. J. (2009). Genetics of anxiety and trauma-related disorders. *Neuroscience, 164*(1), 272-287. doi: S0306-4522(09)01061-6 [pii]

Nutt, D., King, L. A., Saulsbury, W., & Blakemore, C. (2007). Development of a rational scale to assess the harm of drugs of potential misuse. *The Lancet, 369*(9566), 1047–1053. doi: 10.1016/s0140-6736(07)60464-4

Nyman, A. L., Taylor, T. M., & Biener, L. (2002). Trends in cigar smoking and perceptions of health risks among Massachusetts adults. *Tobacco Control, 11*(suppl. 2), ii25–ii28. doi: 10.1136/tc.11.suppl_2.ii25

O'Brien, W. T., Harper, A. D., Jove, F., Woodgett, J. R., Maretto, S., Piccolo, S., & Klein, P. S. (2004). Glycogen synthase kinase-3{beta} haploinsufficiency mimics the behavioral and molecular effects of lithium. *Journal of Neuroscience,*

24(30), 6791–6798. doi: 10.1523/jneurosci.4753-03.2004

Ochoa, E., Li, L., & McNamee, M. (1990). Desensitization of central cholinergic mechanisms and neuroadaptation to nicotine. *Molecular Neurobiology, 4*(3), 251–287. doi: 10.1007/bf02780343

O'Donnell, J. M., Marek, G. J., & Seiden, L. S. (2005). Antidepressant effects assessed using behavior maintained under a differential-reinforcement-of-low-rate (DRL) operant schedule. *Neuroscience and Biobehavioral Reviews, 29*(4–5), 785–798. doi: S0149-7634(05)00047-3 [pii]

Okun, M. S., Boothby, L. A., Bartfield, R. B., & Doering, P. L. (2001). GHB: An important pharmacologic and clinical update. *Journal of Pharmaceutical Sciences, 4*(2), 167–175.

Oldendorf, W. H., Hyman, S., Braun, L., & Oldendorf, S. Z. (1972). Blood–brain barrier: Penetration of morphine, codeine, heroin, and methadone after carotid injection. *Science, 178*(4064), 984–986. doi: 10.1126/science.178.4064.984

Olds, J. (1956). Pleasure center in the brain. *Scientific American, 195*, 105–116.

Olds, J., & Milner, P. (1954). Positive reinforcement produced by electrical stimulation of septal area and other regions of rat brain. *Journal of Comparative and Physiological Psychology, 47*(6), 419–427.

Oliveto, A., Gentry, W. B., Pruzinsky, R., Gonsai, K., Kosten, T. R., Martell, B., & Poling, J. (2010). Behavioral effects of gamma-hydroxybutyrate in humans. *Behavioral Pharmacology, 21*(4), 332–342. doi: 10.1097/FBP.0b013e32833b3397

Oliveto, A., Poling, J., Mancino, M. J., Feldman, Z., Cubells, J. F., Pruzinsky, R., . . . Kosten, T. R. (2011). Randomized, double blind, placebo-controlled trial of disulfiram for the treatment of cocaine dependence in methadone-stabilized patients. *Drug and Alcohol Dependence, 113*(2–3), 184–191. doi: 10.1016/j.drugalcdep.2010.07.022

Olivier, B., Pattij, T., Wood, S. J., Oosting, R., Sarnyai, Z., & Toth, M. (2001). The 5-HT(1A) receptor knockout mouse and anxiety. *Be-*

havioral Pharmacolology, 12(6–7), 439–450.

Omelchenko, N., & Sesack, S. R. (2010). Periaqueductal gray afferents synapse onto dopamine and GABA neurons in the rat ventral tegmental area. *Journal of Neuroscience Research, 88*, 981–991.

Ordway, G. A., Gambarana, C., Tejani-Butt, S. M., Areso, P., Hauptmann, M., & Frazer, A. (1991). Preferential reduction of binding of 125I-iodopindolol to beta-1 adrenoceptors in the amygdala of rat after antidepressant treatments. *Journal of Pharmacology and Experimental Therapeutics, 257*(2), 681–690.

Oscar-Berman, M., & Marinković, K. (2007). Alcohol: Effects on neurobehavioral functions and the brain. *Neuropsychology Review, 17*(3), 239–257. doi: 10.1007/s11065-007-9038-6

Ossipov, M. H., Lai, J., King, T., Vanderah, T. W., Malan, T. P., Jr., Hruby, V. J., & Porreca, F. (2004). Antinociceptive and nociceptive actions of opioids. *Journal of Neurobiology, 61*(1), 126–148. doi: 10.1002/neu.20091

Owens, D. G. C. (1999). *A guide to the extrapyramidal side-effects of antipsychotic drugs.* Cambridge, UK: Cambridge University Press.

Pacifici, R., Zuccaro, P., Pichini, S., Roset, P. N., Poudevida, S., Farré, M., . . . de la Torre, R. (2003). Modulation of the immune system in cannabis users. *Journal of the American Medical Association, 289*(15), 1929–1931. doi: 10.1001/jama.289.15.1929-b

Pan, D., Gatley, S. J., Dewey, S. L., Chen, R., Alexoff, D. A., Ding, Y. S., & Fowler, J. S. (1994). Binding of bromine-substituted analogs of methylphenidate to monoamine transporters. *European Journal of Pharmacology, 264*(2), 177–182.

Panlilio, L. V., & Schindler, C. W. (2000). Self-administration of remifentanil, an ultra-short acting opioid, under continuous and progressive-ratio schedules of reinforcement in rats. *Psychopharmacology, 150*(1), 61–66. doi: 10.1007/s002130000415

Papakostas, G. I., Thase, M. E., Fava, M., Nelson, J. C., & Shelton, R. C. (2007). Are antidepressant drugs that combine serotonergic and noradrenergic mechanisms of action more effective than the selective serotonin reuptake inhibitors in treating major depressive disorder? A meta-analysis of studies of newer agents. *Biological Psychiatry, 62*(11), 1217–1227. doi: 10.1016/j.biopsych.2007.03.027

Papp, L. A., Klein, D. F., Martinez, J., Schneier, F., Cole, R., Liebowitz, M. R., . . . Gorman, J. M. (1993). Diagnostic and substance specificity of carbon-dioxide-induced panic. *American Journal of Psychiatry, 150*(2), 250–257.

Park, S., Knopick, C., McGurk, S., & Meltzer, H. Y. (2000). Nicotine impairs spatial working memory while leaving spatial attention intact. *Neuropsychopharmacology, 22*(2), 200–209. doi: S0893-133X(99)00098-6 [pii]

Parrott, A. C. (2001). Human psychopharmacology of Ecstasy (MDMA): A review of 15 years of empirical research. *Human Psychopharmacology: Clinical and Experimental, 16*(8), 557–577. doi: 10.1002/hup.351

Passie, T., Halpern, J. H., Stichtenoth, D. O., Emrich, H. M., & Hintzen, A. (2008). The pharmacology of lysergic acid diethylamide: A review. *CNS Neuroscience and Therapeutics, 14*, 295–314.

Paulus, M. P., Tapert, S. F., Pulido, C., & Schuckit, M. A. (2006). Alcohol attenuates load-related activation during a working memory task: relation to level of response to alcohol. *Alcoholism: Clinical and Experimental Research, 30*(8), 1363–1371. doi: 10.1111/j.1530-0277.2006.00164.x

Pavlov, I. P., & Anrep, G. V. (1927). *Conditioned reflexes: An investigation of the physiological activity of the cerebral cortex.* London: Oxford University Press.

Paz, R. D., Tardito, S., Atzori, M., & Tseng, K. Y. (2008). Glutamatergic dysfunction in schizophrenia: From basic neuroscience to clinical psychopharmacology. *European Neuropsychopharmacol, 18*(11), 773–786. doi: S0924-977X(08)00167-3 [pii]

Pehrson, A. L., Philibin, S. D., Gross, D., Robinson, S. E., Vann, R. E., Rosecrans, J. A., & James, J. R.

(2008). The effects of acute and repeated nicotine doses on spontaneous activity in male and female Sprague Dawley rats: Analysis of brain area epibatidine binding and cotinine levels. *Pharmacology Biochemistry and Behavior, 89*(3), 424–431. doi: 10.1016/j.pbb.2008.01.018

Pellow, S., & File, S. E. (1986). Anxiolytic and anxiogenic drug effects on exploratory activity in an elevated plus-maze: A novel test of anxiety in the rat. *Pharmacology Biochemistry and Behavior, 24*(3), 525–529. doi: 0091-3057(86)90552-6 [pii]

Pennartz, C. M., Ito, R., Verschure, P. F., Battaglia, F. P., & Robbins, T. W. (2011). The hippocampal-striatal axis in learning, prediction, and goal-directed behavior. *Trends in Neuroscience, 34*(10), 548–559. doi: 10.1016/j.tins.2011.08.001

Pentney, A. R. (2001). An exploration of the history and controversies surrounding MDMA and MDA. *Journal of Psychoactive Drugs, 33*, 213–221.

Pérez-Stable, E. J., Herrera, B., Jacob, P., & Benowitz, N. L. (1998). Nicotine metabolism and intake in black and white smokers. *Journal of the American Medical Association, 280*(2), 152–156. doi: 10.1001/jama.280.2.152

Perkins, K., Epstein, L., Stiller, R., Fernstrom, M., Sexton, J., Jacob, R., & Solberg, R. (1991). Acute effects of nicotine on hunger and caloric intake in smokers and non-smokers. *Psychopharmacology, 103*(1), 103–109. doi: 10.1007/bf02244083

Perkins, K. A., Grobe, J. E., Fonte, C., Goettler, J., Caggiula, A. R., Reynolds, W. A., . . . Jacob, R. G. (1994). Chronic and acute tolerance to subjective, behavioral and cardiovascular effects of nicotine in humans. *Journal of Pharmacology and Experimental Therapeutics, 270*(2), 628–638.

Pertwee, R. G. (2001). Cannabinoid receptors and pain. *Progress in Neurobiology, 63*(5), 569–611. doi: 10.1016/s0301-0082(00)00031-9

Philibin, S. D., Walentiny, D. M., Vunck, S. A., Prus, A. J., Meltzer, H. Y., & Porter, J. H. (2009).

Further characterization of the discriminative stimulus properties of the atypical antipsychotic drug clozapine in C57BL/6 mice: Role of 5-HT(2A) serotonergic and alpha (1) adrenergic antagonism. *Psychopharmacology (Berl), 203*(2), 303–315. doi: 10.1007/s00213-008-1385-3

PHS (Public Health Service). (2002). *Public health service policy on humane care and use of laboratory animals.* Washington, DC: Department of Health and Human Services.

Pifl, C., Drobny, H., Reither, H., Hornykiewicz, O., & Singer, E. A. (1995). Mechanism of the dopamine-releasing actions of amphetamine and cocaine: Plasmalemmal dopamine transporter versus vesicular monoamine transporter. *Molecular Pharmacology, 47*(2), 368–373.

Pistis, M., Muntoni, A. L., Pillolla, G., Perra, S., Cignarella, G., Melis, M., & Gessa, G. L. (2005). Gammahydroxybutyric acid (GHB) and the mesoaccumbens reward circuit: Evidence for GABA(B) receptor-mediated effects. *Neuroscience, 131*(2), 465–474. doi: 10.1016/j.neuroscience.2004.11.021

Pitman, R. K., & Orr, S. P. (1990). Twenty-four hour urinary cortisol and catecholamine excretion in combat-related posttraumatic stress disorder. *Biological Psychiatry, 27*(2), 245–247. doi: 0006-3223(90)90654-K [pii]

Placzek, E. A., Okamoto, Y., Ueda, N., & Barker, E. L. (2008). Mechanisms for recycling and biosynthesis of endogenous cannabinoids anandamide and 2-arachidonylglycerol. *Journal of neurochemistry, 107*(4), 987–1000.

Platt, D. M., Rowlett, J. K., Izenwasser, S., & Spealman, R. D. (2004). Opioid partial agonist effects of 3-o-methylnaltrexone in rhesus monkeys. *Journal of Pharmacology and Experimental Therapeutics, 308*(3), 1030–1039. doi: 10.1124/jpet.103.060962

Pletscher, A. (2006). The dawn of the neurotransmitter era in neuropsychopharmacology. In T. A. Ban & R. U. Udabe (Eds.), *The neurotransmitter era in neuropsychopharmacology.* Buenos Aires: Editorial Polemos.

Poling, A. D., & Byrne, T. (2000). *Introduction to behavioral pharmacology.* Reno, NV: Context Press.

Polissidis, A., Galanopoulos, A., Naxakis, G., Papahatjis, D., Papadopoulou-Daifoti, Z., & Antoniou, K. (2012). The cannabinoid CB1 receptor biphasically modulates motor activity and regulates dopamine and glutamate release region dependently. *The International Journal of Neuropsychopharmacology, FirstView,* 1–11. doi: 10.1017/S1461145712000156

Polo, M. (1871). *The book of Ser Marco Polo, the Venetian: concerning the kingdoms and marvels of the East; newly translated and edited with notes, by Colonel Henry Yule with maps and other illustrations* (H. Yule, Trans.). London: John Murray.

Polosa, R., & Benowitz, N. L. (2011). Treatment of nicotine addiction: present therapeutic options and pipeline developments. *Trends in Pharmacological Sciences, 32*(5), 281–289. doi: 10.1016/j.tips.2010.12.008

Pompili, M., Amador, X. F., Girardi, P., Harkavy-Friedman, J., Harrow, M., Kaplan, K., . . . Tatarelli, R. (2007). Suicide risk in schizophrenia: Learning from the past to change the future. *Annals of General Psychiatry, 6,* 10. doi: 1744-859X-6-10 [pii]

Popik, P., & Kolasiewicz, W. (1999). Mesolimbic NMDA receptors are implicated in the expression of conditioned morphine reward. *Naunyn-Schmiedeberg's Archives of Pharmacology, 359*(4), 288–294. doi: 10.1007/pl00005354

Porcella, A., Casellas, P., Gessa, G. L., & Pani, L. (1998). Cannabinoid receptor CB1 mRNA is highly expressed in the rat ciliary body: Implications for the antiglaucoma properties of marihuana. *Molecular Brain Research, 58,* 240–245.

Porcella, A., Maxia, C., Gessa, G. L., & Pani, L. (2000). The human eye expresses high levels of CB1 cannabinoid receptor mRNA and protein. *European Journal of Neuroscience, 12,* 1123–1127.

Porcella, A., Maxia, C., Gessa, G. L., & Pani, L. (2001). The synthetic cannabinoid WIN52212-2 decreases the intraocular pressure in human glaucoma resistant to conventional therapies. *European Journal of Neuroscience, 13,* 409–412.

Porsolt, R. D., Le Pichon, M., & Jalfre, M. (1977). Depression: A new animal model sensitive to antidepressant treatments. *Nature, 266*(5604), 730–732.

Potkin, S. G., Cohen, M., & Panagides, J. (2007). Efficacy and tolerability of asenapine in acute schizophrenia: A placebo- and risperidone-controlled trial. *Journal of Clinical Psychiatry, 68*(10), 1492–1500.

Powell, A. G., Apovian, C. M., & Aronne, L. J. (2011). New drug targets for the treatment of obesity. [Review]. *Clinical Pharmacology and Therapy, 90*(1), 40–51. doi: 10.1038/clpt.2011.82

Pozzi, L., Invernizzi, R., Garavaglia, C., & Samanin, R. (1999). Fluoxetine increases extracellular dopamine in the prefrontal cortex by a mechanism not dependent on serotonin: A comparison with citalopram. *Journal of Neurochemistry, 73*(3), 1051–1057.

Pradhan, S. N. (1984). Phencyclidine (PCP): Some human studies. *Neuroscience and Biobehavioral Reviews, 8*(4), 493–501. doi: 10.1016/0149–7634(84)90006-x

Prat, G., Adan, A., & Sanchez-Turet, M. (2009). Alcohol hangover: A critical review of explanatory factors. *Human Psychopharmacology, 24*(4), 259–267. doi: 10.1002/hup.1023

Pratt, L. A., Brody, D. J., & Gu, Q. (2011). Antidepressant use in persons aged 12 and over: United States, 2005–2008. *NCHS Data Brief, 76.*

Preston, K. L., Bigelow, G. E., & Liebson, I. A. (1988). Buprenorphine and naloxone alone and in combination in opioid-dependent humans. *Psychopharmacology, 94*(4), 484–490. doi: 10.1007/bf00212842

Pretlow, R. A. (2011). Addiction to highly pleasurable food as a cause of the childhood obesity epidemic: A qualitative Internet study. *Eating Disorders, 19*(4), 295–307. doi: 10.1080/10640266.2011.584803

Primeaux, S. D., Wilson, S. P., Bray, G. A., York, D. A., & Wilson, M. A. (2006). Overexpression of neuropeptide Y in the central nucleus of the amygdala decreases ethanol self-administration in "anxious" rats. *Alcoholism: Clinical and Experimental Research, 30*(5), 791–801.

Pritchett, D. B., Luddens, H., & Seeburg, P. H. (1989). Type I and type II GABA$_A$-benzodiazepine receptors produced in transfected cells. *Science, 245*(4924), 1389–1392.

Pritchett, D. B., Sontheimer, H., Shivers, B. D., Ymer, S., Kettenmann, H., Schofield, P. R., & Seeburg, P. H. (1989). Importance of a novel GABAA receptor subunit for benzodiazepine pharmacology. *Nature, 338*(6216), 582–585. doi: 10.1038/338582a0

ProCon. (2012). Seventeen legal medical marijuana states and DC. Retrieved from http://medicalmarijuana.procon.org/view.resource.php?resourceID=000881

Prus, A. J., Maxwell, A. T., Baker, K. M., Rosecrans, J. A., & James, J. R. (2007). Acute behavioral tolerance to nicotine in the conditioned taste aversion paradigm. *Drug Development Research, 68*(8), 522–528. doi: 10.1002/ddr.20219

Purnell, W. D., & Gregg, J. M. (1975). Delta (9)-tetradydrocannabinol, euphoria, and intraocular pressure in man. *Annals of Ophthalmology, 7,* 921–923.

Rafla, F. K., & Epstein, R. L. (1979). Identification of cocaine and its metabolites in human urine in the presence of ethyl alcohol. *Journal of Analytical Toxicology, 3*(2), 59–63. doi: 10.1093/jat/3.2.59

Rainey, C. L., Conder, P. A., & Goodpaster, J. V. (2011). Chemical characterization of dissolvable tobacco products promoted to reduce harm. *Journal of Agricultural and Food Chemistry, 59*(6), 2745–2751. doi: 10.1021/jf103295d

Ramaekers, J. G., Berghaus, G., van Laar, M., & Drummer, O. H. (2004). Dose-related risk of motor vehicle crashes after cannabis use. *Drug and Alcohol Dependence,*

73(2), 109–119. doi: 10.1016/j.drugalcdep.2003.10.008

Ramirez-Latorre, J., Yu, C. R., Qu, X., Perin, F., Karlin, A., & Role, L. (1996). Functional contributions of [alpha]5 subunit to neuronal acetylcholine receptor channels. [10.1038/380347a0]. *Nature, 380*(6572), 347–351.

Ratiu, P., & Talos, I. (2004). The tale of Phineas Gage, digitally remastered. *New England Journal of Medicine, 351*(23), e21.

Ravnborg, M., Jensen, F. M., Jensen, N.-H., & Holk, I. K. (1987). Pupillary diameter and ventilatory CO_2 sensitivity after epidural morphine and buprenorphine in volunteers. *Anesthesia & Analgesia, 66*(9), 847–851.

Rees, D. C., Knisely, J. S., Jordan, S., & Balster, R. L. (1987). Discriminative stimulus properties of toluene in the mouse. *Toxicology and Applied Pharmacology, 88*(1), 97–104.

Regier, D. A., Narrow, W. E., Rae, D. S., Manderscheid, R. W., Locke, B. Z., & Goodwin, F. K. (1993). The de facto U.S. mental and addictive disorders service system. Epidemiologic catchment area prospective 1-year prevalence rates of disorders and services. *Archives of General Psychiatry, 50*(2), 85–94.

Reissig, C. J., Carter, L. P., Johnson, M. W., Mintzer, M. Z., Klinedinst, M. A., & Griffiths, R. R. (2012). High doses of dextromethorphan, an NMDA antagonist, produce effects similar to classic hallucinogens. *Psychopharmacology (Berl) 223*(1), 1–15.

Resnick, H. S., Yehuda, R., Pitman, R. K., & Foy, D. W. (1995). Effect of previous trauma on acute plasma cortisol level following rape. *American Journal of Psychiatry, 152*(11), 1675–1677.

Reynolds, G. P., Hill, M. J., & Kirk, S. L. (2006). The 5-HT2C receptor and antipsychoticinduced weight gain: Mechanisms and genetics. *Journal of Psychopharmacology, 20*(4 suppl), 15–18. doi: 10.1177/1359786806066040

Richardson, N. R., & Roberts, D. C. (1996). Progressive ratio schedules in drug self-administration studies in rats: A method to evaluate reinforcing efficacy. *Journal of Neuroscience Methods, 66*(1), 1–11. doi: 0165027095001530 [pii]

Richelson, E., & Nelson, A. (1984). Antagonism by neuroleptics of neurotransmitter receptors of normal human brain in vitro. *European Journal of Pharmacology, 103*(3–4), 197–204.

Richelson, E., & Souder, T. (2000). Binding of antipsychotic drugs to human brain receptors focus on newer generation compounds. *Life Sciences, 68*(1), 29–39.

Ridenour, T. A., Bray, B. C., & Cottler, L. B. (2007). Reliability of use, abuse, and dependence of four types of inhalants in adolescents and young adults. *Drug and Alcohol Dependence, 91*(1), 40–49. doi: 10.1016/j.drugalcdep.2007.05.004

Riegel, A. C., Zapata, A., Shippenberg, T. S., & French, E. D. (2007). The abused inhalant toluene increases dopamine release in the nucleus accumbens by directly stimulating ventral tegmental area neurons. *Neuropsychopharmacology, 32*(7), 1558–1569. doi: 1301273 [pii]

Ritz, M. C., Cone, E. J., & Kuhar, M. J. (1990). Cocaine inhibition of ligand binding at dopamine, norepinephrine and serotonin transporters: A structure-activity study. *Life Sciences, 46*(9), 635–645.

Roberts, R. C. (2007). Schizophrenia in translation: Disrupted in schizophrenia (*DISC1*): Integrating clinical and basic findings. *Schizophrenia Bulletin, 33*(1), 11–15. doi: 10.1093/schbul/sbl063

Robinson, T. E., & Becker, J. B. (1986). Enduring changes in brain and behavior produced by chronic amphetamine administration: A review and evaluation of animal models of amphetamine psychosis. *Brain Research, 396*(2), 157–198. doi: S0006-8993(86)80193-7 [pii]

Robinson, T. E., & Berridge, K. C. (2003). Addiction. *Annual Review of Psychology, 54*, 25–53. doi: 10.1146/annurev.psych.54.101601.145237

Rochester, J. A., & Kirchner, J. T. (1999). Ecstasy (3,4-methylenedioxyamphetamine): History, neurochemistry and toxicology. *Journal of the American Board of Family Practice, 12*, 137–142.

Roiko, S. A., Felmlee, M. A., & Morris, M. E. (2012). Brain uptake of the drug of abuse gamma-hydroxybutyric acid in rats. *Drug Metabolism and Disposposition, 40*(1), 212–218. doi: 10.1124/dmd.111.041749

Rook, E. J., Hillebrand, M. J. X., Rosing, H., van Ree, J. M., & Beijnen, J. H. (2005). The quantitative analysis of heroin, methadone and their metabolites and the simultaneous detection of cocaine, acetylcodeine and their metabolites in human plasma by high-performance liquid chromatography coupled with tandem mass spectrometry. *Journal of Chromatography B, 824*(1–2), 213–221. doi: 10.1016/j.jchromb.2005.05.048

Rose, A. K., & Grunsell, L. (2008). The subjective, rather than the disinhibiting, effects of alcohol are related to binge drinking. *Alcoholism: Clinical and Experimental Research, 32*(6), 1096–1104. doi: 10.1111/j.1530-0277.2008.00672.x

Rosecrans, J. A. (1995). The psychopharmacological basis of nicotine's differential effects on behavior: Individual subject variability in the rat. *Behavioral Genetics, 25*(2), 187–196.

Rosecrans, J. A., Stimler, C. A., Hendry, J. S., & Meltzer, L. T. (1989). Nicotine-induced tolerance and dependence in rats and mice: Studies involving schedule-controlled behavior. *Progress in Brain Research, 79*, 239–248.

Rosenbaum, C. D., Carreiro, S. P., & Babu, K. M. (2012). Here today, gone tomorrow . . . and back again? A review of herbal marijuana alternatives (K2, Spice), synthetic cathinones (bath salts), kratom, *Salvia divinorum*, methoxetamine, and piperazines. *Journal of Medical Toxicology, 8*(1), 15–32. doi: 10.1007/s13181-011-0202-2

Rosenberg, N. L., Grigsby, J., Dreisbach, J., Busenbark, D., & Grigsby, P. (2002). Neuropsychologic impairment and MRI abnormalities associated with chronic solvent abuse. *Journal of Toxicology—Clinical Toxicology, 40*(1), 21–34.

Rosenheck, R., Leslie, D., Keefe, R., McEvoy, J., Swartz, M., Perkins, D., . . . Lieberman, J. (2006). Barriers to employment for people with schizophrenia. *American*

Journal of Psychiatry, 163(3), 411–417. doi: 10.1176/appi.ajp.163.3.411

Ross, C. A., Margolis, R. L., Reading, S. A. J., Pletnikov, M., & Coyle, J. T. (2006). Neurobiology of schizophrenia. *Neuron, 52,* 139–153.

Roth, B. L., Baner, K., Westkaemper, R., Siebert, D., Rice, K. C., Steinberg, S., . . . Rothman, R. B. (2002). Salvinorin A: A potent naturally occurring nonnitrogenous kappa opioid selective agonist. *Proceedings of the National Academy of Sciences of the USA, 99*(18), 11934–11939. doi: 10.1073/pnas.182234399

Roy, S., & Loh, H. (1996). Effects of opioids on the immune system. *Neurochemical Research, 21*(11), 1375–1386. doi: 10.1007/bf02532379

Rudnick, G., & Wall, S. C. (1992). The molecular mechanism of "Ecstasy" [3,4-methylenedioxymethamphetamine (MDMA)]: Serotonin transporters are targets for MDMA-induced serotonin release. *Proceedings of the National Academy of Sciences of the USA, 89*(5), 1817–1821.

Rusanen, M., Kivipelto, M., Quesenberry, C. P., Jr., Zhou, J., & Whitmer, R. A. (2011). Heavy smoking in midlife and long-term risk of Alzheimer disease and vascular dementia. *Archives of Internal Medicine, 171*(4), 333–339. doi: 10.1001/archinternmed.2010.393

Russell, W. M. S., & Burch, R. L. (1959). *Principles of humane animal experimentation.* Springfield, IL: Charles C. Thomas.

Russell-Mayhew, S., von Ranson, K. M., & Masson, P. C. (2010). How does overeaters anonymous help its members? A qualitative analysis. *European Eating Disorders Review, 18*(1), 33–42. doi: 10.1002/erv.966

Rutledge, P. C., Park, A., & Sher, K. J. (2008). Twenty-first birthday drinking: Extremely extreme. *Journal of Consulting and Clinical Psychology, 76*(3), 511–516. doi: 2008-06469-015 [pii]

Saccone, S. F., Hinrichs, A. L., Saccone, N. L., Chase, G. A., Konvicka, K., Madden, P. A. F., . . . Bierut, L. J. (2007). Cholinergic nicotinic receptor genes implicated in a nico-tine dependence association study targeting 348 candidate genes with 3713 SNPs. *Human Molecular Genetics, 16*(1), 36–49. doi: 10.1093/hmg/ddl438

Sahay, A., & Hen, R. (2007). Adult hippocampal neurogenesis in depression. *Nature Neuroscience, 10*(9), 1110–1115. doi: nn1969 [pii]

Sams-Dodd, F. (1998). Effects of continuous D-amphetamine and phencyclidine administration on social behaviour, stereotyped behaviour, and locomotor activity in rats. *Neuropsychopharmacology, 19*(1), 18–25. doi: S0893133X97002005 [pii]

Sanger, D. J. (2004). The pharmacology and mechanisms of action of new generation, non-benzodiazepine hypnotic agents. *CNS Drugs, 18,* 9–15.

Santamaria, J., Tolosa, E., & Valles, A. (1986). Parkinson's disease with depression: A possible subgroup of idiopathic parkinsonism. *Neurology, 36*(8), 1130–1133.

Sapolsky, R. M. (1992). Cortisol concentrations and the social significance of rank instability among wild baboons. *Psychoneuroendocrinology, 17,* 702–709.

Sartor, C. E., Grant, J. D., Lynskey, M. T., McCutcheon, V. V., Waldron, M., Statham, D. J., . . . Nelson, E. C. (2012). Common heritable contributions to low-risk trauma, high-risk trauma, posttraumatic stress disorder, and major depression. *Archives of General Psychiatry, 69*(3), 293–299. doi: 10.1001/archgenpsychiatry.2011.1385

Satel, S. (2006). Is caffeine addictive?—a review of the literature. *American Journal of Drug and Alcohol Abuse, 32*(4), 493–502. doi: 10.1080/00952990600918965

Saunders, J. C., Radinger, N., Rochlin, D., & Kline, N. S. (1959). Treatment of depressed and regressed patients with iproniazid and reserpine. *Diseases of the Nervous System, 20,* 31–39.

Savitz, J., & Drevets, W. C. (2009). Bipolar and major depressive disorder: Neuroimaging the developmental-degenerative divide. *Neuroscience and Biobehavioral Reviews, 33*(5), 699–771. doi: 10.1016/j.neubiorev.2009.01.004

Sayette, M. A., Shiffman, S., Tiffany, S. T., Niaura, R. S., Martin, C. S., & Shadel, W. G. (2000). The measurement of drug craving. *Addiction, 95*(suppl. 2), S189–210.

Schilt, T., Koeter, M., Smal, J., Gouwetor, M., van den Brink, W., & Schmand, B. (2010). Long-term neuropsychological effects of Ecstasy in middle-aged Ecstasy/polydrug users. *Psychopharmacology, 207*(4), 583–591. doi: 10.1007/s00213-009-1688-z

Schlaepfer, T. E., Cohen, M. X., Frick, C., Kosel, M., Brodesser, D., Axmacher, N., . . . Sturm, V. (2008). Deep brain stimulation to reward circuitry alleviates anhedonia in refractory major depression. *Neuropsychopharmacology, 33*(2), 368–377. doi: 1301408 [pii]

Schotte, A., Janssen, P. F., Gommeren, W., Luyten, W. H., Van Gompel, P., Lesage, A. S., . . . Leysen, J. E. (1996). Risperidone compared with new and reference antipsychotic drugs: In vitro and in vivo receptor binding. *Psychopharmacology, 124*(1–2), 57–73.

Schroeder, J. P., Cooper, D. A., Schank, J. R., Lyle, M. A., Gaval-Cruz, M., Ogbonmwan, Y. E., . . . Weinshenker, D. (2010). Disulfiram attenuates drug-primed reinstatement of cocaine seeking via inhibition of dopamine beta-hydroxylase. *Neuropsychopharmacology, 35*(12), 2440–2449. doi: 10.1038/npp.2010.127

Schulte, T., Müller-Oehring, E. M., Strasburger, H., Warzel, H., & Sabel, B. A. (2001). Acute effects of alcohol on divided and covert attention in men. *Psychopharmacology, 154*(1), 61–69. doi: 10.1007/s002130000603

Schultes, R. E. (1969). Hallucinogens of plant origin. *Science, 163*(3864), 245–254.

Schulz, R., Wüster, M., Duka, T., & Herz, A. (1980). Acute and chronic ethanol treatment changes endorphin levels in brain and pituitary. *Psychopharmacology, 68*(3), 221–227. doi: 10.1007/bf00428107

Schweizer, T. A., & Vogel-Sprott, M. (2008). Alcohol-impaired speed and accuracy of cognitive functions: A review of acute tolerance and recovery of cognitive performance. *Experimental and Clinical*

Psychopharmacology, 16(3), 240–250. doi: 2008-06716-007 [pii]

Sdao-Jarvie, K., & Vogel-Sprott, M. (1991). Response expectancies affect the acquisition and display of behavioral tolerance to alcohol. *Alcohol, 8*(6), 491–498.

Seeman, P. (2001). Antipsychotic drugs, dopamine receptors, and schizophrenia *Clinical Neuroscience Research, 1*(1–2), 53–60.

Seeman, P., Chau-Wong, M., Tedesco, J., & Wong, K. (1975). Brain receptors for antipsychotic drugs and dopamine: Direct binding assays. *Proceeding of the National Academy of Sciences of the USA, 72*(11), 4376–4380.

Seeman, P. (2005). An update of fast-off dopamine D2 atypical antipsychotics. *American Journal of Psychiatry, 162*(10), 1984–1985.

Seeman, P., & Lee, T. (1975). Antipsychotic drugs: Direct correlation between clinical potency and presynaptic action on dopamine neurons. *Science, 188*(4194), 1217–1219.

Seidel, S., Singer, E. A., Just, H., Farhan, H., Scholze, P., Kudlacek, O., . . . Sitte, H. H. (2005). Amphetamines take two to tango: An oligomer-based counter-transport model of neurotransmitter transport explores the amphetamine action. *Molecular Pharmacology, 67*(1), 140–151. doi: 67/1/140 [pii]

Selvaraj, S., Hoshi, R., Bhagwagar, Z., Murthy, N. V., Hinz, R., Cowen, P., . . . Grasby, P. (2009). Brain serotonin transporter binding in former users of MDMA ("Ecstasy"). *British Journal of Psychiatry, 194*(4), 355–359. doi: 10.1192/bjp.bp.108.050344

Selye, H. (1950). Stress and the general adaptation syndrome. *British Medical Journal, 1*, 1383–1392.

Serretti, A., Kato, M., De Ronchi, D., & Kinoshita, T. (2007). Meta-analysis of serotonin transporter gene promotor polymorphism (5-HTTLPR) association with selective reuptake inhibitor efficacy in depressed patients. *Molecular Psychiatry, 12*, 247–257.

Sesack, S. R., Carr, D. B., Omelchenko, N., & Pinto, A. (2003). Anatomical substrates for glutamate-dopamine interactions: Evidence for specificity of connections and extrasynaptic actions.

Annals of the New York Academy of Sciences, 1003, 36–52.

Sharp, T., Zetterstrom, T., Ljungberg, T., & Ungerstedt, U. (1987). A direct comparison of amphetamine-induced behaviours and regional brain dopamine release in the rat using intracerebral dialysis. *Brain Research, 401*(2), 322–330.

Shelton, K. L., & Balster, R. L. (2004). Effects of abused inhalants and GABA-positive modulators in dizocilpine discriminating inbred mice. *Pharmacology Biochemistry and Behavior, 79*(2), 219–228. doi: 10.1016/j.pbb.2004.07.009

Shen, X. Y., Orson, F. M., & Kosten, T. R. (2012). Vaccines against drug abuse. *Clinical Pharmacology and Therapy, 91*(1), 60–70. doi: 10.1038/clpt.2011.281

Shervette, R. E., Schydlower, M., Fearnow, R. G., & Lampe, R. M. (1979). Jimson "loco" weed abuse in adolescents. *Pediatrics, 63*(4), 520–523.

Shiffman, S. (1989). Tobacco "chippers"—individual differences in tobacco dependence. *Psychopharmacology (Berl) 97*(4), 539–547.

Shimizu, E., Hashimoto, K., & Iyo, M. (2004). Ethnic difference of the BDNF 196G/A (val66met) polymorphism frequencies: The possibility to explain ethnic mental traits. *American Journal of Medical Genetics Part B: Neuropsychiatric Genetics, 126B*(1), 122–123. doi: 10.1002/ajmg.b.20118

Shin, L. M., & Liberzon, I. (2010). The neurocircuitry of fear, stress, and anxiety disorders. *Neuropsychopharmacology, 35*(1), 169–191. doi: npp200983 [pii]

Shoemaker, J. L., Joseph, B. K., Ruckle, M. B., Mayeux, P. R., & Prather, P. L. (2005). The endocannabinoid noladin ether acts as a full agonist at human CB2 cannabinoid receptors. *Journal of Pharmacology and Experimental Therapeutics, 314*(2), 868–875. doi: 10.1124/jpet.105.085282

Shook, J. E., Lemcke, P. K., Gehrig, C. A., Hruby, V. J., & Burks, T. F. (1989). Antidiarrheal properties of supraspinal mu and delta and peripheral mu, delta and kappa opioid receptors: Inhibition of diarrhea without constipation. *Journal*

of Pharmacology and Experimental Therapeutics, 249(1), 83–90.

Shorter, E. (1997). *A history of psychiatry: From the era of the asylum to the age of Prozac.* New York: John Wiley & Sons.

Shu, H., Hayashida, M., Arita, H., Huang, W., Zhang, H., An, K., . . . Hanaoka, K. (2011). Pentazocine-induced antinociception is mediated mainly by μ-opioid receptors and compromised by κ-opioid receptors in mice. *Journal of Pharmacology and Experimental Therapeutics, 338*(2), 579–587. doi: 10.1124/jpet.111.179879

Siebert, D. J. (1994). *Salvia divinorum* and Salvinorin A: New pharmacologic findings. *Journal of Ethnopharmacology, 43*, 53–56.

Siegel, R. K. (1978). Phencyclidine use among youth: History, epidemiology, and acute and chronic intoxication. *NIDA Research Monographs, 21*, 272–288.

Siegel, S. (1984). Pavlovian conditioning and heroin overdose: Reports by overdose victims. *Psychonomic Bulletin and Review, 22*(5), 428–430.

Siegel, S., Hinson, R. E., Krank, M. D., & McCully, J. (1982). Heroin "overdose" death: Contribution of drug-associated environmental cues. *Science, 216*(4544), 436–437.

Sigel, E., & Buhr, A. (1997). The benzodiazepine binding site of GABAA receptors. *Trends in Pharmacological Sciences, 18*(11), 425–429.

Sigmon, S. C., Herning, R. I., Better, W., Cadet, J. L., & Griffiths, R. R. (2009). Caffeine withdrawal, acute effects, tolerance, and absence of net beneficial effects of chronic administration: Cerebral blood flow velocity, quantitative EEG, and subjective effects. *Psychopharmacology (Berl), 204*(4), 573–585. doi: 10.1007/s00213-009-1489-4

Silver, H., Feldman, P., Bilker, W., & Gur, R. C. (2003). Working memory deficit as a core neuropsychological dysfunction in schizophrenia. *American Journal of Psychiatry, 160*(10), 1809–1816.

Silver, J., & Miller, J. H. (2004). Regeneration beyond the glial scar. *National Review of*

Neuroscience, 5(2), 146–156. doi: 10.1038/nrn1326

Simpson, D. D., & Marsh, K. L. (1986). Relapse and recovery among opioid addicts 12 years after treatment. *National Institute on Drug Abuse Research Monograph Series, 72,* 86–103.

Singer, P. (1975). *Animal liberation: A new ethics for our treatment of animals.* New York: New York Review.

Skinner, B. F. (1938). *The behavior of organisms: An experimental analysis.* New York: D. Appleton-Century.

Skolnick, P., & Basile, A. S. (2006). Triple reuptake inhibitors as antidepressants. *Drug Discovery Today: Therapeutic Strategies, 3,* 489–494.

Smith, R. C., & Davis, J. M. (1977). Comparative effects of d-amphetamine, l-amphetamine, and methylphenidate on mood in man. *Psychopharmacology, 53*(1), 1–12. doi: 10.1007/bf00426687

Smith, R. C., Meltzer, H. Y., Arora, R. C., & Davis, J. M. (1977). Effects of phencyclidine on [3H]catecholamine adn [3H]serotonin uptake in synaptosomal preparations from rat brain. *Biochemical Pharmacology, 26,* 1435–1439.

Soine, W. H. (1986). Clandestine drug synthesis. *Medicinal Research Reviews, 6,* 41–74.

Sokol, R. J., Delaney-Black, V., & Nordstrom, B. (2003). Fetal alcohol spectrum disorder. *Journal of the American Medical Association, 290*(22), 2996–2999. doi: 10.1001/jama.290.22.2996

Sokoloff, P., Andrieux, M., Besancon, R., Pilon, C., Martres, M. P., Giros, B., & Schwartz, J. C. (1992). Pharmacology of human dopamine D3 receptor expressed in a mammalian cell line: Comparison with D2 receptor. *European Journal of Pharmacology, 225*(4), 331–337.

Solomon, R. L., & Corbit J. D. (1974). An opponent-process theory of motivation: 1. Temporal dynamics of affect. *Psychology Review, 81,* 119–145.

Spanagel, R., Montkowski, A., Allingham, K., Shoaib, M., Holsboer, F., & Landgraf, R. (1995). Anxiety: A potential predictor of vulnerability to the initiation of ethanol self-administration in rats. *Psychopharmacology, 122*(4), 369–373. doi: 10.1007/bf02246268

Spohn, H. E., & Strauss, M. E. (1989). Relation of neuroleptic and anticholinergic medication to cognitive functions in schizophrenia. *Journal of Abnormal Psychology, 98*(4), 367–380.

Sporer, K. A. (1999). Acute heroin overdose. *Annals of Internal Medicine, 130*(7), 584–590.

Spyraki, C., Fibiger, H. C., & Phillips, A. G. (1983). Attenuation of heroin reward in rats by disruption of the mesolimbic dopamine system. *Psychopharmacology, 79*(2), 278–283. doi: 10.1007/bf00427827

Starr, C., & Taggart, R. (1989) Biology: The unity and diversity of life. Pacific Grave, CA: Brooks/Cole.

Stedman, T. L. (1999). *Stedman's medical dictionary* (27th ed.). Baltimore, MA: Lippincott Williams & Wilkins.

Steele, T. D., Nichols, D. E., & Yim, G. K. W. (1987). Stereochemical effects of 3,4-methylenedioxymethamphetamine (MDMA) and related amphetamine derivatives on inhibition of uptake of [3H]-monoamines into synaptosomes from different regions of rat brain. *Biochemical Pharmacology, 36,* 2297–2303.

Stefanis, C. N., Alevizos, B. H., & Papadimitriou, G. N. (1982). Antidepressant effect of Ro 11-1163, a new MAO inhibitor. *International Pharmacopsychiatry, 17*(1), 43–48.

Stefater, M. A., Wilson-Perez, H. E., Chambers, A. P., Sandoval, D. A., & Seeley, R. J. (2012). All bariatric surgeries are not created equal: Insights from mechanistic comparisons. *Endocrine Reviews.* doi: 10.1210/er.2011-1044

Stein, C., Schafer, M., & Hassan, A. H. (1995). Peripheral opioid receptors. *Annals of Medicine, 27*(2), 219–221.

Steinberg, H., & Sykes, E. A. (1985). Introduction to symposium on endorphins and behavioural processes; review of literature on endorphins and exercise. *Pharmacology, Biochemistry, and Behavior, 23*(5), 857–862.

Stern, R. S., Rosa, F., & Baum, C. (1984). Isotretinoin and pregnancy. *Journal of the American Academy of Dermatology, 10*(5 Pt 1), 851–854.

Sternbach, H. (1991). The serotonin syndrome. *American Journal of Psychiatry, 148*(6), 705–713.

Stolerman, I. P., Pratt, J. A., Garcha, H. S., Giardini, V., & Kumar, R. (1983). Nicotine cue in rats analysed with drugs acting on cholinergic and 5-hydroxytryptamine mechanisms. *Neuropharmacology, 22*(9), 1029–1037.

Stollberger, C., Huber, J. O., & Finsterer, J. (2005). Antipsychotic drugs and QT prolongation. *International Clinical Psychopharmacology, 20*(5), 243–251.

Stone, J. M., Day, F., Tsagaraki, H., Valli, I., McLean, M. A., Lythgoe, D. J., . . . McGuire, P. K. (2009). Glutamate dysfunction in people with prodromal symptoms of psychosis: Relationship to gray matter volume. *Biological Psychiatry, 66,* 533–539.

Subramanya, S. B., Subramanian, V. S., & Said, H. M. (2010). Chronic alcohol consumption and intestinal thiamin absorption: Effects on physiological and molecular parameters of the uptake process. *American Journal of Physiology—Gastrointestinal and Liver Physiology, 299*(1), G23–G31. doi: 10.1152/ajpgi.00132.2010

Substance Abuse and Mental Health Services Administration. (2010). *Results from the 2009 National Survey on Drug Use and Health: Vol. I. Summary of national findings.* Rockville, MD: Office of Applied Studies.

Svingos, A. L., Moriwaki, A., Wang, J. B., Uhl, G. R., & Pickel, V. M. (1997). μ-opioid receptors are localized to extrasynaptic plasma membranes of GABAergic neurons and their targets in the rat nucleus accumbens. *Journal of Neuroscience, 17*(7), 2585–2594.

Swerdlow, P. S. (2000). Use of humans in biomedical experimentation. In F. L. Marina (Ed.), *Scientific integrity: An introductory text with cases* (2nd ed.). Washington, DC: ASM Press.

Swift, R., & Davidson, D. (1998). Alcohol hangover: Mechanisms and mediators. *Alcohol Health and Research World, 22*(1), 54–60.

Szymański, P., Markowicz, M., & Mikiciuk-Olasik, E. (2012). Adaptation of high-throughput screening in drug discovery—toxicological screening tests. *International Journal of Molecular Sciences, 13*(1), 427–452. doi: 10.3390/ijms13010427.

Takeda, S., Jiang, R., Aramaki, H., Imoto, M., Toda, A., Eyanagi, R., . . . Watanabe, K. (2010). Δ⁹-tetrahydrocannabinol and its major metabolite Δ9-tetrahydrocannabinol-11-oic acid as 15-lipoxygenase inhibitors. *Journal of Pharmaceutical Sciences, 100*(3), 1206–1211. doi: 10.1002/jps.22354

Takeuchi, T., Owa, T., Nishino, T., & Kamei, C. (2010). Assessing anxiolytic-like effects of selective serotonin reuptake inhibitors and serotonin-noradrenaline reuptake inhibitors using the elevated plus maze in mice. *Methods and Findings in Experimental and Clinical Pharmacology, 32*(2), 113–121. doi: 1428741 [pii]

Tan, W. C., Lo, C., Jong, A., Xing, L., Fitzgerald, M. J., Vollmer, W. M., . . . Sin, D. D. (2009). Marijuana and chronic obstructive lung disease: A population-based study. *Canadian Medical Association Journal, 180*(8), 814–820. doi: 10.1503/cmaj.081040

Tancer, M., & Johanson, C.-E. (2003). Reinforcing, subjective, and physiological effects of MDMA in humans: A comparison with d-amphetamine and mCPP. *Drug and Alcohol Dependence, 72*(1), 33–44. doi: 10.1016/s0376-8716(03)00172-8

Taylor, D. P., & Hyslop, D. K. (1991). Chronic administration of buspirone down-regulates 5-HT2 receptor binding sites. *Drug Development Research, 24*(1), 93–105. doi: 10.1002/ddr.430240108

Temple, J. L. (2009). Caffeine use in children: What we know, what we have left to learn, and why we should worry. *Neuroscience and Biobehavioral Reviews, 33*(6), 793–806. doi: 10.1016/j.neubiorev.2009.01.001

Thiel, C. M., Zilles, K., & Fink, G. R. (2005). Nicotine modulates reorienting of visuospatial attention and neural activity in human parietal cortex. *Neuropsychopharmacology, 30*(4), 810–820.

Thomas, B. F., Gilliam, A. F., Burch, D. F., Roche, M. J., & Seltzman, H. H. (1998). Comparative receptor binding analyses of cannabinoid agonists and antagonists. *Journal of Pharmacology and Experimental Therapeutics, 285*(1), 285–292.

Thompson, R. F. (1999). James Olds. *Biographical Memoirs 77*. Retrieved from www.nap.edu/html/biomems/jolds.html

Ticku, M. K., Burch, T. P., & Davis, W. C. (1983). The interactions of ethanol with the benzodiazepine-GABA receptor-ionophore complex. *Pharmacology Biochemistry and Behavior, 18*(Supplement 1), 15–18.

Tiwari, A. K., Souza, R. P., & Muller, D. J. (2009). Pharmacogenetics of anxiolytic drugs. *Journal of Neural Transmission, 116*(6), 667–677. doi: 10.1007/s00702-009-0229-6.

Tobin, J. M., Lorenz, A. A., Brousseau, E. R., & Conner, W. R. (1964). Clinical evaluation of oxazepam for the management of anxiety. *Diseases of the Nervous System, 25*, 689–696.

Todaro, B. (2012). Cannabinoids in the treatment of chemotherapy-induced nausea and vomiting. *Journal of the National Comprehensive Cancer Network, 10*(4), 487–492.

Toennes, S. W., Harder, S., Schramm, M., Niess, C., & Kauert, G. F. (2003). Pharmacokinetics of cathinone, cathine, and norephedrine after the chewing of khat leaves. *British Journal of Clinical Pharmacology, 56*(1), 125–130. doi: 10.1046/j.1365-2125.2003.01834.x

Tohen, M., Vieta, E., Calabrese, J., Ketter, T. A., Sachs, G., Bowden, C., . . . Breier, A. (2003). Efficacy of olanzapine and olanzapine-fluoxetine combination in the treatment of bipolar I depression. *Archives of General Psychiatry, 60*(11), 1079–1088. doi: 10.1001/archpsyc.60.11.1079

Tone, A. (2005). Listening to the past: History, psychiatry, and anxiety. *Canadian Journal of Psychiatry, 50*(7), 373–380.

Trigo, J. M., Martin-García, E., Berrendero, F., Robledo, P., & Maldonado, R. (2010). The endogenous opioid system: A common substrate in drug addiction. *Drug and Alcohol Dependence, 108*(3), 183–194. doi: 10.1016/j.drugalcdep.2009.10.011

Trivedi, M. H., Rush, A. J., Wisniewski, S. R., Nierenberg, A. A., Warden, D., Ritz, L., . . . Fava, M. (2006). Evaluation of outcomes with citalopram for depression using measurement-based care in STAR*D: Implications for clinical practice. *American Journal of Psychiatry, 163*(1), 28–40. doi: 163/1/28 [pii]

Trollor, J. N., Chen, X., & Sachdev, P. S. (2009). Neuroleptic malignant syndrome associated with atypical antipsychotic drugs. *CNS Drugs, 23*(6), 477–492. doi: 3 [pii]

Tropea, D., Caleo, M., & Maffei, L. (2003). Synergistic effects of brain-derived neurotrophic factor and chondroitinase ABC on retinal fiber sprouting after denervation of the superior colliculus in adult rats. *Journal of Neuroscience, 23*(18), 7034–7044.

Tschoner, A., Engl, J., Rettenbacher, M., Edlinger, M., Kaser, S., Tatarczyk, T., . . . Ebenbichler, C. F. (2009). Effects of six second generation antipsychotics on body weight and metabolism: Risk assessment and results from a prospective study. *Pharmacopsychiatry, 42*(1), 29–34. doi: 10.1055/s-0028-1100425

Tsuang, M. (2000). Schizophrenia: Genes and environment. *Biological Psychiatry, 47*(3), 210–220. doi: 10.1016/s0006-3223(99)00289-9

Uhr, M., Tontsch, A., Namendorf, C., Ripke, S., Lucae, S., Ising, M., . . . Holsboer, F. (2008). Polymorphisms in the drug transporter gene ABCB1 predict antidepressant treatment response in depression. *Neuron, 57*(2), 203–209. doi: 10.1016/j.neuron.2007.11.017

United Nations Office of Drugs and Crime. (2010). *World drug report 2010*. New York: Author.

USDA. (2006). 9 CFR 1A. (Title 9, Chapter 1, Subchapter A): Animal Welfare. *Federal Register*.

Valzelli, L. (1980). An approach to neuroanatomical and neurochemical psychology. Torino, Italy: C. G. Edizioni Medico Scientifiche.

Vann, R. E., Gamage, T. F., Warner, J. A., Marshall, E. M., Taylor, N. L., Martin, B. R., & Wiley, J. L. (2008). Divergent effects of cannabidiol on the discriminative stimulus and place conditioning effects of Δ^9-tetrahydrocannabinol. *Drug and Alcohol Dependence, 94*(1–3), 191–198. doi: S0376-8716(07)00490-5 [pii]

van Os, J., Kenis, G., & Rutten, B. P. F. (2010). The environment and schizophrenia. *Nature, 468*(7321), 203–212.

van Vliet, I. M., den Boer, J. A., Westenberg, H. G., & Pian, K. L. (1997). Clinical effects of buspirone in social phobia: a double-blind placebo-controlled study. *Journal of Clinical Psychiatry, 58*(4), 164–168.

van Zessen, R., Phillips, J. L., Budygin, E. A., & Stuber, G. D. (2012). Activation of VTA GABA neurons disrupts reward consumption. *Neuron, 73*(6), 1184–1194. doi: 10.1016/j.neuron.2012.02.016

Varela, M., Nogue, S., Oros, M., & Miro, O. (2004). Gamma hydroxybutirate use for sexual assault. *Emergency Medicine Journal, 21*, 255–256.

Vearrier, D., Greenberg, M. I., Miller, S. N., Okaneku, J. T., & Haggerty, D. A. (2012). Methamphetamine: History, pathophysiology, adverse health effects, current trends, and hazards associated with the clandestine manufacture of methamphetamine. *Disease-a-Month, 58*(2), 38–89. doi: 10.1016/j.disamonth.2011.09.004

Veliskova, J., Velisek, L., & Moshe, S. L. (1996). Subthalamic nucleus: A new anticonvulsant site in the brain. *Neuroreport, 7*(11), 1786–1788.

Veliskova, J., Velisek, L., Nunes, M. L., & Moshe, S. L. (1996). Developmental regulation of regional functionality of substantial nigra $GABA_A$ receptors involved in seizures. *European Journal of Pharmacology, 309*(2), 167–173. doi: 001429999600341X [pii]

Vicentic, A., & Jones, D. C. (2007). The CART (cocaine- and amphetamine-regulated transcript) system in appetite and drug addiction. *Journal of Pharmacology and Experimental Therapeutics, 320*(2), 499–506. doi: 10.1124/jpet.105.091512

Vieta, E., Locklear, J., Günther, O., Ekman, M., Miltenburger, C., Chatterton, M. L., . . . Paulsson, B. (2010). Treatment options for bipolar depression: A systematic review of randomized, controlled trials. *Journal of Clinical Psychopharmacology, 30*(5), 579–590. 10.1097/JCP.0b013e3181f15849

Villégier, A.-S., Lotfipour, S., McQuown, S. C., Belluzzi, J. D., & Leslie, F. M. (2007). Tranylcypromine enhancement of nicotine self-administration. *Neuropharmacology, 52*(6), 1415–1425. doi: 10.1016/j.neuropharm.2007.02.001

Virk, M. S., Arttamangkul, S., Birdsong, W. T., & Williams, J. T. (2009). Buprenorphine is a weak partial agonist that inhibits opioid receptor desensitization. *Journal of Neuroscience, 29*(22), 7341–7348. doi: 10.1523/jneurosci.3723-08.2009

Vogel, J. R., Beer, B., & Clody, D. E. (1971). A simple and reliable conflict procedure for testing anti-anxiety agents. *Psychopharmacologia, 21*(1), 1–7.

Volkow, N. D., & O'Brien, C. P. (2007). Issues for DSM-V: Should obesity be included as a brain disorder? [Editorial]. *American Journal of Psychiatry, 164*(5), 708–710. doi: 10.1176/appi.ajp.164.5.708

Volkow, N. D., Wang, G. J., Fowler, J. S., Tomasi, D., & Baler, R. (2011). Food and drug reward: Overlapping circuits in human obesity and addiction. *Current Topics in Behavioral Neurosciences.* doi: 10.1007/7854_2011_169

Volkow, N. D., Wang, G. J., Fischman, M. W., Foltin, R., Fowler, J. S., Franceschi, D., . . . Pappas, N. (2000). Effects of route of administration on cocaine induced dopamine transporter blockade in the human brain. *Life Sciences, 67*(12), 1507–1515. doi: 10.1016/s0024-3205(00)00731-1

Volkow, N. D., & Wise, R. A. (2005). How can drug addiction help us understand obesity? [Review]. *Nature Neuroscience, 8*(5), 555–560. doi: 10.1038/nn1452

Vollenweider, F. X., Leenders, K. L., Scharfetter, C., Maguire, P., Stadelmann, O., & Angst, J. (1997). Positron emission tomography and fluorodeoxyglucose studies of metabolic hyperfrontality and psychopathology in the psilocybin model of psychosis. *Neuropsychopharmacology, 16*(5), 357–372. doi: S0893-133X(96)00246-1 [pii]

Volpi, R., Chiodera, P., Caffarra, P., Scaglioni, A., Saccani, A., & Coiro, V. (1997). Different control mechanisms of growth hormone (GH) secretion between gamma-amino- and gamma-hydroxy-butyric acid: neuroendocrine evidence in Parkinson's disease. *Psychoneuroendocrinology, 22*(7), 531–538.

Volpicelli, J. R., Alterman, A. I., Hayashida, M., & O'Brien, C. P. (1992). Naltrexone in the treatment of alcohol dependence. *Archives of General Psychiatry, 49*(11), 876–880.

Volpicelli, J. R., Sarin-Krishnan, S., & O'Malley, S. S. (2002). Alcoholism pharmacotherapy. In K. L. Davis, D. Charney, J. T. Coyle, & C. Nemeroff (Eds.), *Neuropsychopharmacology: The fifth generation of progress.* Brentwood, NJ: American College of Neuropsychopharmacology.

Vos, J. W., Ufkes, J. G. R., Wilgenburg, H., Geerlings, P. J., & Brink, W. (1995). Pharmacokinetics of methadone and its primary metabolite in 20 opiate addicts. *European Journal of Clinical Pharmacology, 48*(5), 361–366. doi: 10.1007/bf00194951

Wade, D. (2012). Evaluation of the safety and tolerability profile of Sativex: Is it reassuring enough? *Expert Review of Neurotherapeutics, 12*(4 Suppl), 9–14. doi: 10.1586/ern.12.12

Wallis, G. G., McHarg, J. F., & Scott, O. C. A. (1949). Acute psychosis caused by dextro-amphetamine. *British Medical Journal, 2*(4641), 1394.

Walter, H. J., & Messing, R. O. (1999). Regulation of neuronal voltage-gated calcium channels by ethanol. *Neurochemistry International, 35*(2), 95–101.

Warburton, D. (2002). [Without title]. *Psychopharmacology, 162*(4), 345–348. doi: 10.1007/s00213-002-1087-1

Ware, M. A., Wang, T., Shapiro, S., Robinson, A., Ducruet, T., Huynh, T., . . . Collet, J. P. (2010). Smoked cannabis for chronic neuropathic pain: A randomized controlled trial. *Canadian Medical Association Journal, 182*(14), E694–701. doi: 10.1503/cmaj.091414

Warzak, W. J., Evans, S., Floress, M. T., Gross, A. C., & Stoolman, S. (2011). Caffeine consumption in young children. *Journal of Pediatrics, 158*(3), 508–509. doi: 10.1016/j.jpeds.2010.11.022

Watanabe, A. M., McConnaughey, M. M., Strawbridge, R. A., Fleming, J. W., Jones, L. R., & Besch, H. R. (1978). Muscarinic cholinergic receptor modulation of beta-adrenergic receptor affinity for catecholamines. *Journal of Biological Chemistry, 253*(14), 4833–4836.

Watkins, L. R., Milligan, E. D., & Maier, S. F. (2001). Glial activation: A driving force for pathological pain. *Trends in Neuroscience, 24*(8), 450–455.

Wechsler, H., Lee, J. E., Kuo, M., Seibring, M., Nelson, T. F., & Lee, H. (2002). Trends in college binge drinking during a period of increased prevention efforts: Findings from 4 Harvard School of Public Health College Alcohol Study surveys, 1993–2001. *Journal of American College Health, 50*(5), 203–217.

Wee, S., Hicks, M. J., De, B. P., Rosenberg, J. B., Moreno, A. Y., Kaminsky, S. M., . . . Koob, G. F. (2012). Novel cocaine vaccine linked to a disrupted adenovirus gene transfer vector blocks cocaine psychostimulant and reinforcing effects. *Neuropsychopharmacology, 37*(5), 1083–1091. doi: 10.1038/npp.2011.200

Weese, H., & Scharpff, W. (1932). Evipan, ein neuartiges Einschlafmittel. *Deutsche Medizinische Wochenschrift, 58*, 12051207.

Weil, A. T., Zinberg, N. E., & Nelsen, J. M. (1968). Clinical and psychological effects of marihuana in man. *Science, 162*(859), 1234–1242.

Weinberger, D. R. (1996). On the plausibility of "the neurodevelopmental hypothesis" of schizophrenia. *Neuropsychopharmacology, 14*(3 Suppl), 1S–11S. doi: 10.1016/0893-133X(95)00199-N

Welkowitz, L. A., Papp, L., Martinez, J., Browne, S., & Gorman, J. M. (1999). Instructional set and physiological response to CO_2 inhalation. *American Journal of Psychiatry, 156*(5), 745–748.

Wesnes, K., & Warburton, D. M. (1983). Effects of smoking on rapid information processing performance. *Neuropsychobiology, 9*(4), 223–229.

Wesnes, K., & Warburton, D. M. (1984). Effects of scopolamine and nicotine on human rapid information processing performance. *Psychopharmacology, 82*(3), 147–150. doi: 10.1007/bf00427761

Westgate, H. D., & Stiebler, H. J. (1964). Barbiturate abstinence syndrome. *Anesthesiology, 25*, 403–405.

White, A. M., Kraus, C. L., & Swartzwelder, H. S. (2006). Many college freshmen drink at levels far beyond the binge threshold. *Alcoholism: Clinical and Experimental Research, 30*(6), 1006–1010. doi: 10.1111/j.1530-0277.2006.00122.x

Wieland, H. A., & Luddens, H. (1994). Four amino acid exchanges convert a diazepam-insensitive, inverse agonist-preferring $GABA_A$ receptor into a diazepam-preferring $GABA_A$ receptor. *Journal of Medicinal Chemistry, 37*(26), 4576–4580.

Wiese, J. G., Shlipak, M. G., & Browner, W. S. (2000). The alcohol hangover. *Annals of Internal Medicine, 132*(11), 897–902.

Wildmann, J., Niemann, J., & Matthaei, H. (1986). Endogenous benzodiazepine receptor agonist in human and mammalian plasma. *Journal of Neural Transmission, 66*(3–4), 151–160.

Wilk, C. M., Gold, J. M., Humber, K., Dickerson, F., Fenton, W. S., & Buchanan, R. W. (2004). Brief cognitive assessment in schizophrenia: Normative data for the Repeatable Battery for the Assessment of Neuropsychological Status. *Schizophrenia Research, 70*(2–3), 175–186. doi: 10.1016/j.schres.2003.10.009

Williams, C. M., & Kirkham, T. C. (1999). Anandamide induces overeating: Mediation by central cannabinoid (CB1) receptors. *Psychopharmacology, 143*(3), 315–317. doi: 10.1007/s002130050953

Williams, J. F., & Storck, M. (2007). Inhalant abuse. *Pediatrics, 119*(5), 1009–1017. doi: 10.1542/peds.2007-0470

Willis, W. D., & Westlund, K. N. (1997). Neuroanatomy of the pain system and of the pathways that modulate pain. *Journal of Clinical Neurophysiology, 14*(1), 2–31.

Winstock, A. R., Mitcheson, L. R., Deluca, P., Davey, Z., Corazza, O., & Schifano, F. (2011). Mephedrone, new kid for the chop? *Addiction, 106*(1), 154–161. doi: 10.1111/j.1360-0443.2010.03130.x

Winter, J. C., Rice, K. C., Amorosi, D. J., & Rabin, R. A. (2007). Psilocybin-induced stimulus control in the rat. *Pharmacology Biochemistry and Behavior, 87*(4), 472–480. doi: 10.1016/j.pbb.2007.06.003

Wirshing, D. A., Wirshing, W. C., Kysar, L., Berisford, M. A., Goldstein, D., Pashdag, J., . . . Marder, S. R. (1999). Novel antipsychotics: comparison of weight gain liabilities. *Journal of Clinical Psychiatry, 60*(6), 358–363.

Wisden, W., Laurie, D. J., Monyer, H., & Seeburg, P. H. (1992). The distribution of 13 $GABA_A$ receptor subunit mRNAs in the rat brain. I. Telencephalon, diencephalon, mesencephalon. *Journal of Neuroscience, 12*(3), 1040–1062.

Wise, R. A. (1989). Opiate reward: Sites and substrates. *Neuroscience and Biobehavioral Reviews, 13*(2–3), 129–133.

Wise, R. A., Yokel, R. A., & Wit, H. D. (1976). Both positive reinforcement and conditioned aversion from amphetamine and from apomorphine in rats. *Science, 191*(4233), 1273–1275.

Wish, E. D., Fitzelle, D. B., O'Grady, K. E., Hsu, M. H., & Arria, A. M. (2006). Evidence for significant polydrug use among Ecstasy-using college students. *Journal of American College Health, 55*(2), 99–104. doi: 10.3200/jach.55.2.99–104

Wong, A. H. C., & Van Tol, H. H. M. (2003). Schizophrenia: From phenomenology to neurobiology. *Neuroscience and Biobehavioral Reviews, 27*, 269–306.

Wood, D. M., Greene, S. L., & Dargan, P. I. (2011). Clinical pattern of toxicity associated with the novel synthetic cathinone mephedrone. *Emergency Medicine Journal, 28*(4), 280–282. doi: 10.1136/emj.2010.092288

Woods, J. H., & Winger, G. 1995 Current benzodiazepine issues. *Psychopharmacology, 118*, 107–115.

Woodward, N. D., Purdon, S. E., Meltzer, H. Y., & Zald, D. H. (2005). A meta-analysis of neuropsychological change to clozapine, olanzapine, quetiapine, and risperidone in schizophrenia. *International Journal of Neuropsychopharmacology, 8*(3): 457–472.

Woodworth, T. (1999). Date rape drugs. DEA congressional testimony, before the House Commerce Committee, Subcommittee on Oversight and Investigations. Retrieved from www.gpo.gov/fdsys/pkg/CHRG-106hhrg55638/pdf/CHRG-106hhrg55638.pdf

Woolf, N. J. (1991). Cholinergic systems in mammalian brain and spinal cord. Progress in Neurobiology, 37, 475–524.

Woolverton, W. L., Kandel, D., & Schuster, C. R. (1978). Tolerance and cross-tolerance to cocaine and d-amphetamine. *Journal of Pharmacology and Experimental Therapeutics, 205*(3), 525–535.

World Health Organization. (2011). *Global status report on alcohol and health.* Geneva: Author. Retrieved from www.who.int/substance_abuse/publications/global_alcohol_report/en/index.html

World Health Organization. (2012). Alcohol. Retrieved from www.who.int/topics/alcohol_drinking/en

World Health Organization. (2012). Health topics: Substance abuse. Retrieved from www.who.int/topics/substance_abuse/en/

Wu, C. Y., & Wittick, J. J. (1977). Separation of five major alkaloids in gum opium and quantitation of morphine, codeine, and theba-

ine by isocratic reverse phase high performance liquid chromatography. *Analytical Chemistry, 49*(3), 359–363.

Wu, H., Zink, N., Carter, L. P., Mehta, A. K., Hernandez, R. J., Ticku, M. K., . . . Coop, A. (2003). A tertiary alcohol analog of γ-hydroxybutyric acid as a specific γ-hydroxybutyric acid receptor ligand. *Journal of Pharmacology and Experimental Therapeutics, 305*(2), 675–679. doi: 10.1124/jpet.102.046797

Wyndham, C. H. (1977). Heat stroke and hyperthermia in marathon runners. *Annals of the New York Academy of Sciences, 301*(1), 128–138. doi: 10.1111/j.1749-6632.1977.tb38192.x

Xiao, C., & Ye, J. H. (2008). Ethanol dually modulates GABAergic synaptic transmission onto dopaminergic neurons in ventral tegmental area: Role of [mu]-opioid receptors. *Neuroscience, 153*(1), 240–248. doi: 10.1016/j.neuroscience.2008.01.040

Xiao, C., Zhou, C., Li, K., & Ye, J.-H. (2007). Presynaptic GABAA receptors facilitate GABAergic transmission to dopaminergic neurons in the ventral tegmental area of young rats. *Journal of Physiology, 580*(3), 731–743. doi: 10.1113/jphysiol.2006.124099

Yanagisawa, N., Morita, H., & Nakajima, T. (2006). Sarin experiences in Japan: Acute toxicity and long-term effects. *Journal of the Neurological Sciences, 249*(1), 76–85.

Yang, J., Jamei, M., Heydari, A., Yeo, K. R., de la Torre, R., Farré, M., . . . Rostami-Hodjegan, A. (2006). Implications of mechanism-based inhibition of CYP2D6 for the pharmacokinetics and toxicity of MDMA. *Journal of Psychopharmacology, 20*(6), 842–849. doi: 10.1177/0269881106065907

Yang, K., Buhlman, L., Khan, G. M., Nichols, R. A., Jin, G., McIntosh, J. M., . . . Wu, J. (2011). Functional nicotinic acetylcholine receptors containing α6 subunits are on GABAergic neuronal boutons adherent to ventral tegmental area dopamine neurons. *Journal of Neuroscience, 31*(7), 2537–2548. doi: 10.1523/jneurosci.3003-10.2011

Yeh, S. Y., & Woods, L. A. (1970). Isolation of morphine-3-glucuronide from urine and bile of rats injected with codeine. *Journal of Pharmacology and Experimental Therapeutics, 175*(1), 69–74.

Yehuda, R., Southwick, S. M., Nussbaum, G., Wahby, V., Giller, E. L., Jr., & Mason, J. W. (1990). Low urinary cortisol excretion in patients with posttraumatic stress disorder. *Journal of Nervous and Mental Disease, 178*(6), 366–369.

Yoshimoto, K., McBride, W. J., Lumeng, L., & Li, T. K. (1992). Ethanol enhances the release of dopamine and serotonin in the nucleus accumbens of HAD and LAD lines of rats. *Alcoholism: Clinical and Experimental Research, 16*(4), 781–785. doi: 10.1111/j.1530-0277.1992.tb00678.x

Youdim, M. B. H. (2006). Monoamine oxidases, their inhibitors, and the opening of the neurotransmitter era in neuropsychopharmacology. In T. A. Ban & R. U. Udabe (Eds.), *The neurotransmitter era in neuropsychopharmacology.* Buenos Aires: Editorial Polemos.

Yusof, W., & Gan, S. H. (2009). High prevalence of CYP2A6*4 and CYP2A6*9 alleles detected among a Malaysian population. *Clinica Chimica Acta, 403*(1–2), 105–109. doi: 10.1016/j.cca.2009.01.032

Zakhari, S. (1997). Alcohol and the cardiovascular system: Molecular mechanisms for beneficial and harmful action. *Alcohol Health and Research World, 21*(1), 21–29.

Zangrossi, H., Viana, M. B., & Graeff, F. G. (1999). Anxiolytic effect of intra-amygdala injection of midazolam and 8-hydroxy-2-(di-n-propylamino)tetralin in the elevated T-maze. *European Journal of Pharmacology, 369*(3), 267–270.

Zarate, C. A., Jr., Singh, J. B., Carlson, P. J., Brutsche, N. E., Ameli, R., Luckenbaugh, D. A., . . . Manji, H. K. (2006). A randomized trial of an N-methyl-D-aspartate antagonist in treatment-resistant major depression. *Archives of General Psychiatry, 63*(8), 856–864. doi: 10.1001/archpsyc.63.8.856

Zhao-Shea, R., Liu, L., Soll, L. G., Improgo, M. R., Meyers, E. E., McIntosh, J. M., . . . Tapper, A. R. (2011). Nicotine-mediated activation of dopaminergic neurons in distinct regions of the ventral tegmental area. *Neuropsychopharmacology, 36*(5), 1021–1032. doi: 10.1038/npp.2010.240

Zhou, F. C., Lesch, K.-P., & Murphy, D. L. (2002). Serotonin uptake into dopamine neurons via dopamine transporters: A compensatory alternative. *Brain Research,* 942(1–2), 109–119. doi: 10.1016/s0006-8993(02)02709-9

Zimatkin, S. M., Liopo, A. V., & Deitrich, R. A. (1998). Distribution and kinetics of ethanol metabolism in rat brain. *Alcoholism: Clinical and Experimental Research, 22*(8), 1623–1627. doi: 10.1111/j.1530-0277.1998.tb03958.x

Zvosec, D. L., & Smith, S. W. (2009). Response to "Cognitive, psychomotor and subjective effects of sodium oxybate and triazolam in healthy volunteers" (2009), *206*(1), 141–154. *Psychopharmacology (Berl), 207*(3), 509–510; author reply 511-502. doi: 10.1007/s00213-009-1662-9

SUBJECT INDEX/GLOSSARY

Distal, 35

Distillation, 227–229, 230

Distilled alcoholic beverages (spirits) *Alcoholic beverages produced through distillation; have a higher alcohol content than beer and wine,* 228

Distribution *Passage of a drug through the circulatory system,* 106–107

Disulfiram *Treatment for alcohol addiction that inhibits acetaldehyde dehydrogenase enzyme activity, causing noxious effects,* 187, 249–250

Divided attention *Sustained attention on a stimulus despite the presence of distracters,* 241–242

Diviner's sage, 349

Dizocilpine, 341, 342

DNA (deoxyribonucleic acid), 31, 55

Dolophine (methadone), 278, 281–282, 297

Dopamine, 4, 84–87, 173, 287, 369–370

Dopamine hypothesis *Hypothesis for schizophrenia stating that positive symptoms arise from excessive dopamine release in the limbic system,* 415–416

Dopamine neurotransmission
MDMA and, 332–334
phencyclidine and, 343–344
in schizophrenia, 425–427

Dopamine receptors *Receptors activated by dopamine, consisting of subtypes D_1, D_2, D_3, D_4 and D_5,* 86

Dopamine transporter *Membrane transporter for dopamine reuptake,* 86

Dorsal, 35

Dorsal horn, 37

Dorsal root, 37

Dorsal striatum, 147, 149

Dorsolateral prefrontal cortex, 147

Dose *Ratio of the amount of drug per an organism's body weight,* 7–10

Dose-effect curve *Depicts the level of a drug effect by dose,* 7–10

Double-blind procedure *When neither participants nor investigators know the treatment assignments during a study,* 14

Downers, 392

Drinking, 237–238. *See also* Alcohol

Drive theory, 136, 139–142

Dronabinol, 302

Drug *Administered substance that alters physiological functioning*
about, 4
assessing in carefully controlled laboratory environments, 18–19
classification, 131–134
effects of, 7–10, 18
passage through body, 103–111
neurotoxins and damage to nervous system, 122–123
physiological adaptations to chronic drug use, 123–125
psychoactive drugs and receptors, 115–122

Drug abuse
about, 6
with benzodiazepines, 396–397
changes to learning and memory systems and, 147–149
clinical definitions, 134–136
drug addiction diagnosis, 134–136
drug classification, 131–134
neurobiology and stages of drug addiction, 150–151
opioids, 280–282
potential of SSRIs/SNRIs and benzodiazepine, 401

psychological and pharmacological therapies for treating, 151–155
regulatory agencies, 131–134
reward circuitry and, 142–147
theoretical models of drug addiction, 136–142

Drug addiction
diagnosis of, 134–136
Drive theory, 139–142
Incentive-salience model, 139–142
neurobiology and stages of, 150–151
Opponent-process theory, 139–142
theoretical models of, 136–142

Drug development *Multistep process of developing an effective, safe, and profitable therapeutic drug,* 8–9

Drug dispositional tolerance, 123

Drug Enforcement Administration (DEA), 301–302

Drug metabolism *Process of converting a drug into one or more metabolites,* 108–109

Drug properties. *See* Pharmacodynamic properties; Pharmacokinetic properties

Drug synthesis, 26

Drug-discrimination procedure *Procedure that trains an organism to recognize or discriminate between the subjective effects of a particular drug when compared to noticeably different effects,* 180, 181, 272–273, 312

Drug-replacement therapy *Exchanging the addictive drug with a similar but less harmful drug,* 152

Drunken stupor, 243

Dry mouth, 182

D-serene, 82

Duloxetine (Cymbalta), 400

Duragesic (fentanyl), 278

Dynorphin, 283

Dysphoria, 295

Dysthymic disorder *Disorder consisting of a depressed mood that occurs nearly every day for at least 2 years,* 355

E

Ecstasy. *See* MDMA (Ecstasy)

ED_{50} **value** *Represents the dose at which 50% of an effect was observed,* 8

EEG. *See* Electroencephalography (EEG)

Effector enzyme *Enzyme that usually activates a second messenger,* 78

Efferent neurons, 32

Effexor (venlafaxine), 366, 400

Efficacy, on SSRIs/SNRIs and benzodiazepine, 401

18th Amendment *Amendment to U.S. Constitution that banned the sale and distribution of alcohol,* 231

Electrical events, 65–66

Electrical potential *Difference between the electrical charge within a neuron versus the electrical charge of the environment immediately outside the neuron,* 65

Electrical transmission *Series of electrical events that begin at an axon hillock and proceed down the length of an axon,* 65

Electroencephalography (EEG) *Method for recording the electrical activity of brain areas through electrodes placed on the scalp,* 264–265

Electrophysiology, 66

Electrostatic attraction *Attraction of ions with opposite charges,* 69

Elevated plus maze *Most commonly used model in assessing anxiety in mice and rats,* 402–403

Elimination *Process for how a drug leaves the body,* 109–111, 232, 269, 342–343

Elimination rate *Amount of drug eliminated from the body over time,* 109

Embryo, 53, 54

Emotional behaviors, 43–44

Empathogen *Term referring to enhanced empathy; usually in reference to mixed stimulant-psychedelic drugs,* 341

Emphysema *Type of chronic obstructive pulmonary disorder caused by irreversible lung damage,* 210, 211

Emsam (selegiline), 362

Endocannabinoid system, 236–237

Endocrine disruptors, 122

Endogenous opioid system, 282–284

Endoplasmic reticulum, 31

Endozepines *Endogenous or naturally occurring benzodiazepines,* 399

Energy drinks, 216–217

Entacapone, 113

Entactogen *Term meaning "touching within" usually in reference to mixed stimulant-psychedelic drugs,* 341

Environmental neurotoxicology *A field devoted to the study of neurotoxins in the environment,* 122

Ephedra, 162

Ephedrine, 162

Epinephrine, 84–85, 87–88

Episodic memory, 242

EPSP. *See* Excitatory postsynaptic potential (EPSP)

Essential amino acid *Amino acid that is not produced in the body and must come from diet,* 84

Ethanol, 226

Ethical cost *Assessment that weighs the value of potential research discoveries against the potential pain and distress experienced by research subjects,* 20

Ethics, 17, 22–24

Ethyl alcohol (ethanol) *An alcohol that functions as a central nervous system depressant,* 226

Ethylene gas, 268

Euphoria, 295

Event-related potential *EEG recording during a behavioral or cognitive activity,* 264

Everclear, 228–229

Evipal (hexobarbital), 391

Evoked potential *EEG recording during a specific stimulus presentation,* 264

Excitatory amino acid neurotransmitters *An amino acid neurotransmitter family that tends to elicit excitatory effects on neurons,* 81

Excitatory postsynaptic potential (EPSP) *Stimulus that depolarizes a local potential,* 65–66, 346

Excitotoxicity, 98, 375

Exhaustion stage, of general adaptation syndrome, 388–389

Exocytosis *Fusing of synaptic vesicles to the axon membrane and release of stored neurotransmitters into the synaptic cleft,* 75

Experiment, 13

Experimental study *Study in which investigators alter an independent variable to determine if changes occur to the dependent variable,* 13

compounds such as tyramine, 362

Marco Polo, 303

Marijuana, 7, 300. *See also* Cannabinoids

Master gland, 95

Mathylphenidate, 161

MATRICS (Measurement and Treatment Research to Improve Cognition in Schizophrenia), 410

MDMA (Ecstasy) *Mixed stimulant-psychedelic drug; chemically, 3,4-methylenedioxyethamphetamine*
about, 6–7, 12, 134, 341
dopamine neurotransmission and, 332–334
length of psychedelic drug effects, 330–331
metabolism of, 330–331
psychedelic effects of, 334–337
psychostimulant actions, 338–339
psychostimulant effects of, 334–337
serotonin neurotransmission and, 332–334
therapeutic and recreational use, 329–330
tolerance and dependence during chronic use of, 341
use in psychotherapy, 339–340

Measurement and Treatment Research to Improve Cognition in Schizophrenia (MATRICS), 410

Medial, 35

Medical cannabis *Use of cannabis for treating medical conditions such as cancer, weight gain, pain, intraocular pressure, and autoimmune diseases*, 300, 316–317

Medulla *Structure that controls the autonomic nervous system and is situated where the spinal cord meets the hindbrain*, 40–42

Melatonin *Sleep-inducing hormone that plays an important role in circadian rhythm, our natural sleep cycle*, 42, 95

Mellaril (thioridazine), 417

Memory processes, 46–47, 147–149

Mental disorder *Impairment in normal behavioral, cognitive, or emotional function*, 355

Meprobamate (Miltown), 382

Merck, 329–330

Mescaline, 321–322

Mesocortical dopamine pathway *Set of dopamine neurons with somas in the ventral tegmental area and axons terminating in the cerebral cortex, particularly the prefrontal cortex*, 86

Mesolimbic dopamine pathway *Set of dopamine neurons with somas in the ventral tegmental area and axons terminating in the limbic system*, 86

Messenger RNA, 57

Metabolic tolerance to alcohol *Increase in liver alcohol dehydrogenase enzymes resulting in an increased rate of alcohol metabolism*, 246

Metabolism
about, 108–109
benzodiazepines and, 395–396
of MDMA, 330–331
of nicotine, 199–200
of opioids, 280–281

Metabolite *Product resulting of enzymatic transformation of a drug*, 108

Metabotropic receptors *Receptors physically separated from parts of the neurons where the receptors exert its effects*, 78

Met-enkephalin, 283

Meth mouth *Tooth decay caused by methamphetamine use*, 182

Methadone (Dolophine), 278, 281–282, 297

Methamphetamine, 7, 161, 163, 172–173

Methanol, 226

Methcathinone, 161

Methyl alcohol, 226

Methylecgonidine *Byproduct of the freebase synthesis process for cocaine that is harmful to the heart, lungs, and liver*, 171

Methylphenidate, 164, 167, 173–175

Michael I, Russian Tsar, 198

Microdialysis *Procedure used to sample neurochemicals within a brain structure*, 66, 67, 270, 426–427

Microelectrode *Electrode used in electrophysiology that records the activity of only a few neurons or a single neuron*, 66, 67

Midbrain, 39

Migration *Neurodevelopment phase involving the moving of newly generated cells to parts of the nervous system*, 54

Milner, Peter, 142–143

Miltown (meprobamate), 382

Miosis *Pupil constriction that can occur after opioid administration*, 295

Misuse, 5–6

Mitochondrion, 31

Mixed opioid receptor agonist-antagonists *Drugs that exhibit agonist actions at some opioid receptors while exhibiting antagonist actions at other opioid receptors*, 285

R

Radioligand binding *Research technique used to study the affinity and efficacy that drugs have for receptors*, 114

Rapid detoxification *Detoxification process lasting as long as 10 days and using opioid antagonist administration in a treatment facility*, 296, 297

Rate dependent effects *Differences in a drug's behavioral effects as a function of predrug administration response rates*, 178

Rate-limiting step *Slowest conversion rate in a synthesis process*, 86

Rave *Large organized party held in a dance club or warehouse where electronic dance music is played with a light show*, 338, 341

Rebound, 338, 341

Receptive area, 32

Receptor action, opioid drug classification by, 284–286

Receptor agonists, 289–294

Receptor antagonism, 112

Receptor binding affinity *Drug's strength of binding to a receptor*, 114, 115

Receptor efficacy *Drug's ability to alter the activity of receptor*, 115

Receptor knock-out mice, 186

Receptors *Proteins located in neuron membranes that can be bound to and activated by neurotransmitters*
about, 31–32
neurotransmitters binding to, 75–80
psychoactive drugs and, 115–122

Recreational drug *Drug taken by a user to experience its physical or mental effects*
about, 5–6, 130

of MDMA, 329–330
of psychostimulants, 166–170

Reefer, 301

Reference memory, 46

Refractory period *Period following an action potential when the neuron resists producing another action potential*, 71

Regulatory agencies, 131–134

Reinforcement *Process in which the resulting consequence from a response increases the frequency of future responses*, 137, 289–296, 349

Reinstatement, 141, 294

Relapse *Return to a chronic drug use state that meets the clinical features of addiction*, 136, 151

Relative refractory period *Second phase of the refractory period, during which greater depolarization is necessary to reach threshold and produce another action potential*, 71

Relaxation, 295

Remifentanil, 290–291

Reserpine, 354, 359

Residual schizophrenia, 409

Resistance stage, of general adaptation syndrome, 388–389

Respiratory depression, 295, 392

Respiratory functioning
alcohol and, 238–239
opioid drugs and, 295

Response time
of antidepressant drugs, 367
on SSRIs/SNRIs and benzodiazepine, 401

Resting potential, 67–70, 284

Restlessness, 295

Reticular activating system *System of structures that support arousal in the cerebral cortex*, 46

Reticular formation, 46

Reuptake, 75

Reversible inhibitor of MAO$_A$ (RIMA) *Antidepressant drug that selectively inhibits MAO$_A$ but allows for displacement from MAO$_A$ by other compounds such as tyramine*, 362

Reversible MAO inhibitor *Antidepressant drug that either temporarily binds to MAO or allows other compounds to displace the drug from MAO*, 362

Reward, 44, 286–289

Reward center, 44

Reward circuit, 44, 142–147

Ribosomes, 57

Risperidone (Risperdal), 376, 417

Ritaline, 167

Robo-tripping, 276, 349

Rolfe, John, 198

Romans, 279

Rubbing alcohol, 226

Runge, Friedlieb, 218

Rush phase, 289

S

Sabril (vigabatrin), 188, 399

Safety pharmacology *Screening process that identifies the adverse effects of drugs*, 26

Sagittal plane, 35

Salt forms, of psychostimulants, 170–171

Saltatory conduction, 73

Salvinorin A *Psychoactive constituent of the psychedelic plant Salvia divinorum*, 283, 349

Saphris (asenapine), 417

Sativex *Cannabinoid medication that consists of a one-to-one ratio of cannabidiol and Δ^9-THC*, 317

Schizophrenia *Severe, life-long mental illness consisting of disturbed thought processes and poor emotional responsiveness*

Schizophrenia (*contiued*)
about, 408–412
antipsychotic drugs for,
408–417, 425–427
dissociative anesthetics for, 342
history of, 414
neurobiological profile of,
412–413
prevalence, 410–412
Schizophrenia-like effects,
dissociative anesthetics
and, 347–348
Scopolamine *Muscarinic
receptor antagonist that
produces true visual
hallucinations, delusional
thinking, and disorienta-
tion about time and place,*
349–350
Second messenger, 78
Second-generation antipsychotic drugs, 417
Secondhand smoking, 196
Selective MAO$_B$ inhibitors
*Antidepressant drugs that
primarily inhibit MAO$_B$
enzymes and exhibit
weaker inhibition of MAO$_A$
enzymes,* 362
**Selective serotonin reuptake
inhibitor (SSRI)** *Antidepressant drug that blocks
serotonin transporters
resulting in greater serotonin levels within synapses,*
331, 359, 364–365, 400
Selegiline (Emsam), 362
Self-administration, 140–141,
290, 293–294
Semantic memory, 242
Semisynthetic opioids *Opioids
synthesized from morphine
or codeine,* 278
Senile plaques *Degenerated
neurons formed from
overproduction of amyloid
beta 42 peptides, causing
cell death,* 98
Sensitization *Increased
responsiveness to a drug's
effects,* 124, 183–185

Sensitization to alcohol
*Increase in alcohol's
efficacy, especially its
reinforcing effects,* 247
Sensory neuron *Neuron that
conveys sensory informa-
tion via axons to the
central nervous system,*
32–33
Sensory-gating deficit *A
schizophrenic's
diminished capacity to
filter out unimportant
stimuli in his or her
environment,* 410
Seroquel (quetiapine), 376, 377,
417
Serotonin, 84–85, 88–89,
235–236, 368–369.
See also Anxiety disorders
**Serotonin discontinuation
syndrome** *Syndrome
caused by abrupt with-
drawal of an antidepressant
drug, resulting in sensory
disturbances, sleeping
disturbances, disequilib-
rium, flulike symptoms,
and gastrointestinal effects,*
365
Serotonin neurotransmitter
system
LSD and, 324–326
MDMA and, 332–334
phencyclidine and, 343–344
**Serotonin norepinephrine
reuptake inhibitors (SNRIs)**
*Antidepressant drugs that
enhance levels of serotonin
and norepinephrine by
blocking serotonin and
norepinephrine transport-
ers,* 359, 365–366, 400
Serotonin syndrome *Antidepressant drug-induced
life-threatening condition
characterized by agitation,
restlessness, disturbances in
cognitive functioning, and
possibly hallucinations,*
365

Serotonin-transporter-gene-
linked polymorphic region,
378
Sexual side effects *Sexual
dysfunction, including
erectile dysfunction,
inability to achieve orgasm,
and loss of sexual drive
caused by antidepressant
drugs,* 365
Short route, for sensory
information from thalamus,
385
Short-acting barbiturate, 391, 392
Short-acting benzodiazepines,
395–396
**Short-term opioid detoxifica-
tion** *Detoxification process
that lasts as long as 30
days and usually uses
opioid receptor agonists,*
296, 297
Shrooms, 321
Shulgin, Alexander, 329–330
Siegel, Shepard, 102, 125
Singer, Peter, 22
Single-blind procedure *When
researchers do not inform
study participants which
treatment or placebo they
received,* 14
Sky, 164
Smoking, 214–215. *See also*
Cannabis
Smokless tobacco, 193
Sniffing, 267–269
Snorting, 171
SNRIs. *See* Serotonin norepinephrine reuptake inhibi-
tors (SNRIs)
Social interaction tests, 337
Social phobia *Fear of being in
or performing in social or
public situations,* 383
Social therapies *Therapies that
consist of group therapy
sessions where individuals
interact with a group
therapist as well as other
individuals also struggling
with addiction,* 153

Wine, 228
Withdrawal, 124, 150
Working memory *Consists of short-term verbal or nonverbal memories employed to carry out a task,* 46
Wyden, Ron, 192

X

Xanax (alprazolam), 395, 396
Xylene, 267
Xyrem, 257

Z

Zectran, 330

Zeff, Leo, 330
Zeprexa (olanzapine), 376, 417, 423
Zero-order kinetics, 232
Zimelidine (Zelmid), 364
Ziprasidone (Geodon), 417
Zygote, 53